AIDS and
Heart Disease

AIDS and
Heart Disease

edited by
Ronald Ross Watson
University of Arizona
Tucson, Arizona, U.S.A.

MARCEL DEKKER, INC.   NEW YORK · BASEL

Library of Congress Cataloging-in-Publication Data
A catalog record for this book is available from the Library of Congress.

ISBN: 0-8247-4115-3

This book is printed on acid-free paper.

Headquarters
Marcel Dekker, Inc., 270 Madison Avenue, New York, NY 10016, U.S.A.
tel: 212-696-9000; fax: 212-685-4540

Distribution and Customer Service
Marcel Dekker, Inc., Cimarron Road, Monticello, New York 12701, U.S.A.
tel: 800-228-1160; fax: 845-796-1772

Eastern Hemisphere Distribution
Marcel Dekker AG, Hutgasse 4, Postfach 812, CH-4001 Basel, Switzerland
tel: 41-61-260-6300; fax: 41-61-260-6333

World Wide Web
http://www.dekker.com

The publisher offers discounts on this book when ordered in bulk quantities. For more information, write to Special Sales/Professional Marketing at the headquarters address above.

Preface

Although heart disease should not be a problem among AIDS patients, since most are children or relatively young adults, more than 50% have significant signs of cardiac damage upon autopsy. As antiretroviral drugs prolong their survival, the importance and prevalence of heart disease in AIDS patients will only increase as they age and enter the time in life when heart disease is frequent. Even so, dilated cardiomyopathy and associated symptoms of congestive heart failure are being recognized with increasing frequency in retrovirus-infected people. Estimates are that 25% of HIV-seropositive individuals will eventually manifest evidence of left ventricular dysfunction, giving rise to as many as 50,000 new cases of symptomatic heart failure each year among these patients. Despite this clinical recognition, the pathogenesis of AIDS-related cardiomyopathy remains unclear, limiting application of both specific treatments and preventive strategies. This book defines, in several chapters, the role of retroviruses in heart disease occurring in murine, primate, and human systems. Limitations in the understanding of the relationship between HIV infection and the development of dilated cardiomyopathy are confounded by the use of illicit drugs and antiretroviral agents, which may be cardiotoxic. Therefore we emphasize the role of drug abuse and alcohol as immunodulatory substances that have a role in AIDS-related heart disease. The current therapeutic drugs, protein inhibitors, promote the accumulation of fat and longer survival, increasing the contributory factors and allowing more time for the development of damage to the heart. Very recent work shows that retroviruses cause direct heart damage as well as weakening of the immune system, so that opportunistic pathogens can take hold, persist, and eventually damage the heart. Accumulation of fat and dramatically increased levels of serum fatty acids and cholesterol—as often happens during protease inhibitor treatment of AIDS—are well-known risk factors for cardiovascular disease. Improved nutrition remains a mild and readily available approach to modifying these changes and their actions on heart function during retroviral infection. A number of chapters describe the roles of fat, antioxidants, and other nutritional and dietary materials that can modify or affect heart disease. The potential synergisms with the modifications made by the retroviral infection are defined.

This book provides vital, up-to-date reviews of the mechanisms by which HIV infects target cells (endothelial cells), damages the heart and related vascular systems, and facilitates the destructive effects of other pathogens. In addition, the cardiotoxic side effects of current AIDS therapies, such as changes in body fat, need to be explained and ideas for their mediation must be carefully reviewed. This book, then, will serve as a desk reference for AIDS and cardiovascular researchers as well as primary care physicians and AIDS patients themselves. It will stimulate research while educating both health-oriented lay people as well as scientists and health care professionals.

ACKNOWLEDGMENTS

The National Heart, Lung, and Blood Institute (NHLBI) and supplement grants (HL 59794 and HL 63667) from the National Institute of Drug Abuse (NIDA) to Ronald Ross Watson funded the research that stimulated this book. Assistance by Thom Eagan and Allyson Beste is greatly appreciated, as it facilitated communication with the contributors. Finally, appreciation is extended to Jag H. Khalsa, Ph.D., of NIDA, and Lan-Hsiang Wang, Ph.D., of NHLBI, who have encouraged research on AIDS-related heart disease for years.

Ronald Ross Watson

Contents

Contributors

Brian G. Abbott, M.D.   Assistant Professor, Section of Cardiovascular Medicine, Department of Internal Medicine, Yale University School of Medicine, New Haven, Connecticut, U.S.A.

Charles E. Alpers, M.D.   Professor, Department of Pathology, University of Washington Medical Center, Seattle, Washington, U.S.A.

Mohsen Araghi-Niknam, Ph.D.   Research Associate, Department of Psychiatry, University of Minnesota, Minneapolis, Minnesota, U.S.A.

Giuseppe Barbaro, M.D.   Chief, Cardiology Unit, Department of Medical Pathophysiology, University La Sapienza, Rome, Italy

Kelly J. Blackstock, M.S.   College of Veterinary Medicine and Biomedical Science, Colorado State University, Fort Collins, Colorado, U.S.A.

Simin Bourchi-Vaghefi, Ph.D.   Professor, Department of Public Health, College of Health, University of North Florida, Jacksonville, Florida, U.S.A.

Angela A. L. Carville, B.V.M.S.   Veterinary Surgeon, Department of Primate Medicine, New England Primate Research Center, Southborough, Massachusetts, U.S.A.

Changyi (Johnny) Chen, M.D., Ph.D.   Professor of Surgery and Molecular and Cellular Biology, Michael E. DeBakey Department of Surgery, Baylor College of Medicine, Houston, Texas, U.S.A.

Yinhong Chen, M.D., Ph.D.   Institute of Molecular Medicine, University of California, La Jolla, California, U.S.A.

David S. Chi, Ph.D.   Professor and Chief, Division of Biomedical Research, Department of Internal Medicine, James H. Quillen College of Medicine, East Tennessee State University, Johnson City, Tennessee, U.S.A.

Jean Ducobu, M.D.   Head, Department of Medicine, CHU Tivoli, La Louvière, Belgium

Milan Fiala, M.D.   Associate Researcher, Department of Medicine, David Geffen School of Medicine at UCLA, and Greater Los Angeles VA Medical Center, Los Angeles, California, U.S.A.

Sander G. Genser, M.D., M.P.H.   Associate Clinical Professor (Adjunct), Department of Psychiatry, Uniformed Services University of the Health Sciences, Bethesda, Maryland, U.S.A.

Zaher Hanna, Ph.D.   Senior Researcher, Laboratory of Molecular Biology, Clinical Research Institute of Montreal, Montreal, Quebec, Canada

Raxit J. Jariwalla, Ph.D.   Principal Investigator, Department of Viral, Immune and Metabolic Diseases, California Institute for Medical Research, San Jose, California, U.S.A.

Paul Jolicoeur, M.D., Ph.D.   Scientist, Clinical Research Institute of Montreal, Montreal, Quebec, Canada

Denis G. Kay, Ph.D.   Associate Researcher, Laboratory of Molecular Biology, Clinical Research Institute of Montreal, Montreal, Quebec, Canada

Jag H. Khalsa, Ph.D.   Acting Head, Medical Consequences Unit, Center on AIDS and Other Medical Consequences of Drug Abuse, National Institute on Drug Abuse, National Institutes of Health, Bethesda, Maryland, U.S.A.

Kwang Sik Kim, M.D.   Professor and Director, Division of Pediatric Infectious Diseases, Department of Pediatrics, Johns Hopkins Medical Institutions, Baltimore, Maryland, U.S.A.

Guha Krishnaswamy, M.D., F.A.C.P., F.C.C.P.   Professor, Department of Internal Medicine, James H. Quillen College of Medicine, East Tennessee State University, and James H. Quillen VA Medical Center, Johnson City, Tennessee, U.S.A.

Shenghan Lai, M.D., M.P.H.   Associate Professor, Departments of Epidemiology and Medicine, Johns Hopkins Medical Institutions, Baltimore, Maryland, U.S.A.

Heather L. LaMarca, B.S.   Interdisciplinary Program in Molecular and Cellular Biology, Department of Microbiology and Immunology, Tulane University Health Sciences Center, New Orleans, Louisiana, U.S.A.

Chuangfu Li, M.D. Associate Professor, Department of Surgery, James H. Quillen College of Medicine, East Tennessee State University, Johnson City, Tennessee, U.S.A.

João A. C. Lima, M.D., M.B.A. Associate Professor, Division of Cardiology, Department of Medicine, Johns Hopkins Medical Institutions, Baltimore, Maryland, U.S.A.

Peter H. Lin, M.D. Assistant Professor, Department of Surgery, Baylor College of Medicine, Houston, Texas, U.S.A.

Kai Liu, M.D. Visiting Research Faculty, Department of Medicine, James H. Quillen College of Medicine, East Tennessee State University, Johnson City, Tennessee, U.S.A.

Yingying Liu, M.S. Researcher/Nutritionist, Department of Health Promotion Sciences, College of Public Health, University of Arizona, Tucson, Arizona, U.S.A.

Albert S. Lossinsky, Ph.D. Head, Laboratories of Immunohistochemistry and Scanning Electron Microscopy, Neural Engineering Department, Huntington Medical Research Institutes, Pasadena, California, U.S.A.

Alan B. Lumsden, M.D., F.A.C.S. Professor and Chief, Division of Vascular Surgery and Endovascular Therapy, Michael E. DeBakey Department of Surgery, Baylor College of Medicine, Houston, Texas, U.S.A.

William R. MacLellan, M.D. Assistant Professor, Cardiology Division, Department of Medicine, David Geffen School of Medicine at UCLA, Los Angeles, California, U.S.A.

Zeina Makhoul, M.S. Teaching Assistant, Department of Nutritional Sciences, University of Arizona, Tucson, Arizona, U.S.A.

Arthur Margolin, Ph.D. Research Scientist, Department of Psychiatry, Yale University School of Medicine, New Haven, Connecticut, U.S.A.

Jaclyn Maurer, M.S., R.D. Senior Research Specialist, Department of Nutritional Sciences, University of Arizona, Tucson, Arizona, U.S.A.

Harris E. McFerrin, M.S. Interdisciplinary Program in Molecular and Cellular Biology, Department of Microbiology and Immunology, Tulane University Health Sciences Center, New Orleans, Louisiana, U.S.A.

Qingyi Meng, M.D., Ph.D. Department of Emergency Medicine, Chinese PLA General Hospital, Beijing, China

James P. Morgan, M.D., Ph.D.   Professor, Cardiovascular Division, Department of Medicine, Harvard Medical School, and Beth Israel Deaconess Medical Center, Boston, Massachusetts, U.S.A.

Cindy A. Morris, Ph.D.   Associate Professor, Interdisciplinary Program in Molecular and Cellular Biology, Department of Microbiology and Immunology, Tulane Cancer Center, Tulane University Health Sciences Center, New Orleans, Louisiana, U.S.A.

Anja S. Mühlfeld, M.D.   Department of Nephrology and Immunology, Rheinisch Westfälisch Technische Hochschule Aachen, Aachen, Germany

Anne B. Nelson, Ph.D.   Postdoctoral Fellow, Department of Microbiology and Immunology, Tulane University Health Sciences Center, New Orleans, Louisiana, U.S.A.

Hiren B. Patel, M.D.   Department of Internal Medicine, Holston Valley Medical Center, Kingsport, Tennessee, U.S.A.

M. C. Payen, M.D.   Chief, Department of Infectious Diseases, Saint-Pierre Hospital, Université Libre de Bruxelles, Brussels, Belgium

Jennifer J. Ravia, M.S.   Instructor, Department of Nutritional Sciences, University of Arizona, Tucson, Arizona, U.S.A.

Kenneth P. Roos, Ph.D.   Professor, Department of Physiology, David Geffen School of Medicine at UCLA, Los Angeles, California, U.S.A.

Stephan Segerer, M.D.   Medizinische Poliklinik, Klinikum-Innenstadt, University of Munich, Munich, Germany

Ramón Tomás Sepulveda, M.S., Ph.D.   Research Specialist, Department of Microbiology and Immunology and Health Promotion Science, University of Arizona, Tucson, Arizona, U.S.A.

John F. Setaro, M.D.   Associate Professor, Section of Cardiovascular Medicine, Department of Internal Medicine, Yale University School of Medicine, New Haven, Connecticut, U.S.A.

Richard P. Shannon, M.D.   Claude R. Joyner Professor and Chairman, Department of Medicine, Allegheny General Hospital, Pittsburgh, Pennsylvania, U.S.A.

Bryan D. Shelby, M.S.P.H.   Interdisciplinary Program in Molecular and Cellular Biology, Department of Microbiology and Immunology, Tulane University Health Sciences Center, New Orleans, Louisiana, U.S.A.

Elizabeth H. Sheppard, M.S., C.H.E.S.   Health Educator and Private Nutritional Consultant, Tucson, Arizona, U.S.A.

Daniel Sijipunda Dube, M.D., B.Sc. Postdoctoral Fellow, Department of Pulmonary and Critical Care Medicine, Stanford University, Palo Alto, California, U.S.A.

Marie-Chantal Simard, Ph.D. Laboratory of Molecular Biology, Clinical Research Institute of Montreal, Montreal, Quebec, Canada

George G. Sokos, D.O. Chief Resident, Department of Medicine, Allegheny General Hospital, Pittsburgh, Pennsylvania, U.S.A.

William L. Stone, Ph.D. Professor, Department of Pediatrics, James H. Quillen College of Medicine, East Tennessee State University, Johnson City, Tennessee, U.S.A.

Deborah E. Sullivan, Ph.D. Research Assistant Professor, Department of Microbiology and Immunology, Tulane University Health Sciences Center, New Orleans, Louisiana, U.S.A.

Lance S. Terada, M.D. Professor, Division of Pulmonary and Critical Care Medicine, Department of Internal Medicine, University of Texas Southwestern Medical Center, and Dallas Veterans Administration Medical Center, Dallas, Texas, U.S.A.

Jufeng Wang, M.D., Ph.D. Instructor, Cardiovascular Division, Department of Medicine, Harvard Medical School, and Beth Israel Deaconess Medical Center, Boston, Massachusetts, U.S.A.

Ronald Ross Watson, Ph.D. Professor, Department of Health Promotion Sciences, College of Public Health and School of Medicine, University of Arizona, Tucson, Arizona, U.S.A.

Aurea Westrick-Thompson, M.S., R.D., L.D./N. Pediatric Clinical Dietician, Baptist Medical Center/Wolfson Children's Hospital, Jacksonville, Florida, U.S.A.

Ru Feng Wu, M.D., Ph.D. Instructor, Department of Internal Medicine, University of Texas Southwestern Medical Center, and Dallas Veterans Administration Medical Center, Dallas, Texas, U.S.A.

Qizhi (Cathy) Yao, M.D., Ph.D. Associate Professor of Surgery and Molecular Virology and Microbiology, Michael E. DeBakey Department of Surgery, Baylor College of Medicine, Houston, Texas, U.S.A.

Qianli Yu, Ph.D. Department of Medical Pharmacology, University of Arizona, Tucson, Arizona, U.S.A.

Ping Yue, M.D., Ph.D. Research Associate, Animal Physiology Core Laboratory, Clinical Research Institute of Montreal, Montreal, Quebec, Canada

Jin Zhang, Ph.D. Postdoctoral Fellow, Department of Pathology, Brigham and Women's Hospital, and Harvard Medical School, Boston, Massachusetts, U.S.A.

AIDS and Heart Disease

1

Heart Disease in AIDS

Qianli Yu and Ronald Ross Watson
University of Arizona, Tucson, Arizona, U.S.A.

INTRODUCTION

Acquired immunodeficiency syndrome (AIDS) is caused by infection with human immunodeficiency virus (HIV). According to the Joint United Nations Programme on HIV/AIDS and the World Health Organization, 36.1 million adults and 1.4 million children were living with HIV at the end of 2000 (1). AIDS deaths since the beginning of the epidemic total 21.8 million. During 2000, some 5.3 million people became infected with HIV, with 3 million deaths from HIV/AIDS. Deaths among those already infected will continue to increase (1). In the United States, about 40,000 new HIV infections occurred in the year 2000, with 688,000 cases of AIDS reported since 1981 (2).

In recent years, our understanding of AIDS as a dynamic viral infection has evolved. AIDS-associated heart lesions are often unrecognized, even in the initial diagnosis of AIDS in a given patient (3). In retrospective studies, about 50% of AIDS cases reported showed cardiac abnormalities (4,5). In the United States, more than 5000 patients per year are estimated to have cardiac complications resulting from HIV infection (3). The present review provides information on heart disease in AIDS, including its cause and pathogenesis.

DESCRIPTION

AIDS is characterized by an acquired, profound, irreversible immunosuppression that predisposes the patient to multiple opportunistic infections, malignant neoplasms, and a progressive dysfunction of multiple organ systems. The first cardiac involvement in AIDS patients was reported in 1983 (6), describing myocardial Kaposi's sarcoma at autopsy. Symptomatic and asymptomatic cardiac involvement in AIDS patients ranges between 28 and 73% (7). Epstein et al. (8) reported that cardiovascular disease was the fourth leading cause of dilated cardiomyopathy in the United States. Congestive heart failure has become the leading cause of death in pediatric patients with AIDS; half of them die within 6 to 12 months (9).

HEART DISEASES IN AIDS

Cardiac disease in AIDS patients may occur coincidentally; as a complication of AIDS or the treatment of AIDS; or as the direct result of HIV infection of the heart (10). As the AIDS epidemic spreads, heart disease problems resulting from AIDS become more prominent due to increased numbers of newly diagnosed patients with AIDS. In addition, the highly active antiretroviral therapy (HAART) that has enhanced the survival rate in HIV/AIDS patients facilitates manifestation of late-stage HIV infection, including HIV-related cardiac diseases. These cardiac diseases mainly include myocarditis, dilated cardiomyopathy, pericardial effusion, nonbacterial endo-carditis, pulmonary hypertension, cardiac neoplasm, and drug-induced cardiotoxic-ity. Heart disease can occur in various AIDS stages, but it is more common to detect cardiac abnormalities in the later stages. Some of those cardiac abnormalities can occur without any clinical manifestation, and they can complicate the course of the disease severely (11). Myocarditis is an inflammatory heart disease. Autopsy statistics indicate that approximately one-third of all AIDS patients had myocardial compli-cations, but the specific cause was found in only 20% of patients with myocarditis. Organisms such as *Toxoplasma gondii*, *Mycobacterium tuberculosis*, and *Cryptococcus neoformans* are common pathogens that can cause AIDS myocarditis, while *Myoco-bacterium avium intracellulare* complex, *Coccidioides immitis*, and cytomegalovirus have been reported as rarely infectious pathogens of myocarditis in AIDS patients (12). A recent review reported that HIV itself, in the absence of opportunistic pathogens, causes myocarditis in AIDS patients (13). HIV and its protein components were found in AIDS patients' heart tissue with myocarditis, suggesting that HIV and its components might be the cause of myocarditis (14,15). Myocarditis may also play a role in the development of ventricular dysfunction in HIV patients (16).

Dilated cardiomyopathy involves dilation of ventricular cavities and increased heart weight. The first case of AIDS-related dilated cardiomyopathy was described in 1986, followed by some other reported cases (17). Dilated cardiomyopathy is one of the most common cardiac complications of HIV infection; it occurs in the later stages of HIV infection, usually with a significantly low CD4 cell count (17). Dilated cardiomyopathy can enlarge all four chambers of the heart, causing diffuse left ventricular hypokinesis, increase fractional shortening, and eventually myocardial dysfunction. Survival of patients with myocardial dysfunction is extremely low, approximately 30% of HIV-related deaths being due to myocardial dysfunction (18,19). The pathogenesis of cardiomyopathy remains obscure; Barbaro reported that dilated cardiomyopathy was associated with infective endocarditis and pericardial effusion (20). Some case studies have shown that HIV itself can cause cardiac injury (21,22). Animal studies using murine AIDS have shown that immune dysfunction facilitated coxsackievirus infection, cardiomyopathy, and premature death (23); cocaine injection accentuated both.

Pericardial effusion is another common form of cardiovascular involvement in HIV infection. *M. tuberculosis hominis* and *M. avium intracellulare* pericarditis had a greater prevalence (20). The clinical manifestations of pericarditis include pericardial effusion, pericarditis, cardiac tamponade, and constrictive pericarditis. Approximately 20% of AIDS patients have pericardial effusion (24,25). Most of these cases are indio-pathic, but the etiology can be infection, lymphoma, Kaposi's sarcoma, myocardial infarction, or fibrinous exudates (19).

Endocarditis in AIDS patients is relatively uncommon and usually nonbacterial; the incidence rate is 3 to 5% in AIDS patients; *Staphylococcus aureus* and *Candida albicans* endocarditis are usually prevalent (20). It often occurs in drug addicts older than 50 years. HIV infection may increase the risk of infective endocarditis among intravenous drug users and homosexuals. The major organisms that cause endocarditis in AIDS patients are *S. aureus* (75%) and *Streptococcus viridans* (20%) (26). The symptoms of these patients are fever, sweats, weight loss, pneumonia, and/or meningitis (13). The mortality from infective endocarditis increases significantly in the late stages of HIV infection (26).

The first case of pulmonary hypertension in AIDS patients was reported in 1987 (21). The incidence of pulmonary hypertension in AIDS patients is much higher than in the general public, and mainly male and young patients are associated with it (27). Its common symptom is dyspnea; intravenous drug abuse, homosexuality, and hemophilia are the risk factors (27). Half of those AIDS patients who had pulmonary hypertension died within a year because of right-sided heart failure and respiratory failure. The pathogenesis of pulmonary hypertension in AIDS patients is unclear. A study performed by Mette (28) revealed that HIV is not directly associated with pulmonary hypertension in AIDS patients; however, increases of endothelin 1, tumor necrosis factor alpha (TNF-α), and platelet-derived growth factor due to HIV are associated with pulmonary hypertension (29).

Two types of cardiac-associated malignant neoplasms are common in patients with AIDS: Kaposi's sarcoma involves the heart and is usually metastatic; lymphomas are extremely rare in the heart even though they are the commonest cancer in AIDS. The incidence of Kaposi's sarcoma involving the heart ranges from 12 to 28% in retrospective autopsies (30) of patients who were, for the most part, homosexual or bisexual. Kaposi's sarcoma involves the visceral layer, serous pericardium, or sub-epicardial fat. Lymphomas are usually unsuspected clinically. Presentation with cardiac symptoms includes congestive heart failure, pericardial effusion, and heart block (13), while asymptomic lymphomas in AIDS progress rapidly and lead to cardiac dysfunction. The prognosis of patients with HIV-associated cardiac lymphoma is generally poor (14). Although there are several reports of coronary artery abnormalities in AIDS patients (31,32), their incidence is relatively uncommon. Through autopsy of the abnormal coronary artery in AIDS patients, significant coronary lesions were found as atherosclerosis, fibrosis, sclerohyalinosis, and myocardial interstitial fibrosis. However, the cause of these lesions is not clear. Given the absence of other cardiovascular risk factors, atherosclerosis or angiitis may be related to an opportunistic viral infection (13).

Medications taken by AIDS patients may cause cardiovascular toxicities such as dilated cardiomyopathy, ventricular tachycardia, myocardial infarction or ischemia, and congestive heart failure. AIDS patients treated with amphotericin B, interferon alpha, zidovudine or azidothymidine (AZT), and doxorubicin have shown cardiotoxicities (13).

ALCOHOL USE, DRUG ABUSE, AND HEART DISEASE IN AIDS

Alcohol use and drug abuse can increase the morbidity from heart disease in AIDS patients (7). Alcohol (ethanol) consumption alters cardiac contractile function and is a leading cause of cardiomyopathy in the United States (26). Alcoholic cardiomyopathy enlarges the heart and induces endocardial thickening, remodeling, interstitial fibrosis, myocyte hypertrophy and atrophy, and focal necrotic mycocytes (21). In murine AIDS, ethanol consumption has been shown to promote cardiomyopathy (unpublished data).

Cocaine abuse also may contribute to the development of heart disease in murine (23) and human AIDS. Cocaine can be a cardiotoxin to myocardial cells and also has vascular effects on AIDS patients. Myocardial effects of cocaine administration include cardiomegaly and left ventricular hypertrophy (27). Cocaine injection and increased heart disease in murine AIDS, especially with coxsackievirus B3 infection, correlate with significant heart lesions (23).

A recent review concluded that the heart is very sensitive to methamphetamine and can easily be damaged by this drug. Heart problems from methamphetamine abuse include tachycardia, dilated cardiomyopathy, and even heart failure (33).

Heart disease in AIDS may also be associated with low levels of tissue nutrients, resulting from poverty-induced malnutrition. Low levels of selenium or L-carnitine can cause heart failure in AIDS patients. Selenium content in hearts from AIDS patients has been found to be substantially diminished; selenium supplementation reversed the cardiomyopathy (7). Combined selenium and vitamin E deficiency cause fatal myopathy in guinea pigs (34). In African AIDS patients, lower socioeconomic status was a significant risk factor for mortality from heart disease (35).

DIAGNOSIS AND TREATMENT

The assessment methods of heart disease in AIDS patients include physical examination, electrocardiography (ECG), two-dimensional echocardiography, and Doppler echocardiography. Pathological examinations include autopsy and routine techniques with hematoxylin and eosin, Ziehl-Neelsen, Gomori, and Grocott stains (36).

Except for anecdotal evidence, no particular reports of treatment for AIDS patients with heart disease exist (19). Though anti-HIV drugs can reduce viral replication, delay disease progression, and prolong survival, the prevalence of cardiac involvement cannot be significantly influenced by anti-HIV therapy. The treatment regimen should avoid cardiotoxic drugs and supplement with nutrients such as vitamin E and selenium.

CONCLUSION

Cardiac diseases in AIDS patients have become more prominent, primarily presenting as myocarditis, dilated cardiomyopathy, pericardial effusion, nonbacterial endocarditis, pulmonary hypertension, cardiac neoplasm, and drug-induced cardiotoxicity. In some cases opportunistic infections, HIV protein components, Kaposi's sarcoma, cardiac lymphoma, and antiretroviral drugs may cause cardiac disease in AIDS patients. However, the cause and pathogenesis of some heart diseases in AIDS is not clear. Alcohol use, drug abuse, and malnutrition can increase the morbidity of AIDS patients with heart disease.

ACKNOWLEDGMENTS

The preparation of this chapter was supported and stimulated by research as well as its NIDA Supplements, NIH grants HL59794 and HL63667.

REFERENCES

1. http://www.avert.org/worldstatinfo.htm.
2. http://www.unaids.org/wac/2000/wad00/files/WAD_epidemic_report.htm.
3. Milei J, Grana D, FernanDez Alonso G, Matturri L. Cardiac involvement in acquired immunodeficiency syndrome. Clin Cardiol 1998; 21:465–472.
4. DeCastro S, Migliau G, Silvestri A. Heart involvement in AIDS: a prospective study during various stages of the disease. Eur Heart J 1992; 13:1452–1459.
5. Fong IW, Howard R, Elzawi A, Simbul M, Chiasson D. Cardiac involvement in human immunodeficiency virus infected patients. J AIDS 1993; 6:380–385.
6. Autran B, Gorin I, Leibowith M, et al. AIDS in a Haitian woman with cardiac Kaposi's sarcoma and Whipple's disease. Lancet 1983; 1:767–768.
7. Lewis W. Cardiomyopathy in AIDS. Prog Cardiovasc Dis 2000; 43:151–170.
8. Epstein JE, Eichbaum QG, Lipshultz SE. Cardiovascular manifestations of HIV infection. Comp Ther 1996; 22:485–489.
9. Johann-Liang R, Cervia JS, Noel GJ. Characteristics of human immunodeficiency virus-infected children at the time of death. Pediatr Infect Dis J 1997; 16:1145–1150.
10. Patel RC, Fishman WH. Cardiac involvement in HIV infection. Med Clin North Am 1996; 80:1493–1512.
11. De Castro S, Mibliau G, Silvestri A, D'Amati G, Giannantoni P, Cartón D, Kol A, Vullo V, Circlli A. Heart involvement in AIDS. Eur Heart J 1992; 13:1452–1459.
12. Kaul S, Fishbei MC, Sigel RJ. Cardiac manifestations of acquired immune deficiency syndrome. Am Heart J 1991; 122:535–544.
13. Rerkpattanapipat P, Wongpraparut N, Jacobs EL, Kotler NM. Cardiac manifestations of acquired immunodeficiency syndrome. Arch Intern Med 2000; 160:602–608.
14. Cotton P. AIDS giving rising to cardiac problems [letter]. JAMA 1990; 263:2149.
15. Grody WW, Cheng L, Lewis W. Infection of the heart by the human immunodeficiency virus. Am J Cardiol 1990; 66:203–206.
16. Anderson DW, Virmani F, Reilly JM. Prevalent myocarditis at necropsy in acquired immunodeficiency syndrome. J Am Coll Cardiol 1988; 11:792–799.
17. Cohen IS, Anderson DW, Virmani R. Congestive cardiomyopathy in association with the acquired immunodeficiency syndrome. N Engl J Med 1986; 315:628–630.
18. Herskowits A. Cardiomyopathy and other symptomatic heart diseases associated with HIV infection. Curr Opin Cardiol 1996; 11:325–331.
19. Acierno LJ. Cardiac complications in acquired immunodeficiency syndrome. J Am Coll Cardiol 1989; 13:1144–1154.
20. Barbaro G, Di Lorenzo G, Grisorio B, Barbarini G. Cardiac involvement in the acquired immunodeficiency syndrome: a multicenter clinical-pathological study. Gruppo Italiano per lo Studio Cardiologico dei Pazienti Affetti da AIDS Investigators. AIDS Res Hum Retrovir 1998; 14:1071–1077.
21. Ho DD, Pomerants FJ, Kaplan JC. Pathogenesis of infection with human immuno-deficiency virus. N Engl J Med 1987; 317:278–286.
22. Nathan PE, Arsura EL, Zappi M. Pericarditis with tamponade due to cytomegalovirus in the acquired immunodeficiency syndrome. Chest 1991; 99:765–766.
23. Sepulveda RT, Jiang S, Beischel J, Bellamy WT, Watson RR. Cocaine injection and

coxsackievirus B3 infection increase heart disease during murine AIDS. J AIDS 2000; 25:S19–S26.

24. Fink L, Reichek N, Sutton MG. Cardiac abnormalities in acquired immune deficiency syndrome. Am J Cardiol 1984; 54:1161–1163.

25. Stang JI, Kakaza HH, Gibson DG, Girling DJ, Numm AJ, Fox W. Controlled trial of prednisolone as adjuvant in treatment of tuberculous constrictive pericarditis in Transkei. Lancet 1987; 2:1418–1422.

26. Nahass RG, Weinstein MP, Bartels J, Gocke DJ. Infective endocarditis in intravenous drug users. J Infect Dis 1990; 162:967–970.

27. Mesa RA, Edell ES, Dunn WF, Edwards WD. Human immunodeficiency virus infection and pulmonary hypertension. Mayo Clin Proc 1998; 73:37–44.

28. Mette SA, Palevsky HI, Pietra GG, Willians TM, Bruder E, Prestipina AJ, Patrick AM, Wirth JA. Primary pulmonary hypertension in association with human immunodeficiency virus infection. Am Rev Respir Dis 1992; 145:1196–1200.

29. Humbert M, Monti G, Fartoukh M, Magna A, Brenot F, Rain B, Capron F, Galanaud P, Duoux P, Simonneau G, Emilie D. Platelet-derived growth factor expression in primary pulmonary hypertension. Eur Respir J 1998; 11:554–559.

30. Lewis W. AIDS: cardiac findings from 115 autopsies. Prog Cardiovasc Dis 1989; 32:207–215.

31. Paton P, Tabib A, Loire R, Tete R. Coronary artery lesions and human immunodeficiency virus infection. Res Virol 1993; 144:225–231.

32. Tabib A, Greenland T, Mercier I, Loire R, Mornex JF. Coronary lesions in young HIV-positive subjects at necropsy. Lancet 1992; 340:730.

33. Eagan T, Watson RR. Methamphetamine in Heart Disease. Cardiovasc Review Report 2002; 23:320–324.

34. Hill KE, Motley AK, Li X, May MJ, Burk FK. Combined selenium and vitamin E deficiency causes fatal myopathy in guinea pigs. J Nutr 2001; 131:1798–1802.

35. Longo-Mbenza B, Seghers KV, Phuati M, Bikangi FN, Mubagawa K. Heart involvement and HIV infection in African patients. Int J Cardiol 1998; 64:63–73.

36. Volga G, Herdy H. Cardiac abnormalities in the acquired immunodeficiency syndrome. Arq Gras Cardiol 1999; 73:45–53.

2

Mechanisms of Atherogenesis in HIV Infection

Guha Krishnaswamy
James H. Quillen College of Medicine, East Tennessee State University, and James H. Quillen VA Medical Center, Johnson City, Tennessee, U.S.A.

Kai Liu, Chuangfu Li, and David S. Chi
James H. Quillen College of Medicine, East Tennessee State University, Johnson City, Tennessee, U.S.A.

Daniel Sijipunda Dube
Stanford University, Palo Alto, California, U.S.A.

INTRODUCTION

With the increasing life spans of patients infected with the AIDS virus, morbidity and mortality associated with a plethora of cardiovascular complications is becoming more obvious in this population (1,2). HIV infection itself has been associated with the development of dilated cardiomyopathy, pericardial effusions, and vasculopathy. However, recent reports on the appearance of premature atherosclerosis in young patients have raised serious concerns regarding the role of viral and other factors in atherogenesis (1–5). In addition, highly active antiretroviral therapy (HAART) used for the treatment of HIV infection has been associated with dyslipidemia and lipodystrophy, which can further accentuate the development of atherosclerosis (2). Cocaine abuse, which is becoming alarmingly common, has also been associated with the development of atherosclerosis but may also synergize with HIV infection in causing endothelial injury. In the individual patient who is infected with HIV and is abusing cocaine, accelerated development of coronary disease is very likely. Table 1 lists the roles of HIV infection, HAART, and cocaine in the genesis of vascular disease. The molecular mechanisms underlying these complicated interactions are reviewed in this chapter.

ATHEROSCLEROSIS AS AN INFLAMMATORY DISEASE

It is well recognized that human atherosclerosis is a chronic inflammatory fibroproliferative disease involving the blood vessel (6). Besides a role for lipoproteins that is

Table 1 Vasculopathy Associated with HIV Infection and Cocaine Use

Condition	Associated complications
HIV-related disorders	
Tissue affected	
Coronary artery injury	Eccentric vasculopathy, atherosclerosis
	Sclerohyalinosis
Small- to medium-size artery	Aneurysm, vasculitis, atherosclerosis
Pulmonary circulation	Pulmonary hypertension
Protease inhibitor–induced disorders	
Lipodystrophy	Dyslipidemia, accelerated atherosclerosis
Insulin resistance	Hyperglycemia, accelerated atherosclerosis
Cocaine-induced vascular injury	
Hypertension	Accelerated atherosclerosis
Coronary vasoconstriction	Angina pectoris, ischemia
Adrenergic surge	Tachycardia, hypertension, ischemia

well established, a pivotal role for immune activation has been demonstrated (7–9). The atherosclerotic lesion is composed of activated infiltrating cells. These include macrophages/foam cells, T cells, mast cells, endothelial cells, and myofibroblasts (8,9). Nuclear translocation of transcription factors and elaboration of inflammatory proteins lead to chronic vascular inflammatory responses orchestrated by these cells, culminating in atherosclerosis. The following sections provide an introduction to the molecular basis of atherosclerosis and a framework for a better understanding what may happen with HIV infection and cocaine abuse.

Cellular Biology of the Inflammatory Response

Ross and colleagues hypothesized a "response to injury hypothesis" in the early 1970s (10). According to this hypothesis, atherosclerosis is a chronic inflammatory fibro-proliferative response to multiple injurious stimuli. With chronicity, this response may become exuberant, leading to manifestations of vasculopathy. The possibility that the control of genes leading to the elaboration of various cytokines and growth factors incriminated in this exuberant response may lead to amelioration of the disease has led to exciting insights into the molecular biology of atherosclerosis (11).

CD4+ T cells and macrophages tend to accumulate in atheromatous plaques. Schmitz et al. reviewed the role of CD4+ T cells and macrophages in the atheromatous plaque, the expression of class II MHC molecules, and cell-cell contact signaling molecules such as CD40 and CD40 L—molecules pivotal to mononuclear activation and function (6). These events likely occur early in life. For example, Stary demonstrated intimal macrophages and foam cells as early as infancy, and with later involvement of smooth muscle cells, T cells, mast cells, and plasma cells (12). Endothelial cell activation and dysfunction is pivotal to atherogenesis, as reviewed by LaRosa, Ross, and other established investigators (8,13). Endothelial activation may result from infection (HIV, chlamydiae), hypertension, diabetes mellitus, cigarette smoke, dyslipidemia (HAART), or elevated homocysteine levels. Endothelial injury can lead to a sequence of events leading to increased adhesiveness of platelets and leukocytes and the outpouring of proinflammatory cytokines and growth factors. Subsequent proliferation of vascular smooth muscle cells and infiltration by inflammatory cells lead to arterial wall thickening and vascular remodeling (8,10).

Mechanisms Regulating Atherogenesis

In the earliest stages of atherosclerosis, normal resting endothelial cells undergo activation by atherogenic lipids (low-density lipoproteins), nicotine abuse, infection (*Chlamydia pneumoniae* and cytomegalovirus), hypertension, and elevated levels of homocysteine and glucose (diabetes mellitus). The dysfunctional and/or activated endothelium expresses genes for various proteins involved in inflammation, as summarized by us and others (8,13,14). These include adhesion molecules [CAMs such as vascular cell adhesion molecule-1 (VCAM-1) and intercellular adhesion molecule-1 (ICAM-1)] and chemokines [such as monocyte chemotactic protein-1 (MCP-1), growth-related oncogene-alpha (gro-α), regulated upon activation normal T cell–expressed and secreted (RANTES)] that regulate cellular trafficking and the processes involved in mononuclear recruitment to the vascular wall (14). Other cytokines—such as the monokines, interleukin-1 beta (IL-1 β), tumor necrosis factor alpha (TNF-α), and interleukin-6 (IL-6)—activate the acute-phase response, characterized by hepatic synthesis of complement proteins, C-reactive protein (CRP), and fibrinogen (Table 2). These cytokines also make the endothelial surface more adhesive (by inducing CAMs) and procoagulant. Other cytokines—such as IL-2, interferon gamma (IFN-γ), IL-12, and IL-18—may have various facilitatory roles in atherosclerosis, while cytokines such as IL-4 and IL-10 may have inhibitory functions (Table 2).

Growth factors such as transforming growth factor beta (TGF-β) and platelet-derived growth factors A and B (PDGF-A and B) as well as colony-stimulating factors such as granulocyte-macrophage colony-stimulating factor (GM-CSF), macrophage colony-stimulating factor (M-CSF), and granulocyte colony-stimulating factor (G-CSF) can also modulate endothelial-macrophage function and activation. Orchestrated evolution of the inflammatory response can lead to atheroma formation, culminating in plaque rupture and coronary thrombotic disease with a fatal consequence or development of ischemic cardiomyopathy (7–9). The roles of key cytokines in atherogenesis are summarized in Table 2. It is likely that in HIV infection, some or many of these cytokines and growth factors are invoked as part of the aberrant immune activation and dysregulation seen in the disease.

Pivotal Role for Nuclear Factor Kappa B in Atherosclerosis

Nuclear factor kappa B (NF-κB) is a redox-sensitive transcription factor that regulates the expression of a battery of inflammatory genes (15). The NF-κB family consists of the proteins p50, p52, p65 (RelA), c-Rel, and RelB, which exist as dimers within the cytoplasm of the cell coupled to an inhibitory protein called IκBα. This latter protein maintains the dimers in an inactive state. Following cellular activation, IκBα is phosphorylated and undergoes ubiquination and proteolytic degradation. This is mediated by IκB kinases (IKKs) This process results in activation of NF-κB, which subsequently translocates to the nucleus, binds to consensus sequences on the promoter of the specific genes mentioned above, and leads to their transcription (16–18). Hence activation of NF-κB can have profound effects on vascular inflammation and atherogenesis.

Table 2 Role of Selected Cytokines in Atherogenesis

Cytokine	Primary cell sources	Relevance to atherosclerosis
APR		
IL-1 α/β/IL-6/TNF-α[a]	Mast cells, macrophages T cells, endothelium	EC activation, cytokine synthesis, permeability
		Acute-phase response: CRP, fibrinogen
		Monocyte recruitment
Th1 cytokines		
IL-2[a]	T cells	Growth/activation of plaque T cells
IFN γ[a]	T cells, NK cells	Enhances plaque Th1 cell differentiation
		Inhibits Th2 differentiation
		MHC II induction, macrophage activation
		Plaque instability
Th2 cytokines		
IL-4[b]	T cells, mast cells	Enhances Th2 development
		Inhibits plaque Th1 differentiation
		Inhibits macrophage function
		Inhibits fibrinogen synthesis
IL-10[b]	T cells, monocytes Macrophages	Inhibits Th1 cytokine synthesis
		Inhibits macrophage function, adhesion
		Inhibits fibrinogen synthesis
Others		
IL-12[a]	B cells, dendritic cells Macrophages	Proliferation/differentiation of Th1 subset
		Enhances IFN-γ and MCP-1 production
IL-18[a]	Monocytes, macrophages	Increased IFN-γ and GM-CSF production
		Plaque instability
		Synergizes with IL-12 in Th1 differentiation

[a] Proatherogenic.
[b] Antiatherogenic.
Key: APR = acute phase response cytokines; CRP = C-reactive protein; EC, endothelial cell; GM-CSF, granulocyte-macrophage colony stimulating factor; IFN-γ = interferon gamma; IL-1, interleukin 1; MCP-1 = monocyte chemotactic protein-1; MHC = major histocompatibility complex; NK, natural killer; TNF-α, tumor nercrosis factor alpha.

Hypoxemia, reactive oxygen intermediates, bacterial infection (19), bacterial endotoxin, viral infection, thrombin (20), and inflammatory cytokines such as IL-1 and TNF-α are all capable of inducing nuclear translocation of this factor (14,15). NF-κB, in turn, regulates genes involved in both innate and adaptive immunity. These include the adhesion molecules (ICAM-1 and VCAM-1) (21), cytokines (such as IL-1, TNF-α, IL-2, IL-6, IL-8, IL-12, M-CSF, MCP-1, and MIP-1 α) (16) and inducible nitric oxide synthase. NF-κB activation can be pivotal to atherogenesis (22–

24). Recent studies have shown that activated NF-κB is expressed in atheromatous tissue and in the plaque (25). Blood vessels from healthy individuals expressed only minimal amounts on quiescent NF-κB, which was present mainly in the cytosol and not yet translocated to the nucleus. Moreover, medications effective in ameliorating atherosclerotic heart disease, such as the angiotensin converting enzyme (ACE) inhibitors, salicylates, and statins, probably act by inhibiting nuclear translocation of NF-κB (26–28).

CONTRIBUTORS TO HIV-ASSOCIATED VASCULOPATHY

Many factors may participate in the genesis of cardiovascular disease in HIV-infected patients. In any given patient, one or several of these factors may have additive or

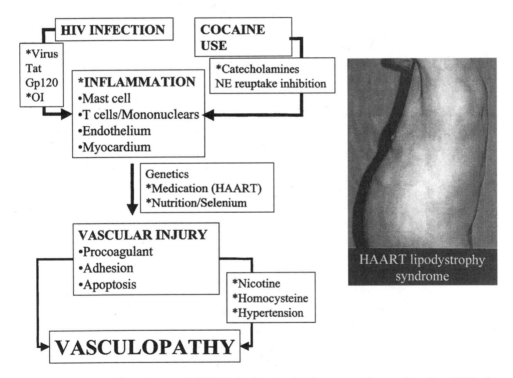

Figure 1   Role of cocaine and HIV infection in development of vasculopathy. HIV—by elaboration of soluble products, direct viral infection, or associated opportunistic infection (OI)—activates an inflammatory cascade. This can be accentuated by the effects of catecholamines induced by cocaine. Associated factors—such as nutritional deficiency, genetic susceptibility, and medications (HAART)—further accentuate immune injury, leading to vascular inflammation and athersclerotic vasculopathy. Other cardiovascular risk factors—such as nicotine abuse, homocysteine, and elevated blood pressure—can accelerate these changes. Dyslipidemia accompanying the lipodystrophic changes (as shown in accompanying photo) induced by the use of protease inhibitors can accelerate atherosclerosis and endothelial dysfunction.

synergistic effects on disease pathogenesis. The various pathogenic mechanisms involved in the genesis of HIV-associated cardiac disease are summarized in Figure 1 (29). It is possible that HIV could infect cardiac tissue directly, leading to dysfunction. Barbaro et al. demonstrated detection of HIV nucleotides in the hearts of 6% of 952 patients (30). In 36 of these patients, an active myocarditis was present, and 6 of these patients were coinfected with coxsackievirus group B, two with cytomegalovirus (CMV), and one with Epstein-Barr virus (EBV). Cardiotoxic cytokines, such as IL-1, TNF-α, and IL-6 are elevated in patients with HIV infection. HIV viral proteins (gp120, tat), coinfection with other cardiotropic viruses, autoimmune responses directed against myocardium, illicit drug use (for example, cocaine), the HIV wasting syndrome with its associated malnutrition and deficiency of micronutrients (antioxidant vitamins, selenium), concurrent cardiovascular risk factors (dyslipidemia, smoking, family history, hypertension), and the effects of antiretroviral drugs may all deleterious undermine myocardial function by the induction of apoptosis and cardiomyocyte injury and by indirect effects on lipid metabolism or immune function. In this regard, highly active antiretroviral drug therapy has been associated with lipodystrophy, dyslipidemias, and the development of insulin resistance (31).

CENTRAL ROLE FOR ENDOTHELIAL DYSFUNCTION IN HIV INFECTION

There is ample clinical evidence for disturbed vascular and endothelial function in HIV infection. Clinicopathological studies of ocular and brain tissue from HIV-1-infected patients have confirmed the presence of increased endothelial permeability and vascular leakage (32,33). Children infected with HIV and/or manifesting AIDS demonstrate a vasculopathy (34). Other instances of accelerated atherosclerosis and vascular injury have been described, suggesting that vascular damage is a feature of HIV infection. Since endothelial injury is an early event in vascular injury (35), it is very likely that vasculopathy in HIV infection is associated with direct or indirect evidence of endothelial dysfunction.

Evidence for Endothelial Injury in HIV Infection

There is indirect evidence for endothelial injury in HIV infection. Various markers of endothelial cell damage—such as von Willebrand factor antigen (vWF), soluble thrombomodulin (sTM), adhesion molecule E-selectin, tissue-type plasminogen activator (t-PA), plasminogen activator inhibitor (PA-I), fibronectin, ACE, and endothelin—are detectable in elevated quantities in the sera of patients infected with HIV-1 (36–39). Of these proteins, t-PA, PA-I, sTM, and vWF induce alterations in the coagulation cascade, leading to atherothrombosis. Janier and colleagues showed that the measurement of vWF antigenemia provided a good measure of endothelial damage (40). Increased levels of vWF antigen are observed in all stages of infection, whereas fibronectin and ACE levels increase only in advanced stages (41). As shown by Lafeuillade et al., levels of vWF antigen increase with disease progression and correlate closely with CD4 T-cell numbers and levels of β_2 microglobulin (37). Seigneur et al. found an increase of vWF, soluble vascular cell adhesion molecule 1 (VCAM-1), sTM, and E-selectin in the serum of HIV-infected patients (39). They also showed that levels of vWF and VCAM-1 significantly correlated with the CD4+ T lymphopenia (39). Strong correlations were also seen between levels of vWF and those of the inflammatory cytokines TNF-α and IFN-α (39).

There is direct evidence of endothelial activation in vivo in HIV-infected individuals. Zietz et al., for example, looked at the effects of HIV infection on endothelial activation by comparing aortic endothelial cells in pre-AIDS and AIDS patients (42). Aortic endothelial cells from infected individuals showed enhanced cell surface expression of human leukocyte antigen (HLA-DR) (expressed in endothelial cells of nearly 50% of infected individuals) and CAMs (including VCAM-1 and E-selectin). Endothelium from HIV-infected individuals also demonstrated enhanced leukocyte adherence and disturbed arrangement of cells as compared to uninfected control individuals (42).

Thus, ample evidence exists from both in vitro and in vivo studies, of endothelial activation in HIV infection. Endothelial activation and dysfunction could initiate a sequence of events culminating in atherosclerosis.

Role of Virus

CD4+ T-helper cells and monocytes are the most common virally infected cells in the bloodstream (43), while macrophages are by far the most abundant HIV-positive cells in the tissues. Since macrophages appear to serve as viral reservoirs in tissues and organ systems, they are thought to be the primary vehicles for HIV dissemination (44). Whether HIV-1 enters endothelium is controversial. Although in vivo evidence for endothelial cell infection by HIV is scant, some studies suggest that endothelial cells may be permissive to HIV infection. Bone marrow microvascular endothelial cells (MVEC) as well as placental, retinal, and brain endothelial cells have shown staining for HIV antigens in tissue obtained from infected individuals (45–49). Human liver sinusoid endothelium may also be permissive to HIV infection and is likely related to expression of CD4 antigen on these cells (50). Virus budding by electron microscopy and in situ persistence can be demonstrated in endothelial cells by double labeling with vWF and gp120 or p24. Virus produced by endothelial cells was also found to be infectious for a human T-cell line, suggesting one mode of viral infection of T cells (50). The expression of p24 antigen, formation of syncytia, viral budding as well as infectivity of released viral particles for a cultured cell line have been demonstrated (51). Infection of human umbilical vein endolethelial cells (HUVEC) probably occurs through a galactosyl ceramide receptor, but replication is restricted and mature virus is undetectable in these cells.

Virally infected endothelial cells can be pathological in several ways. Some investigators have suggested that virus rescue from endothelial cells can occur in the presence of T cells. Infected endothelial cells may also secrete atherogenic cytokines. Coculture of HUVEC possessing HIV DNA with peripheral blood mononuclear cells or CD4+ T cells induces syncytia formation in these T cells (52). Dianzani et al. cocultured HIV-infected HUVEC infected with T cells and showed that treatment with IFN-γ enhanced ICAM-1 expression and HIV-1 yield, while anti-ICAM antibody blocked HIV rescue (53). HIV-infected HUVEC secrete elevated levels of IL-6, and the production of IL-6 appears to be proportional to the size of the viral inoculum (54). IL-6 is a crucial cytokine that mediates the acute-phase response, characterized by the synthesis of acute-phase proteins (C-reactive protein, fibrinogen), neutrophil mobilization from the bone marrow, increased body temperature by stimulation of the hypothalamus, and protein and energy mobilization (14,55).

In summary, several lines of evidence suggest that some endothelial cells are permissive to HIV infection and could serve as a reservoir for virus. Infected endothelial cells may also be more adhesive for mononuclear cells and, by secreting atherogenic cytokines, may promote atherogenesis.

Role of Chemokines in HIV Entry

Several chemokine receptors serve as coreceptors for HIV-1 (56,57). Chemokines have been classified into the C-C and C-X-C groups based on structural characteristics and their binding to unique cell surface receptors. Endothelial cells do not appear to express CC-chemokine receptors but express essentially all known CXC-chemokine receptors (58). Feil et al. determined that the most abundantly expressed chemokine receptor on endothelial cells was the CXCR-4, also called the fusin receptor. CXCR-4 has been proven to be a coreceptor for the infection of CD4 + cells by certain strains of HIV-1 (59). However, it has recently been reported that CXCR-4/fusin was able to function as an alternate receptor for some isolates of HIV-2 in a number of CD4− cell lines, including T and B lymphoid cell lines and a nonlymphoid rhabdomyosarcoma cell line (60). This is supported by the observation that CD4-independent viral infection is inhibited by an antifusin monoclonal antibody. However, whether the expression of CXCR-4 or other chemokine receptors could function as a CD4 and GalCer-independent mechanism for HIV infection of endothelial cells has not been shown yet. Of great interest is the role for chemokines such as MCP-1 in atherogenesis. MCP-1/CCR2 knockout mice do not develop atherosclerosis (61). IL-8, another chemokine, has been detected in atheromatous plaque tissue (62). The relationships between viral entry, chemokine receptors, circulating chemokines, and the appearance of cardiovascular disease need further study.

Effects of Tat Protein on Endothelium

HIV-associated proteins tat and gp120 are detectable in blood and tissues of infected patients and can act as soluble mediators. Tat is normally active after the virus has incorporated its genome into the host's DNA and is a transactivator that, when bound to cellular DNA, allows regulation of certain proteins important to viral replication. The other protein, gp120, is a viral envelope glycoprotein that is directly responsible for entry of the virus into T-helper cells by binding to the CD4 surface marker. These two proteins can be secreted in a soluble form and also demonstrate biological activity when exposed to endothelial cells even in the absence of intact virus. As summarized below, tat protein and gp120 can mediate endothelial activation and allow expression of inflammatory cytokines and adhesion molecules, thereby contributing to pathogenesis of disease.

Tat Induces Cytokine Transcription and Nuclear Factor Kappa B Translocation

Tat, the transactivator of viral transcription, activates human endothelial cells to express inflammatory cytokines and adhesion molecules. Tat also contributes to angiogenesis and possibly to the development of Kaposi's sarcoma (KS) (63,64). Zidovetzki and coworkers studied the effects of tat protein on brain-derived endothelial cells. These investigators demonstrated that tat rapidly induces these cells to express IL-6 mRNA (65). Protein kinase C (PKC) activity was seen within 30 sec of activation of endothelial cells by tat and was essential for protein kinase A (PKA) activation. These changes occurred even with low concentrations of tat at 10 ng/mL. Accordingly, tat-induced IL-6 mRNA expression was inhibited by a PKA inhibitor. Exposure of brain-derived endothelial cells to tat activates IL-6 production and enhances permeability of these cells, allowing cellular emigration. When endothelial cells are activated with exogenous tat protein, these cells express E-selectin and synthesize IL-6, as shown by Hoffman et al. (66). TNF-α appears to synergize with low concentrations of tat to activate IL-6 production from endothelial cells. The same group studied the response of brain capillary endothelial cells to tat protein in combination with TNF-α and transforming growth factor beta (TGF-β) (67). Similarly, a strong upregulation of IL-8 mRNA occurs when endothelial cells are exposed to tat protein at a concentration of 100 ng/mL, and this effect is enhanced by addition of TNF-α (67). On the other hand, TGF-β had inhibitory effects on IL-8 mRNA expression in response to tat (67). Thus, in an environment enriched in TNF-α, tat enhances the production of chemotactic cytokines, further amplifying the inflammatory response.

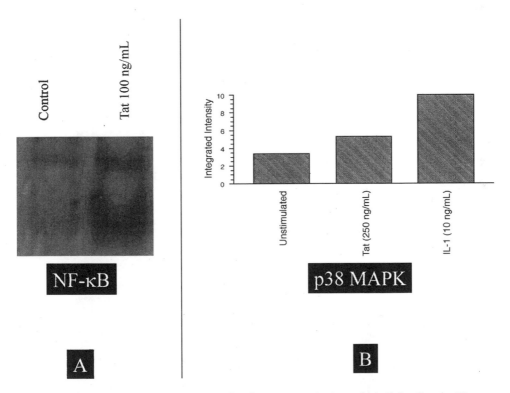

Figure 2 Induction of signaling proteins by tat protein in endothelial cells. A. Human pulmonary artery endothelial cells were activated with tat (250 ng/mL) and nuclear translocation of nuclear factor kappa B was assessed by electrophoresis mobilityshift assay (EMSA). B. Induction of p38 mitogen-activated protein kinases (MAPK) in human endothelial cells by tat protein. Human pulmonary artery endothelial cells were activated with tat (250 ng/mL) or IL-1 β (10 ng/mL) and MAPK phosphorylation was assessed using Western blotting.

We examined the effects of tat protein on endothelial cell signaling and cytokine secretion. Human pulmonary endothelial cells were activated with either tat protein (100 to 250 ng/mL) or IL-1 β (10 ng/mL) for varying periods of time. Cytoplasmic and nuclear membrane protein was isolated and assayed for p38 MAPK by Western blotting and for NF-κB nuclear translocation by electrophoresis mobility shift assay. Supernatants of stimulated cells were collected after 24 hr and assayed for cytokines by enzyme-linked immunosorbent assay (ELISA). Our data are shown in Figures 2 and 3. Tat induced nuclear translocation of NF-κB by 1 hr (Fig. 2A), while tat also induced p38 mitogen-activated protein kinases (MAPK) within 45 min (Fig. 2B). Tat was not nearly as efficient as IL-1 β but was definitely associated with activation of both NF-κB and MAPK. By ELISA, tat at 250 and 500 ng/mL induced a significant and dose-dependent secretion of IL-6 into the supernatant (Fig. 3). The induction of these transcription factors and signaling proteins as well as IL-6 secretion suggest on additional mechanism by which HIV can influence inflammatory processes in vascular tissues.

Tat Induces Endothelial Cell Adhesion Molecule Expression

Tat protein influences endothelial cell expression of cell adhesion molecules (CAMs). Dhawan and coworkers exposed HUVEC to tat protein and measured cell surface expression of the CAMs, intercellular adhesion molecule 1 (ICAM-1), Vascular cell adhesion molecule 1 (VCAM-1), and endothelial leukocyte adhesion molecule 1 (ELAM-1) (68). These CAMs were shown to rapidly increase, a process blocked by

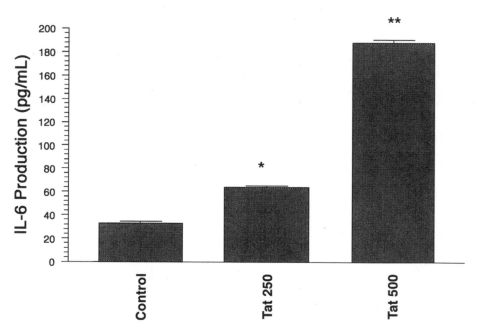

Figure 3 Tat protein induces secretion of interleukin-6 (IL-6) in human pulmonary artery endothelial cells. Endothelial cells were activated by tat at 250- and 500-ng/mL concentrations. Statistically significant enhancement of IL-6 secretion from endothelial cells was seen (*, ** $p < 0.05$ compared to controls).

antitat antibody. Expression of CAMs on endothelial cell surfaces is associated with increased adhesiveness of these cells for leukocytes. Thus, increased adhesiveness of tat-activated endothelium for HL-60 mononuclear cells was shown by the same investigators—a process further amplified by the addition of TNF-α. Tat protein also alters the adhesive properties of monocytes, making them more adherent to endothelial cells through the upregulation of integrins (69). We examined the effects of tat protein on VCAM-1 and ICAM-1 expression in human pulmonary artery endothelial cells (HPAEC). HPAEC were activated with either tat protein alone (100 or 250 ng/ mL) and/or IL-1 β (10 ng/mL). RNA was extracted from activated endothelial cells in 4 hr and subjected to reverse transcription-polymerase chain reaction (RT-PCR) for VCAM-1 and GADPH (housekeeping gene). Then, 24 hr after activation, endothelial cells were incubated with fluorescently labeled antibodies to VCAM-1 or ICAM-1. Both tat protein and IL-1 β induced transcripts for VCAM-1 in HPAEC (Fig. 4a). By flow cytometry, enhanced expression of VCAM-1 on endothelial cell surfaces was seen with both tat protein and IL-1 β (Fig. 4b). Similar upregulation of cell surface ICAM-1 by IL-1 β was seen.

These adhesion molecules are important under normal inflammatory conditions in the adherence of leukocytes to the endothelium, ultimately allowing the immune cells to leave the vasculature and infiltrate the surrounding vascular tissue. Our data as well as the recent observation that tat activates nuclear translocation of NF-κB (70) are significant. NF-κB activates transcription of cytokine and adhesion molecule genes and hence may be pivotal to orchestration of endothelium-dependent inflammatory responses (17). Drugs such as salicylates and/or statins, by blocking NF-κB translocation, may be beneficial in the modulation of endothelial responses (70).

Tat Receptors on Endothelial Cells: Effects on Angiogenesis

Vascular endothelial cells proliferate, migrate, and degrade basement membranes in response to tat protein and inflammatory cytokines (64). Tat specifically binds to the Flk/KDR receptor, which is a vascular endothelial growth factor-A tyrosine kinase receptor (71). Hence, tat-mediated angiogenesis can be inhibited by agents blocking Flk/KDR. The interactions between the $\alpha_5\beta_1$ and $\alpha_v\beta_3$ integrins and tat are also sufficient to mediate vascular migration and also provide the adhesion signals required for Kaposi sarcoma (KS) cell growth and proliferation (72). Tat also appears to assist in angiogenesis by mobilizing basic fibroblast growth factor (bFGF). Tat protein retrieves into soluble form extracellular bFGF bound to heparan sulfate proteoglycans by competing for binding sites (72). bFGF is a true angiogenic factor, which is also required for growth and maintenance of KS. The RGD sequence of tat is also able to induce the expression of a 72-kDa collagenase, a metalloproteinase that is important for mediating the invasive properties of KS.

EFFECTS OF GP120 PROTEIN ON ENDOTHELIUM

The envelope glycoprotein gp120 has several effects relevant to endothelial cell function, some of which could predispose the blood vessel to atherogenesis. Gp120 has been shown to alter endothelial permeability and to induce endothelial cell apoptosis. In addition, findings in our laboratory (discussed later) demonstrate that

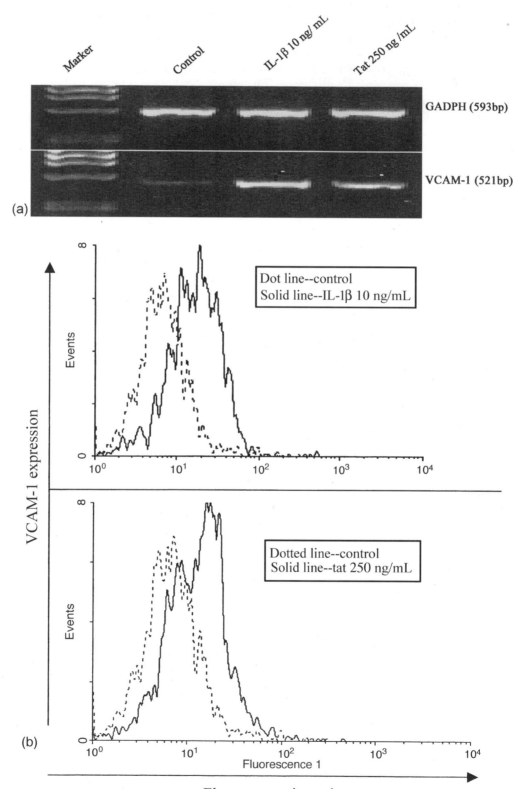

(a)

(b)

Fluorescence intensity

mast cells undergo activation when exposed to a combination of cocaine and gp120. In a recent study, researchers reported that exposure of umbilical vein endothelial cells (HUVEC) to low concentrations of gp120 induced an apoptotic program mediated probably by the chemokine receptors, CCR5 and CXCR4 but not by CD4 (73).

Annunziata et al. showed that gp120 was able to increase the permeability of rat brain endothelium to macromolecules. This effect occurred in a dose-dependent fashion and was blocked by antibody to gp120 (74). The authors also showed that endothelial cells exposed to gp120 showed cell surface immunoreactivity for substance P. Accordingly, this effect of gp120 was also blocked by spantide (a substance P antagonist). The investigators concluded that substance P, which is commonly associated with pain fiber transmission and inflammation-like responses, plays a role in the gp120-mediated stimulation of rat brain endothelial cultures.

Stefano et al. found that by itself gp120 could enhance monocyte adhesion to endothelial cells, a phenomenon crucial to early atherogenesis (75). However, this adhesive event was blocked by the addition of morphine and anadamide to the cell cultures. This suggested the involvement of nitric oxide, since both drugs induce production of nitric oxide (NO), which prevents monocyte adherence, perhaps by reducing expression of the adhesion molecule VCAM-1 on endothelial surfaces. In summary, gp120, a soluble product of HIV infection, can alter endothelial function in several ways, including induction of apoptosis, activating cytokine expression by mononuclear cells, enhancing adhesiveness of mononuclear cells to endothelium, and increasing endothelial permeability.

APOPTOSIS IN HIV INFECTION

Apoptosis, or programmed cell death, plays a pivotal role in CD4+ lymphocyte depletion in HIV infection (76,77). Apoptosis of nonlymphoid cells may also be of pivotal importance to HIV pathogenesis. Thus, apoptosis of neurons, astrocytes, and vascular endothelial cells may contribute to the development of neuronal injury, thrombotic thrombocytopenic purpura (TTP), and even atherogenesis (78,79).

Endothelial cell apoptosis has been observed to occur in a variety of clinical conditions and may predispose to thrombosis. Plasma from HIV-infected patients suffering from TTP-induced enhanced apoptosis in cultured microvascular endothelial cells derived from the skin (78,80). The mechanisms behind these endothelial apoptotic responses are unclear. Some data suggests that lipoproteins may be

Figure 4 (a) Induction of VCAM-1 transcripts in endothelial cells by tat protein. Human pulmonary artery endothelial cells were activated with either IL-1 β (10 ng/mL) or tat (250 ng/mL) for 4 hr, RNA extracted and subjected to reverse transcription polymerase chain reaction (RT-PCR) using primers specific for either GADPH (housekeeping gene) or VCAM-1 genes. Specificity of amplification was confirmed by direct sequencing of the amplified products. (b) Induction of VCAM-1 on endothelial cell surface by tat protein. Human pulmonary artery endothelial cells were activated with either IL-1 β or with tat protein (250 ng/mL) for 24 hr and expression of VCAM-1 on cell surfaces assessed by flow cytometry using fluorescent-tagged antibodies specific for VCAM-1.

involved in endothelial cell apoptosis and may involved in the vasculopathy of AIDS (1,2,81). The newer protease inhibitors have been linked to dyslipidemia-related accelerated atherosclerosis, and endothelial cell apoptosis may be occurring in this condition (2,82,83). Galle et al. showed that both oxidized low-density lipoproteins (oxLDL) and oxidized lipoprotein (a) [oxLp (a)] increased the rate of apoptosis in endothelial cells and in rabbit aorta (84,85). This occurred in a dose-dependent manner (84,85). Oxidized lipoprotein-mediated induction of apoptosis was enhanced by inhibition of superoxide dismutase (SOD) (a scavenger of reactive oxygen species) and antioxidants, suggesting a role for oxidative stress in this process. Apoptotic endothelial cells can predispose to thrombus formation. Bombeli et al. have shown that exposure of cultured endothelial cells to apoptosis-inducing agents such as staurosporin resulted in a significant increase in thrombin formation in recalcified citrated plasma (86). Enhancement of monocyte adhesion, increased procoagulant properties, and other mechanisms can lead apoptotic endothelial cells to accentuate atherogenesis.

A MONOCYTE-ENDOTHELIAL AXIS IN HIV-INDUCED VASCULOPATHY

Monocyte activation in HIV infection can lead to the elaboration of several cytokines that can influence endothelial function and adhesiveness. Both HIV glycoprotein gp120 and tat protein can activate monocytes to secrete inflammatory cytokines. Wahl and coworkers activated monocytes with purified HIV gp120 protein and found a dose-dependent upregulation of prostaglandin E_2 and IL-1 synthesis (87). Gp120 blocked the binding of OKT4 antibody to CD4 on monocytes. Since both IL-1 and prostanoids can have profound effects on endothelial adhesive function, this interactions may have significance for atherogenesis (88,89). Tat protein has been shown to activate monocytes to express integrins, thereby modulating monocyte-endothelial adhesion and interactions (69). This monocyte adhesion was associated with disruption of endothelial monolayers, probably mediated by elaboration of MMP-9 from monocytes (69). Lafrenie and colleagues demonstrated that tat protein itself has chemotactic properties. Pretreatment of monocytes with minute amounts of tat protein (10 ng/mL) increased their ability to invade matrigel-coated filters even in the absence of a chemoattractant (90). In a checkerboard analysis, monocytes were shown to migrate in response to a tat chemotactic gradient (90). Treatment of monocytes with tat protein is associated with expression of IL-1 β and TNF-α, cytokines known to activate endothelium (91). Thus one can envision a HIV-monocyte-endothelial axis that may be pivotal to the development of atherosclerotic vasculopathy.

OXIDANT INJURY AND ENDOTHELIAL FUNCTION

In HIV-infected individuals there is compelling evidence for an enhanced production of reactive oxygen species (ROS) and reactive nitrogen oxide species (RNOS) as well as a depletion of many antioxidant defense systems by mechanisms involving the synthesis of HIV gp120 and tat proteins (92–95). Patients with AIDS have decreased

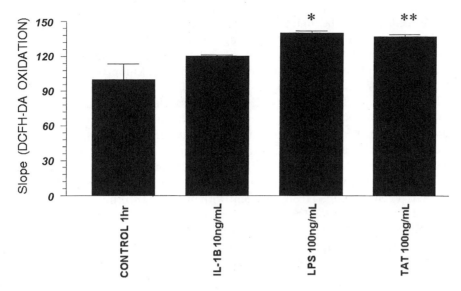

Figure 5 Induction of reactive oxygen species in endothelial cells by tat protein. The oxidation of dihydrohydrochlorofluorescein to dicholorofluorescein was assessed using a fluorescent plate reader. *, ** indicate $p < 0.05$ compared to control.

levels of plasma glutathione, ascorbate, and vitamin E as well as increased plasma levels of lipid peroxidation products. The decrease in antioxidant nutrients is related to the severity of the disease (96). We activated endothelial cells with tat protein, lipopolysaccharide (LPS), or IL-1β and measured oxidation of nonfluorescent 2′,7′-dichlorohydrofluorescein (DCHF) to dichlorofluorescein (DCF), which emits fluorescence. The fluorescence microplate reader was used to monitor fluorescence. The results are shown in Figure 5. Tat and LPS induced significant increases in DCHF oxidation ($p < 0.05$ compared to control). Endothelial dysfunction, monocyte activation, and worsening of vascular disease may follow production of ROS. This may be accentuated by nutritional deficiencies of antioxidants in patients infected with HIV.

EVIDENCE FOR MAST CELL ACTIVATION BY COCAINE

Human mast cells may play a role in atherogenesis and plaque rupture (9). The human mast cell is found around blood vessels and beneath the epithelium of the skin and mucous membranes (97). Traditionally, mast cells have been classified into two types based on their expression of proteases in granules. Thus, MC_T cells (also regarded as immune cell–associated) contain tryptase in their granules, and are dominantly located in respiratory and intestinal mucosa. These cells colocalize around T cells. The granule morphology in MC_T cells is described as scroll-rich. On the other hand, MC_{TC} cells contain both tryptase and chymase in their granules. They are dominantly found in connective tissue areas such as skin, conjunctiva, and synovium and their granule morphology is described as lattice or grating structures. Typically, mast cells stain metachromatically, due to the presence of the sulfated glycosaminoglycan heparin. Mast cells express the high-affinity receptor for immunoglobulin E (IgE) or FcεRI on their cell surfaces. This receptor belongs to a group of immunoreceptors that express a common gamma chain, including the T-cell receptor for antigen. Following cross-linkage of FcεRI by antigen, mast cell activation occurs. Lipoproteins, bacteria, complement products and neuropeptides can all induce mast cell degranulation without the need for the high-affinity IgE receptor–associated signaling. Mast cell activation, in turn, results in signaling events and the elaboration of inflammatory mediators, which are then secreted into the microenvironment. These cytokines, prostanoids, leukotrienes, and histamine can have a major impact on the development of vascular inflammation. Mast cells are increased in the adventitia of blood vessels from persons dying of cocaine-associated coronary thrombotic disease (98). We activated HMC-1 cells (obtained from a patient with mast cell leukemia) with cocaine and gp120 and assayed for NF-κB translocation to the nucleus. The results are shown in Figure 6. Nuclear translocation of NF-κB was seen most clearly with cocaine and gp120 together. Mast cells primed with IL-1 β or TNF-α produce more proinflammatory cytokines than mast cells activated via the FcεRI alone. In patients with HIV infection, monocyte activation induces production of IL-1 and TNF-α, and a monocyte–mast cell axis may exist that potentiates inflammatory responses. These data suggest that this in vitro phenomenon may have important in vivo biological consequences. In recent studies, we have seen enhanced tryptase secretion from mast

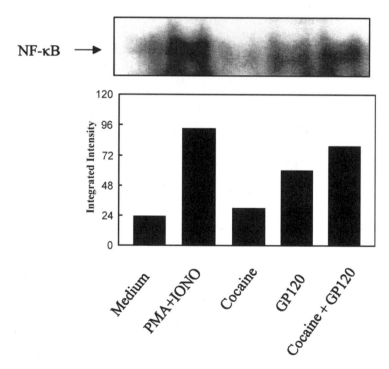

Figure 6 Induction of nuclear factor kappa B in human mast cells (HMC-1) by a combination of gp120 protein and cocaine. Significant enhancement of nuclear translocation of nuclear factor kappa B in HMC-1 cell line was seen in response to a phorbol ester (PMA) and calcium ionophore as well as to a combination of cocaine and gp120.

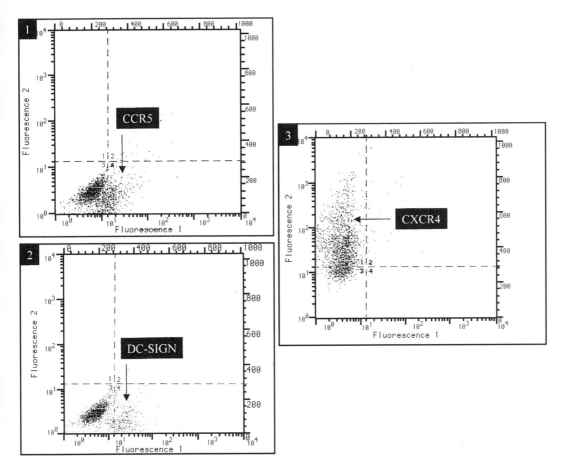

Figure 7 HMC-1 mast cells express several HIV coreceptors, including CCR5, CXCR4, and DC-SIGN. This suggests that direct infection of mast cells by virus is likely and may contribute to vascular pathology given the role played by mast cells in atherosclerosis. (Kelley JL, Chi DS, Abou-Auda W, Smith JK, Krishnaswamy G. The molecular role of mast cells in atherosclerotic cardiovascular disease. Mol Med Today 2000; 6(8):304–308.)

cells activated with cocaine. Moreover, human mast cells express many HIV coreceptors, such as CCR5, CXCR4, and DC-SIGN, raising the possibility that they may serve as reservoir for virus (Fig. 7). These studies, taken together, suggest a possible role for mast cells and a mast cell–monocyte axis in vascular disease complicating cocaine abuse and HIV infection.

SYNERGISTIC ROLE OF HIV INFECTION AND COCAINE IN POTENTIATING VASCULAR DISEASE

Endothelial or mast cell activation by HIV infection or cocaine can initiate vascular injury and signaling via the translocation of nuclear transcription factors, such as nuclear factor kappa B (NF-κB) and protein kinase C (PKC). Both of these signaling proteins have been implicated in atherogenesis (99–101). Since NF-κB undergoes nuclear translocation and binding to the promoter sites of cytokine, chemokine, and adhesion molecule genes, this can initiate an inflammatory cascade characterized by mononuclear cell recruitment and the subsequent macrophage foam cell formation (102–105) (Fig. 8). Endothelial dysfunction and injury have been considered pivotal early events in atherogenesis (35) and can lead to the initiation of a cascade of inflammatory events in HIV infection that can predispose the patient to the development of cardiovascular disease. Besides direct infection and the effects of secreted tat and gp120, endothelial activation may also be due to HIV-1–associated complement pathway activation and circulating immune complexes with HIV-1 antigens (106,107). Other factors include coinfection with other cardiotropic viruses, autoimmune responses directed against myocardium, illicit drug use (for example, cocaine), the HIV wasting syndrome with its associated malnutrition and deficiency of micronutrients (antioxidant vitamins, selenium), concurrent cardiovascular risk factors—hemodynamic stress, hypertension, smoking, ageing and metabolic factors such as homocysteine and dyslipidemia (13,55)—and the effects of retroviral drugs (such as reverse transcriptase and protease inhibitors), which may all have deleterious effects on endothelial function. Some of these interactions are summarized in Figure 8.

Endothelial activation and the effects of circulating cytokines such as TNF-α, IL-1, and IFN-γ induce the expression of adhesion molecules such as intercellular

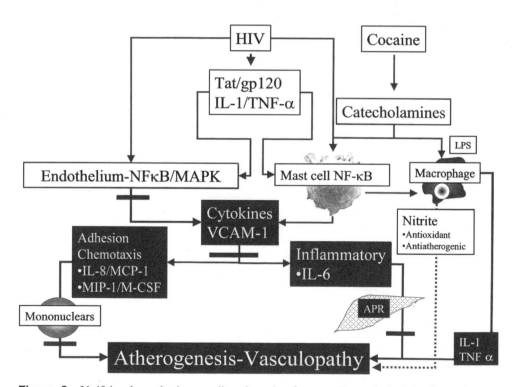

Figure 8 Unifying hypothesis regarding the role of mast cells, endothelial cells, and macrophages in the pathogenesis of HIV- and cocaine-associated atherogenesis and vasculopathy. Refer to text for detailed discussions.

adhesion molecule-1 (ICAM-1), VCAM-1, and endothelial leukocyte adhesion molecule 1 (ELAM-1) and enhance the adhesion of leukocytes to the endothelium (Fig. 8). Interactions between the very late activating antigen-4 (VLA-4) and VCAM-1 could lead to the recruitment of mononuclears to vascular sites, leading to foam cell formation. The human endothelium is a rich source of inflammatory mediators itself and could contribute to the inflammatory milieu (14,55). IL-6 can modulate production of acute-phase proteins, such as CRP, from the liver. Atherogenic chemokines and cytokines such as IL-1, IL-8, and MCP-1 attract more leukocytes to the locally restricted/infected site resulting in an "inflammatory cascade" (Fig. 8). This may result in patches of adherent leukocytes, which release toxic products to damage the endothelium. This is supported by the report that a positive correlation exists between the number of adherent cells and the degree of endothelial disturbance (42). The apoptosis of endothelial cells can lead to a procoagulant environment, leading to atherothrombotic disease and vasculopathy. Mononuclear infiltration and foam cell formation may ensue, leading to progressive vascular remodeling and atherosclerotic plaque formation. Cardiac ischemia can lead to ventricular remodeling and the development of cardiomyopathy with ventricular dysfunction. Cocaine, by virtue of catecholamine elaboration and mast cell activation, can further accentuate endothelial injury and leukocyte adhesion. Hence, in an ever-progressing vicious cycle, HIV-induced endothelial cell dysfunction can lead to the genesis and maturation of cardiovascular disease, ultimately contributing to enormous morbidity and mortality of the HIV-infected population.

ACKNOWLEDGMENTS

Funded by NIH grants AI-43310 and HL-63070, the Rondal Cole Foundation and the Chair of Excellence in Medicine (State of Tennessee grant 20233), the Cardiovascular Research Institute, and the Research Development Committee, East Tennessee State University.

REFERENCES

1. Kelley J, Chi DS, Henry J, Stone WL, Smith JK, Krishnaswamy G. HIV- and cocaine-induced cardiovascular disease: pathogenesis and clinical implications. Cardiovasc Rev Rep 2000; 21(7):365–370.
2. Krishnaswamy G, Chi DS, Kelley JL, Sarubbi F, Smith JK, Peiris A. The cardiovascular and metabolic complications of hiv infection. Cardiol Rev 2000; 8(5):260–268.
3. Depairon M, Chessex S, Sudre P, Rodondi N, Doser N, Chave JP, Riesen W, Nicod P, Darioli R, Telenti A, Mooser V. Premature atherosclerosis in HIV-infected individuals—focus on protease inhibitor therapy. AIDS 2001; 15(3):329–334.
4. Duong M, Buisson M, Cottin Y, Piroth L, Lhuillier I, Grappin M, Chavanet P, Wolff JE, Portier H. Coronary heart disease associated with the use of human immunodeficiency virus (HIV)-1 protease inhibitors: report of four cases and review. Clin Cardiol 2001; 24(10):690–694.
5. Lewis W. Atherosclerosis in AIDS: potential pathogenetic roles of antiretroviral therapy and HIV. J Mol Cell Cardiol 2000; 32(12):2115–2129.

6.   Schmitz G, Herr AS, Rothe G. T-lymphocytes and monocytes in atherogenesis. Herz 1998; 23:168–177.

7.   Ross R. Rous-Whipple Award Lecture. Atherosclerosis: a defense mechanism gone awry. Am J Pathol 1993; 143:987–1002.

8.   Ross R. Atherosclerosis—an inflammatory disease. N Engl J Med 1999; 340:115–126.

9.   Kelley JL, Chi DS, Abou-Auda W, Smith JK, Krishnaswamy G. The molecular role of mast cells in atherosclerotic cardiovascular disease. Mol Med Today 2000; 6(8):304–308.

10. Ross R. Cellular and molecular studies of atherogenesis. Atherosclerosis 1997; 131(suppl):S3–S4.

11. Ross R. The pathogenesis of atherosclerosis: a perspective for the 1990s. Nature 1993; 362:801–809.

12. Stary HC. The sequence of cell and matrix changes in atherosclerotic lesions of coronary arteries in the first forty years of life. Eur Heart J 1990; 11(suppl E):3–19.

13. LaRosa JC. Atherogenesis and its relationship to coronary risk factors. Clin Cornerstone 1998; 1(1):3–11.

14. Krishnaswamy G, Kelley J, Yerra L, Smith JK, Chi DS. Human endothelium as a source of multifunctional cytokines: molecular regulation and possible role in human disease. J Interferon Cytokine Res 1999; 19:91–104.

15. Krishnaswamy G. Treatment strategies for bronchial asthma: an update. Hosp Pract (Off Ed) 2001; 36(8):25–35.

16. Scheinman RI, Cogswell PC, Lofquist AK, Baldwin A.S. Jr. Role of transcriptional activation of I kappa B alpha in mediation of immunosuppression by glucocorticoids [see comments]. Science 1995; 270:283–286.

17. Barnes PJ. Nuclear factor-kappa B. Int J Biochem Cell Biol 1997; 29:867–870.

18. Adcock IM. Transcription factors as activators of gene transcription: AP-1 and NF-kappa B. Monaldi Arch Chest Dis 1997; 52:178–186.

19. Ebnet K, Brown KD, Siebenlist UK, Simon MM, Shaw S. *Borrelia burgdorferi* activates nuclear factor-kappa B and is a potent inducer of chemokine and adhesion molecule gene expression in endothelial cells and fibroblasts. J Immunol 1997; 158:3285–3292.

20. Maruyama I, Shigeta K, Miyahara H, Nakajima T, Shin H, Ide S, Kitajima I. Thrombin activates NF-kappa B through thrombin receptor and results in proliferation of vascular smooth muscle cells: role of thrombin in atherosclerosis and restenosis. Ann N Y Acad Sci 1997; 811:429–436.

21. Shu HB, Agranoff AB, Nabel EG, Leung K, Duckett CS, Neish AS, Collins T, Nabel GJ. Differential regulation of vascular cell adhesion molecule 1 gene expression by specific NF-kappa B subunits in endothelial and epithelial cells. Mol Cell Biol 1993; 13:6283–6289.

22. Brand K, Page S, Walli AK, Neumeier D, Baeuerle PA. Role of nuclear factor-kappa B in atherogenesis. Exp Physiol 1997; 82:297–304.

23. Navab M, Fogelman AM, Berliner JA, Territo MC, Demer LL, Frank JS, Watson AD, Edwards PA, Lusis AJ. Pathogenesis of atherosclerosis. Am J Cardiol 1995; 76:18C–23C.

24. Collins T. Endothelial nuclear factor-kappa B and the initiation of the atherosclerotic lesion. Lab Invest 1993; 68:499–508.

25. Brand K, Page S, Rogler G, Bartsch A, Brandl R, Knuechel R, Page M, Kaltschmidt C, Baeuerle PA, Neumeier D. Activated transcription factor nuclear factor-kappa B is present in the atherosclerotic lesion. J Clin Invest 1996; 97:1715–1722.

26. Hernandez-Presa MA, Bustos C, Ortego M, Tunon J, Ortega L, Egido J. ACE inhibitor quinapril reduces the arterial expression of NF- kappaB- dependent proinflammatory factors but not of collagen I in a rabbit model of atherosclerosis. Am J Pathol 1998; 153:1825–1837.

27. Bustos C, Hernandez-Presa MA, Ortego M, Tunon J, Ortega L, Perez F, Diaz C,

Hernandez G, Egido J. HMG-CoA reductase inhibition by atorvastatin reduces neo-intimal inflammation in a rabbit model of atherosclerosis. J Am Coll Cardiol 1998; 32(7):2057–2064.

28. Pierce JW, Read MA, Ding H, Luscinskas FW, Collins T. Salicylates inhibit I kappa B-alpha phosphorylation, endothelial-leukocyte adhesion molecule expression, and neutrophil transmigration. J Immunol 1996; 156:3961–3969.

29. Thornton FJ, Schaffer MR, Witte MB, Moldawer LL, MacKay SL, Abouhamze A, Tannahill CL, Barbul A. Enhanced collagen accumulation following direct transfection of the inducible nitric oxide synthase gene in cutaneous wounds. Biochem Biophys Res Commun 1998; 246:654–659.

30. Schaffer MR, Fuchs N, Proksch B, Bongartz M, Beiter T, Becker HD. Tacrolimus impairs wound healing: a possible role of decreased nitric oxide synthesis. Transplantation 1998; 65:813–818.

31. Schaffer MR, Tantry U, Efron PA, Ahrendt GM, Thornton FJ, Barbul A. Diabetes-impaired healing and reduced wound nitric oxide synthesis: a possible pathophysiologic correlation. Surgery 1997; 121:513–519.

32. Gariano RF, Rickman LS, Freeman WR. Ocular examination and diagnosis in patients with the acquired immunodeficiency syndrome. West J Med 1993; 158(3):254–262.

33. Rhodes RH. Evidence of serum-protein leakage across the blood-brain barrier in the acquired immunodeficiency syndrome. J Neuropathol Exp Neurol 1991; 50(2):171–183.

34. Joshi VV, Pawel B, Connor E, Sharer L, Oleske JM, Morrison S, Marin-Garcia J. Arteriopathy in children with acquired immune deficiency syndrome. Pediatr Pathol 1987; 7(3):261–275.

35. Liao JK. Endothelium and acute coronary syndromes. Clin Chem 1998; 44:1799–1808.

36. Schved JF, Gris JC, Arnaud A, Martinez P, Sanchez N, Wautier JL, Sarlat C. von Willebrand factor antigen, tissue-type plasminogen activator antigen, and risk of death in human immunodeficiency virus 1–related clinical disease: independent prognostic relevance of tissue-type plasminogen activator. J Lab Clin Med 1992; 120(3):411–419.

37. Lafeuillade A, Alessi MC, Poizot-Martin I, Boyer-Neumann C, Zandotti C, Quilichini R, Aubert L, Tamalet C, Juhan-Vague I, Gastaut JA. Endothelial cell dysfunction in HIV infection. J AIDS 1992; 5:127–131.

38. Rolinski B, Geier SA, Sadri I, Klauss V, Bogner JR, Ehrenreich H, Goebel FD. Endothelin-1 immunoreactivity in plasma is elevated in HIV-1 infected patients with retinal microangiopathic syndrome. Clin Invest 1994; 72(4):288–293.

39. Seigneur M, Constans J, Blann A, Renard M, Pellegrin JL, Amiral J, Boisseau M, Conri C. Soluble adhesion molecules and endothelial cell damage in HIV infected patients. Thromb Haemost 1997; 77:646–649.

40. Janier M, Flageul B, Drouet L, Scrobohaci ML, Villette JM, Palangie A, Cottenot F. Cutaneous and plasma values of von Willebrand factor in AIDS: a marker of endothelial stimulation? J Invest Dermatol 1988; 90:703–707.

41. Drouet L, Scrobohaci ML, Janier M, Baudin B. Endothelial cells: target for the HIV1 virus? Nouv Rev Fr Hematol 1990; 32:103–106.

42. Zietz C, Hotz B, Sturzl M, Rauch E, Penning R, Lohrs U. Aortic endothelium in HIV-1 infection: chronic injury, activation, and increased leukocyte adherence. Am J Pathol 1996; 149:1887–1898.

43. Lane HC, Fauci AS. Immunologic abnormalities in the acquired immunodeficiency syndrome. Annu Rev Immunol 1985; 3:477–500.

44. Meltzer MS, Skillman DR, Hoover DL, Hanson BD, Turpin JA, Kalter DC, Gendelman HE. Macrophages and the human immunodeficiency virus. Immunol Today 1990; 11(6):217–223.

45. Moses AV, Williams S, Heneveld ML, Strussenberg J, Rarick M, Loveless M, Bagby G, Nelson JA. Human immunodeficiency virus infection of bone marrow endothelium

reduces induction of stromal hematopoietic growth factors [see comments]. Blood 1996; 87:919–925.

46. Canque B, Marandin A, Rosenzwajg M, Louache F, Vainchenker W, Gluckman JC. Susceptibility of human bone marrow stromal cells to human immunodeficiency virus (HIV). Virology 1995; 208:779–783.

47. Faulk WP, Labarrere CA. HIV proteins in normal human placentae. Am J Reprod Immunol 1991; 25:99–104.

48. Skolnik PR, Pomerantz RJ, de la Monte SM, Lee SF, Hsiung GD, Foos RY, Cowan GM, Kosloff BR, Hirsch MS, Pepose JS. Dual infection of retina with human immunodeficiency virus type 1 and cytomegalovirus. Am J Ophthalmol 1989; 107:361–372.

49. Pumarola-Sune T, Navia BA, Cordon-Cardo C, Cho ES, Price RW. HIV antigen in the brains of patients with the AIDS dementia complex. Ann Neurol 1987; 21(5):490–496.

50. Steffan AM, Lafon ME, Gendrault JL, Schweitzer C, Royer C, Jaeck D, Arnaud JP, Schmitt MP, Aubertin AM, Kirn A. Primary cultures of endothelial cells from the human liver sinusoid are permissive for human immunodeficiency virus type 1. Proc Natl Acad Sci USA 1992; 89:1582–1586.

51. Steffan AM, Lafon ME, Gendrault JL, Smedsrod B, Nonnenmacher H, Koehren F, Gut JP, de Monte M, Martin JP, Royer C, Kirn A. Productive infection of primary cultures of endothelial cells from the cat liver sinusoid with the feline immunodeficiency virus. Hepatology 1996; 23:964–970.

52. Scheglovitova O, Capobianchi MR, Antonelli G, Guanmu D, Fais S, Dianzani F. CD4 positive lymphoid cells rescue HIV-1 replication from abortively infected human primary endothelial cells. Int Conf AIDS 1993; 9:142.

53. Dianzani F, Scheglovitova O, Gentile M, Scanio V, Barresi C, Ficociello B, Bianchi F, Fiumara D, Capobianchi MR. Interferon gamma stimulates cell-mediated transmission of HIV type 1 from abortively infected endothelial cells. AIDS Res Hum Retrovir 1996; 12:621–627.

54. Corbeil J, Evans LA, McQueen PW, Vasak E, Edward PD, Richman DD, Penny R, Cooper DA. Productive in vitro infection of human umbilical vein endothelial cells and three colon carcinoma cell lines with HIV-1. Immunol Cell Biol 1995; 73:140–145.

55. Krishnaswamy G, Smith JK, Mukkamala R, Hall K, Joyner W, L Y, Chi DS. Multifunctional cytokine expression by human coronary endothelium and regulation by monokines and glucocorticoids. Microvasc Res 1998; 55:189–200.

56. Banks WA, Akerstrom V, Kastin AJ. Adsorptive endocytosis mediates the passage of HIV-1 across the blood-brain barrier: evidence for a post-internalization coreceptor. J Cell Sci 1998; 111:533–540.

57. Cohen OJ, Kinter A, Fauci AS. Host factors in the pathogenesis of HIV disease. Immunol Rev 1997; 159:31–48.

58. Feil C, Augustin HG. Endothelial cells differentially express functional CXC-chemokine receptor-4 (CXCR-4/fusin) under the control of autocrine activity and exogenous cytokines. Biochem Biophys Res Commun 1998; 247(1):38–45.

59. Gupta SK, Lysko PG, Pillarisetti K, Ohlstein E, Stadel JM. Chemokine receptors in human endothelial cells. Functional expression of CXCR4 and its transcriptional regulation by inflammatory cytokines. J Biol Chem 1998; 273(7):4282–4287.

60. Endres MJ, Clapham PR, Marsh M, Ahuja M, Turner JD, McKnight A, Thomas JF, Stoebenau-Haggarty B, Choe S, Vance PJ, Wells TN, Power CA, Sutterwala SS, Doms RW, Landau NR, Hoxie JA. CD4-independent infection by HIV-2 is mediated by fusin/CXCR4. Cell 1996; 87(4):745–756.

61. Boring L, Gosling J, Cleary M, Charo IF. Decreased lesion formation in CCR2-/- mice reveals a role for chemokines in the initiation of atherosclerosis. Nature 1998; 394:894–897.

62. Simonini A, Moscucci M, Muller DW, Bates ER, Pagani FD, Burdick MD, Strieter RM.

IL-8 is an angiogenic factor in human coronary atherectomy tissue. Circulation 2000; 101(13):1519–1526.

63. Mitola S, Soldi R, Zanon I, Barra L, Gutierrez MI, Berkhout B, Giacca M, Bussolino F. Identification of specific molecular structures of human immunodeficiency virus type 1 Tat relevant for its biological effects on vascular endothelial cells. J Virol 2000; 74(1):344–353.

64. Albini A, Barillari G, Benelli R, Gallo RC, Ensoli B. Angiogenic properties of human immunodeficiency virus type 1 Tat protein. Proc Natl Acad Sci USA 1995; 92(11):4838–4842.

65. Zidovetzki R, Wang JL, Chen P, Jeyaseelan R, Hofman F. Human immunodeficiency virus Tat protein induces interleukin 6 mRNA expression in human brain endothelial cells via protein kinase C- and cAMP-dependent protein kinase pathways. AIDS Res Hum Retrovir 1998; 14:825–833.

66. Hofman FM, Wright AD, Dohadwala MM, Wong-Staal F, Walker SM. Exogenous tat protein activates human endothelial cells [see comments]. Blood 1993; 82:2774–2780.

67. Hofman FM, Chen P, Incardona F, Zidovetzki R, Hinton DR. HIV-1 tat protein induces the production of interleukin-8 by human brain-derived endothelial cells. J Neuro-immunol 1999; 94:28–39.

68. Dhawan S, Puri RK, Kumar A, Duplan H, Masson JM, Aggarwal BB. Human immunodeficiency virus-1-tat protein induces the cell surface expression of endothelial leukocyte adhesion molecule-1, vascular cell adhesion molecule-1, and intercellular adhesion molecule-1 in human endothelial cells. Blood 1997; 90:1535–1544.

69. Lafrenie RM, Wahl LM, Epstein JS, Hewlett IK, Yamada KM, Dhawan S. HIV-1-Tat modulates the function of monocytes and alters their interactions with microvessel endothelial cells A mechanism of HIV pathogenesis. J Immunol 1996; 156(4):1638–1645.

70. Demarchi F, d'Adda di Fagagna F, Falaschi A, Giacca M. Activation of transcription factor NF-kappaB by the Tat protein of human immunodeficiency virus type 1. J Virol 1996; 70:4427–4437.

71. Albini A, Soldi R, Giunciuglio D, Giraudo E, Benelli R, Primo L, Noonan D, Salio M, Camussi G, Rockl W, Bussolino F. The angiogenesis induced by HIV-1 tat protein is mediated by the Flk-1/KDR receptor on vascular endothelial cells. Nat Med 1996; 2:1371–1375.

72. Barillari G, Sgadari C, Fiorelli V, Samaniego F, Colombini S, Manzari V, Modesti A, Nair BC, Cafaro A, Sturzl M, Ensoli B. The Tat protein of human immunodeficiency virus type-1 promotes vascular cell growth and locomotion by engaging the alpha5beta1 and alphavbeta3 integrins and by mobilizing sequestered basic fibroblast growth factor. Blood 1999; 94:663–672.

73. Huang MB, Hunter M, Bond VC. Effect of extracellular human immunodeficiency virus type 1 glycoprotein 120 on primary human vascular endothelial cell cultures. AIDS Res Hum Retrovir 1999; 15(14):1265–1277.

74. Annunziata P, Cioni C, Toneatto S, Paccagnini E. HIV-1 gp120 increases the permeability of rat brain endothelium cultures by a mechanism involving substance P. AIDS 1998; 12:2377–2385.

75. Stefano GB, Salzet M, Bilfinger TV. Long-term exposure of human blood vessels to HIV gp120, morphine, and anandamide increases endothelial adhesion of monocytes: uncoupling of nitric oxide release. J Cardiovasc Pharmacol 1998; 31:862–868.

76. Finkel TH, Tudor-Williams G, Banda NK, Cotton MF, Curiel T, Monks C, Baba TW, Ruprecht RM, Kupfer A. Apoptosis occurs predominantly in bystander cells and not in productively infected cells of HIV- and SIV-infected lymph nodes [see comments]. Nat Med 1995; 1(2):129–134.

77. Ameisen JC, Estaquier J, Idziorek T, De Bels F. Programmed cell death and AIDS pathogenesis: significance and potential mechanisms. Curr Top Microbiol Immunol 1995; 200:195–211.

78. Laurence J, Mitra D, Steiner M, Staiano-Coico L, Jaffe E. Plasma from patients with idiopathic and human immunodeficiency virus- associated thrombotic thrombocytopenic purpura induces apoptosis in microvascular endothelial cells. Blood 1996; 87: 3245–3254.

79. Shi B, De Girolami U, He J, Wang S, Lorenzo A, Busciglio J, Gabuzda D. Apoptosis induced by HIV-1 infection of the central nervous system. J Clin Invest 1996; 98:1979–1990.

80. Dang CT, Magid MS, Weksler B, Chadburn A, Laurence J. Enhanced endothelial cell apoptosis in splenic tissues of patients with thrombotic thrombocytopenic purpura. Blood 1999; 93(4):1264–1270.

81. Yunis NA, Stone VE. Cardiac manifestations of HIV/AIDS: a review of disease spectrum and clinical management. J AIDS Retrovir 1998; 18:145–154.

82. Periard D, Telenti A, Sudre P, Cheseaux JJ, Halfon P, Reymond MJ, Marcovina SM, Glauser MP, Nicod P, Darioli R, Mooser V. Atherogenic dyslipidemia in HIV-infected individuals treated with protease inhibitors. The Swiss HIV Cohort Study. Circulation 1999; 100(7):700–705.

83. Behrens G, Schmidt H, Meyer D, Stoll M, Schmidt RE. Vascular complications associated with use of HIV protease inhibitors [letter; comment]. Lancet 1998; 351:1958.

84. Galle J, Heermeier K, Wanner C. Atherogenic lipoproteins, oxidative stress, and cell death. Kidney Int 1999; 71(suppl):S62–S65.

85. Galle J, Schneider R, Heinloth A, Wanner C, Galle PR, Conzelmann E, Dimmeler S, Heermeier K. Lp(a) and LDL induce apoptosis in human endothelial cells and in rabbit aorta: role of oxidative stress. Kidney Int 1999; 55(4):1450–1461.

86. Bombeli T, Karsan A, Tait JF, Harlan JM. Apoptotic vascular endothelial cells become procoagulant. Blood 1997; 89(7):2429–2442.

87. Wahl LM, Corcoran ML, Pyle SW, Arthur LO, Harel-Bellan A, Farrar WL. Human immunodeficiency virus glycoprotein (gp120) induction of monocyte arachidonic acid metabolites and interleukin-1. Proc Natl Acad Sci USA 1989; 86:621–625.

88. Frenette PS, Wagner DD. Adhesion molecules—part II: blood vessels and blood cells. N Engl J Med 1996; 335(1):43–45.

89. Frenette PS, Wagner DD. Adhesion molecules—part 1. N Engl J Med 1996; 334(23): 1526–1529.

90. Lafrenie RM, Wahl LM, Epstein JS, Hewlett IK, Yamada KM, Dhawan S. HIV-1-Tat protein promotes chemotaxis and invasive behavior by monocytes. J Immunol 1996; 157:974–977.

91. Lafrenie RM, Wahl LM, Epstein JS, Yamada KM, Dhawan S. Activation of monocytes by HIV-Tat treatment is mediated by cytokine expression. J Immunol 1997; 159:4077–4083.

92. Roberts CR. Is asthma a fibrotic disease? Chest 1995; 107:111S–117S.

93. Roberts WC. Factors involved in the development of symptom-producing atherosclerotic plaques. Am J Cardiol 1995; 75:1B–2B.

94. Tewari M, Tuncay OC, Milchman A, Reddy PJ, Reddy CD, Cressman DE, Taub R, Newton RC, Tewari DS. Association of interleukin-1-induced, NF kappa B DNA-binding activity with collagenase gene expression in human gingival fibroblasts. Arch Oral Biol 1996; 41:461–468.

95. Yokoo T, Kitamura M. Dual regulation of IL-1 beta-mediated matrix metalloproteinase-9 expression in mesangial cells by NF-kappa B and AP-1. Am J Physiol 1996; 270:F123–F130.

96. Arsura M, Wu M, Sonenshein GE. TGF beta 1 inhibits NF-kappa B/Rel activity inducing apoptosis of B cells: transcriptional activation of I kappa B alpha. Immunity 1996; 5:31–40.

97. Krishnaswamy G, Kelley J, Johnson D, Youngberg G, Stone W, Huang SK, Bieber J, Chi

DS. The human mast cell: functions in physiology and disease. Front Biosci 2001; 6:D1109–D1127.

98. Chen GJ, Pillai R, Erickson JR, Martinez F, Estrada AL, Watson RR. Cocaine immunotoxicity: abnormal cytokine production in Hispanic drug users. Toxicol Lett 1991; 59:81–88.

99. Lindner V, Collins T. Expression of NF-kappa B and I kappa B-alpha by aortic endothelium in an arterial injury model. Am J Pathol 1996; 148:427–438.

100. Kane A, Hane L, Dangou JM, Diop IB, Thiam S, Sarr M, Ba SA, Ndiaye PD, Diouf SM. [Left ventricular aneurysm in human immunodeficiency virus infection: a case report]. Arch Mal Coeur Vaiss 1998; 91:419–423.

101. Telasky C, Tredget EE, Shen Q, Khorramizadeh MR, Iwashina T, Scott PG, Ghahary A. IFN-alpha2b suppresses the fibrogenic effects of insulin-like growth factor-1 in dermal fibroblasts. J Interferon Cytokine Res 1998; 18:571–577.

102. Howarth PH. The airway inflammatory response in allergic asthma and its relationship to clinical disease. Allergy 1995; 50:13–21.

103. Southern PJ, Berg P. Transformation of mammalian cells to antibiotic resistance with a bacterial gene under control of the SV40 early region promoter. J Mol Appl Genet 1982; 1:327–341.

104. Bird JL, Tyler JA. Tumour necrosis factor alpha, interferon gamma and dexamethasone regulate IGF-I-maintained collagen production in cultured human fibroblasts. J Endocrinol 1995; 147:167–176.

105. Fan J, Char D, Bagby GJ, Gelato MC, Lang CH. Regulation of insulin-like growth factor-I (IGF-I) and IGF- binding proteins by tumor necrosis factor. Am J Physiol 1995; 269:R1204–R1212.

106. James TN. Normal and abnormal consequences of apoptosis in the human heart (review). Annu Rev Physiol 1998; 60:309–325.

107. Marschang P, Gurtler L, Totsch M, Thielens NM, Arlaud GJ, Hittmair A, Katinger H, Dierich MP. HIV-1 and HIV-2 isolates differ in their ability to activate the complement system on the surface of infected cells. AIDS 1993; 7(7):903–910.

3

Role of HIV-1 Macropinocytosis and Cardiomyocyte Apoptosis in the Pathogenesis of HIV Cardiomyopathy

Milan Fiala
David Geffen School of Medicine at UCLA and Greater Los Angeles VA Medical Center, Los Angeles, California, U.S.A.

Kenneth P. Roos and William R. MacLellan
David Geffen School of Medicine at UCLA, Los Angeles, California, U.S.A.

Albert S. Lossinsky
Huntington Medical Research Institutes, Pasadena, California, U.S.A.

INTRODUCTION

HIV-1 cardiomyopathy (HIVCM) is an increasing cause of cardiovascular morbidity and mortality in young and middle-aged HIV-1–positive adults surviving acute complications of AIDS (1,2). It is controversial whether HIV-1 per se, opportunistic viral infections, substance abuse, and/or highly active antiretroviral therapy (HAART) is primarily responsible for HIVCM. Although HIV-1 is clearly an etiological factor in HIVCM, the role of HIV-1 proteins, which are considered important in HIV-1 encephalitis [i.e. gp120 (3,4), Tat (5), and Nef (4)] have not been clarified in HIVCM. We have investigated HIV-1 entry and apoptosis in human coronary artery endothelial cells and neonatal rat myocytes in vitro and in heart tissues of patients with AIDS ex vivo. Our data indicate that HIV-1 invades the heart and brain by a transcellular route through coronary artery endothelial cells (CAECs) or brain microvascular endothelial cells (BMVECs), respectively, using the mechanism of macropinocytosis. In the myocardium, HIV-1 infects macrophages and lymphocytes and induces cardiomyocyte apoptosis and heart failure.

CELL-FREE VIRUS INVADES THE HEART AND BRAIN BY MACROPINOCYTOSIS

In advanced stages of AIDS, HIV-1 enters into target organs, such as the brain and the heart, by "Trojan horse" transport in infected monocytes/macrophages. However, early after the infection, cell-free HIV-1 could be the first to enter through

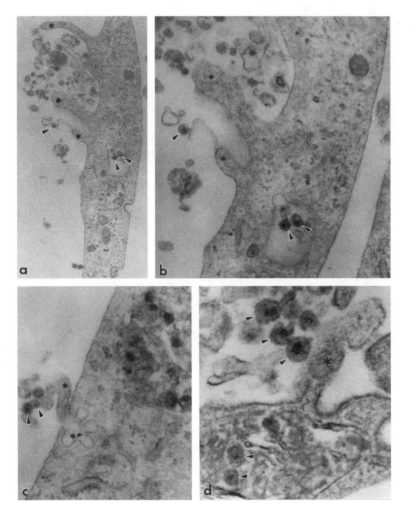

Figure 1 (a,b) Endothelial cell with microvilli (∗) and binding virions (▶). Note an intracellular vacuole containing two virions. (c) Note the group of racemic caveolae (∗∗) underlying the microvillus with several virions. (d) Higher magnification of an endothelial cell with a microvillus entangling extracellular virions. Some virions are located within a large vacuole (▶). Original magnifications: (a) 10,000×, (b) 20,000×, (c) 20,000×, (d) 50,000×.

endothelial cells and induce the chemokines necessary for transmigration of monocytes and lymphocytes (6). The mechanism by which cell-free HIV-1 penetrates the blood-brain and coronary endothelial barriers has been controversial. In brain tissue, HIV-1 DNA was identified in brain endothelial cells by polymerase chain reaction (PCR) in situ hybridization (7). We have analyzed cell-free virus invasion through cultured brain microvascular endothelial cells (BMVECs) (8) and CAECs (9) by PCR as well as electron and confocal microscopy. Our studies were performed in tissue culture inserts with BMVEC monolayers completely covering a porous membrane dividing the upper and lower chambers in the wells of a 24-well plate (6). In these endothelial cells, HIV does not cause productive infection; therefore, virus does not penetrate by replication and budding from the abluminal surface of endothelial cells. Virus exposure does not disrupt endothelial tight junctions, as shown by measuring the permeability coefficient of tight endothelial monolayers for up to 48 hr postinfection. Rather, HIV-1 exposure induces microvilli on endothelial cell surfaces, which entangle the virions and deliver them through surface craters into cytoplasmic vesicles (Fig. 1). This endocytic entry is defined as macropinocytosis (10) according to the presence of microvilli on the surface of infected cells, inhibition of virus endocytosis by the Na^+/K^+ channel blocker dimethylamiloride, and variable but occasionally giant size of the cytoplasmic vesicles. Later (16 hr postinfection), approximately 95 to 99% of these intracytoplasmic virions become inactivated in the vesicles fused with lysosomes, as shown by electron microscopy (Fig. 2), PCR,

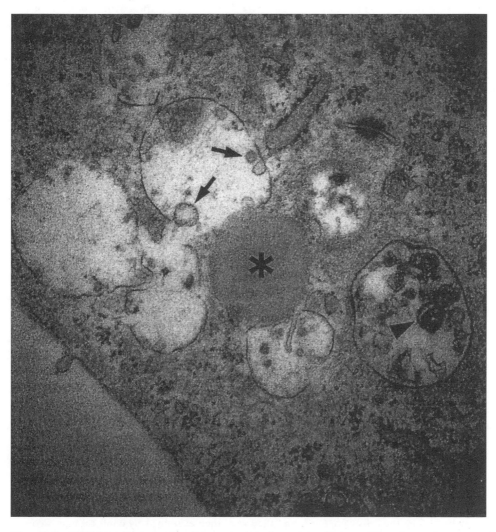

Figure 2 HIV-1 virions are lysed in cytoplasmic vesicles fusing with primary lysosomes (BMVECs 16 hr postinfection, ×30,000). (From Ref. 8.)

and infectious assays of the virus. However, the small fraction escaping lysis is undoubtedly more than sufficient in vivo to infect susceptible macrophages patrolling perivascular spaces, as suggested in an in vitro model of the blood-brain barrier, where susceptible lymphoblastoid cells in the lower chamber were infected by the virus penetrating from the upper chamber (8).

The virus plays an active role in endothelial cell remodeling by activation of mitogen-activated protein kinase (MAPK) signaling pathways, and virus entry is dependent upon this signaling, since U0126, an upstream MAPK kinase blocker, inhibits virus entry (8). The endothelial cell entry is also dependent upon ganglioside GM1 (with which it colocalizes) and intact lipid rafts (cholesterol-extracting agents block virus entry). Virus entry is, however, independent of classical receptors for HIV-1, since neither anti-CD4 nor AOP-RANTES blocks its entry, whereas HIV-1 without an envelope is able to efficiently enter these cells. Additionally, the polysaccharide heparin completely blocks virus entry (Fig. 3), indicating the role of cell membrane glycosaminoglycans in virus entry, as shown with HIV-1 invasion of macrophages (11).

These results show that cell-free virus can penetrate the blood-brain and coronary endothelial barriers by nonspecific binding and transcellular endocytic (macropinocytotic) transport, which is induced by MAPK signaling through a receptor in lipid rafts. HIV-1 infection of perivascular macrophages is then able to induce the chemokines attracting monocyte migration into the brain or the heart, as shown by our experiments in the blood-brain barrier model (Table 2 in Ref. 6).

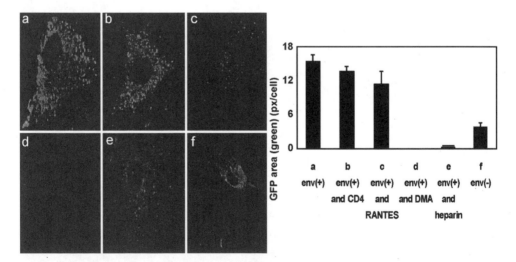

Figure 3 HIV-1 enters into BMVECs by macropinocytosis. BMVECs were either not pretreated (a) and (f), or were pretreated with anti-CD4 (b), AOP-RANTES (c), dimethyl-amiloride (DMA) (d), or heparin (e). HIV-1-Vpr-GFP with envelope (a to e) or HIV-1-Vpr-GFP without envelope (f) was placed on the cells, cholera toxin B-Texas Red was added 2.5 hr postinfection, the cells were fixed, and they were then examined by confocal microscopy 3 hr postinfection. (×95.) The bar graph indicates intracellular GFP density (pixels/cell). (From Ref. 8.)

COCAINE PROMOTES HIV-1 INVASION BY A PARACELLULAR ROUTE

Exposure of endothelial cells to HIV-1 does not open a paracellular route (permeability does not change for 48 hr postinfection). However, tumor necrosis factor-α (TNF-α and cocaine may disrupt the endothelial barrier's function and increase paracellular invasion by HIV-1, as may occur in inflammatory states (6) and cocaine abuse (12), respectively. Our previous studies concerning upregulation by cocaine of adhesion molecules (13) and induction of oxidative stress (14), and our recent microarray analysis of gene expression in BMVECs treated with cocaine, suggest that cocaine abuse has far-reaching consequences for human health. BMVECs treated with cocaine become more permissive for monocyte migration (13), which could enhance Trojan transport of HIV-1 and promote coronary and brain vessel atherosclerosis noted in HIV-1-positive patients who abuse cocaine and are treated with highly active antiretroviral therapy (HAART). In patients abusing cocaine, the balance of Th1- and Th2-type cytokines is modulated, as demonstrated in human volunteers who received cocaine infusion (15). The effects of cocaine on endothelial cells are mediated by several mechanisms. Cocaine induces oxidative injury with activation of the transcription factors nuclear factor κB (NF-κB) and activator protein 1 (AP-1) (14).Cocaine also stimulates expression of adhesion molecules on endothelial cells, in particular intercellular adhesion molecule 1 (ICAM-1), vascular cell adhesion molecule 1 (VCAM-1), and endothelial leukocyte adhesion molecule 1 (ELAM-1) (13). Furthermore, this drug stimulates TNF-α secretion in cocultures of endothelial cells with monocytes (13). Cocaine could, therefore, disrupt the endothelial barriers by several mechanisms.

HIV-1 INFECTS INFLAMMATORY CELLS, MACROPHAGES, AND T CELLS BUT NOT CARDIOMYOCYTES AND INDUCES CARDIOMYOCYTE APOPTOSIS

In our studies of hearts from AIDS patients, HIVCM was diagnosed by clinical history, elevated plasma level of brain natriuretic peptide (BNP), dilated left ventricle, and myocardial fibrosis (16). The mean heart weight in the group with cardiomyopathy was increased compared to HIV-1-infected hearts without cardiomyopathy. In situ hybridization studies initially suggested that in HIVCM the virus infects a limited number of myocytes (17). However, without identification of these virus-positive cells by immunocytochemistry, the cellular localization of the positive signal was unclear. We have found, using double immunocytochemical staining of HIV-1-infected hearts with anti-gp120 and anti-CD68 or anti-CD3, that the viral proteins gp120 and Nef are strongly expressed on infiltrating macrophages and T cells but only weakly or not at all on cardiomyocytes (Fig. 4), and the degree of inflammatory infiltration with cyclo-oxygenase–2 (COX-2)–activated macrophages correlates with HIVCM (16). The importance of HIV-1–infected macrophages in HIVCM was not realized in previous studies (2), probably due to differences in the techniques. In our study (16), CD68- and gp120-positive macrophages were detected only after treatment of the heart tissues using an "antigen retrieval technique,"

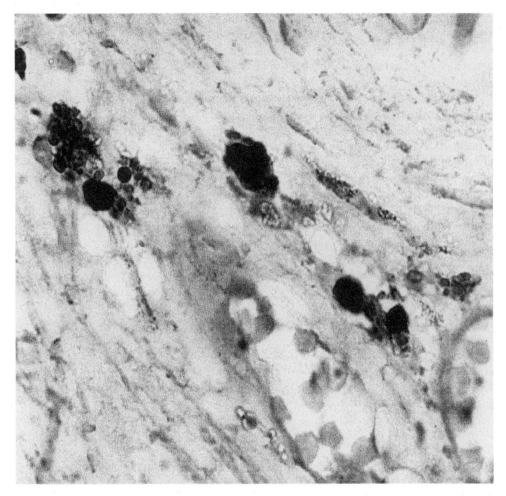

Figure 4 HIV-1 envelope protein gp120 is expressed on perivascular inflammatory cells (macrophages and lymphocytes) but not on cardiomyocytes (anti-gp120 immunocytochemistry of an AIDS heart with cardiomyopathy) (×100).

which unmasks cell antigens. Our recent data from a larger study of AIDS heart tissues confirm the strong association of HIVCM with COX-2–positive macrophage infiltration and the expression of gp120, but not Nef, by these inflammatory cells. The results of TUNEL staining of HIVCM-positive and HIVCM-negative hearts also show that HIVCM is significantly associated with cardiomyocyte apoptosis, and apoptosis is related to gp120 and TNF-α expression. Recently, we have induced apoptosis of rat neonatal cardiomyocytes by infectious HIV-1 or gp120; strengthening the hypothesis that gp120 is one of the viral proteins causing HIVCM. Our data do not exclude a role of Tat, which also produces rat cardiomyocyte apoptosis in vitro.

OTHER PATHOGENETIC MECHANISMS INVOLVED IN HIV-1 CARDIOMYOPATHY

The pathogenesis of cardiomyopathy is in general complex and poorly understood. Cardiac hypertrophy precedes decompensation. The hypertrophy is linked to induction of fetal genes, such as atrial natriuretic factor (ANF). Histochemistry of the heart tissues with HIVCM shows moderate to heavy fibrosis and TUNEL-positive apoptosis of cardiomyocytes, but there is no correlation between these pathological alterations. Thus ANF induction and/or other mechanisms, in addition to apoptosis, may play a role in cardiac hypertrophy.

CONCLUSIONS CONCERNING THE PATHOGENESIS OF HIV CARDIOMYOPATHY

HIV-1 induces HIVCM by the following mechanisms (Fig. 5): HIV-1 penetrates the endothelial barrier by macropinocytosis and Trojan transport. In the heart, HIV infects perivascular macrophages and lymphocytes, inducing chemokines and thus attracting migration of additional inflammatory cells, macrophages, and T cells. Infected macrophages and lymphocytes produce virions, gp120 and TNF-α which induce cardiomyocyte apoptosis and heart failure.

ACKNOWLEDGMENTS

This work was supported in part by NIH grants HL63065 and HL63639 to MF and Laubish endowment to KPR and WRM. We thank Amir Korkouri for assistance with the preparation of the manuscript.

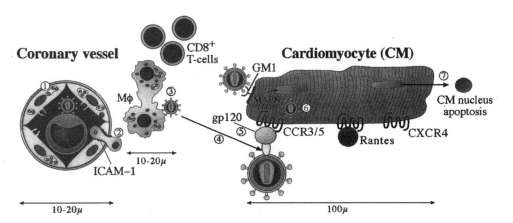

Figure 5 Pathogenesis of HIV-1 cardiomyopathy. HIV-1 invades the myocardium through endothelial cells by macropinocytosis or "Trojan horse" transport and infects perivascular macrophages, which produce additional virus and cytokines, such as TNF-α. The virus produces cardiomyocyte apoptosis either by signaling through CCR3, CCR5, or CXCR4, by entry into cardiomyocytes (after binding to ganglioside GM1), or through TNF-α.

REFERENCES

1. Barbaro G, Di Lorenzo G, Grisorio B, Barbarini G. Incidence of dilated cardiomyopathy and detection of HIV in myocardial cells of HIV-positive patients. Gruppo Italiano per lo Studio Cardiologico dei Pazienti Affetti da AIDS [see comments]. N Engl J Med 1998; 339:1093–1099.
2. Barbaro G, Lipshultz SE. Pathogenesis of HIV-associated cardiomyopathy. Ann N Y Acad Sci 2001; 946:57–81.
3. Jones MV, Bell JE, Nath A. Immunolocalization of HIV envelope gp120 in HIV encephalitis with dementia. AIDS 2000; 14:2709–2713.
4. Mankowski J, Flaherty M, Spelman J, et al. Pathogenesis of SIV encephalitis: viral determinants of neurovirulence. J Virol 1997; 71:6055–6060.
5. Bonwetsch R, Croul S, Richardson MW, et al. Role of HIV-1 Tat and CC chemokine MIP-1alpha in the pathogenesis of HIV associated central nervous system disorders. J Neurovirol 1999; 5:685–694.
6. Fiala M, Looney DJ, Stins M, et al. TNF-alpha opens a paracellular route for HIV-1 invasion across the blood-brain barrier. Mol Med 1997; 3:553–564.
7. An SF, Groves M, Gray F, ScaravilliF. Early entry and widespread cellular involvement of HIV-1 DNA in brains of HIV-1 positive asymptomatic individuals. J Neuropathol Exp Neurol 1999; 58:1156–1162.
8. Liu NQ, Lossinsky AS, Popik W, et al. Human immunodeficiency virus type 1 enters brain microvascular endothelia by macropinocytosis dependent on lipid rafts and the mitogen-activated protein kinase signaling pathway. J Virol 2002; 76:6689–6700.
9. Gujuluva C, Burns AR, Pushkarsky T, et al. HIV-1 penetrates coronary artery endothelial cells by transcytosis. Mol Med 2001; 7:169–176.
10. Marsh M. Endocytosis. In: Hames B, ed. Frontiers in Molecular Biology. Oxford, UK: Oxford University Press, 2001.
11. Saphire AC, Bobardt MD, Zhang Z, David G, Gallay PA. Syndecans serve as attachment receptors for human immunodeficiency virus type 1 on macrophages. J Virol 2001; 75:9187–9200.
12. Zhang L, Looney D, Taub D, et al. Cocaine opens the blood-brain barrier to HIV-1 invasion. J Neurol Virol 1998; 4:619–626.
13. Gan X, Zhang L, Taub D, et al. Cocaine enhances endothelial adhesion molecules and leukocyte migration. Clin Immunol 1999; 91:68–76.
14. Lee YW, Hennig B, Fiala M, Kim KS, Toborek M. Cocaine activates redox-regulated transcription factors and induces TNF-alpha expression in human brain endothelial cells. Brain Res 2001; 920:125–133.
15. Gan X, Zhang L, Newton T, et al. Cocaine infusion increases interferon-gamma and decreases interleukin-10 in cocaine-dependent subjects. Clin Immunol Immunopathol 1998; 89:181–190.
16. Liu QN, Reddy S, Sayre JW, Pop V, Graves MC, Fiala M. Essential role of HIV type 1–infected and cyclooxygenase 2–activated macrophages and T cells in HIV type 1 myocarditis. AIDS Res Hum Retrovir 2001; 17:1423–1433.
17. Grody W, Cheng L, Lewis W. Infection of the human heart by the human immunodeficiency virus. Am J Cardiol 1990; 66:203–206.

4

HIV-1 and the Blood-Brain Barrier

Kwang Sik Kim
Johns Hopkins Medical Institutions, Baltimore, Maryland, U.S.A.

INTRODUCTION

Central nervous system (CNS) dysfunction represents a common and serious manifestation of HIV-1 infection. Approximately one-third of adults and one-half of children with AIDS have neurological complications, which are directly attributable to infection of the CNS by HIV-1 (1,2). Neurological manifestations of primary HIV-1 infection are associated with an accelerated progression of disease (3), and the presence of progressive encephalopathy has been correlated with poor outcome (4). The exact timing of HIV-1 infection of the CNS is unknown. Several studies have shown entry of HIV-1 into the CNS early after infection (5–13); however, how HIV-1 enters the CNS is unclear. HIV-1–associated neurological dysfunction occurs in the absence of opportunistic infections, implying the limited role of coinfection in the pathogenesis of HIV-1 encephalopathy. In addition, neurological impairment has been shown to be the first signs of HIV-1–related diseases in some cases (6,9).

Under physiological conditions, the blood-brain barrier selectively regulates the exchange of macromolecules and cells between circulation and CNS. Several investigators have shown that structural and functional perturbations of the blood-brain barrier occur commonly during HIV-1 infection, as shown by increased cerebrospinal fluid (CSF)–serum albumin ratios, demonstration of serum protein extravasation in the brains of patients with HIV-1 infection, increased matrix metalloproteinases, and disruption of tight junctions as determined by the altered patterns of zonula occludens 1 (ZO-1) and occludins (14–20). But the mechanisms contributing to these permeability changes in the blood-brain barrier during HIV-1 infection remain incompletely understood. The availability of human brain microvascular endothelial cells (HBMEC), which constitute the blood-brain barrier, have made it possible to examine and characterize their role in the development of HIV-1 encephalopathy and dysfunction of the blood-brain barrier.

BLOOD-BRAIN BARRIER

An in vitro blood-brain barrier model has been constructed with HBMEC with or without astrocytes (21–23), but the contribution of astrocyte cocultivation to the blood-brain barrier model's permissiveness to HIV-1 invasion is not clear. For example, our previous studies indicate that HBMEC represent the main barrier to HIV-1 invasion of the blood-brain barrier, which is not affected by astrocyte cocultivation (22).

HBMEC have been successfully isolated and cultivated in vitro and purified by fluorescent activated sorting (FACS) using fluorescently labeled DiI-AcLDL. Upon cultivation on collagen-coated Transwell inserts, HBMEC exhibited morphological and functional properties of tight junction formation as well as polar monolayer, as shown by the development of high transendothelial electrical resistance equal to 300 to 600 Ω/cm^2 (24–26), a unique property of the brain microvascular endothelial cell monolayer compared to systemic vascular endothelium.

HIV-1 enters susceptible cells by fusion of its envelope with the plasma membrane after binding to the cell surface CD4 molecule and interaction with the chemokine coreceptors (CXCR4 or CCR5). HIV-1 strains that infect macrophages and primary T cells use CCR5 (R5 for CCR5-tropic virus), whereas HIV-1 strains that infect transformed T-cell lines and activated primary T cells use CXCR4 (X4 for CXCR4-tropic virus); HIV-1 strains that use CCR5 and CXCR4 are called R5X4 for dual-tropic virus. HIV-1 strains with R5 tropism are shown to be present during the early acute phase of infection, and viral strains with X4 or R5X4 tropism usually arise later in the course of infection (26).

HIV-1 Receptor CD4

It is widely accepted that CD4 is not shown to be present on HBMEC derived from adults and nonbrain endothelial cells such as human umbilical vein endothelial cells (HUVEC). In contrast, HBMEC derived from children are found to possess CD4 (23). For example, the presence of CD4 on children's HBMEC was demonstrated by RT-PCR using specific primers for CD4 as well as by FACS analysis and immunocytochemistry of purified HBMEC with anti-CD4 monoclonal antibody and Western blotting of HBMEC membrane proteins with anti-CD4 monoclonal antibody. In addition, CD4 was shown to be present on microvessels of children's brain cryosections (Fig. 1). Children's HBMEC were shown to be responsive to gp120

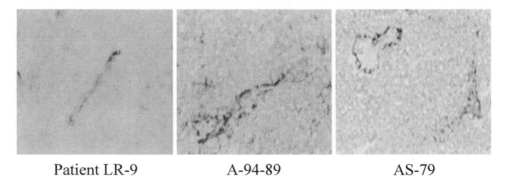

Patient LR-9   A-94-89   AS-79

Figure 1 Immunocytochemistry for CD4 on microvessels in frozen sections of three different pediatric brains. The dark precipitates indicate the presence of CD4.

in their expression of cell adhesion molecules (e.g., VCAM-1, ICAM-1), IL-6 secretion, and monocyte transmigration, which were inhibited by anti-CD4 antibodies as well as by anti-gp120 antibodies (23). In contrast, adults' HBMEC and HUVEC are not responsive to gp120. These findings indicate that CD4 on children's HBMEC is functional.

HIV-1 Coreceptors and Chemokine Receptors

The expression patterns of α- and β-chemokine receptors (e.g., CXCR4 and CCR3/CCR5, respectively) are shown to vary depending upon the source of HBMEC and types of endothelial cells. For example, Berger et al. reported that CCR3 and CXCR4 are highly expressed, but CCR5 is expressed at a low density in adults' HBMEC (27). We have shown the expression of CXCR4 in both children's and adults' HBMEC, but the expression of CCR3 and CCR5 is more evident in children's HBMEC (Fig. 2). It is important to note that CD4-independent entry

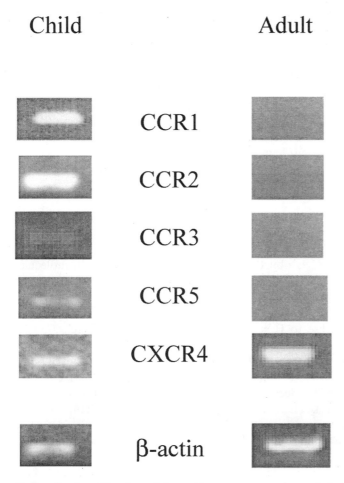

Figure 2 Amplification of chemokine receptors and β-actin by RT-PCR from children's and adults' HBMEC.

of HIV-1 has been documented, but there are no reports of HIV-1 infection independent of chemokine receptors (26). Of interest, the role of CD4 in HIV-1 interactions with chemokine receptors may differ between CCR5 and CXCR4. For example, gp120 from an X4 strain was shown to bind CXCR4 in the absence of CD4, whereas the binding to CCR5 of gp120 from R5 strains requires its prior binding to CD4 (26) (see "HIV-1 Invasion of the Blood-Brain Barrier," below). The biological functions of chemokines are also shown to be affected by their association with cellular or matrix extracellular glycoaminoglycans (28) (see "Other Receptors for HIV-1," below), but the relevance of this concept to HIV-1 neuropathogenesis is unclear.

Other Receptors for HIV-1

Children and adults' HBMEC are shown to possess sulfatide, another receptor molecule for HIV-1 and gp120, whereas no galactosylceramide was demonstrated from HBMEC (29). Sulfatide and galactosylceramide have been identified as the receptor molecules for HIV-1 and gp120, but the contribution of sulfatide to HIV-1–associated encephalopathy and the blood-brain barrier dysfunction remains unclear. DC/L-SIGNs (*S*pecific *I*CAM-3 *G*rabbing *N*onintegrin) are type II membrane proteins with external mannose-binding, C-type lectin domains and have been shown to bind the glycan-rich HIV-1 envelope in a CD4-independent manner (30,31). Commercial adults' HBMEC have been shown to express DC-SIGN and L-SIGN (31), but it is unclear whether these glycoproteins contribute to HIV-1 neuropathogenesis and blood-brain barrier dysfunction. Cell surface heparan sulfate proteoglycans such as the syndecans have been shown to efficiently mediate HIV-1 attachment to macrophages (28,32), but their role in HIV-1 neuropathogenesis remains unclear.

Other Characteristics of HBMEC

It is important to note the responsiveness of HBMEC to proinflammatory cytokines such as TNF-α and IFN-γ, since these cytokines have been shown to be elevated in the sera, CSF, and brains of HIV-1-infected patients (32–35). For example, both children's and adults' HBMEC exhibit the upregulation of cell adhesion molecules (e.g., VCAM-1 and ICAM-1) in response to TNF-α, and these patterns of response were similar to those obtained with HUVEC (36). Both children's and adults' HBMEC have been shown to exhibit the upregulation of β-chemokine receptors (CCR3 and CCR5) in response to IFN-γ. However, expression of E-selection on HBMEC varies depending upon the cell type and source of HBMEC. For example, expression of E-selectin has shown to be negligible with and without TNF-α stimulation on children's HBMEC as well as on microvessels in situ (36). In contrast, TNF-α–induced expression of E-selectin was shown to be evident in HUVEC as well as in adults' HBMEC (36–40). The constitutive expression of E-selectin has been shown to be negligible or low in both children's and adults' HBMEC (36,38) except for commercially available adults' HBMEC (39,40). However, these commercial HBMEC were specifically selected from a pool of endothelial cells for the presence of E-selectin and thereafter expanded. These results suggest that the activation patterns of brain microvascular endothelial cells in response to cytokines may vary depending upon the source of cells (Table 1).

Table 1 Comparison of Characteristics of Human Brain Microvascular Endothelial Cells (HBMEC) Derived from Children and Adults Versus Human Umbilical Vein Endothelial Cells (HUVEC)

Characteristics	Children's HBMEC	Adults' HBMEC	HUVEC
Presence of CD4	Yes	No	No
Presence of sulfatide	Yes	Yes	No
Presence of chemokine receptors	Yes (α- and β-chemokine receptors)	Yes (α-chemokine receptor, negligible β-chemokine receptor)	Yes (α-chemokine receptor)
DC/L-SIGN	Unknown	Yes	Unknown
Heparan sulfate preoteoglycans	Yes	Yes	Yes
VCAM-1/ICAM-1 upregulation by gp120	Yes	No	No
VCAM-1/ICAM-1 upregulation by cytokines or LPS	Yes	Yes	Yes
E-selectin expression by cytokines	No	Yes	Yes
Cytotoxicity by cytokines and gp120	Yes	No	No
KDR upregulation by cytokines and ethanol	Yes	Yes	Unknown

HIV-1 INVASION OF THE BLOOD-BRAIN BARRIER

HIV-1 may pass through the blood-brain barrier either through HBMEC or inside infected CD4+ T cells and monocytes. Several lines of evidence suggest that HIV-1 invasion into the brain is mediated through cell-associated HIV-1 in CD4+ T cells and monocytes that traffic across the blood-brain barrier (1,2,21). The cells chiefly infected by HIV-1 in the brain are cells for macrophage/microglia lineages (2,21,41). These findings suggest that the passage of virus-infected monocytes across HBMEC contributes to the HIV-1 infection of the CNS and subsequent development of HIV-1 encephalopathy and blood-brain barrier dysfunction by producing cytokines, chemokines, arachidonic acid metabolites, and other neurotoxic substances. The upregulation of VCAM-1 and ICAM-1 expression in HBMEC by HIV-1, HIV-1 proteins (e.g., gp120), and cytokines (e.g., TNF-α) may facilitate the binding of circulating HIV-1–infected monocytes to HBMEC via VCAM-1/VLA-1 and ICAM-1/LFA-1 interactions, resulting in enhanced trafficking into the CNS. In addition, microglia and astrocyte-derived chemokines such as macrophage chemotactic protein (MCP)-1 and SDF-1 affect monocyte and lymphocyte migration across the blood-brain barrier (42).

At present, there is a great deal of controversy concerning whether HBMEC are permissive for HIV-1 infection. For example, Moses et al. showed that adults' HBMEC were permissive for HIV-1 infection, but they failed to demonstrate the presence of CD4 and galactosylceramide on adults HBMEC (43). In contrast, several investigators have shown that HIV-1 does not productively infect adults' HBMEC

(44,45). As described above, we have shown that children's HBMEC processes CD4 and chemokine receptors and are responsive to gp120 in the upregulation of VCAM-1 and ICAM-1, which are inhibited by anti-CD4 antibody, but they are not permissive for productive infection with HIV-1. We and others have shown that HIV-1 infection of children's and adults' HBMEC resulted in abortive infection (23,45). Liu et al. have shown that HIV-1 enters adults' HBMEC by macro-pinocytosis involving lipid rafts, mitogen-activated protein kinase (MAPK) signaling, and glycosylaminoglycans, while chemokine receptors play limited roles in HIV-1 entry of adults' HBMEC (45). This mechanism is similar to that described with HIV-1 entry into monocytes (46), suggesting that cell-free HIV-1 and cell-associated HIV-1 may gain access to the CNS by a similar route/mechanism (45). This concept, however, differs from that obtained with rhesus macaque brain capillary endothelial cells, which were found to express chemokine receptors and exhibited CD4-inde-pendent, chemokine receptor–dependent entry of HIV-1 into the CNS (47).

EFFECTS OF HIV-1 PROTEINS ON HBMEC

Several HIV-1 proteins—such as the envelope protein gp120 and the regulatory proteins Tat and Nef—have been implicated in the pathogenesis of HIV-1 encepha-lopathy and blood-brain barrier dysfunction. Nef protein has been shown to recruit leukocytes into the subarachnoid space and induce blood-brain disruption in the rat (48), but its effect on HBMEC is not clear.

Gp120

In HIV-1 infected patients, HIV-1 or viral proteins such as gp120 or Tat or virally induced cytokines (e.g., TNF-α and IFN-α) may act on HBMEC and allow the entry of HIV-1-infected monocytes/macrophages into the CNS and/or result in blood-brain barrier dysfunction. HIV-1 gp120 is capable of altering and activating in vivo the blood-brain barrier. This was shown in the brains of HIV-1 gp120 transgenic mice by the demonstration of albumin extravasation and upregulation of ICAM-1 and VCAM-1 in cerebral vessels (49). We have previously shown that gp120 activates children's HBMEC in upregulating ICAM-1 and VCAM-1 expression, IL-6 secretion, and increased monocyte transmigration across HBMEC monolayers, which were inhibited by anti-gp120 and anti-CD4 antibodies. In contrast, adults' HBMEC failed to exhibit any responses to gp120. These findings indicate that gp120 activates children's HBMEC via CD4 (23).

As described earlier, structural and functional perturbations of the blood-brain barrier are shown to occur commonly during HIV-1 infection (14–20), but the mechanisms contributing to the blood-brain barrier dysfunction remain incom-pletely understood. HIV-1–associated blood-brain barrier dysfunction has been shown to involve many viral and host factors. For example, both M- and T-tropic gp120 in the presence of IFN-γ exhibited increased permeability and cytotoxicity in children's HBMEC (Fig. 3). In contrast, gp120/IFN-γ failed to exhibit such proper-ties in adults' HBMEC. These responses in children's HBMEC to gp120/IFN-γ were inhibited by anti-CD4 antibody (Fig. 4), indicating the importance of gp120-CD4 interaction, but this did not explain the requirement of IFN-γ in gp120-mediated

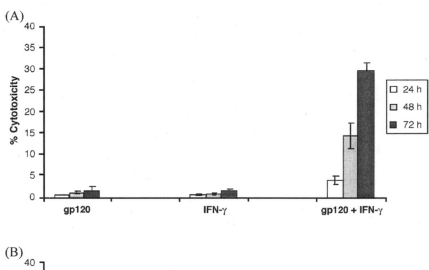

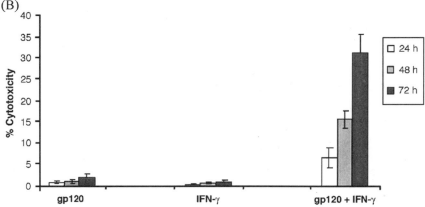

Figure 3 M- and T-tropic gp120-mediated cytotoxicity in the presence of IFN-γ in children's HBMEC.

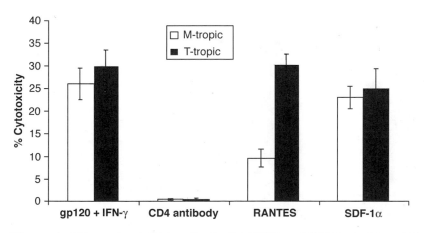

Figure 4 Effects of anti-CD4 antibody, RANTES, and SDF-1α in M- and T-tropic gp120/IFN-γ-mediated cytotoxicity of children's HBMEC.

cytopathic changes in children's HBMEC. As described earlier, IFN-γ upregulated the expression of β-chemokine receptors (CCR3 and CCR5) in HBMEC. RANTES inhibited M-tropic gp120/IFN-γ mediated cytopathic changes in children's HBMEC (Fig. 4), indicating the relevance of β-chemokine receptors in M-tropic gp120-mediated blood-brain barrier dysfunction. Similarly, synthetic peptides representing CD4- and chemokine-binding domains of gp120 inhibited both M- and T-tropic gp120/IFN-γ–mediated cytopathic changes in children's HBMEC, indicating the importance of CD4 and chemokine receptors in M- and T-tropic gp120-mediated cytopathic changes in children's HBMEC. Of interest, SDF-1α and CXCR4 inhibitors failed to exhibit any inhibitory activity in T-tropic gp120/IFN-γ mediated cytopathic changes in children's HBMEC (Fig. 4), suggesting the existence of non-CXCR4 receptor for T-tropic gp120 in children's HBMEC.

A similar concept was established for the involvement of p38 MAP kinase activation in M- and T-tropic gp120/IFN-γ–mediated cytopathic changes in children's HBMEC. For example, SB 202190 (p38 MAP kinase inhibitor) inhibited M- and T-tropic gp120/IFN-γ–mediated cytotoxicity in children's HBMEC, while PD 98059 (ERK1/ERK2 inhibitor) had no inhibitory effect (Fig. 5). The relevance of p38 MAP kinase activation was further shown by the demonstration that M- and T-tropic gp120 in the presence of IFN-γ stimulated p38 MAP kinase activation. Anti-CD4 antibody inhibited p38 MAP kinase activation in response to both M- and T-tropic gp120 and RANTES inhibited M-tropic gp120-mediated p38 MAP kinase activation. In contrast, SDF-1α and CXCR4 inhibitors failed to exhibit any inhibition of T-tropic gp120-mediated p38 MAP kinase activation. As shown above for gp120-mediated cytopathic changes, peptides representing CD4 and chemokine receptor binding domains of gp120 were effective in inhibiting p38 MAP kinase activation in response to both M- and T-tropic gp120. Pertussis toxin (100 ng/mL) also was effective in blocking both cytotoxicity and p38 MAP kinase activation in response to M- and T-tropic gp120/IFN-γ in children's HBMEC, supporting the

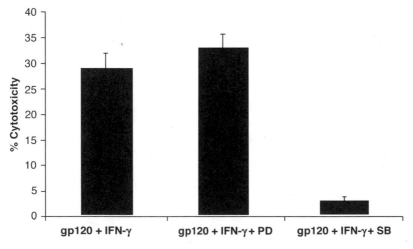

Figure 5 SB 202190 inhibited M- and T-tropic gp120-mediated cytotoxicity of children's HBMEC, while PD98059 had no inhibitory effect.

concept that chemokine receptor coupling to Gαi receptor is relevant to M- and T-tropic gp120-mediated activation and injury of children's HBMEC.

Tat

Tat protein of HIV-1 is a transcriptional activator essential for viral replication. Tat is secreted by the HIV-1–infected cells, and picomolar concentrations of Tat have been detected in the supernatant of HIV-1–infected cells as well as in the sera of some HIV-1–infected individuals (50–52). Extracellular Tat acts as a pleiotropic molecule affecting expression of host cellular genes and contributes to HIV-1–associated neuropathogenesis and blood-brain barrier dysfunction (53–56). Tat consists of 86 to 104 amino acids encoded by two exons and can be divided into five domains termed N-terminal, cysteine-rich, core, basic, and C-terminal. The C-terminal domain contains an RGD sequence, which represents the major cell attachment moiety mostly recognized by integrin receptors $\alpha5\beta_1$ and $\alpha v\beta_3$ for fibronectin and vitronectin, respectively (57). The basic domain (42–64aa) is similar to the basic sequence of VEGF-A and has been shown to bind $\alpha v\beta_5$ and KDR, while the cysteine domain interacts with chemokine receptors CCR2 and CCR3. Thus, different domains of Tat are shown to interact with at least three classes of cell surface receptors present on different target cells such as cell adhesion receptors of the integrin family, VEGF receptors of KDR and Flt-1, and chemokine receptors CCR2 and CCR3.

IFN-γ treatment has been shown to upregulate *kdr* and *ccr3* mRNA in both children's and adults' HBMEC. Tat in the presence of IFN-γ activates KDR (i.e., tyrosine phophorylation) in both children's and adults' HBMEC and anti-KDR antibody blocks Tat-mediated permeability and cytotoxicity in IFN-γ–treated HBMEC (Fig. 6). Of interest, the basic domain–deleted Tat was still able to exhibit some cytopathic changes in HBMEC. These findings suggest that Tat is another HIV-1 protein contributing to blood-brain barrier dysfunction but required IFN-γ treatment, involving perhaps the basic and cysteine domains representing their interactions with KDR and CCR3, respectively. These findings are consistent with

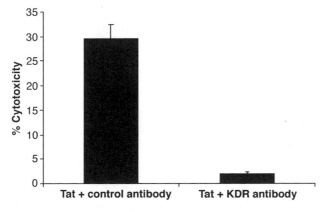

Figure 6 Tat-mediated cytotoxicity of children's and adults' HBMEC in the presence of IFN-γ is mediated by its interaction with KDR.

those of others who have shown that vascular endothelial cells become responsive to Tat after exposure to inflammatory cytokines such as TNF-α and IFN-γ (58,59). In contrast, other investigators have shown in HUVEC that Tat activates KDR, leading to angiogenic effect or apoptosis, and this activation does not require IFN-γ (60,61). This difference (priming versus no priming with inflammatory cytokines) may be due to different cell types (HBMEC versus HUVEC) or different phenotypes (permeability and cytotoxicity versus angiogenesis) or involvement of different domains of Tat (basic region versus cysteine region versus C-terminal region).

EFFECTS OF ALCOHOL AND COCAINE ON THE HIV-1 AND HBMEC INTERACTIONS

Because of the similarities of the clinical and pathological features of alcohol abuse and HIV-1 encephalitis (62,63), alcohol has been postulated as a cofactor that adversely affects HIV-1 encephalopathy and blood-brain barrier dysfunction. It is, however, unclear whether alcohol in conjunction with HIV-1 and viral proteins affects HBMEC. Alcohol has been shown to both enhance and inhibit nitric oxide production in a number of cell types, such as rat brain endothelial cells, aortic smooth muscle cells, and hepatic endothelial cells (64–66). Free radical formation has also been shown to be associated with tissue injury in alcoholic liver disease (67). Our recent studies have shown that clinically relevant concentrations of alcohol (10 to 100 nM) primed HBMEC for the upregulation of vascular endothelial growth factor receptor 2 (VEGFR2 or KDR), resulting in increased cytotoxicity and permeability changes in response to Tat, which were inhibited by anti-KDR antibody. These findings indicate that alcohol and HIV-1 proteins such as Tat contribute to the blood-brain barrier dysfunction.

Cocaine is the most commonly abused drug. Its abuse has been associated with vasculitis and stroke, and cocaine is suspected to affect HIV-1 encephalopathy and blood-brain barrier dysfunction. Cocaine at 10^{-5} and 10^{-6} M has been shown to increase blood-brain barrier permeability and M-tropic HIV-1 traversal across HBMEC monolayer via a paracellular route (68). Cocaine upregulated the expression of ICAM-1 and VCAM-1 in HBMEC and cocaine of 10^{-4} to 10^{-8} M enhanced monocyte transmigration across HBMEC monolayer (69). Cocaine also increased secretion of chemokines (e.g. IL-8, interferon-inducible protein 10, macrophage inflammatory protein 1α, and monocyte chemoattractant protein 1) and cytokines (e.g., TNFα) from human monocytes (68). Thus, cocaine can increase HIV-1 invasion into the CNS by its direct effect on HBMEC, by its upregulation of cell adhesion molecule expression (which facilitates trafficking cell-associated HIV into the CNS), and by its paracrine effects of proinflammatory cytokines and chemokines on the blood-brain barrier.

ACKNOWLEDGMENTS

This work was supported by NIH grants RO1-HL 61951 and AA 13858. The figures were generated by Monique Stins, Naveed Khan, and Francescopaolo Dicello; the author thanks them for their help.

REFERENCES

1. Bacellar H, Munoz A, Miller EN, Cohen BA, Besley D, Selnes OA, Becker JT, McArthur JC. Temporal trends in the incidence of HIV-1 related neurologic diesases: multicenter AIDS Cohort Study, 1985 1992. Neurology 1994; 44:1892–1900.
2. Lipton SA, Gendelman HE. Dementia associated with the acquired immunodeficiency syndrome. N Engl J Med 1995; 332:934–940.
3. Boufassa F, Bachmeyer C, Carre N, Deveau C, Persoz A, Jadand C, Sereni D, Bucquet D. Influence of neurologic manifestations of primary HIV infection on disease progression. J Infect Dis 1995; 171:1190–1195.
4. Belman AL, Diamond G, Dickson D, Horoupian D, Llena J, Lantos G, Rubinstein A. Pediatric acquired immunodeficiency syndrome. Am J Dis Child 1988; 142:29–35.
5. Grant I, Atkinson JH, Hesselink JR, Kennedy CJ, Richman DD, Spector SA, McCutchan JA. Evidence for early central nervous system involvement in the acquired immunodeficiency syndrome (AIDS) and other human immunodeficiency virus (HIV) infections. Ann Intern Med 1987; 107:828–836.
6. Berger JR, Moskowitz L, Fischi M, Kelley RE. Neurologic disease as the presenting manifestation of acquired immunodeficiency syndrome. South Med J 1987; 80:683–686.
7. Davis LE, Hjelle BL, Miller VE, et al. Early viral brain invasion in iatrogenic human immunodeficiency virus infection. Neurology 1992; 42:1736–1739.
8. Diederich N, Ackermann R, Jurgens R, et al. Early involvement of the nervous system by human immunodeficiency virus. Eur Neurol 1988; 28:93–105.
9. Scoff GB, Hutto C, Makuch RW, Mastrucci MT, O'Connor T, Mitchell CD, Trapido EJ, ParksWP. Survival in children with perinatally acquired human immunodeficiency virus type I infection. N Engl J Med 1990; 321:1791–1796.
10. Navia BA, Price RW. The acquired immunodeficiency dementia complex as the presenting or sole manifestation of human immunodeficiency virus infection. Arch Neurol 1987; 44:65–69.
11. Cooper DA, Gold J, Maclean P, Donovan B, Finlayson R, Barnes TG, Michelmore HMN, Brooke P, Penny R. Acute AIDS retrovirus infection: definition of a clinical illness associated with seroconversion. Lancet 1985; 1:537–540.
12. Resnick L, DiMarzo-Veronese F, Schupbach J, Tourtellotte WW, Ho DD, Muller F, Shapshak P, Bogt M, Groopman JE, Markham PD, Gallo RC. Intra-blood-brain barrier synthesis of HTLV-111 specific IgG in patients with neurologic symptoms associated with AIDS or AIDS-related complex. N Engl J Med 1985; 313:1498–1504.
13. Goudsmit J, Wolters EC, Bakker M, Smit K, van der Noorda J, Hische EAH, Tutuarima JA, van der Heim HJ. Intrathecal synthesis of antibodies to HTLV-111 in patients without AIDS or AIDS related complex. Br Med J 1986; 292:1231.
14. Dallasta LM, Pisarov LA, Esplen JE, Werley JV, Moses AV, Nelson JA, Achim CL. Blood-brain barrier tight junction disruption in human immunodeficiency virus-1 encephalitis. Am J Pathol 1999; 155:1915–1927.
15. Power C, Kong PA, Crawford CO, Wesselingh S, Glass JD, McArthur JC, Trapp BD. Cerebral white matter changes in acquired immunodeficiency syndrome dementia: alterations of the blood-brain barrier. Ann Neurol 1993; 34:339–350.
16. Rhodes RH. Evidence of serum-protein leakage across the blood-brain barrier in the acquired immunodeficiency syndrome. J Neuropathol Exp Neurol 1991; 50:171–183.
17. Petito CK, Cash KS. Blood-brain barrier abnormalities in the acquired immunodeficiency syndrome: immunohistochemical localization of serum proteins in postmortem brain. Ann Neurol 1992; 32:658–666.
18. Tran Dinh YR, Mamo H, Cervoni J, Caulin C, Saimot AC. Disturbances in the cerebral perfusion of human immune deficiency virus-1 seropositive asymptomatic subjects: a quantitative tomography study of 18 cases. J Nucl Med 1990; 10:1601–1607.

19. Marshall DW, Brey RL, Butzin CA, Lucey DR, Abbadessa SM, Boswell RN. CSF changes in a longitudinal study of 124 neurologically normal HIV-1-infected US Air Force personnel. J AIDS 1991; 4:777–781.

20. Sporer B, Paul R, Koedel U, Grimm R, Wick M, Goebel FD, Pfister HW. Presence of matrix metalloproteinase-9 activity in the cerebrospinal fluid of human immunodeficiency virus–infected patients. J Infect Dis 1998; 178:854–857.

21. Persidsky Y, Stins M, Way D, Witte MH, Weinand M, Kim KS, Bock P, Gendelman HE, Fiala M. A model for monocyte migration through the blood-brain barrier during HIV-1 encephalitis. J Immunol 1997; 158:3499–3510.

22. Fiala M, Looney DJ, Stins M, Way DD, Zhang L, Gan X, Chiappelli F, Schweitzer ES, Shapshak P, Weinand M, Graves MC, Witte M, Kim KS. TNF-α opens a paracellular route for HIV-1 invasion across the blood-brain barrier. Mol Med 1997; 3:553–564.

23. Stins MF, Shen Y, Huang SH, Gilles F, Kalra VK, Kim KS. Gp120 activates children's brain endothelial cells via CD4. J Neurovirol 2001; 7:125–134.

24. Stins MF, Badger JL, Kim KS. Bacterial invasion and transcytosis in transfected human brain microvascular endothelial cells. Microb Pathog 2001; 30:19–28.

25. Zhang GW, Khan NA, Kim KJ, Stins M, Kim KS. TGF-β increases *E. coli* K1 adherence, invasion and transcytosis in human brain microvascular endothelial cells. Cell Tissue Res 2002; 309:281–286.

26. Littman DR. Chemokine receptors: keys to AIDS pathogenesis. Cell 1998; 93:677–680.

27. Berger O, Gan X, Gujuluva C, Burns AR, Sulur G, Stins M, Way D, Witte M, Weinand M, Said J, Kim KS, Taub D, Graves MC, Fiala M. CXC and CC chemokine receptors on coronary and brain endothelia. Mol Med 1999; 5:795–805.

28. Valenzuela-Fernandez A, Palanche T, Amara A, Magerus A, Altmeyer R, Delaunay T, Virelizier J-L, Baleux F, Galzi J-L, Arenzana-Seisdedos F. Optimal inhibition of X4 HIV isolates by the CXC chemokine stromal cell–derived factor 1α requires interaction with cell surface heparan sulfate proteoglycans. J Biol Chem 2001; 276:26550–26558.

29. Nemani PV, Wass CA, Hacker J, Jann K, Kim KS. Adhesion of S-fimbriated *Escherichia coli* to brain glycolipids mediated by sfaA gene encoded protein of S-fimbriae. J Biol Chem 1993; 268:10356–10363.

30. Curtis BM, Scharnowske S, Watson AJ. Sequence and expression of a membrane-associated C-type lectin that exhibits CD-4-independent binding of human immunodeficiency virus envelope glycoprotein gp120. Proc Natl Acad Sci USA 1992; 89:8356–8360.

31. Mukhtar M, Harley S, Chen P, BouHamdan M, Patel C, Acheampong E, Pomerantz RJ. Primary isolated human brain microvascular endothelial cells express diverse HIV-SIV-associated chemokine co-receptors and DC-SIGN and L-SIGN. Virology 2002; 297:78–88.

32. Saphire ACS, Bobardt MD, Zhang Z, David G, Gallay P. Syndecans serve as attachment receptors for human immunodeficiency virus type 1 on macrophages. J Virol 2001; 75:9187–9200.

33. Lahdevirta J, Maury CPJ, Teppo AM, Repo H. Elevated levels of circulating cachectin/tumor necrosis factor in patients with acquired immunodeficiency syndrome. Am J Med 1988; 85:289–291.

34. Graziosi C, Gantt KR, Vaccarezza M, Demarest JF, Daucher M, Saag MS, Shaw GM, Quinn TC, Cohen OJ, Welbon CC, Pantaleo G, Fauci AS. Kinetics of cytokine expression during primary human immunodeficiency virus type 1 infection. Proc Natl Acad Sci USA 1996; 93:4386–4391.

35. Fan J, Bass HZ, Fahey JL. Elevated IFN-γ and decreased IL-2 gene expression are associated with HIV infection. J Immunol 1993; 151:5031–5040.

36. Stins MF, Gilles F, Kim KS. Selective expression of adhesion molecules on human brain microvascular endothelial cells. J Neuroimmunol 1997; 76:81–90.

37. Bevilacqua MP, Pober JS, Mendrick DL, Cotran RS, Gimbrone MA. Identification

of an inducible leukocyte adhesion molecule. ELAM-1. Proc Natl Acad Sci USA 1987; 84:9238–9242.

38. Wong D, Dorovini-Zis K. Regulation of cytokines and lipopolysaccharide of E-selectin expression by human brain microvessel endothelial cells in primary culture. J Neuropathol Exp Neurol 1996; 55:225–235.

39. Dhawan S, Weeks SW, Soderland C, Schnaper HW, Toto LA, Asthana SP, Hewlett IK, Stetler-Stevenson WG, Yamada SS, Yamada KM, Meltzer MS. HIV-1 infection alters monocyte interactions with human microvascular endothelial cells. J Immunol 1995; 154:422–432.

40. Nottet HS, Persidsky Y, Sasseville VG, Nukuna AN, Bock P, Zhai QH, Sharer LR, McComb RD, Swindels S, Soderland C, Gendelman HE. Mechanisms for the trans-endothelial migration of HIV-1 infected monocytes into the brain. J Immunol 1996; 156:1284–1295.

41. Merrill JE, Chen IS. HIV-1, macrophages, glial cells, and cytokines in AIDS nervous system disease. FASEB J 1991; 5:2391.

42. Persidsky Y, Ghorpade A, Rasmussen J, Limoges J, Liu XJ, Stins M, Fiala M, Way D, Kim KS, Witte MH, Weinand M, Carhart L, Gendelman HE. Microglial and astrocyte chemokines regulate monocyte migration through the blood-brain barrier in human immunodeficiency virus-1 encephalitis. Am J Pathol 1999; 155:1599–1611.

43. Moses AV, Blood FE, Pauza CD, Nelson JA. Human immunodeficiency virus infection of human brain capillary endothelial cells occurs via a CD4/galactosylceramide-independent mechanism. Proc Natl Acad Sci USA 1993; 90:10474–10478.

44. Poland SD, Rice GPA, Dekaban GA. HIV-1 infection of human brain-derived microvascular endothelial cells in vitro. J AIDS Hum Retrovirol 1995; 8:437–445.

45. Liu NQ, Lossinsky AS, Popik W, Li X, Gujuluva C, Kriederman B, Roberts J, Pushkarsky T, Bukrinsky M, Witte M, Weinand M, Fiala M. Human immunodeficiency virus type 1 enters brain microvascular endothelia by macropinocytosis dependent on lipid rafts and the mitogen-activated protein kinase signaling pathway. J Virol 2002; 76:6689–6700.

46. Marechal V, Prevost M-C, Petit C, Perret E, Heard J-M, Schwartz O. Human immunodeficiency virus type 1 entry into macrophages mediated by macropinocytosis. J Virol 2001; 75:11166–11177.

47. Edinger AL, Mankowski JL, Doranz BJ, Margulies BJ, Lee B, Rucker J, Hoffman TL, Berson JF, Zink MC, Hirsch VM, Clements JE, Doms RW. CD4-independent, CCR5-dependent infection of brain capillary endothelial cells by a neurovirulent simian immunodeficiency: VI. Proc Natl Acad Sci USA 1997; 94:14742–14747.

48. Sporer B, Koedel U, Paul R, Kohleisen B, Erfle V, Fontana A, Pfister HW. Human immunodeficiency virus type −1 Nef protein induces blood-brain barrier disruption in the rat: role of matrix metalloproteinase-9. J Neuroimmunol 2000; 102:125–130.

49. Toneatto S, Finco O, van der Putten H, Abrignani S, Annunziata P. Evidence of blood-brain barrier alteration and activation in HIV-1 gp120 transgenic mice. AIDS 1999; 13:2343–2348.

50. Ensoli B, Buonaguro L, Barillari G, Fiorelli V, Gendelman R, Morgan RA, Wingfield P, Gallo RC. Release, uptake and effects of extracellular human immunodeficiency virus type 1 Tat protein on cell growth and viral transactivation. J Virol 1993; 67:277–287.

51. Thomas CA, Dobkin J, Weinberger OK. Tat-mediated transcellular activation of HIV-1 long terminal repeat directed gene expression by HIV-1 infected peripheral blood mononuclear cells. J Immunol 1994; 153:3831–3839.

52. Westendorp MO, Frank R, Ochsenbauer C, Stricker K, Dhein J, Walczak H, Debatin KM, Krammer PH. Sensitization of T cells to CD45-mediated apoptosis by HIV-1 Tat and gp120. Nature 1995; 375:497–500.

53. Wesselingh SL, Power C, Glass JD, Tyor WR, McArthur JC, Farber JM, Griffin JW,

Griffin DE. Intracerebral cytokine messenger RNA expression in acquired immunodeficiency syndrome dementia. Ann Neurol 1993; 33:576–582.

54. Wiley CA, Baldwin M, Achim CL. Expression of regulatory and structural mRNA in the central nervous system. AIDS 1996; 10:843–847.

55. Hofman FM, Dohadwala MM, Wright AD, Hinton DR, Walker SM. Exogenous tat protein activates central nervous system–derived endothelial cells. J Neuroimmunol 1994; 53:1–10.

56. Rappaport J, Joseph J, Groul S, Alexander G, Del Valle L, Amini S, Khalili K. Molecular pathway involved in HIV-1-induced CNS pathology: role of viral regulatory protein, Tat. J Leuk Biol 1999; 65:458–465.

57. Barillari G, Ensoli B. Angiogenic effects of extracellular human immunodeficiency virus type 1 Tat protein and its role in the pathogenesis of AIDS-associated Kaposi's sarcoma. Clin Microbiol Rev 2002; 15:310–326.

58. Fiorelli V, Barillari G, Toschi E, Sgadari C, Monini P, Sturzl M, Ensoli B. IFN-γ induces endothelial cells to proliferate and to invade the extracellular matrix in response to the HIV-1 Tat protein: implications for AIDS-Kaposi's sarcoma pathogenesis. J Immunol 1999; 162:1165–1170.

59. Barillari G, Sgadari C, Palladino C, Gendelman R, Caputo A, Morris CB, Nair BC, Markham P, Andre N, Sturzl M, Ensoli B. Inflammatory cytokines synergize with the HIV-1 Tat protein to promote angiogenesis and Kaposi's sarcoma via induction of basic fibroblast growth factor and the $\alpha_v\beta_3$ integrin. J Immunol 1999; 163:1929–1935.

60. Albini A, Soldi R, Giunciuglio D, Giraudo E, Benelli R, Primo L, Noonan D, Salio M, Camussi G, Rocki W, Bussolino F. The angiogenesis induced by HIV-1 Tat protein is mediated by the Flk-1/KDR receptor on vascular endothelial cells. Nat Med 1996; 2:1371–1375.

61. Jia H, Lohr M, Jezequel S, Davis D, Shaikh S, Selwood D, Zachary I. Cysteine-rich and basic domain HIV-1 Tat peptides inhibit angiogenesis and induce endothelial cell apoptosis. Biochem Biophys Res Commun 2001; 283:469–479.

62. Fein G, Fletcher DJ, DiSclafani V. Effect of chronic alcohol abuse on the CNS morbidity of HIV disease. Alcohol Clin Exp Res 1998; 22:196S–200S.

63. Tyor WR, Middaugh LD. Do alcohol and cocaine abuse alter the course of HIV-associated dementia complex? J Leuk Biol 1999; 65:475–481.

64. Durante W, Cheng K, Sunahara RK, Schafer AJ. Ethanol potentiates interleukin-1 beta-stimulated inducible nitric oxide synthese expression in cultured vascular smooth muscle cells. Biochem J 1995; 308:231–236.

65. Naassila M, Roux F, Daust M. Ethanol potentiates lipopolysaccharide- or interleukin-1β-induced nitric oxide generation in RBE4 cells. Eur J Pharmacol 1996; 313:273–277.

66. Wang JF, Greenberg SS, Spitzer JJ. Chronic alcohol administration stimulates nitric oxide formation in the rat liver with or without pre-treatment by lipopolysaccharide. Alcohol Clin Exp Res 1995; 19:387–393.

67. Bautista AP. Serial review: alcohol, oxidative stress and cell injury. Free Radic Biol Med 2001; 31:1527–1532.

68. Zhang L, Looney D, Taub D, Chang SL, Way D, Witte MH, Graves MC, Fiala M. Cocaine opens the blood-brain barrier to HIV-1 invasion. J Neurovirol 1998; 4:619–626.

69. Gan X, Zhang L, Berger O, Stins MF, Way D, Taub DD, Chang SL, Kim KS, House SD, Weinand M, Witte M, Graves MC, Fiala M. Cocaine enhances brain endothelial adhesion molecules and leukocyte migration. Clin Immunol 1999; 91:68–76.

5

HIV, Cocaine, and the Heart: Pathophysiology and Clinical Implications

John F. Setaro, Brian G. Abbott, and Arthur Margolin
Yale University School of Medicine, New Haven, Connecticut, U.S.A.

INTRODUCTION: TWO EPIDEMICS

The twin contemporary epidemics of HIV/AIDS and cocaine abuse have conspired to produce a population of individuals who manifest cardiac abnormalities, the pathophysiology and proper treatment of which have yet to be fully defined (1,2). Both HIV/AIDS and cocaine use independently can promote cardiac dysfunction, and whether both etiologies in concert can demonstrate synergistic effects represents an important question. Potential cardiac side effects of antiretroviral therapy complicate this issue further (3), although recent reports suggest that therapeutic benefits significantly outweigh risks (4–6). Yet adverse cardiovascular effects of simultaneous cocaine use and HIV disease may have significant health consequences for individual patients as well as for the health care system at large, particularly if specialized and costly cardiac care is required as these patients survive and extend their lives. In the following section, pathophysiological and therapeutic implications of the combined HIV/AIDS and cocaine disorders will be considered.

HIV AND THE HEART

Cardiac involvement in human immunodeficiency virus (HIV) infection and the acquired immunodeficiency syndrome (AIDS) is well characterized, with abnormalities noted in virtually all heart structures including pericardium, valves, and myocardium. Symptomatic heart disease is often progressive and fatal. Patients typically succumb to biventricular dysfunction in the context of worsening dilated cardiomyopathy (7–11). Pericarditis, myocarditis, and endocarditis have been observed (12–14). Cytokines may play a role in HIV-associated myocarditis, with studies demonstrating abnormally high levels of interleukin-6 (IL-6) in cases of biopsy-proven HIV-related myocarditis (2). Elevated concentrations of tumor necrosis factor alpha (TNF-α) have been noted in general studies of cardiomyopathy and myocarditis (15).

While most patients with AIDS do not manifest overt clinical evidence of cardiac disease until the later stages, approximately half of all patients with HIV infection harbor evidence of abnormalities by echocardiography despite a lack of cardiac symptoms (16–19). This incipient cardiac dysfunction may result from opportunistic infections but more recently been has linked to HIV infection itself. Enhanced survival with newer treatments for HIV infection may lead to a wider prevalence of HIV-related cardiac abnormalities. Because advancing cardiac involvement is usually clinically silent, it is conceivable that earlier detection of subtle cardiac derangements could forestall progression.

COCAINE AND THE HEART

Substance abuse is frequent in patients with HIV and AIDS, and a percentage of patients using cocaine are likely to have occult HIV infection (1,20). Cocaine use in HIV-infected individuals may represent an additional potent risk factor for the development of heart disease. Acutely, cocaine administration has been correlated with a wide range of effects, including rises in heart rate and blood pressure, coronary vasoconstriction, increases in myocardial contractility, and deterioration in left ventricular ejection fraction. Cocaine can produce nonischemic global hypokinesis in some users, and transient congestive heart failure following cocaine use has been witnessed (21). Cocaine use can also stimulate vasospasm, cardiac rhythm disturbances, myocardial ischemia, and infarction (22,23). Left ventricular hypertrophy, reflected in significantly abnormal left ventricular mass index and wall thickness by ultrasound, has been cited in chronic cocaine users (24,25). Clinically silent reductions in left ventricular systolic performance appear in as many as 7% of cocaine users (26). One report employing two-dimensional Doppler echocardiography noted significant preclinical dysfunction in diastolic cardiac filling in asymptomatic cocaine-addicted subjects as compared with controls (27).

INTERACTION OF COCAINE AND HIV IN PROMOTING CARDIAC DISEASE

Although previous echocardiographic assessments have observed abnormalities in both systolic and diastolic function in subjects with either HIV disease or cocaine use, the degree of left ventricular dysfunction in asymptomatic patients with both HIV infection and cocaine abuse has not been elucidated. Mechanisms for a synergistic action have been proposed and include a role for catecholamines, abnormal platelet behavior, and the influence of chemokines, cytokines, and endothelial cells.

Influence of Catecholamines

It is plausible that catecholamines exert a major influence in the progression of cocaine cardiotoxicity. Pathological studies of cocaine subjects who experienced ventricular arrhythmias revealed contraction bands in 93%, consistent with catecholamine excess, thereby providing the substrate for lethal rhythm disorders (28). Catecholamines may exacerbate endothelial cell damage and thereby facilitate progression of HIV disease. Soodini and Morgan have proposed that cocaine-based catecholamine stimuli could amplify viral toxicity once the HIV virus has penetrated the cellular membrane, perhaps by enhancing viral replication through alterations in cellular pH, osmolarity, or depletion of energy stores required for protective enzyme activity—all catecholamine-related effects unlikely to be witnessed with non-catecholamine drugs of abuse such as opioids, cannabis, caffeine, alcohol, nicotine, or phencyclidine (2). Murine models suggest that elevated catecholamine states can aggravate myocarditis (29,30), and subjects with acute cocaine cardiotoxicity typically have high levels of catecholamines such as epinephrine and norepinephrine (31).

Role of Platelet Behavior

Cocaine may foster the tendency of platelets to adhere, creating a prothrombotic milieu. In addition to possible direct effects on platelet release (32), cocaine may also indirectly prime platelets for activation, raising the number of circulating activated platelets (33). Acute myocardial infarction caused by platelet-rich clot in otherwise normal coronary arteries is temporally linked to cocaine use. Platelet-rich thrombi may intensify the vasoconstrictive properties of cocaine to produce ischemic syndromes (34,35). Increased platelet activation is also correlated with HIV infection. Platelet activation may also contribute to enhanced clearance of platelets: survival of platelets in nonthrombocytopenic HIV-positive subjects is abnormally low (36).

Beyond adverse effects upon platelets, both cocaine and HIV infection may injure the vascular endothelium. Healthy endothelial cells competently inhibit platelet activation and adhesion to vessel walls. These protective mechanisms are partly mediated by bradykinin, which catalyzes endothelial release of prostacyclin and nitric oxide, both of which are strong platelet inhibitors and vasodilators (37). Activation of the renin-angiotensin system (RAS) in patients with HIV infection stimulates bradykinin degradation, promoting platelet adhesion (38). Cocaine directly activates endothelial cells to generate endothelin-1, an extremely potent vasoconstrictor, through angiotensin-mediated pathways (39,40). Therefore, in both HIV infection and cocaine use, loss of endothelial cell antithrombotic and vasodilatory behavior is linked to upregulation of the RAS.

Effects of Chemokines, Cytokines, and Endothelial Cells

Several investigations have supported the concept of cocaine-facilitated HIV involvement in vascular tissue of the brain and potentially the heart. Even limited exposures to cocaine can damage endothelial cells (41,42). Cocaine's widespread effects on the neuroendocrine (hypothalamic-pituitary-adrenal axis) and immune systems cause an upregulation of proinflammatory cytokines, and cocaine-related vascular pathological effects may lead to derangement in endothelial cell function, including function at the blood-brain barrier, with progressive neurological consequences in HIV-infected patients (43,44). Experimental blood-brain barrier assays have revealed that cocaine increases permeability and monocyte migration across the barrier and that cocaine enhances the expression of endothelial cell adhesion molecules (45). These molecules include intercellular adhesion molecule 1 (ICAM-1), vascular cell adhesion molecule 1 (VCAM-1), and platelet/endothelial cell adhesion molecule 1 (PECAM-1). Further studies suggest a possible role in HIV-cocaine disorder for chemokine receptors situated on brain endothelial cells (46).

Zhang and associates have provided additional insights into the question of cocaine-mediated enhancement of HIV-related vascular effects in the brain, which theoretically could be extended to cardiac tissue as well (47). These authors observed, in an experimental preparation, multiple cocaine- related effects including greater molecular permeability of the blood-brain barrier, enhanced viral invasion by macrophage-tropic HIV-1, increased apoptosis (programmed cell death) of brain endothelial cells and monocytes, and augmented production of diverse chemokines. These chemokines included IL-8, interferon-inducible protein 10, macrophage inflammatory protein 1 alpha, and monocyte chemoattractant protein 1. The cytokine TNF-α was also generated in greater concentration, and it facilitated brain invasion by multiple HIV-1 strains (47). Nair and colleagues further defined mechanisms of cocaine-related immunopathogenesis in HIV infection through cocaine's inhibition of HIV protective chemokines and upregulation of HIV-entry coreceptors (48). In a murine model of severe combined immunodeficiency (SCID), Roth and associates demonstrated that human peripheral blood leukocytes injected into the mice had twice the propensity to become HIV-infected when exposed to the virus in the setting of cocaine versus virus alone (49). Lower CD4:CD8 ratios and a significantly augmented viral load were found in the cocaine-exposed group. Cytokine activation in congestive heart failure in general (50), as well as HIV/AIDS cardiomyopathy specifically (3,9) has been well described, and the above studies underscore a similar role for these substances when cocaine and HIV combine to attack vascular tissue, likely irrespective of anatomical location.

TREATMENT OF BOTH ADDICTION AND CARDIAC COMPONENTS IN THE HIV/COCAINE POPULATION: ANGIOTENSIN CONVERTING ENZYME INHIBITORS

Treatment options for cocaine addiction are presently limited, and no pharmacological compound has yet demonstrated overall effectiveness for therapy of this disorder in controlled prospective randomized trials. Most drugs analyzed to date have been psychotropic in origin. Even if found to be effective, a compound's interactions with cocaine—which could magnify its stimulatory or cardiotoxic aspects—may limit usefulness (51). The development of a safe and effective agent to treat both cocaine addiction and its cardiovascular sequelae, and that is also well tolerated by HIV patients, would constitute a major therapeutic advance. Underlying the development of such a drug would be the recognition that the behavioral and cardiovascular effects of cocaine are modulated through diverse, albeit related, pharmacological pathways. In this section we provide background for the investigation of angiotensin converting enzyme (ACE) inhibitors, commonly used to treat hypertension and congestive heart failure, in treating cocaine-addicted cohorts. Primarily, ACE inhibitors may prove desirable by modulating levels of dopamine and corticotropin-releasing factor in the brain and by their ability to reverse cardiovascular and platelet dysfunction. Several available ACE inhibitors differ in the functional group (sulfhydryl, carboxyl, or phosphinyl) used to inhibit ACE through binding to its zinc ion as well as in several other respects, including lipophilicity, tissue penetration, and route of elimination. These differences may influence selection of an ACE inhibitor in the study of cocaine addiction. The general properties of the RAS and its pharmacological inhibition with respect to renal, vascular, and cardiac systems have been reviewed recently (52). Of particular interest in the HIV-cocaine group, increased rates of left ventricular hypertrophy as well as diastolic dysfunction have been found in both cocaine abusers and in HIV-positive individuals. The potential utility of ACE inhibitors in these populations is suggested by findings that ACE-inhibitor therapy is associated with regression of left ventricular hypertrophy (53,54) as well as improvements in diastolic function (55).

ACE Inhibitors and Thrombotic Effects

Other potential benefits favoring ACE inhibition in HIV-cocaine disease relate to antithrombotic properties and the reversal of acute toxic cardiac effects of cocaine. Angiotensin II directly enhances platelet aggregation and release, and ACE inhibitors downregulate the platelet metabolic pathways that promote reactivity. ACE inhibition may also block platelet thromboxane synthesis and stimulate prostacyclin formation, with consequent decrements in shear- and agonist-induced platelet reactivity (56). In cocaine users, ACE inhibitors may also limit procoagulant endothelial cell effects of RAS activation by preventing the degradation of bradykinin (57), restoring vasodilatation in constricted atherosclerotic vessels under sympathetic stress, and improving fibrinolytic function (58). In a rodent model, Trouve and colleagues (59) increased survival with administration of enalaprilat, the active metabolite of the ACE inhibitor enalapril, after administering an otherwise lethal dose of cocaine. ACE inhibitors may also protect against adverse cardiac events, such as myocardial ischemia, that can occur acutely with cocaine administration or in a withdrawal context when cocaine users are newly abstinent (60).

ACE Inhibitors and Psychotropic Effects

Although the presence of angiotensin II in the brain was suggested over 40 years ago (61), specific characterization of the loci and potential function of ACE and angiotensin receptors in the central nervous system (CNS) is as yet imperfect. However, the existence in the brain of a complete, intrinsic RAS, with local expression of mRNA for renin, angiotensinogen, and ACE, has been confirmed (62). It is likely that angiotensin II is a neurotransmitter that interacts with catecholamines, serotonin, and other peptides and possesses receptors in diverse regions—including the locus coeruleus, hypothalamus, and subfornical organ—and dopaminergic regions such as the striatum and substantia nigra (63,64). In rodentia, high levels of ACE activity have been discovered in the striatum, cerebellum, pituitary gland, caudate nucleus, area postrema, choroid plexus, and locus coeruleus (65). ACE plays a key part in the metabolism of brain neuropeptides, including [Met]- and [Leu]-enkephalin, dopamine, substance P, and dynorphin (62,66).

In seeking a useful therapy for cocaine addiction, investigators have recognized the role played by the mesoaccumbens dopaminergic reward system in drug-taking behaviors (67). Agents with dopaminergic properties may diminish cocaine use by reversing or compensating for the downregulation in dopaminergic systems resulting from chronic cocaine habituation, a condition linked to dysphoric states that maintain addictive behavior (68,69). ACE inhibitors are potentially useful in this instance because they are capable of stimulating dopamine release in the CNS. Jenkins and associates (66) found that ACE inhibitors elevate dopamine levels in the striatum and suggest that this dopaminergic activity may be modulated via the endogenous opioid system—for example, the enkephalin system—by augmenting concentrations of preproenkephalin mRNA. This possibility is particularly interesting in light of findings that the endogenous opioid system in cocaine abusers is disrupted (70). Therefore it is arguable that ACE inhibitors may normalize dopaminergic systems by a mechanism not previously recognized or analyzed in cocaine-addicted patients.

Additional CNS effects of ACE inhibitors are suggested in experimental studies that describe activation of the hypothalamic-pituitary-adrenal axis by drugs of abuse, creating positive behavioral reinforcement. Withdrawal from cocaine causes activation of corticotropin-releasing factor (CRF) (71). CRF release may mediate the dysphoria of abstinence as well as stress-related relapse to cocaine use. Of major interest, ACE inhibitors suppress CRF release (72) and angiotensin II stimulates CRF release (73). In this fashion ACE inhibitors could ameliorate stress-related relapse to cocaine. HIV-positive cocaine users may harbor greater vulnerability to stress-related relapse than HIV-negative cocaine users, given the combined influence of cocaine and HIV-linked neuroendocrine activation. Beyond dopaminergic and CRF-lowering properties, ACE inhibitors may also show benefit in this population because of antidepressant (74) as well as cognitive-enhancing effects (75).

Preliminary Studies

As a preliminary assessment, we evaluated the cardiac status of asymptomatic HIV infected cocaine users employing two-dimensional echocardiography and Doppler examinations to determine the prevalence of structural and functional abnormalities. Evaluation of platelet function was conducted as well.

Clinical Evaluation of Subjects

Enrollment consisted of 16 asymptomatic HIV-positive cocaine-using individuals. Previously, each had tested positive for HIV and was maintained on oral methadone treatment. Clinical history and physical examination were obtained. Active cardio-pulmonary disease (dyspnea, chest pain, orthopnea, syncope) or established diabetes or treated hypertension represented exclusionary criteria. Previously published normative echocardiographic data from healthy individuals under the age of 50 ($n = 61$) were used as control comparisons (76). Experienced observers collected demographic and biophysical data including height, weight, body surface area (BSA), heart rate, blood pressure, and 12-lead electrocardiography.

There were 10 male and 6 female subjects with a mean age of 42 (range 28 to 50). Of these, 4 (25%) were noted to be hypertensive (>140/90 mmHg). Mean years since first testing HIV positive was 8.2 (range 0.5 to 14 years), and 50% were administered antiretroviral therapy with protease inhibitors at study entry. Mean CD4 count was $254/mm^3$ (range 45 to 548). Average RNA viral load measured by quantitative polymerase chain reaction was 96,713 copies per milliliter (range 220 to 690,000).

All reported cocaine ingestion in the 30 days prior to study, using the drug an average of 12.2 ± 14 days during the prior month. The majority of subjects (11 of 16) reported cocaine use during the week prior to the echocardiographic study, averaging 4.9 ± 2.1 days on which they used cocaine. Subjects overall had been using cocaine for an average of 17.6 ± 7.7 years. Of the 16 patients, 5 (31.5%) used cocaine intravenously, 1 (6%) took it intranasally, and 10 (62.5%) inhaled the free-based form of cocaine. All subjects had been enrolled in a methadone maintenance program, and the mean daily methadone dose was 76 ± 14 mg.

Imaging of Cardiac Structure and Function

All participants then underwent transthoracic echocardiography conducted by a dedicated ultrasonographer, consisting of routine time-motion, two-dimensional, and Doppler echocardiographic examinations. Images were acquired using a Sequoia model C256 ultrasonoscope with 2.5- ansd 3.5-mHz transducers (Acuson, Mountainview, CA). Standard parasternal long-axis and apical two-, four-, and five-chamber views were acquired. M-mode echocardiograms were accomplished in the parasternal window, and Doppler recordings were obtained in the apical views in accordance with the published recommendations of the American Society of Echocardiography (77).

Echocardiographic variables were measured using the 3.5-mHz transducer: left atrial dimension (LA), left ventricular end-diastolic (LVEDD) dimension, end-systolic dimension (LVESD), interventricular septum (IVS), and posterior wall thickness (PW) measured at end diastole. Left ventricular ejection fraction (LVEF) and left ventricular mass (LVm) were computed by the Teicholz formula, with subsequent calculation of left ventricular mass index (LVm/BSA).

Pulsed Doppler recordings of transmitral flow were obtained in the apical two-chamber view during expiration using the 2.5-mHz transducer with the sample volume positioned at the mitral leaflet tips (78). Peak velocities of early (E) and late (A) mitral valve inflow, the corresponding E/A ratio, and the mitral valve early flow deceleration time (MVdt) were ascertained. Continuous-wave Doppler recordings of flow across the tricuspid valve in systole were used to estimate pulmonary artery systolic pressure.

The results of transthoracic echocardiography in our 16 study subjects were compared with normative data from 61 healthy controls subjects (76). No serious cardiac abnormalities were noted in the study sample with regard to systolic behavior, valve function, or the pericardium. The HIV-positive cocaine abuse subset, compared with normative data from the age-matched healthy control group, was similar with respect to left ventricular end diastolic (LVEDD) and left ventricular end systolic (LVESD) dimensions (LVEDD 50 ± 5 mm versus 49 ± 4 mm and LVESD 31 ± 4 mm versus 31 ± 3 mm, respectively; neither *p* value significant). The thicknesses of the interventricular septum (IVS) and posterior wall (PW) were similar (IVS 9.9 ± 1.8 mm versus 9.3 ± 1.1 mm; PW 9.6 ± 1.3 mm versus 9.1 ± 0.9 mm, respectively; neither *p* value significant). There was no difference in left ventricular ejection fraction (LVEF) between the two groups (LVEF 63 ± 8% versus 60 ± 5%, respectively, *p* value not significant).

However, study subjects compared with controls had significantly greater left atrial (LA) size (LA 37 ± 4 mm versus 34 ± 4 mm, respectively), left ventricular mass (LVm) (LVm 212 ± 52 g versus 160 ± 36 g, respectively), and left ventricular mass index (LVm/BSA) in both males (LVm/BSA 120 ± 22 g/m^2 versus 97 ± 14 g/m^2, respectively) and females (LVm/BSA 105 $\pm$ 35 g/m^2 versus 82 $\pm$ 13 g/m^2, respectively; all p values less than 0.05). In respect to diastolic function, when study subjects were compared with controls, the E/A ratio was significantly reduced (1.3 $\pm$ 0.3 versus 1.9 $\pm$ 0.6, respectively), and the mitral valve deceleration time (MVdt) was significantly increased in study patients compared with controls (MVdt 278 $\pm$ 96 ms versus 179 $\pm$ 20 ms; all p values less than 0.05).

The results of this study indicate that asymptomatic HIV-positive cocaine abusers have preclinical abnormalities of cardiac function that can be identified by transthoracic echocardiography. Significant changes in the mitral valve filling pattern, as evidenced by reduction of the E/A ratio and increases in the deceleration time, indicate impairment in diastolic function of the left ventricle in cocaine users who are also HIV-positive. This abnormality may be an early manifestation of cardiac involvement of HIV, cocaine cardiomyopathy, or both.

Analysis of Echocardiographic Findings

Prior investigations examining either HIV/AIDS subjects or cocaine users have revealed early impairment of systolic and diastolic function (13,26,79,80). One study employing echocardiography in 69 randomly selected asymptomatic HIV-infected patients described depressed global left ventricular systolic function in 14.5% (13). Other reports confirm asymptomatic left ventricular systolic dysfunction in as many as 67 to 90% of patients with HIV infection. Coudray and colleagues (80) analyzed 28 asymptomatic HIV patients, 23 patients with AIDS, and 25 age- and sex-matched controls using conventional two-dimensional echocardiography and Doppler examinations. Compared with controls, significant increases were noted in both mitral deceleration time (MVdt) and isovolumic relaxation time (IVRT), suggesting abnormal diastolic behavior.

The largest echocardiographic series reported to date was published by the Gruppo Italiano per lo Studio Cardiologico dei Pazienti Affetti da AIDS, comparing echocardiographic and Doppler parameters in 1236 patients with asymptomatic HIV disease with an equal number of unaffected, healthy controls (81). Even in the absence of cardiac symptoms, the HIV cohort showed a 20% mean reduction in LVEF, a 34% reduction in the E/A ratio, and a 20% increase in IVRT compared with healthy controls ($p < 0.001$).

The appearance of left ventricular hypertrophy has also been noted in the setting of chronic cocaine use (24). Om and colleagues (25) studied 58 cocaine users without history of systemic hypertension or HIV disease who underwent echocardiography either to exclude endocarditis, to evaluate left ventricular function, or to assess a history of chest pain. The authors noted significantly greater left ventricular hypertrophy (defined as a left ventricular mass index >125g/m^2 for men and >110 g/m^2 for women) in comparison with age- and sex-matched controls. Both the demographics (74% African American, 60% male) and the echocardiographic findings (mean LV mass index in male cocaine users 112 + 41 g/m^2 versus 83 + 23 g/m^2 in healthy volunteers) parallel our observation of increased LV mass and impaired diastolic filling in HIV/cocaine-using subjects. Significant differences in cocaine-related hypertrophy have been reported in African-American males compared with Caucasians: these differences are not related to hypertension or to the quantity of cocaine usually ingested (82).

Diastolic dysfunction was noted in a study of 10 normotensive cocaine users (27). Although ventricular mass was normal, subjects demonstrated significant reductions in the E/A ratio compared with normal controls, illustrating early impairment of diastolic filling. Yet not all studies have observed an increased incidence of left ventricular hypertrophy (83,84) or diastolic dysfunction (85) in cocaine-using patients. An echocardiographic study of 85 HIV-negative African-American male intravenous drug users discovered left ventricular hypertrophy in 14%, suggesting that ethnic and lifestyle factors may play a critical part as well (86).

As noted above, cardiac manifestations of AIDS are well described, ranging from end-stage congestive cardiomyopathy (10,2,77,87) to pericardial effusions (14). Left ventricular hypertrophy and diastolic dysfunction have been reported in HIV-positive individuals (13,26,79,80). Thus, it is not surprising that we noted a significant prevalence of ventricular hypertrophy and impaired diastolic filling in HIV-positive subjects who are also cocaine users. Of particular note, in our group of HIV-positive cocaine users, the degree of diastolic dysfunction and the extent of abnormal left ventricular mass was greater than would be expected in age-, sex-, and ethnically matched healthy controls (76,82) and was increased compared with similar cohorts of longstanding cocaine users (22,25–27,82,85) or HIV-positive individuals (12,13,16,22,25,26,79,82,85). Whether this type of preclinical impairment will progress to further symptomatic systolic or diastolic dysfunction remains to be elucidated. Previous studies have outlined such a scenario (88,89).

This study was limited by small sample size and the use of historical controls (90). Newer modalities to quantitate diastolic filling abnormalities (isovolumic relaxation time, interrogation of pulmonary venous flow, tissue Doppler) in future studies may strengthen the ability to detect preclinical diastolic dysfunction. One-quarter of our group had undiagnosed and untreated high blood pressure, a possible confounding variable in cardiac pathophysiology. That 10 of the 16 subjects were African American may represent a limitation as well.

Platelet Assays

Platelet assays in 16 HIV-positive/cocaine-using subjects versus 16 HIV-negative, non-cocaine-using sex- and age-matched controls included (1) percentage circulating activated (CD62P+) platelets, (2) CD62P response to the platelet agonist adenosine diphosphate (ADP), (3) platelet dense granule release (aggregation) in response to ADP, and (4) platelet kinetics (91,92). Baseline percentage activated platelets in HIV-positive cocaine users were significantly greater than in controls (10.3 ± 4.2% versus 5.7 ± 3.9%, respectively, $p < 0.05$), a finding consistent with our prior report of enhanced platelet activation in HIV-negative cocaine users (33).

Under ADP stimulation, study subjects compared to controls consistently demonstrated increased platelet reactivity in respect to both percentage and mean CD62P release and aggregation. Study subjects had a rate of platelet aggregation 74 ± 21% higher in response to low dose ADP, and 54 ± 12% higher at high ADP doses ($p < 0.01$, for both comparisons). Baseline CD62P values did not correlate with agonist response to ADP ($r = 0.61$, $p > 0.05$), indicating that circulating platelets in HIV-positive cocaine users are primed to undergo α- or dense-granule release in reaction to physiological agonists. Platelet kinetics studies were performed, with the youngest circulating platelets easily identifiable using fluorescent nucleic acid binding dyes, to measure the percentage of circulating reticulating platelets (RP) (93). HIV-positive cocaine-using subjects had significantly greater RP values, 19.4 ± 8.4%, compared with controls, 10.1 ± 3.0% ($p < 0.05$), despite similar platelet counts, suggesting more rapid platelet turnover. Although RP values did not correlate with baseline platelet activation ($r = 0.55, p > 0.05$), the RP% correlated well with response to ADP ($r = 0.81, p < 0.05$), suggesting that higher platelet reactivity may lead to increased platelet turnover.

Preliminary Effect of Fosinopril Treatment on Addiction

ACE inhibition was employed first in a preliminary study of HIV-negative cocaine users on methadone maintenance, then in a group of HIV-positive cocaine users. Fosinopril was selected for cocaine addiction therapy because, as a highly lipophilic agent, it crosses the blood-brain barrier well and, compared with other ACE inhibitors, creates in the brain an immediate and long-lasting inhibition of ACE over a wide dose spectrum (94). Fosinopril also has a number of other potential advantages: (1) it contains a phosphinyl group as the zinc ligand, possibly explaining its beneficial cardiovascular effects; (2) it inhibits platelet reactivity and proaggregatory behavior (95); (3) it can normalize endothelin-1 levels (96); and (4) it is eliminated by both liver and kidneys—potentially a benefit in HIV/AIDS patients who may have hepatic or renal dysfunction (97).

In the HIV-negative cocaine group using fosinopril 15 mg versus placebo, there were 5 patients: 4 male, 1 female; 2 white, 2 African American, 1 Hispanic; average age 43 (range 34 to 48). All reported using cocaine the week before study entry: 2 injected the drug intravenously, 2 smoked it, and 1 used cocaine intranasally. They reported cocaine use on an average of 3.6 (±1.7) days during that week. Fosinopril was well tolerated, without any significant alterations in blood pressure. While receiving fosinopril, 2 of the 5 patients attained cocaine abstinence, proven by cocaine-free urine studies. Each subject self-reported no cocaine ingestion during the final week of the study, when they were taking 15 mg/day fosinopril. One patient, who had been using intravenous cocaine for 20 years, achieved 4 cocaine-free weeks while taking fosinopril. The second patient, who had been smoking cocaine for a year, achieved 3 weeks of cocaine abstinence while taking fosinopril. Cocaine craving ratings and self-reported quantitative use were significantly reduced during the course of the study (51).

In the HIV-positive cocaine group, the target dose of fosinopril was increased to 20 mg daily, with weekly titration. A total of 6 HIV-positive subjects (3 African-American males, 2 white males, and 1 white female) entered the protocol. They had been using cocaine for an average of 14 years (range 10 to 20), 5 patients by smoking and 1 by injecting the drug intravenously. The average number of years since the HIV diagnosis was 9.9 (±5.2) years. Average viral load (RNA by polymerase chain reaction) and CD4 cell counts were 20,937 copies per milliliter (range 220 to 68,000) and 270/mm^3 (range 89 to 560), respectively. Of the 6 patients, 4 achieved the goal dose of 20 mg/day, which was well tolerated with respect to symptoms and blood pressure changes. The 2 remaining patients left the study for reasons unrelated to medication. Two of the four patients cited no cocaine use after 1 week at 20 mg/day, verified by urine study. Cocaine craving was absent in 3 patients at this dose and reduced in the fourth patient.

Future Directions

Our preliminary analysis of a small group of HIV-positive cocaine-using subjects yielded evidence of enhanced platelet reactivity, including priming of both α-granule and dense granule release, supporting a role for ACE-inhibitor treatment. Although the echocardiographic study disclosed no serious cardiac abnormalities, we found differences from normal reference values with regard to diastolic function, the abnormality of which may respond to treatment at an early stage. Alternatively, patients with the level of diastolic dysfunction revealed in our preliminary examination may suffer accelerated progression under the pathological stimulation of both cocaine use and HIV disease. Nonetheless, HIV-positive individuals who use cocaine may be at heightened risk for the development of left ventricular hypertrophy and diastolic dysfunction despite a lack of symptoms. Echocardiography is useful to detect these abnormalities and may play a part in screening asymptomatic patients with early HIV disease, who may receive benefit from lifestyle changes and specific preventive medications.

The respective contributions of cocaine and HIV disease to the pathophysiology of diastolic dysfunction cannot be determined in our study and may indeed be extremely challenging to disentangle even under ideal trial conditions. In addition, limited sample size did not allow analysis of echocardiographic data by race, an important variable in prior cocaine related studies (82). Larger studies of cocaine using individuals controlled for HIV status, severity of addiction, presence of hypertension, ethnicity, and gender will be required to address this issue fully.

The preliminary analysis of fosinopril use in HIV-positive and HIV-negative cocaine patients suggests good tolerance and reduced cocaine use and craving in some patients. A larger placebo-controlled trial has now been established to assess cardiovascular and psychological responses to ACE inhibition in the HIV/cocaine cohort. In particular, these patients manifest a constellation of preclinical cardiovascular disorders that are potentially reversible with ACE inhibitors, with early indications that the ACE inhibitor fosinopril may be capable of alleviating the problem of cocaine addiction in this population. Further investigations are needed to delineate the effects of therapy and determine which anti-HIV drugs or specific cardioactive agents are most beneficial in improving clinical status, echocardiographic findings, and long-term outcomes in this patient group. Present and future studies promise to deepen our understanding of the role of the renin-angiotensin system in cocaine addiction disorders, HIV disease, or both when they coexist.

ACKNOWLEDGMENTS

Supported in part by National Institutes of Health grants DA09250 and DA00277 from the National Institute on Drug Abuse; HL63063 and HL02660 from the National Heart, Lung, and Blood Institute; and Bristol Myers Squibb, who provided study drug and placebo compounds.

REFERENCES

1. Tardiff K, Marzuk PM, Leon AC, et al. Human immunodeficiency virus among trauma patients in New York City. Ann Emerg Med 1998; 32:151–154.
2. Soodini G, Morgan JP. Can cocaine abuse exacerbate the cardiac toxicity of human immunodeficiency virus? Clin Cardiol 2001; 24:177–181.

3. Barbaro G, Lipshultz SE. Pathogenesis of HIV-associated cardiomyopathy. Ann N Y Acad Sci 2001; 946:57–81.

4. Hoffman C, Jaeger H. Cardiology and AIDS-HAART (highly active anti-retroviral therapy). Ann N Y Acad Sci 2001; 946:130–144.

5. Bozzette SA, Ake CF, Tam HK, Chang SW, Louis TA. Cardiovascular and cerebrovascular events in patients treated for human immunodeficiency virus infection. N Engl J Med 2003; 348:702–710.

6. Kuritzkes DR, Currier J. Cardiovasular risk factors and antiretroviral therapy. N Engl J Med 2003; 348:679–680.

7. Calabrese LH, Proffitt MR, Yen-Lieberman B, Hobbs RE, Ratliff NB. Congestive cardiomyopathy and illness related to the acquired immunodeficiency syndrome (AIDS) associated with isolation of retrovirus from myocardium. Ann Intern Med 1987; 107:691–692.

8. Webb JG, Chan-Yan C, Kiess MC. Cardiac dysfunction associated with the acquired immunodeficiency syndrome (AIDS). Clin Cardiol 1988; 11:423–426.

9. Lewis W. Cardiomyopathy in AIDS: a pathophysiological perspective. Prog Cardiovasc Dis 2000; 43:151–170.

10. Cohen I, Anderson D, Virmani R, Reen BM, Macher A. Congestive cardiomyopathy in association with the acquired immunodeficiency syndrome. N Engl J Med 1986; 315:628–630.

11. Kaminski HJ, Katzman M, Wiest PM, Ellner JJ, Gifford DR, Rackley R, et al. Cardiomyopathy associated with the acquired immune deficiency syndrome. J AIDS 1988; 1:105–110.

12. Levy WS, Simon GL, Rios JC, Ross AM. Prevalence of cardiac abnormalities in human immunodeficiency virus infection. Am J Cardiol 1989; 63:86–89.

13. Herskowitz A, Vlahov D, Willoughby S, Chaisson RE, Schulman SP, Neumann DA. Prevalence and incidence of left ventricular dysfunction in patients with human immunodeficiency virus infection. Am J Cardiol 1993; 71:955–958.

14. Heidenreich PA, Eisenberg MJ, Kee LL, Somelofski CA, Hollander H. Pericardial effusion in AIDS: incidence and survival. Circulation 1995; 92:3229–3234.

15. Matsumori A, Yamada T, Suzuki H, et al. Increased circulating cytokines in patients with myocarditis and cardiomyopathy. Br Heart J 1994; 72:561–566.

16. Milei J, Grana D, Fernandez Alonso G, Matturi L. Cardiac involvement in acquired immunodeficiency syndrome—a review to push action. The Committee for the Study of Cardiac Involvement in AIDS. Clin Cardiol 1998; 21:465–472.

17. Corallo S, Mutinelli MR, Moroni M, Lazzarin A, Celano V, Repossini A, et al. Echocardiography detects myocardial damage in AIDS: prospective study in 102 patients. Eur Heart J 1988; 9:887–892.

18. Raffanti SP, Chiaramida AJ, Sen P, Wright P, Middleton JR, Chiaramida S. Assessment of cardiac function in patients with the acquired immunodeficiency syndrome. Chest 1988; 93:592–594.

19. Longo-Mbenza B, Seghers LV, Vita EK, Tonduangu K, Bayekula M. Assessment of ventricular diastolic function in aids patients from Congo: a Doppler echocardiographic study. Heart 1998; 80:184–189.

20. Compton WM. Cocaine use and HIV risk in out of treatment drug abusers. Drug Alcohol Depend 2000; 58:215–218.

21. Boehrer JD, Moliterno DJ, Willard JE, Snyder RWD, Horton RP, Glamann D, et al. Hemodynamic effects of intranasal cocaine in humans. J Am Coll Cardiol 1992; 20:90–93.

22. Kloner RA, Hale S, Alker K, Rezkalla S. The effects of acute and chronic cocaine use on the heart. Circulation 1992; 85:407–419.

23. Lange RA, Hillis LD. Cardiovascular complications of cocaine use. N Engl J Med 2001; 345:351–358.

24. Brickner ME, Willard JE, Eichhorn EJ, Black J, Grayburn PA. Left ventricular hypertrophy associated with chronic cocaine abuse. Circulation 1991; 84:1130–1135.

25. Om A, Ellaham S, Vetrovec G, Guard C, Reese S, Nixon J. Left ventricular hypertrophy in normotensive cocaine users. Am Heart J 1993; 125:1441–1443.

26. Bertolet B, Freund G, Martin C, Perchalski D, Williams C, Pepine C. Unrecognized left ventricular dysfunction in an apparently healthy cocaine abuse population. Clin Cardiol 1990; 13:323–328.

27. Mondillo S, Agricola E, D'Aprile N, Nicoletti A, Palazzuoli V. Evaluation of diastolic function in patients addicted to recreational cocaine. Minerva Cardioangiol 1997; 45:489–493.

28. Tazelaar HD, Karch SB, Stephens BG, Billingham ME. Cocaine and the heart. Hum Pathol 1987; 18:195–199.

29. Kammermeier M, Grobecker HF. Cardiotoxicity of catecholamines after application of L-dopa in Wistar-Kyoto (WKY) and spontaneously hypertensive rats (SHR). Hypertens Res 1995; 18(suppl 1):S165–S168.

30. Seta Y, Kanda T, Yokoyama T, et al. Effect of amrinone on murine viral myocarditis. Res Commun Mol Pathol Pharmacol 1997; 95:57–66.

31. Karch SB. Serum catecholamines in cocaine intoxicated patients with cardiac symptoms [abstr]. Ann Emerg Med 1987; 16:481.

32. Kugelmass AD, Oda A, Monahan K, Cabral C, Ware JA. Activation of human platelets by cocaine. Circulation 1993; 88:876–883.

33. Rinder HM, Ault KA, Jatlow PI, Kosten TR, Smith BR. Platelet alpha-granule release in cocaine users. Circulation 1994; 90:1162–1167.

34. Minor RL, Scott BD, Brown DD, Winniford MD. Cocaine-induced myocardial infarction in patients with normal coronary arteries. Ann Intern Med 1991; 115:797–806.

35. Vitullo JC, Karam R, Mekhail M, Wicker P, Engelmann GL, Khairallah PA. Cocaine-induced small vessel spasm in isolated rat hearts. Am J Pathol 1989; 135:85–91.

36. Ballem PJ, Belzberg A, Devine DV, Lyster D, Spruston B, Chambers H, Doubroff P, Mikulash K. Kinetic studies of the mechanism of thrombocytopenia in patients with human immunodeficiency virus infection. N Engl J Med 1992; 327:1779–1784.

37. Hornig B, Kohler C, Drexler H. Role of bradykinin in mediating vascular effects of angiotensin-converting enzyme inhibitors in humans. Circulation 1997; 95:1115–1118.

38. Mombouli JV. ACE inhibition, endothelial function and coronary artery lesions. Role of kinins and nitric oxide. Drugs 1997; 54:12–22.

39. Drexler H, Kurz S, Jeserich M, Munzel T, Hornig B. Effect of chronic angiotensin-converting enzyme inhibition on endothelial function in patients with chronic heart failure. Am J Cardiol 1995; 76(suppl):13E–18E.

40. Hendricks-Munoz KD, Gerrets RP, Higgins RD, Munoz JL, Caines VV. Cocaine-stimulated endothelin-1 release is decreased by angiotensin-converting enzyme inhibitors in cultured endothelial cells. Cardiovasc Res 1996; 31:117–123.

41. Kolodgie FD, Virmani R, Cornhill JF, Herderick EE, Smialek J. Increase in atherosclerosis and adventitial mast cells in cocaine abusers: an alternative mechanism of cocaine-associated coronary vasospasm and thrombosis. J Am Coll Cardiol 1991; 17:1553–1560.

42. Egashira K, Pipers FS, Morgan JP. Effects of cocaine on epicardial coronary artery reactivity in miniature swine after endothelial injury and high cholesterol feeding. In vivo and in vitro analysis. J Clin Invest 1991; 88:1307–1314.

43. Fiala AM, Gan XH, Newton T, Chiappelli F, Shapshak P, Kermani V, Kung MA, Diagne A, Martinez O, Way D, Weinand M, Witte M, Graves M. Divergent effects of cocaine on cytokine production by lymphocytes and monocyte/macrophages: HIV-1 enhancement by cocaine within the blood-brain barrier. Adv Exp Med Biol 1996; 402:145–156.

44. Shapshak P, Crandall KA, Xin KQ, et al. HIV-1 neuropathogenesis and abused drugs: current reviews, problems, and solutions. Adv Exp Biol 1996; 402:171–186.

45. Fiala M, Gan XH, Zhang L, House SD, Newton T, Graves MC, Shapshak P, Stins M, Kim KS, Witte M, Chang SL. Cocaine enhances monocyte migration across the blood-brain barrier: cocaine's connection to AIDS dementia and vasculitis? Adv Exp Med Biol 1998; 437:199–205.

46. Fiala M, Gujuluva C, Berger O, Bukrinsky M, Kim KS, Graves MC. Chemokine receptors on brain endothelia—keys to HIV-1 neuroinvasion. Adv Exp Med Biol 2001; 493:35–40.

47. Zhang L, Looney D, Taub D, Chang SL, Way D, Witte MH, Graves MC, Fiala M. Cocaine opens the blood-brain barrier to HIV-1 invasion. J Neurovirol 1998; 4:619–626.

48. Nair MP, Mahajan S, Chadha KC, Nair NM, Hewitt RG, Pillai SK, Chadha P, Sukumaran PC, Schwartz SA. Effect of cocaine on chemokine and CCR-5 gene expression by mononuclear cells from normal donors and HIV-1 infected patients. Adv Exp Med Biol 2001; 493:235–240.

49. Roth MD, Tashkin DP, Choi R, Jamieson BD, Zack JA, Baldwin GC. Cocaine enhances human immunodeficiency virus replication in a model of severe combined immunodeficient mice implanted with human peripheral blood leukocytes. J Infect Dis 2002; 185:701–705.

50. Clark DJ, Cleman MW, Pfau SE, Rollins SA, Ramahi TM, Mayer C, Caulin-Glaser T, Daher E, Kosiborod M, Bell L, Setaro JF. Serum complement activation in congestive heart failure. Am Heart J 2001; 141:684–690.

51. Margolin A, Avants SK, Setaro JF, Rinder HM, Grupp L. Cocaine, HIV, and their cardiovascular effects: is there a role for ACE-inhibitor therapy? Drug Alcohol Depend 2000; 61:35–45.

52. Perazella M, Setaro JF. Renin-angiotensin-aldosterone system: Fundamental aspects and clinical implications in renal and cardiovascular disorders. J Nucl Cardiol 2003; 10:184–196.

53. Brunner HR, Waeber B, Nussberger J. Angiotensin-converting enzyme inhibitors. In: Messerili FH, ed. Cardiovascular Drug Therapy. 2d ed. Philadelphia: Saunders, 1996: 690–711.

54. Schmeider RE, Martus P, Klingbeil A. Reversal of left ventricular hypertrophy in essential hypertension: a meta-analysis of randomized double-blind studies. JAMA 1996; 275: 1507–1513.

55. Sagastagoitia JD, Morillas M, Martinez A, et al. Improvement in diastolic function in hypertensive patients with left ventricular hypertrophy with inhibitors of the angiotensin converting enzyme. Rev Clin Esp 1998; 198:15–22.

56. Mezei Z, Kis B, Gecse A, Telegdy G, Abraham G, Sonkodi S. Platelet eicosanoids and the effect of captopril in blood pressure regulation. Eur J Pharmacol 1997; 340:67–73.

57. Giugliano D, Marfella R, Acampora R, Giunta R, Coppola L, D'Onofrio F. Effects of perindopril and carvedilol on endothelium-dependent vascular functions in patients with diabetes and hypertension. Diabetes Care 1998; 21:631–636.

58. Tomiyama H, Kimura Y, Mitsuhashi H, Kinouchi T, et al. Relationship between endothelial function and fibrinolysis in early hypertension. Hypertension 1998; 31:321–327.

59. Trouve R, Latour C, Nahas G. Cocaine and the renin-angiotensin system. Adv Biosci 1991; 80:165–176.

60. Nademanne K, Gorelick D, Josephson MA, Ryan MA, Wilkins JA, Robertson HA, Vaghaiwalla F, Intarachot V. Myocardial ischemia during cocaine withdrawal. Ann Intern Med 1989; 111:876–880.

61. Bickerton RK, Buckley JP. Evidence for a central mechanism in angiotensin-induced hypertension. Proc Soc Exp Biol Med 1961; 106:834.

62. Unger T, Baldoer E, Ganten D, Lang RE, Rettig R. Brain angiotensin: pathways and pharmacology. Circulation 1988; 77:40–54.

63. Phillips MI. Functions of angiotensin in the central nervous system. Annu Rev Physiol 1987; 49:413–435.

64. Jenkins TA, Allen AM, Chai DP, Paxinos G, Mendelsohn FAO. Interactions of angiotensin II with central dopamine. In: Raizada MK, ed. Recent Advances in Cellular and Molecular Aspects of Angiotensin Receptors. New York: Plenum Press, 1996:93–103.

65. Skidgel RA, Defendini R, Erdos EG. Angiotensin I converting enzyme and its role in neuropeptide metabolism. In: Turner AJ, ed. Neuropeptides and Their Peptidases. New York: Ellis Horwood, 1987:165–182.

66. Jenkins TA, Mendelsohn FAO, Chai SY. Angiotensin converting enzyme modulates dopamine turnover in the striatum. J Neurochem 1997; 68:1304–1311.

67. Beitner-Johnson D, Nestler EJ. Basic neurobiology of cocaine: Actions within the mesolimbic dopamine system. In: Kosten TR, Kleber HD, eds. Clinician's Guide to Cocaine Addiction. New York: Guilford Press, 1992.

68. Parsons LH, Smith AD, Justice JB. Basal extracellular dopaine is decreased in the rat nucleus accumbens during abstinence from chronic cocaine. Synapse 1991; 9:60–65.

69. Gold MS, Miller NS, Jonas JM. Cocaine (and crack) neurobiology. In: Lowinson JH, Ruiz P, Millman RB, eds. Substance Abuse: A Comprehensive Textbook. Baltimore: Williams & Wilkins, 1992:222–235.

70. Kreek MJ. Cocaine, dopamine and endogenous opioid system. J Addict Dis 1996; 15:73–96.

71. DeVries AC, Pert A. Conditioned increases in anxiogenic-like behavior following exposure to contextual stimuli associated with cocaine are mediated by corticotropin-releasing factor. Psychopharmacology 1998; 137:333–340.

72. Zacharieva S, Matrozov P, Stoeva I, Andonova K. The effect of angiotensin converting enzyme inhibition on ACTH response to corticotropin releasing hormone (CRH) in normal men. Horm Metal Res 1991; 23:245–254.

73. Aguilera G, Young WS, Kiss A, Bathis A. Direct regulation of hypothalamic corticotropin releasing hormone neurons by angiotensin II. Neuroendocrinology 1995; 61:437–444.

74. Bisio A, Rosola R, Abbati CDC, Sorlini L. Antidepressant activity of angiotensin-converting enzyme inhibitors. Curr Ther Res 1990; 48:191–197.

75. Barnes JM, Barnes NM, Costall B, Coughlan J, Kelly ME, Naylor RJ, Tomkins DM, Williams TJ. Angiotensin-converting enzyme inhibition, angiotensin and cognition. J Cardiovasc Pharmacol 1989; 19(suppl):S63–S71.

76. Klein A, Burstow DJ. Effects of age on left ventricular dimensions and filling dynamics in 117 normal persons. Mayo Clin Proc 1994; 69:212–224.

77. Schiller NB, Shah PM, Crawford M. Recommendations for quantitation of the left ventricle by two-dimensional echocardiography. J Am Soc Echocardiogr 1989; 2:83–88.

78. De Zuttere D, Touche TGS. Doppler echocardiographic measurement of mitral flow volume: validation of a new method in adult patients. J Am Coll Cardiol 1988; 11:343–350.

79. Barbaro G, Di Lorenzo G, Grisorio B, Barbarini G. Cardiac involvement in the acquired immunodeficiency syndrome: a multicenter clinical-pathological study. Gruppo Italiano per lo Studio Cardiologico dei Pazienti Affetti da AIDS Investigators. AIDS Res Hum Retrovir 1998; 14:1071–1077.

80. Coudray N, de Zuttere D, Force G, Champetier de Ribes D, Pourny JC, Antony I, et al. Left ventricular diastolic function in asymptomatic and symptomatic human immunodeficiency virus carriers: an echocardiographic study. Eur Heart J 1995; 16:61–67.

81. Barbaro G, Barbarini G, Di Lorenzo G. Early impairment of systolic and diastolic function in asymptomatic HIV-positive patients: a multicenter echocardiographic and echo-Doppler study. Gruppo Italiano per lo Studio Cardiologico dei Pazienti Affetti da AIDS Investigators. AIDS Res Hum Retrovir 1996; 12:1559–1563.

82. Willett DL, Brickner ME, Cigarroa CG, de Filippi CR, Eichhorn EJ, Grayburn PA. Racial differences in the prevalence of left ventricular hypertrophy among chronic cocaine abusers. Am J Cardiol 1995; 76:937–940.

83. Eisenberg MJ, Jue J, Mendelson J, Jones RT, Schiller NB. Left ventricular morphologic features and function in nonhospitalized cocaine users: a quantitative two-dimensional echocardiographic study. Am Heart J 1995; 129:941–946.

84. Hoegerman GS, Lewis CE, Flack J, Raczynski JM, Caveny J, Gardin JM. Lack of association of recreational cocaine and alcohol use with left ventricular mass in young adults: the coronary artery risk development in young adults (cardia) study. J Am Coll Cardiol 1995; 25:895–900.

85. Chakko S, Fernandez A. Cardiac manifestations of cocaine abuse: a cross sectional study of asymptomatic men with a history of long-term abuse of "crack" cocaine. J Am Coll Cardiol 1992; 20:1168–1174.

86. Willoughby SB, Vlahov D, Herskowitz A. Frequency of left ventricular dysfunction and other echocardiographic abnormalities in human immunodeficiency virus seronegative intravenous drug users. Am J Cardiol 1993; 71:446–447.

87. De Castro S, d'Amati G, Gallo P, Cartoni D, Santopadre P, Vullo V, et al. Frequency of development of acute global left ventricular dysfunction in human immunodeficiency virus infection. J Am Coll Cardiol 1994; 24:1018–1024.

88. Vasan RS, Benjamin EJ, Levy D. Prevalence, clinical features and prognosis of diastolic heart failure: an epidemiologic perspective. J Am Coll Cardiol 1995; 25:281–288.

89. Litwin SE, Grossman W. Diastolic dysfunction as a cause of heart failure. J Am Coll Cardiol 1993; 22:49A–55A.

90. Abbott BG, Larson MS, Margolin A, Avants SK, Jaffe CC, Setaro JF. Cardiac systolic performance and diastolic filling in subjects with both HIV disease and chronic cocaine use: demographic and echocardiographic assessment. In press.

91. Rinder CS, Student LA, Bonan JL, Rinder HM, Smith BR. Aspirin does not inhibit adenosine diphosphate-induced platelet a-granule release. Blood 1993; 82:505–512.

92. Peterec SM, Brennan SA, Rinder HM, Wnek JL, Beardsley DS. Reticulated platelet values in normal and thrombocytopenic neonates. J Pediatr 1996; 129:269–274.

93. Rinder HM, Munz U, Ault KA, Bonan JL, Smith BR. Utility of reticulated platelets in the evaluation of thrombopoietic disorders. Arch Pathol Lab Med 1993; 117:606–610.

94. Cushman DW, Wang FL, Fung CM, Grover CM, Harvey CM, Scalese RJ, Mitch SL, DeForrest JM. Comparisons, in vitro, ex vivo, and in vivo, of the actions of seven structurally diverse inhibitors of angiotensin-converting enzyme (ACE). Br J Clin Pharmacother 1989; 28(suppl):115S–131S.

95. Keidar S, Oiknine J, Leiba A, Shapira C, Leiba M, Aviram M. Fosinopril reduces ADP-induced platelet aggregation in hypertensive patients. J Cardiovasc Pharmacol 1996; 27:183–186.

96. Galatius-Jensen S, Wroblewski H, Emmeluth C, et al. Plasma endothelin in congestive heart failure: effect of the ACE inhibitor, fosinopril. Cardiovasc Res 1996; 32:1148–1154.

97. Sica DA, Fosinopril. Messerli FH, ed. Cardiovascular Drug Therapy. Philadelphia: Saunders, 1996:801–809.

6

HIV-Associated Thrombotic Microangiopathy

Anja S. Mühlfeld
Rheinisch Westfälisch Technische Hochschule Aachen, Achen, Germany

Stephan Segerer
University of Munich, Munich, Germany

Charles E. Alpers
University of Washington Medical Center, Seattle, Washington, U.S.A.

INTRODUCTION

The term *thrombotic microangiopathy* (TMA) was first introduced by Symmers in 1952 (1). It defines a pathological lesion characterized by thickened walls of small arteries and arterioles with mucinous swelling of the intima and endothelial cells, which at times detach from the basement membrane. Poorly defined material accumulates in the subendothelial space and together, with intraluminal platelet and fibrin thrombi, can cause obstruction of vessels. The kidney appears to be an organ particularly vulnerable to TMA injury, with characteristic morphological alterations involving the glomeruli and microvasculature; this organ is the particular focus of this review. TMA occurs in a variety of clinical settings as a result of multiple types of initiating injuries (Table 1). Among these, two important and closely related syndromes—which have as their basis the pathological lesions of TMA—are referred to as thrombotic thrombocytopenic purpura (TTP) and hemolytic uremic syndrome (HUS). The classical symptom constellation of these entities consists of microangiopathic hemolytic anemia, thrombocytopenia, fever, neurological abnormalities, and renal insuffiency. Patients with TTP primarily present with neurological symptoms, whereas renal involvement is the hallmark of HUS (2). The association between TMA and infection with the human immune deficiency virus (HIV) was first described by Boccia et al. in 1984 (3). Since then, thrombotic microangiopathy, typically manifest as HUS or TTP, has been established as a common form of HIV associated disease (4).

Table 1   Etiolological and Predisposing Factors for Thrombotic Microangiopathy

Triggers of vascular injury	Congenital predisposing conditions
Bacteria/bacterial toxins	Decreased levels of factor H
Escherichia coli (verotoxin)	Decreased levels of C3
Shigella dysenteriae (shigatoxin)	Abnormal von Willebrand factor (vWF)
Campylobacter jejuni	Abnormal vWF-cleaving protease
Salmonella typhi	
Yersinia enterocolitica	
Mycoplasma pneumoniae	
Streptococcus pneumoniae	
Viruses	
HIV	
Coxsackie B	
Echovirus	
Influenza virus	
Epstein-Barr virus	
Parvovirus B19	
Herpes simplex virus	
Antibodies and immune complexes	
Anti–endothelial-cell antibodies	
Antiplatelet antibodies	
Drugs	
Mitomycin C, doxorubicin (Adriamycin), vinblastine	
Cyclosporine, FK506	
Ticlopidine, clopidrogel	
Quinine	
Oral contraceptives	
Autoimmune disease	
Lupus erythematodes	
Still's disease	
Scleroderma	
Cardiolipin/phospholipid antibodies	
Various	
Malignant hypertension	
Radiation	
Postpartum renal failure	

Source: Adapted and expanded from Ref. 2.

ETIOLOGY

TMA represents a somewhat nonspecific pathological finding associated with a variety of etiological factors and predisposing conditions (see Table 1). The spectrum ranges from infectious disease, pregnancy (5–7), and autoimmune disorders (8–10) to cancer and drug toxicities (11,12).

Different genetic mutations with autosomal recessive or dominant traits also have been described in families with familial TTP/HUS. In some of these cases a deficiency in the von Willebrand factor–cleaving protease has been described (13–15). Another genetic defect has been localized to the gene encoding complement factor H. Patients with mutations in this gene often have low C3 levels due to persistent activation of the alternative complement pathway and may develop TTP at some time during their lives (16–21).

Infections appear to play an important role in a significant proportion of cases. In particular, childhood HUS has a strong association with Shiga toxin–producing strains of *Escherichia coli*, primarily serotype O157:H7. In these cases the onset of HUS is preceded by an episode of gastroenteritis (22–24). Other bacteria—such as *Campylobacter jejuni*, *Salmonella typhi*, *Yersinia enterocolitica*, *Mycoplasma pneumoniae*, and *Streptococcus pneumoniae*—have also been described as predisposing infectious agents (25–32). Viral infections like coxsackie B, echovirus, influenza virus, Epstein-Barr virus, parvovirus B19, and herpes simplex virus have been implicated in the pathogenesis of TTP/HUS as well (33,34). The role for each of these viruses in the initiation of TMA via direct infection with the virus or exposure to viral particles versus the altered host cytokine milieu occurring as a result of virus infection has yet to be established. In recent years, HIV infection has also been identified as an infectious etiological factor for nonfamilial thrombotic microangiopathies. There is evidence indicating that HIV-associated TMA represents one of the most common forms of HIV-associated kidney diseases (35).

EPIDEMIOLOGY

The exact incidence and prevalence of TMA in HIV-infected patients is currently unknown. However, some data are available that provide an outline of the prevalence of HIV infection in patients with TMA. Torok et al. reviewed U.S. national mortality data between 1968 and 1991 and found HIV or HIV-related conditions listed in 61 (1.3%) mortality certificates from patients who died from TMA (36). Of these cases, 51 occurred in the years 1988 to 1991. In a retrospective study of 50 serum specimens from patients treated for thrombotic microangiopathy at the University of Miami, 7 contained antibodies against HIV-1 (37). Hymes et al. reported that 4 out of 14 patients admitted to the New York Medical Center between 1985 and 1987 with thrombotic microangiopathy tested seropositive for HIV (4). In the years from 1990 to 1996 an additional 27 patients were treated for the same condition: of these 16 were HIV-infected (4), indicating the rising importance of HIV infection in patients with thrombotic microangiopathy.

Two studies assessed the incidence of TMA-like syndromes in series of HIV-positive patients with and without AIDS (38,39). Out of 350 patients admitted to the John Hopkins Hospital HIV inpatient service, 7% had a TMA-like syndrome (thrombocytopenia, schistocytosis, and anemia plus renal dysfunction or neurological symptoms) (38). Gadallah reviewed the charts of 214 patients who were hospitalized and died of AIDS at the medical center of Louisiana State University (39), finding that 15 patients (7%) had evidence of TMA at the time of their death. Of these patients, 7 had no direct cause of death other than TMA. These results indicate that, although TMA seems to be a rare condition in the general population, it may be of great importance among those who are infected with HIV.

CLINICAL FEATURES

The clinical features of HIV-associated TMA resemble those of idiopathic TMA. Multiple studies report thrombocytopenia as the most common clinical feature, with a mean platelet count of about 16,000/mm^3 (40,41). Despite these low platelet counts, bleeding complications seem to be uncommon. Hymes et al. described only four episodes of hemorrhage in their series of 14 patients (4). Another review revealed bleeding symptoms in 3 of 18 patients, ranging from cutaneous bruising and gingival hemorrhage to hematochezia (41). Coagulation parameters are usually within the normal range.

Fever is the second most prevalent clinical symptom, occurring in 75 to 100% of affected individuals (4,40,42), but it is of limited diagnostic value in immunocompromised patients. Another characteristic laboratory finding is hemolytic anemia with severely decreased hematocrit [mean 19% (37)] and hemoglobin (42). Fragmented erythrocytes in the form of schistocytes and helmet cells can be found in the peripheral blood smear (38). At the same time, lactate dehydrogenase (LDH) and indirect bilirubin, a metabolic product of hemoglobin breakdown, are elevated, both being markers of red blood cell destruction (4). Most patients have elevated reticulocyte counts (a marker of compensatory increased production of red blood cells) ranging from 1.4 to 16% (41), and the bone marrow shows signs of activation of erythro- and thrombopoiesis.

Patients presenting with neurological symptoms are classified as having TTP. Symptoms can range from mild temporary confusion or headache to focal neurological signs focal as well as generalized seizures and ultimately coma or death (42–45).

About 20 to 30% of the patients with HIV-associated TMA are suffering from renal failure, and many of these have been classified as HUS (4,43). Impaired excretory renal function, reflected by increased serum creatinine and blood urea nitrogen (BUN), is the most common presentation. Urinalysis may reveal microscopic hematuria, few casts, and mild proteinuria (46,47).

PATHOLOGY

Pathological features of TMA in HIV-infected patients are indistinguishable from those in noninfected individuals (3,48,49). In the kidney, glomeruli demonstrate thickening of the capillary walls. This is caused by swelling of the endothelial cells and expansion of the subendothelial space. Separation of the endothelium from the basement membrane and production of new basement membrane like material by endothelial or interposed mesangial cells may give rise to a typical double-contoured appearance ("split basement membranes") of the capillary walls. Capillary lumina may be substantially reduced or even completely occluded. The glomerular capillaries can also be filled with thrombi composed of fragmented red blood cells, fibrin and platelets (50–52) (Fig. 1).

Mesangial cells are usually not increased in number but appear swollen and hypertrophic. Mesangiolysis is frequent (53), and these lesions can result in proliferative or sclerosing changes of the mesangium.

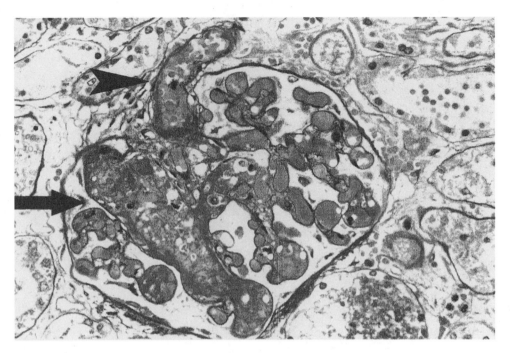

Figure 1 Kidney of patient with HIV-associated thrombotic microangiopathy. The glomerulus contains thrombi in most glomerular capillaries, associated with mesangiolysis (thick arrow). There is also a thrombus in a hilar arteriole (arrowhead). (PAS stain.)

Electron microscopic findings confirm the results of light microscopy. The capillary walls are thickened, resulting from swelling of the endothelial cells and widening of the subendothelial space by electron-lucent and/or finely granulated material (53). This material is composed of a mixture of fibrin, insudated plasma, and cell debris. There may be newly formed glomerular basement membrane underlying endothelial cells detached from the original basement membrane (50). The mesangial matrix is swollen, with a reticular appearance produced by accumulation of an ill-defined electron-lucent material, similar to that seen in the subendothelial space. In areas of mesangiolysis, adjacent capillary loops may form large dilated aneurysms filled with red blood cells, platelets, leukocytes, and fibrin. In the arterioles and arteries, the endothelium shows similar changes as in the glomerulus, with cell swelling and focal detachment from the underlying structures. The intima appears widened and has a lucent appearance. Reduplication of elastic membranes with multilayering of intimal smooth muscle cells can be a distinctive finding. Fibrin may be found in the vascular wall as well as in intraluminal thrombi consisting of platelets and electron-dense material. These characteristic structural and ultrastructural changes have recently been demonstrated in a nonhuman primate model of HIV associated thrombotic microangiopathy (54). About 20% of macaques infected with a strain of HIV-2 demonstrated the typical pathological changes of TMA (see Fig. 2). This may, in the future, serve as a useful model for HIV-associated TMA and allow further investigation of the underlying pathophysiology, as discussed below.

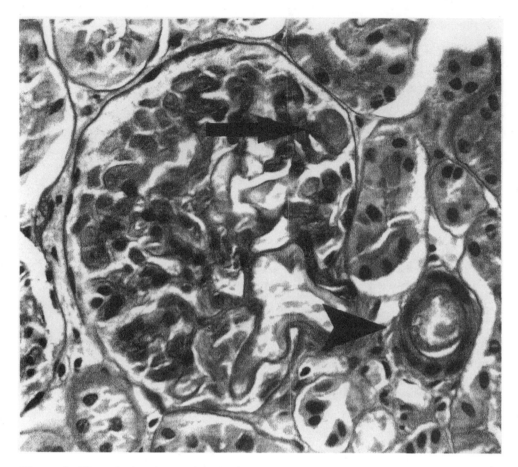

Figure 2 Thrombotic microangiopathy in macaque infected with a strain of HIV-2. (PAS stain.) A thick arrow marks intraglomerular thrombus, while the arrowhead points to thrombus in a hilar arteriole.

PATHOPHYSIOLOGY

The pathogenesis of TMA, independent of the multiple etiological or predisposing factors, involves a common pathway of endothelial cell injury. Various causes for this injury have been proposed in the last decades, ranging from indirect activation of endothelial cells by cytokines to direct cellular damage by various toxins and infectious agents.

The mechanism by which HIV mediates endothelial cell injury remains unknown. An obvious mechanism would be endothelial cell injury consequent to direct viral infection, but endothelial cell infection has been difficult to establish. An important obstacle to HIV infection is that endothelial cells in vivo typically do not express the principal receptor (CD4) utilized for viral entry into the cells. Endothelial cells also do not express one of the principal coreceptors (chemokine receptor CCR5) utilized for this purpose and express the other major coreceptor (chemokine receptor CXCR4) utilized for viral entry into cells only under limited circumstances. Nevertheless, there has been limited evidence that HIV is able to infect CD4-negative human microvascular endothelial cells in vitro and in vivo (55–58). Endothelial cells derived from adipose tissue have been demonstrated to have phagocytic vacuoles containing virus-like particles and to release infectious particles into the supernatant. This process was partially inhibited by cycloheximide, suggesting the de novo synthesis of viral protein (55). Similar results of HIV infection with a very low viral reproduction rate were confirmed for brain-derived microvascular endothelial cells in vitro (56). Another group has shown the presence of p24 antigen in bone marrow microvascular endothelial cells of HIV-infected patients. Supernatant of these cells contained infectious virus, as shown by a focal infectivity assay using HeLa CD4 cells (57). P24 antigen has been revealed in bone marrow endothelial cells of an HIV-infected patient with thrombotic thrombocytopenic purpura (58). Productive HIV-1 infection was also reported in human umbilical vein endothelial cells (59,60). Using in situ hybridization to detect viral RNA, we have been unable to demonstrate endothelial cell infection by HIV-2 in HIV-2–infected macaques with renal and systemic TMA (54,61).

Aside from direct infection of endothelial cells by HIV, HIV infection in general may create a vascular milieu favoring coagulation. Increased levels of von Willebrand factor have been shown in 125 HIV-positive patients and were found to be closely correlated with disease progression, CD4 + cell count, and levels of β2 microglobulin. Levels of plasminogen activator inhibitor were increased in infected patients, while protein S was decreased (62,63). However, these studies did not indicate that these changes were associated with TMA. In one study focused on the acute phase of HUS, PAI-1 levels were not changed, indicating that altered fibrinolysis involving PAI-1 was unlikely to be an important mechanism underlying HIV-associated TMA (64). Another potentially relevant cause of HIV-associated TMA might be increased production of circulating antiphospholipid/anticardiolipin antibodies, known to induce TMA syndromes in the non-HIV-infected population. Such antibodies are relatively common in HIV-infected patients, but their presence does not correlate with TMA or other manifestations of AIDS (65,66).

Despite the inability to identify a specific mechanism, studies have indicated that endothelial cell damage may be a key factor in the pathogenesis of TMA. Dang et al. have demonstrated enhanced, probably Fas-mediated endothelial cell apoptosis in splenic tissue from patients with TTP undergoing splenenectomy (67). There is evidence that this kind of damage to microvascular endothelial cells (MVEC) can be induced by plasma from patients with idiopathic and HIV-associated thrombotic thrombocytopenic purpura (68). Jimenez et al. have shown that plasma from patients with TTP activates and damages renal and brain microvascular endothelial cells (69). Activated MVEC had increased procoagulatory activity as measured by Russell viper venom assay and also demonstrated upregulated expression of the leukocyte adhesion molecules ICAM-1 and VCAM-1. Exposure of these cells to plasma obtained from patients with TTP led to a large increase in endothelial microparticles (EMP), a marker of endothelial cell damage. A similar increase in EMPs could be seen in patients in the acute phase of TTP (69).

Another group has demonstrated that plasma from patients suffering from idiopathic or HIV-associated TTP induces apoptosis in endothelial cells of microvascular origin (MVEC) but not of large vessel origin (70). They also showed that endothelial cells derived from areas that are not classically involved in the clinical course of the disease, such as the hepatic and pulmonary microvasculature, are not susceptible to plasma-induced apoptosis (71). The apoptotic process appeared to be mediated by the induction of Fas (CD95) in these cells, while inhibitors of caspases 1 and 3 were able to block TTP/HUS plasma-mediated apoptosis (72). Gene expression studies have indicated that regional difference in the resistance to cell death might be due to differential gene expression. In contrast to skin-derived MVEC, pulmonary microvascular endothelial cells are able to maintain higher baseline prosurvival signals, like TRAIL antagonist osteoprotegerin and vascular endothelial growth factors VEGF/VEGF-C and their receptors VEGF-2/VEGF-3, when exposed to TTP plasma (73).

The cellular injury of TMA in the HIV-2–infected macaque model has recently been further characterized in whole tissue sections in an attempt to clarify issues of endothelial cell injury and death in the setting of HIV infection (74). Large areas of cellular damage, with DNA strand breaks, have been identified in kidneys from these animals, which correspond to areas of morphological TMA injury (Fig. 3). These areas demonstrate a common injury process involving cells of the arterial walls and adjacent veins, adjacent tubular epithelium, and whole glomeruli. Morphologically, the injured cells show characteristic nuclear swelling with a distinctive ultrastructural correlate of a pattern of dispersed nuclear chromatin. These results are remarkable for the fact that the involved cells demonstrated features of apoptotic cell death

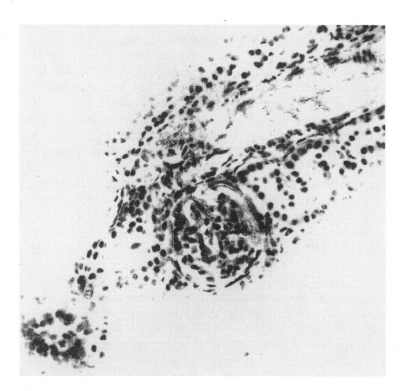

Figure 3 TUNEL stain in kidney from HIV-2–infected macaque with thrombotic microangiopathy. The dark nuclear stain identifies demarcated areas of renal injury with apoptotic features. The affected area includes blood vessels, tubules, and glomeruli, while the adjacent tissue remains unaffected.

(reacting with relative specific markers of apoptosis such as TUNEL and ssDNA stains and lack of inflammation) in combination with features of oncotic necrosis (distribution pattern over broad areas, with involvement of different cell types and nuclear swelling). Kidneys from affected animals have demonstrated decreased numbers of Ki67-positive glomerular cells, representing decreased cellular proliferation. In contrast to the marked histological changes, the animals had no significant changes in renal function, suggesting a sublethal insult (74). As noted above, no evidence of renal parenchymal infection can be detected at these sites of injury, although infection of circulating leukocytes within the peritubular microvasculature can be demonstrated. This leads to the supposition that the thrombotic microangiopathic injury is caused by changes in circulating cytokines or in the local or circulating vascular milieu, rather than occurring secondary to direct infection of tissues of affected organs.

Recent studies have identified a potential link between endothelial cell damage and apoptosis and increased procoagulatory properties. These changes included depressed prostacyclin production, decreased clotting time in the Russell viper venom assay, increased tissue factor activity, and decreased expression of thrombomodulin, heparan sulfates, and tissue factor pathway inhibitor in microvascular endothelial cells (71,75,76). In conjunction with the above-mentioned studies on microvascular endothelial cells and the HIV-2–infected nonhuman primates, these features illustrate the need to better understand how HIV infection might cause cell death or sublethal injury to endothelial cells and whether such injury is a likely causative mechanism of HIV-associated TMA.

PROGNOSIS

The prognosis of HIV-associated thrombotic microangiopathy in the acute setting may be similar to that of patients with idiopathic forms (resolution of the acute episode in 87 and 83%, respectively) (77). The long-term prognosis of HIV-infected patients with TMA is not clearly established but appears to be grave. Reports of HIV-infected patients with TMA surviving for longer than 2 years are lacking. Gadallah et al. reported that patients with HIV-associated TMA and overt AIDS had a significantly worse acute outcome than patients with TMA and asymptomatic HIV-infection, who had a good prognosis (39). A different study showed that HIV-positive patients presenting with thrombotic microangiopathy are more likely to have a low CD4 lymphocyte count and Centers for Disease Control stage C disease, which may indicate that patients tend to develop TMA in a later stage of the HIV infection (38). The authors also demonstrated that these patients had an earlier mortality than HIV-positive patients without the disease.

SUMMARY AND OUTLOOK

During the last two decades the role of HIV as a cause of TMA has become increasingly apparent. Clinicians must be aware of the relatively high incidence of TMA in patients infected with HIV. The therapeutic approach for these patients does not differ from the therapy of adults with TMA who are uninfected by HIV. The prognosis seems to be related to the stage of the HIV infection and seems to be poor in patients with overt AIDS. Although there are several hypotheses about the pathophysiology of HIV-associated TMA, the role of direct HIV infection in the pathogenesis of the disease remains unproven. Studies to date indicate an indirect injury to microvascular endothelium as the leading pathogenic mechanism for this disease process. Future studies are required to define the impact of antiretroviral treatment on the incidence and outcome of HIV-associated TMA.

REFERENCES

1. Symmers WSC. Thrombotic microangiopathic haemolytic anemia (thrombotic micro-angiopathy). Br Med J 1952; 2:897–903.
2. Ruggenenti P, Noris M, Remuzzi G. Thrombotic microangiopathy, hemolytic uremic syndrome, and thrombotic thrombocytopenic purpura. Kidney Int 2001; 60:831–846.
3. Boccia RV, Gelmann EP, Baker CC, Marti G, Longo DL. A hemolytic-uremic syndrome with the acquired immunodeficiency syndrome. Ann Intern Med 1984; 101:716–717.
4. Hymes KB, Karpatkin S. Human immunodeficiency virus infection and thrombotic microangiopathy. Semin Hematol 1997; 34:117–125.
5. Takahashi Y, Imai A, Hayasaki Y, Kawabata I, Tamaya T. Postpartum micro-angiopathic hemolytic anemia: cases of successful and dismal outcome assisted with plasma therapy. Eur J Obstet Gynecol Reprod Biol 2000; 89:213–215.
6. Segonds A, Louradour N, Suc JM, Orfila C. Postpartum hemolytic uremic syndrome: a study of three cases with a review of the literature. Clin Nephrol 1979; 12:229–242.
7. Suc JM, Segonds A, Orfila C, Durand D, Louradour N, Counillon F. Post-partum thrombotic microangiopathy. Panminerva Med 1977; 19:423–432.
8. Diamond JR. Hemolytic uremic syndrome/thrombotic thrombocytopenic purpura (HUS/TTP) complicating adult Still's disease: remission induced with intravenous immunoglobulin G. J Nephrol 1997; 10:253–257.
9. Nesher G, Hanna VE, Moore TL, Hersh M, Osborn TG. Thrombotic microangio-graphic hemolytic anemia in systemic lupus erythematosus. Semin Arthritis Rheum 1994; 24:165–172.
10. Musa MO, Nounou R, Sahovic E, Seth P, Qadi A, Aljurf M. Fulminant thrombotic thrombocytopenic purpura in two patients with systemic lupus erythematosus and phospholipid autoantibodies. Eur J Haematol 2000; 64:433–435.
11. Lesesne JB, Rothschild N, Erickson B, Korec S, Sisk R, Keller J, Arbus M, Woolley PV, Chiazze L, Schein PS, et al. Cancer-associated hemolytic-uremic syndrome: analysis of 85 cases from a national registry. J Clin Oncol 1989; 7:781–789.
12. Kwaan HC, Gordon LI. Thrombotic microangiopathy in the cancer patient. Acta Haematol 2001; 106:52–56.
13. Furlan M, Lammle B. Deficiency of von Willebrand factor–cleaving protease in familial and acquired thrombotic thrombocytopenic purpura. Baillieres Clin Haematol 1998; 11:509–514.
14. Galbusera M, Noris M, Rossi C, Orisio S, Caprioli J, Ruggeri ZM, Amadei B, Ruggenenti P, Vasile B, Casari G, Remuzzi G. Increased fragmentation of von Willebrand factor, due to abnormal cleavage of the subunit, parallels disease activity in recurrent hemolytic uremic syndrome and thrombotic thrombocytopenic purpura and discloses predisposition in families. The Italian Registry of Familial and Recurrent HUS/TTP. Blood 1999; 94:610–620.
15. Veyradier A, Obert B, Houllier A, Meyer D, Girma JP. Specific von Willebrand factor–cleaving protease in thrombotic microangiopathies: a study of 111 cases. Blood 2001; 98:1765–1772.

16. Warwicker P, Donne RL, Goodship JA, Goodship TH, Howie AJ, Kumararatne DS, Thompson RA, Taylor CM. Familial relapsing haemolytic uraemic syndrome and complement factor H deficiency. Nephrol Dial Transplant 1999; 14:1229–1233.

17. Warwicker P, Goodship TH, Donne RL, Pirson Y, Nicholls A, Ward RM, Turnpenny P, Goodship JA. Genetic studies into inherited and sporadic hemolytic uremic syndrome. Kidney Int 1998; 53:836–844.

18. Pichette V, Querin S, Schurch W, Brun G, Lehner-Netsch G, Delage JM. Familial hemolytic-uremic syndrome and homozygous factor H deficiency. Am J Kidney Dis 1994; 24:936–941.

19. Carreras L, Romero R, Requesens C, Oliver AJ, Carrera M, Clavo M, Alsina J. Familial hypocomplementemic hemolytic uremic syndrome with HLA-A3, B7 haplotype. JAMA 1981; 245:602–604.

20. Richards A, Buddles MR, Donne RL, Kaplan BS, Kirk E, Venning MC, Tielemans CL, Goodship JA, Goodship TH. Factor H mutations in hemolytic uremic syndrome cluster in exons 18–20, a domain important for host cell recognition. Am J Hum Genet 2001; 68:485–490.

21. Landau D, Shalev H, Levy-Finer G, Polonsky A, Segev Y, Katchko L. Familial hemolytic uremic syndrome associated with complement factor H deficiency. J Pediatr 2001; 138:412–417.

22. Hogan MC, Gloor JM, Uhl JR, Cockerill FR, Milliner DS. Two cases of non-O157:H7 *Escherichia coli* hemolytic uremic syndrome caused by urinary tract infection. Am J Kidney Dis 2001; 38:E22.

23. Richardson SE, Karmali MA, Becker LE, Smith CR. The histopathology of the hemolytic uremic syndrome associated with verocytotoxin-producing *Escherichia coli* infections. Hum Pathol 1988; 19:1102–1108.

24. Banatvala N, Griffin PM, Greene KD, Barrett TJ, Bibb WF, Green JH, Wells JG. The United States National Prospective Hemolytic Uremic Syndrome Study: microbiologic, serologic, clinical, and epidemiologic findings. J Infect Dis 2001; 183:1063–1070.

25. Chamovitz BN, Hartstein AI, Alexander SR, Terry AB, Short P, Katon R. *Campylobacter jejuni*–associated hemolytic-uremic syndrome in a mother and daughter. Pediatrics 1983; 71:253–256.

26. Delans RJ, Biuso JD, Saba SR, Ramirez G. Hemolytic uremic syndrome after *Campylobacter*-induced diarrhea in an adult. Arch Intern Med 1984; 144:1074–1076.

27. Azim T, Rashid A, Qadri F, Sarker MS, Hamadani J, Salam MA, Wahed MA, Albert MJ. Antibodies to Shiga toxin in the serum of children with *Shigella*-associated haemolytic uraemic syndrome. J Med Microbiol 1999; 48:11–16.

28. Bhimma R, Rollins NC, Coovadia HM, Adhikari M. Post-dysenteric hemolytic uremic syndrome in children during an epidemic of *Shigella* dysentery in Kwazulu/Natal. Pediatr Nephrol 1997; 11:560–564.

29. Tsukahara H, Hayashi S, Nakamura K, Nomura Y, Yoshimoto M, Fujisawa S. Haemolytic uraemic syndrome associated with *Yersinia enterocolitica* infection. Pediatr Nephrol 1988; 2:309–311.

30. Flores FX, Jabs K, Thorne GM, Jaeger J, Linshaw MA, Somers MJ. Immune response to *Escherichia coli* O157:H7 in hemolytic uremic syndrome following salmonellosis. Pediatr Nephrol 1997; 11:488–490.

31. Pan CG, Leichter HE, Werlin SL. Hepatocellular injury in *Streptococcus pneumoniae*–associated hemolytic uremic syndrome in children. Pediatr Nephrol 1995; 9:690–693.

32. Bar Meir E, Amital H, Levy Y, Kneller A, Bar-Dayan Y, Shoenfeld Y. *Mycoplasma pneumoniae*–induced thrombotic thrombocytopenic purpura. Acta Haematol 2000; 103:112–115.

33. Larke RP, Preiksaitis JK, Devine RD, Harley FL. Haemolytic uraemic syndrome: evidence of multiple viral infections in a cluster of ten cases. J Med Virol 1983; 12:51–59.

34. Kok RH, Wolfhagen MJ, Klosters G. A syndrome resembling thrombotic thrombocy-topenic purpura associated with human parvovirus B19 infection. Clin Infect Dis 2001; 32:311–312.

35. Peraldi MN, Maslo C, Akposso K, Mougenot B, Rondeau E, Sraer JD. Acute renal failure in the course of HIV infection: a single-institution retrospective study of ninety-two patients anad sixty renal biopsies. Nephrol Dial Transplant 1999; 14:1578–1585.

36. Torok TJ, Holman RC, Chorba TL. Increasing mortality from thrombotic thrombo-cytopenic purpura in the United States—analysis of national mortality data, 1968–1991. Am J Hematol 1995; 50:84–90.

37. Ucar A, Fernandez HF, Byrnes JJ, Lian EC, Harrington WJ Jr. Thrombotic microan-giopathy and retroviral infections: a 13-year experience. Am J Hematol 1994; 45:304–309.

38. Moore RD. Schistocytosis and a thrombotic microangiopathy-like syndrome in hospitalized HIV-infected patients. Am J Hematol 1999; 60:116–120.

39. Gadallah MF, el-Shahawy MA, Campese VM, Todd JR, King JW. Disparate prognosis of thrombotic microangiopathy in HIV-infected patients with and without AIDS. Am J Nephrol 1996; 16:446–450.

40. Kado DM, Korotzer BS, Brass EP. Clinical characterization of thrombotic micro-angiopathy in HIV infection. AIDS 1996; 10:1747–1749.

41. Rarick MU, Espina B, Mocharnuk R, Trilling Y, Levine AM. Thrombotic thrombo-cytopenic purpura in patients with human immunodeficiency virus infection: a report of three cases and review of the literature. Am J Hematol 1992; 40:103–109.

42. Kennedy SS, Zacharski LR, Beck JR. Thrombotic thrombocytopenic purpura: analysis of 48 unselected cases. Semin Thromb Hemost 1980; 6:341–349.

43. Sutor GC, Schmidt RE, Albrecht H. Thrombotic microangiopathies and HIV infection: report of two typical cases, features of HUS and TTP, and review of the literature. Infection 1999; 27:12–15.

44. Hollenbeck M, Kutkuhn B, Aul C, Leschke M, Willers R, Grabensee B. Haemolytic-uraemic syndrome and thrombotic-thrombocytopenic purpura in adults: clinical findings and prognostic factors for death and end-stage renal disease. Nephrol Dial Transplant 1998; 13:76–81.

45. Rooney JC, Anderson RM, Hopkins IJ. Clinical and pathological aspects of central nervous system involvement in the haemolytic uraemic syndrome. Aust Paediatr J 1971; 7:28–33.

46. Remuzzi G. HUS and TTP: variable expression of a single entity. Kidney Int 1987; 32:292–308.

47. Eknoyan G, Riggs SA. Renal involvement in patients with thrombotic thrombocyto-penic purpura. Am J Nephrol 1986; 6:117–131.

48. Sacristan Lista F, Saavedra Alonso AJ, Oliver Morales J, Vazquez Martul E. Nephrotic syndrome due to thrombotic microangiopathy (TMA) as the first manifestation of human immunodeficiency virus infection: recovery before antiretroviral therapy without specific treatment against TMA. Clin Nephrol 2001; 55:404–407.

49. Kelleher P, Severn A, Tomson C, Lucas S, Parkin J, Pinching A, Miller R. The haemolytic uraemic syndrome in patients with AIDS. Genitourin Med 1996; 72:172–175.

50. Asada Y, Sumiyoshi A, Hayashi T, Suzumiya J, Kaketani K. Immunohistochemistry of vascular lesion in thrombotic thrombocytopenic purpura, with special reference to factor VIII related antigen. Thromb Res 1985; 38:469–479.

51. Berkowitz LR, Dalldorf FG, Blatt PM. Thrombotic thrombocytopenic purpura: a pathology review. JAMA 1979; 241:1709–1710.

52. Conlon PJ, Howell DN, Macik G, Kovalik EC, Smith SR. The renal manifestations and outcome of thrombotic thrombocytopenic purpura/hemolytic uremic syndrome in adults. Nephrol Dial Transplant 1995; 10:1189–1193.

53. Churg J, Strauss L. Renal involvement in thrombotic microangiopathies. Semin Nephrol 1985; 5:46–56.

54. Eitner F, Cui Y, Hudkins KL, Schmidt A, Birkebak T, Agy MB, Hu SL, Morton WR, Anderson DM, Alpers CE. Thrombotic microangiopathy in the HIV-2–infected macaque. Am J Pathol 1999; 155:649–661.

55. Cenacchi G, Re MC, Preda P, Pasquinelli G, Furlini G, Apkarian RP. M La Placa, GN Martinelli, Human immunodeficiency virus type-1 (HIV-1) infection of endothelial cells in vitro: a virological, ultrastructural and immuno-cytochemical approach. J Submicrosc Cytol Pathol 1992; 24:155–161.

56. Poland SD, Rice GP, Dekaban GA. HIV-1 infection of human brain-derived microvascular endothelial cells in vitro. J Acquir Immune Defic Syndr Hum Retrovirol 1995; 8:437–445.

57. Moses AV, Williams S, Heneveld ML, Strussenberg J, Rarick M, Loveless M, Bagby G, Nelson JA. Human immunodeficiency virus infection of bone marrow endothelium reduces induction of stromal hematopoietic growth factors. Blood 1996; 87:919–925.

58. del Arco A, Martinez MA, Pena JM, Gamallo C, Gonzalez JJ, Barbado FJ, Vazquez JJ. Thrombotic thrombocytopenic purpura associated with human immunodeficiency virus infection: demonstration of p24 antigen in endothelial cells. Clin Infect Dis 1993; 17:360–363.

59. Corbeil J, Evans LA, McQueen PW, Vasak E, Edward PD, Richman DD, Penny R, Cooper DA. Productive in vitro infection of human umbilical vein endothelial cells and three colon carcinoma cell lines with HIV-1. Immunol Cell Biol 1995; 73:140–145.

60. Conaldi PG, Serra C, Dolei A, Basolo F, Falcone V, Mariani G, Speziale P, Toniolo A. Productive HIV-1 infection of human vascular endothelial cells requires cell proliferation and is stimulated by combined treatment with interleukin-1 beta plus tumor necrosis factor-alpha. J Med Virol 1995; 47:355–363.

61. Eitner F, Cui Y, Hudkins KL, Stokes MB, Segerer S, Mack M, Lewis PL, Abraham AA, Schlondorff D, Gallo G, Kimmel PL, Alpers CE. Chemokine receptor CCR5 and CXCR4 expression in HIV-associated kidney disease. J Am Soc Nephrol 2000; 11:856–867.

62. Lafeuillade A, Alessi MC, Poizot-Martin I, Boyer-Neumann C, Zandotti C, Quilichini R, Aubert L, Tamalet C, Juhan-Vague I, Gastaut JA. Endothelial cell dysfunction in HIV infection. J AIDS 1992; 5:127–131.

63. Karmochkine M, Ankri A, Calvez V, Bonmarchant M, Coutellier A, Herson S. Plasma hypercoagulability is correlated to plasma HIV load. Thromb Haemost 1998; 80:208–209.

64. Peraldi MN, Maslo C, Berrou J, Rondeau E, Rozenbaum W, Sraer JD. Tissue-type plasminogen activator activity in HIV-associated HUS. Nephrol Dial Transplant 1998; 13:919–923.

65. Ankri A, Bonmarchand M, Coutellier A, Herson S, Karmochkine M. Antiphospholipid antibodies are an epiphenomenon in HIV-infected patients. AIDS 1999; 13:1282–1283.

66. Uthman IW, Gharavi AE. Viral infections and antiphospholipid antibodies. Semin Arthritis Rheum 2002; 31:256–263.

67. Dang CT, Magid MS, Weksler B, Chadburn A, Laurence J. Enhanced endothelial cell apoptosis in splenic tissues of patients with thrombotic thrombocytopenic purpura. Blood 1999; 93:1264–1270.

68. Wu XW, Li QZ, Lian EC. Plasma from a patient with thrombotic thrombocytopenic purpura induces endothelial cell apoptosis and platelet aggregation. Thromb Res 1999; 93:79–87.

69. Jimenez JJ, Jy W, Mauro LM, Horstman LL, Ahn YS. Elevated endothelial microparticles in thrombotic thrombocytopenic purpura: findings from brain and renal microvascular cell culture and patients with active disease. Br J Haematol 2001; 112:81–90.

70. Laurence J, Mitra D, Steiner M, Staiano-Coico L, Jaffe E. Plasma from patients with idiopathic and human immunodeficiency virus–associated thrombotic thrombocytopenic purpura induces apoptosis in microvascular endothelial cells. Blood 1996; 87:3245–3254.

71. Mitra D, Jaffe EA, Weksler B, Hajjar KA, Soderland C, Laurence J. Thrombotic thrombocytopenic purpura and sporadic hemolytic-uremic syndrome plasmas induce apoptosis in restricted lineages of human microvascular endothelial cells. Blood 1997; 89:1224–1234.

72. Mitra D, Kim J, MacLow C, Karsan A, Laurence J. Role of caspases 1 and 3 and Bcl-2-related molecules in endothelial cell apoptosis associated with thrombotic micro-angiopathies. Am J Hematol 1998; 59:279–287.

73. Kim J, Wu H, Hawthorne L, Rafii S, Laurence J. Endothelial cell apoptotic genes associated with the pathogenesis of thrombotic microangiopathies: an application of oligonucleotide genechip technology. Microvasc Res 2001; 62:83–93.

74. Segerer S, Eitner F, Cui Y, Hudkins KL, Alpers CE. Cellular injury associated with renal thrombotic microangiopathy in human immunodeficiency virus–infected macaques. J Am Soc Nephrol 2002; 13:370–378.

75. Casciola-Rosen L, Rosen A, Petri M, Schlissel M. Surface blebs on apoptotic cells are sites of enhanced procoagulant activity: implications for coagulation events and antigenic spread in systemic lupus erythematosus. Proc Natl Acad Sci USA 1996; 93:1624–1629.

76. Bombeli T, Karsan A, Tait JF, Harlan JM. Apoptotic vascular endothelial cells become procoagulant. Blood 1997; 89:2429–2442.

77. Thompson CE, Damon LE, Ries CA, Linker CA. Thrombotic microangiopathies in the 1980s: clinical features, response to treatment, and the impact of the human immunodeficiency virus epidemic. Blood 1992; 80:1890–1895.

7

Pathogenesis of HIV-Associated Vasculopathy

Lance S. Terada and Ru Feng Wu
University of Texas Southwestern Medical Center and Dallas Veterans Administration Medical Center, Dallas, Texas, U.S.A.

The vascular endothelium serves numerous diverse functions vital to the proper homeostasis of all organs. Beyond providing a conduit for oxygen delivery, the endothelium directs inflammatory cell traffic, controls thrombosis and macromolecular transport, presents a source of and target for cytokines and growth factors, and co-ordinates angiogenic activity. Accordingly, acute and chronic illnesses that derange endothelial function—such as diabetes mellitus, sepsis, and atherosclerosis—cause widespread, protean, and often severe manifestations of disease. To this list of systemic vascular diseases we add AIDS. The vascular endothelium is a silent target of human immunodeficiency virus-1 (HIV-1), and infection of individuals with HIV-1 results in a series of diffuse vascular processes that frequently progress unrecognized.

AIDS VASCULOPATHY: PHENOTYPES

The endothelium of AIDS patients displays a number of abnormalities consistent with abnormal activation, proliferation, and death. Compared with the highly oriented, monotonously organized endothelium of normal patients, the aortic endothelium of AIDS patients demonstrates marked dysmorphic changes (Fig. 1) with chaotic cell distribution, atypia with giant cell formation, pyknotic nuclei suggestive of apoptotic cells, and bare denuded patches. These findings are common, being found in 94% of HIV-infected patients in one autopsy study (1). In addition, this abnormal endothelium focally expresses increased levels of surface endothelial adhesion proteins such as E-selectin and VCAM-1, with abnormal aggregations of leukocytes (1). Accordingly, AIDS patients frequently develop idiopathic forms of inflammatory conditions such as myocarditis, interstitial pneumonitis, and encephalitis. Systemic vasculitis has also been reported by a number of investigators, with clinical and histological patterns resembling necrotizing and nonnecrotizing arteritis, polyarteritis nodosa, Henoch-Schönlein purpura, and hypersensitivity vasculitis (2,3).

Measurements of microcirculatory blood flow in vivo, assessed by nail-fold microscopy and retinal fluorescein angiography, reveal severely disturbed blood flow

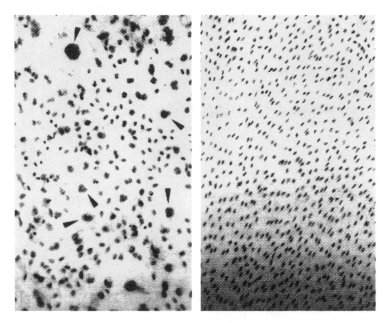

Figure 1   En face preparations of aortic endothelium from normal (right) and HIV-1-infected (left) patients. Normal endothelium presents a continuous, oriented, and orderly monolayer of cells. Aortic endothelium of HIV-1–infected patients displays disorganized structure with multinucleate endothelial cells, pyknotic endothelial cells, and denuded patches. (From Ref. 1.)

(4,5). Indeed, the most frequent finding in AIDS patients' retinas, the organ in which microvascular pathology is most directly observable, is a microangiopathic syndrome marked by loss of retinal capillary cells and focal occlusions of small vessels (5,6). This syndrome may represent a focal manifestation of a systemic syndrome, since its severity correlates highly with positron emission tomography (PET) scan assessments of cerebral perfusion defects and cognitive function (7). Cotton-wool infarcts and retinal hemorrhages are common even in asymptomatic patients (5): in one autopsy study, numerous vascular breaches, infarcts, and telangiectasias were seen in the retinas of HIV-infected patients, with ruptured or unruptured microaneurysms being present in all (Fig. 2) (8). Importantly, the retinal endothelium has been shown to be capable of supporting productive HIV-1 infection in vivo (9), and this proximity to the central nervous system (CNS) has extensive ramifications for HIV-related neurological syndromes.

Arteriolar blood flow may also be compromised through abnormal thrombosis or vascular remodeling. Widespread digital ischemia with gangrene is an uncommon but dramatic presentation of HIV infection (10), and malignant atrophic papulosis, which causes infarctive thrombosis of the skin and viscera, has been reported (11). Thrombotic microangiopathy, the second most common renal lesion seen in AIDS, causes intra- and extraglomerular arteriolar thrombus formation and is the hallmark lesion of hemolytic uremic syndrome and thrombotic thrombocytopenic purpura (12–14), two AIDS-associated syndromes. An etiological connection between this renal lesion and AIDS is strengthened by the finding of renal thrombotic microangiopathy

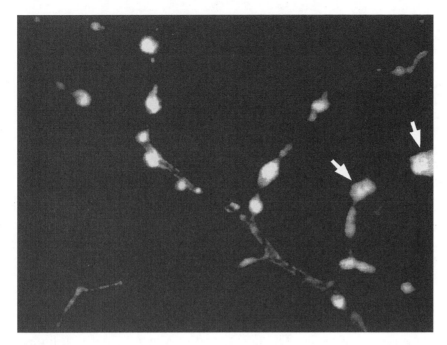

Figure 2   The retinal microvasculature of an AIDS patient was highlighted by perfusion with fluorescent microspheres. Numerous microaneurysms are noted. (From Ref. 8.)

in HIV-2–infected macaque monkeys (12). Nonthrombotic vaso-oclusion is seen in primary pulmonary hypertension, which is increased in the AIDS population. This disease is presently thought to arise from unregulated endothelial cell (EC) proliferation. Most plexiform lesions, for instance, harbor a monoclonal expansion of endothelial cells within the intima of the early plexiform lesion (15), suggesting a growth-dysregulated state, which in AIDS may involve other vascular beds. In support of this speculation, a recent autopsy study of 13 young HIV-infected patients, 23 to 32 years old, revealed proliferative intimal thickening in the coronaries of all hearts examined (16). The neointima was often found to be of unusual morphology and was hyperplastic to the extent of severe luminal encroachment, yet only two patients died a cardiac death, again emphasizing the silent nature of AIDS-associated vasculopathies. Importantly, this impressive neointimal hyperplasia is mirrored by lesions in the coronary arteries of macaque monkeys infected with simian immuno-deficiency virus (SIV) (17), strengthening the etiological tie to lentiviral infection.

Another manifestation of abnormal vascular architecture is seen in the pediatric AIDS population. Cerebrovascular lesions are recognized in 25% of pediatric AIDS autopsies and include a distinct form of fusiform aneurysmal dilation of the large arteries leaving the circle of Willis (18,19). In this highly lethal condition, the arterial intima becomes markedly hyperplastic, the media becomes acellular and fibrotic, and the intervening internal elastic lamina is degraded. Interestingly, the histological features of this vasculopathy are replicated in other tissue beds in a transgenic mouse model, in which an HIV proviral transgene missing *gag*, *pol*, and much of the *env* genes is expressed (20). This model demonstrates the ability of the HIV-1 accessory proteins to derange vascular cell growth and vessel wall architecture.

Finally, an extreme example of vascular cell dysregulation in AIDS can be found in Kaposi's sarcoma (KS). The two hallmarks of this lesion, blood in non-EC-lined spaces and disorganized proliferation of an abnormal, spindle-shaped cell, both suggest a process marked by increased EC proliferation and failed differentiation. In fact, the lineage of origin of the spindle cells is difficult to determine, since they appear to have features of both ECs and mesenchymal cells (21). However, some of the earliest changes to skin parenchymal cells seems to be the appearance of abnormal vascular structures such as thick-walled capillaries and dilated, thin walled blood-filled spaces (22). Spindle cells are absent in such early lesions. Ultrastructurally, ECs appear hyperplastic and hypertrophied to the point of closing off lumina, with the development of poor intercellular junctions and degeneration of basement membranes. ECs then escape capillaries, migrate, and make incomplete attempts to form lumina (23). Of additional interest, uninvolved perilesional skin also displays the same endothelial abnormalities. Taken together, these findings suggest that the EC is a target that responds to soluble mediators, resulting in a field effect. Indeed, KS lesions have been likened in histological appearance to granulation tissue, in which nascent ECs are actively invading matrix in an attempt to form vascular structures.

Consistent with the multicentric nature of KS, some investigators suggest that early KS may arise not from the metastatic spread of a monoclonal transformed spindle cell but rather from a multifocal and polyclonal expansion of endothelial cells responding to abnormal growth signals. For instance, analysis of advanced nodular KS lesions in HIV-infected women suggests a polyclonal inactivation of the highly polymorphic, X-linked human androgen receptor gene, demonstrating that spindle cells from a given lesion may not arise from a common cellular ancestor (24). At a later stage, however, it is likely that a certain subpopulations of spindle cells acquire a malignant phenotype. Indeed, other investigators have found monoclonality of microdissected fragments within KS lesions (25).

In summary, HIV-infected patients manifest a variety of primary vascular disorders marked by phenotypic abnormalities of endothelial proliferation, activation, and morphology and of gross structural derangements of both macrovascular and microvascular architecture.

PATHOGENESIS: ROLE OF HIV-1 TAT

In some instances, AIDS vasculopathy may reflect infection of vascular endothelial cells with HIV-1. However, few human vascular beds can support productive infection with HIV-1. Two notable exceptions exist. The capacity of human brain endothelium to undergo productive infection by HIV-1 has been demonstrated by the expression of viral proteins in the CNS endothelium in vivo (26–28) and by direct infection of cultured human brain endothelium by HIV-1 (29). In addition, the highly specialized bone marrow endothelium, like that of the brain, can and does become infected with HIV-1 (30,31).

The majority of vasculopathic lesions, however, likely arise not from direct endothelial infection but from exposure of the endothelium to viral products, cytokines and growth factors produced in response to the virus, or a combination of both. An intriguing candidate for a vasculopathic factor is the viral accessory protein Tat. Tat is an HIV-1–encoded product best known as a TAR-binding protein necessary for full transactivation of the HIV-LTR (32). Although Tat is a small protein, it contains five structural domains and has pleiotropic effects on a number of human cells (33). Important among its domains is a highly conserved cysteine-rich core necessary for transactivation, a basic domain containing an RKKRRQRR motif, and a C-terminal RGD-containing region.

Although its chief viral function is to act as a transcription factor, Tat can be released from cells and is therefore found circulating in the blood of AIDS patients (34). Tat can be taken up by uninfected cells via integrin-mediated endocytosis (35), where it has protean effects. More importantly, it acts as a protocytokine by recognizing endothelial receptors and initiating outside-in signaling. For instance, the Tat basic domain mimics basic growth factors and ligates and causes autophosphorylation of Flk-1/KDR, one of several cognate receptors for the strongly angiogenic vascular endothelial growth factor (VEGF) (36). Accordingly, Tat promotes endothelial and KS spindle cell proliferation (37,38), causes normal endothelial cells to migrate and invade matrix in vitro (39), and initiates angiogenesis in vivo (40). In addition, the RGD region of Tat binds with high affinity to two important endothelial integrins, $\alpha_v\beta_3$ and $\alpha_5\beta_1$, which normally anchor the cell to fibronectin and vitronectin and facilitate attachment-dependent growth factor signaling (41). Competing RGD tripeptides block the synergistic ability of Tat and bFGF to cause KS lesions in mice, suggesting a functional role for the Tat RGD domain in initiating EC growth signals (42). Interestingly, the Tat protein of HIV-2 lacks an RGD motif; accordingly, HIV-2–infected patients have a 12-fold lower prevalence of KS than HIV-1–infected individuals from the same demographic population and with the same prevalence of HHV8 infection (43). Further, a direct link between KS and HIV-1 Tat was made with the finding that Tat-expressing transgenic mice develop KS-like lesions (44). In the mouse model, expression of the Tat transgene was limited to the skin, yet the spindle cells did not express Tat stably but rather appeared to be paracrine targets of the protein, consistent with the existence of a field effect. In humans, the further progression of precursor KS lesions to a frankly malignant phenotype may be facilitated by infection with human herpesvirus 8, which expresses several potential oncogenes (45).

Besides its potential impact on proliferative pathways, Tat can also activate endothelial inflammatory pathways. Endothelial cells exposed to Tat display increased levels of the inflammatory adhesion proteins ICAM-1, VCAM, and E-selectin (46–48). Tat also increases nuclear translocation and DNA binding of NF-κB (48–50) and causes release of the inflammatory chemokine monocyte chemoattractant protein-1 (MCP-1) from lung endothelial cells (51).

TAT-ACTIVATED SIGNALING PATHWAYS: OXIDANTS AS SIGNALING AGENTS

Despite the marked phenotypic vascular cell changes induced by Tat in vitro and in vivo, little is known about the intracellular signal transduction pathways initiated by this molecule. Within 15 min, extracellular Tat causes marked increases in tyrosine phosphorylation of multiple endothelial proteins (52). In KS 38 cells, Tat specifically causes tyrosine phosphorylation of focal adhesion proteins such as Pyk2, paxillin, and p130^{Cas} as well as activation the tyrosine kinase Src (53). In both immortalized endothelial cells and KS cells, Tat also activates the stress-activated MAP kinase c-Jun amino terminal kinase (JNK), important in both proliferative and apoptotic responses (53,54). Because Tat can transactivate TNF-α and AIDS patients have increased levels of TNF-α, it is notable that Tat and TNF-α appear to synergize at low levels to activate endothelial cell JNK (54). In addition, Tat activates caspase 3 in human microvascular endothelial cells, leading to apoptosis (55), potentially a correlate of endothelial cell pyknosis in AIDS patients (Fig. 1).

A potential clue to the proximal signaling pathways activated by Tat is the observation that Tat-expressing HeLa cells have increased levels of carbonyl proteins, reduced sulfhydryl content, and lowered reduced:oxidized glutathione ratios, all markers of oxidant stress (56,57). Tat appears to increase cellular oxidant levels by at least two mechanisms. Intracellular Tat reduces both activity and mRNA levels of Mn-SOD, a critical endogenous antioxidant (56). The proposed mechanism of this decrease involves binding of Tat to a Tar-like stem-loop structure in the Mn-SOD transcript (56). Indeed, AIDS patients harbor many biochemical footprints of chronic oxidative stress, such as reduced levels of blood cysteine and cellular glutathione (58). In addition, lung lavage fluids of infected patients also have reduced glutathione levels (59), and patients have reduced vitamin E levels (60) and increased malondialdehyde (61). The glutathione deficit progresses as clinical disease advances (62).

Besides reducing antioxidant levels, Tat appears to activate an EC oxidase. Extracellular Tat increases oxidant production by ECV-304 cells within 15 min, and this acute oxidant burst is diminished by inhibitors of an NADPH oxidase but not by inhibitors of xanthine oxidase, NO synthase, or mitochondrial respiration (54). Downstream of this oxidant burst, the JNK MAPK is activated, indicating activation by Tat of a specific signaling oxidase (Fig. 3). The pattern of oxidant-dependent activation of JNK is similar with that initiated by TNF-α, suggesting intersection of the two agonist pathways at or proximal to such an oxidase (63).

The utilization by Tat of evanescent reactive oxidants as specific signaling elements is entirely consistent with Tat's ability to engage basic receptor-mediated signal transduction machinery. In an emerging paradigm, endogenous oxidants are produced as tightly regulated, self-limited physiological signaling elements. Specifically, intracellular oxidant production appears necessary to transmit signals downstream from cytokine and growth factor receptor engagement. Growth factor–stimulated tyrosine phosphorylation, ERK activation, and DNA synthesis, for instance, are accompanied by a transient burst of H_2O_2 (64), and oxidant scavengers diminish both ERK activation and DNA synthesis. Further, TNF-α stimulates oxidant production in vascular cells, and scavengers decrease JNK activation by TNF-α (63,65,66). Oxidants also act as key regulators of growth factor and cytokine-induced activation of NF-κB (67,68). Importantly, Tat potentiates TNFα-mediated activation of NF-kB through an oxidant-dependent mechanism (69).

The specific targets of oxidants have not been established, although a principal mode of action is likely to be the inactivation of protein tyrosine phosphatases (PTP) via oxidation of the conserved active site phosphate-accepting cysteine residue. O_2^- appears to be a highly efficient and specific oxidant in PTP-1B inactivation, attracted by a cationic charge trap in the active site pocket (70). Inactivation of this latter phosphatase by O_2^- is reversible, potentially allowing transient increases in tyrosine kinase-dependent signaling. The rapid tyrosine phosphorylation of multiple endothe-

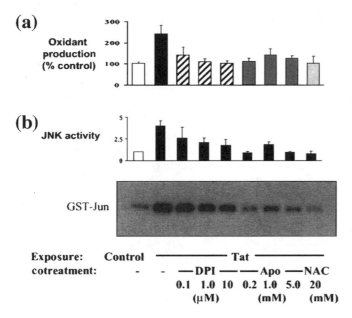

Figure 3 ECV-304 cells were exposed to HIV-1 Tat for 10 min; oxidant production and JNK MAPK activation were measured. (a) Tat increased intracellular oxidant production, measured as fluorescence of the superoxide-sensitive fluorochrome dichlorofluorescin diacetate. Two chemically distinct inhibitors of the NADPH oxidase, diphenylene iodonium (DPI) and apocynin (Apo), and the antioxidant N-acetyl cysteine (NAC) decreased Tat-induced oxidant burst by these cells. (b) Tat rapidly increased activity of the JNK MAPK as well. Again, the NADPH oxidase inhibitors DPI and apocynin and the antioxidant NAC decreased Tat-induced JNK activation. (From Ref. 54.)

lial proteins following exposure to Tat (52) is therefore consistent with Tat-induced oxidant-dependent signaling.

Tat appears to activate an endothelial oxidase with an inhibitor profile much like that of the NADPH oxidase of professional phagocytes. The molecular composition of the NADPH oxidase functioning in vascular cells is incompletely understood. In neutrophils, three cytosolic subunits ($p47^{phox}$, $p67^{phox}$, and $p40^{phox}$) combine with Rac2 and the membrane cytochrome b_{558} ($p22^{phox}$ and $gp91^{phox}$) to constitute an active oxidase. A similar arrangement may exist in vascular cells, with Rac1 substituting for Rac2. For instance, $p22^{phox}$ has been cloned from rat vascular smooth muscle cells (71) and plays a clear physiological role in angiotensin II signaling (72). In addition, five human paralogues of the $gp91^{phox}$ family have been described, now termed Nox1-5, with the phagocyte $gp91^{phox}$ being Nox2 (73). The three anatomical vascular layers appear to express these Nox paralogues differentially. Normal intima expresses $gp91^{phox}$, detected by RT-PCR in cultured endothelial cells and by immunohisto-chemistry in tissues (74–76), whereas endothelial Nox1 expression is low (77). $gp91^{phox}$ from rat endothelium has been cloned and is highly homologous to mouse phagocyte $gp91^{phox}$, but with potentially important differences in putative glycosylation sites suggesting differential subcellular targeting (78). This subunit has been found to be responsible for endothelial oxidant production in postischemic mouse lungs (79).

gp91^{phox} has also been cloned from human endothelial cells, and its sequence is reported to be identical to that of human phagocytes (77). In contrast to endothelial cells, vascular smooth muscle cells express higher levels of Nox1 and Nox4 than gp91^{phox} (77,80). However, immunohistochemical studies suggest that the media of pulmonary artery, and, to a lesser extent, aorta, do express low levels of gp91^{phox} protein (76,81). Similar immunohistochemical studies of the aorta suggest that adventitial fibroblasts also express significant levels of gp91^{phox} (76,82). Recently, p22^{phox} was also cloned from both rat coronary microvascular endothelial cells (78) and human umbilical vein endothelial cells (77), and a partial sequence of the human endothelial protein was noted to be identical to phagocyte p22^{phox}.

Considerably less is known about vascular homologues of the cystosolic NADPH oxidase subunits p47^{phox} and p67^{phox}. Immunohistochemical studies have consistently demonstrated immunoreactive p47^{phox} and p67^{phox} in both endothelial (74,75,79,83) and adventitial (82) cells, with low levels expressed by medial cells (75), similar to the vascular distribution of gp91^{phox}. We recently cloned full-length p47^{phox} from human umbilical vein endothelial cells and found nearly 100% identity with the phagocyte sequence, with conservation of SH3 binding sites and critically phosphorylated serines (63). Further, expression of p47^{phox} containing a W(193)R mutation, which disrupts the first SH3 domain, also decreased JNK activation and oxidant production by TNF-α. Thus, like events in phagocytes, those in endothelial cells also appear to require p47^{phox} to assemble an active oxidase following ligand binding. Further, vascular smooth muscle cells and aortic rings from p47$^{phox-/-}$ mice fail to produce O$_2^-$ upon phorbol ester or diethyldithiocarbamate stimulation, in contrast to cells from wild-type mice (84,85). Finally, electroporation of neutralizing antisera against p47^{phox} diminishes angiotensin II activation of JAK/STAT in rat vascular smooth muscle cells (86), confirming its importance in ligand-initiated oxidant-dependent vascular cell signaling.

A notable difference between the oxidase of vascular cells and phagocytes is the subcellular distribution of p47^{phox}. In endothelial cells, this oxidase subunit is recovered entirely in the particulate, not cytosolic fraction (Ref. 63 and unpublished observations), suggesting that the oxidase may already be tethered at or close to its site of action in unstimulated cells. Further, in both whole cell extracts and membrane preparations, endogenous p47^{phox} is not detergent-extractable, indicating a cytoskeletal and membrane skeletal localization. Immunostains also suggest colocalization with both actin filamentous structures and microtubules (63). In addition, a p47-GFP fusion protein localizes to actin structures in human endothelial cells (87). Even in stimulated phagocytes, there is a rapid association of the active, most heavily phosphorylated oxidase proteins with the neutrophil cytoskeleton (88,89). Further, when vascular cells are stimulated with cytokines or growth factors, p47-GFP migrates avidly to membrane ruffles (Fig. 4) (63), actin-rich structures associated with intense respiratory burst activity in professional phagocytes (90), and oxidant production in migrating endothelial cells (91). These observations reveal some similarities in subcellular targeting of the active oxidase in endothelial cells as in phagocytes.

The association of endothelial cell p47^{phox} with the cytoskeleton carries two important ramifications. First, both the NADPH oxidase and the cytoskeleton are targets for HIV-1 Tat. Tat not only activates an NADPH oxidase in vascular cells but also stimulates cytoskeletal rearrangement and junctional disorganization (52,54). Exogenously added H$_2$O$_2$ also produces similar endothelial gap formation, with

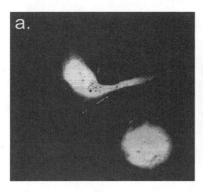 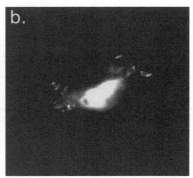

Figure 4 ECV-304 cells were transfected with a fusion between GFP and the NADPH oxidase subunit p47^{phox} (p47-GFP) and live cells were examined. (a) In resting cells, p47-GFP localizes to membrane and reticular internal structures. (b) After stimulation with TNF-α,

disappearance of membrane VE-cadherin (92) and loss of peripheral actin bands (93,94). This may suggest that the oxidase can act upstream of and therefore mediate these particular cytoskeletal rearrangements.

A second reason for the potential importance of a cytoskeletal location of p47^{phox} is that it may place the oxidase close to a number of signaling complexes. The cytoskeleton is not merely a passive target of Tat and cytokine signaling but is a requisite constituent of many if not most signaling pathways. Hence, cytoskeletal integrity is itself necessary for events upstream of oxidase activation. Disruption of microfilaments with cytochalasin B abolishes Tat-induced JNK activation (54), and cytoskeletal integrity is necessary for TNF-α–induced oxidant production as well as JNK activation (63). Although the precise role of the cytoskeleton in mediating signals is not clear, many if not all signaling molecules appear to bind directly or indirectly through scaffolds or adapters to the cytoskeleton, suggesting that it may act as a solid matrix that allows colocalization of signaling factors. Thus, a number of signaling proteins such as MAP kinases, PI3K, Ras-family G proteins, adapters, and Src kinases are associated with the cytoskeletal framework (95). In particular, membrane ruffles, to which endothelial cell p47^{phox} localize, contain large numbers of proximal signaling proteins such as PAK1, c-Ab1, ABI-1, Pyk2, PTPφ, and Rac1. Physical organization of sequential signaling factors may promote efficiency of reactions by increasing local concentrations of reactants and may also increase signal specificity by direct linking of proximal receptor with distal molecular targets. Accurate subcellular targeting would seem to be especially important for a signaling oxidase. A key property of oxidants is their instability, rendering them ideal to transmit biochemically compartmentalized, short-lived signals. Thus, oxidants generated at one site would be expected to target nearby oxidant-sensitive signaling proteins and not distant, accidental intracellular targets.

In further support of the concept that HIV-1 Tat initiates site-directed formation of signaling oxidants within endothelial cells, we recently established that the NADPH oxidase subunit p47^{phox} is a binding partner of the orphan adapter TNF receptor–associated factor 4 (TRAF4). A human endothelial cell library was screened using

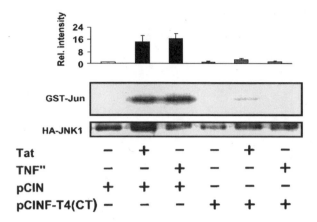

Figure 5   The p47-interacting domain of TRAF4 interferes with ligand-induced JNK activation. Human endothelial cells were cotransfected with HA-JNK1 and either empty vector (pCIN) or vector containing the p47-interacting fragment of TRAF4 [pCINF-T4(CT)]. Disruption of the TRAF4-p47 interaction using the truncated TRAF4 protein greatly reduced

yeast two-hybrid technology, and TRAF4 was recovered and shown to interact with full-length $p47^{phox}$ in vitro and in whole cells (87). Like $p47^{phox}$, TRAF4 was found largely in the cytoskeletal fraction, comparable to the location of its cytokine receptor-associated relatives TRAFs 2, 5, and 6 (96). Overexpression of $p47^{phox}$ and TRAF4 increased oxidant production and JNK activation, whereas each alone had minimal effect. In addition, forced interaction through genetic fusion between $p47^{phox}$ and the TRAF4 C-terminus caused constitutive activation of JNK, and this activation was decreased by the antioxidant *N*-acetyl cysteine. In order to interrupt association of endogenous $p47^{phox}$ and TRAF4, the $p47^{phox}$-binding domain of TRAF4 was over-expressed in endothelial cells. Ectopic expression of this fragment blocked endothelial cell JNK activation by both HIV-1 Tat and TNF-α, suggesting an uncoupling of $p47^{phox}$ from upstream signaling events (Fig. 5). A secondary screen of endothelial cell proteins for TRAF4-interacting partners yielded a number of proteins known to control cell fate through either proliferative or apoptotic pathways (87). These studies again highlight the capacity of HIV-1 Tat to initiate signals which enter basic endothelial cell signaling cassettes at the level of an NADPH oxidase.

CONCLUSION

In summary, HIV-1–infected patients manifest a variety of peripheral vascular abnormalities ranging from gross vessel wall deformities to endothelial cellular derangements of proliferation, apoptosis, and activation. The viral accessory protein Tat is capable of inducing many of these abnormal phenotypic vascular changes, and it likely targets the endothelium in conjunction with other factors such as cytokines. Tat appears capable of activating a number of basic endothelial signaling cassettes at least in part through activation of a specific signaling oxidase, which is shared by cytokine and growth factor pathways. The reason for the pleiotropic vascular response to HIV-1 at this point is unclear and worth further study.

REFERENCES

1. Zietz C, Hotz B, Sturzl M, Rauch E, Penning R, Lohrs U. Aortic endothelium in HIV-1 infection: chronic injury, activation, and increased leukocyte adherence. Am J Pathol 1996; 149:1887–1898.
2. Calabrese LH, Estes M, Yen-Lieberman B, Proffitt MR, Tubbs R, Fishleder AJ, Levin KH. Systemic vasculitis in association with human immunodeficiency virus infection. Arthritis Rheum 1989; 32:569–576.
3. Gherardi R, Belec L, Mhiri C, Gray F, Lescs MC, Sobel A, Guillevin L, Wechsler J. The spectrum of vasculitis in human immunodeficiency virus–infected patients. A clinico-pathologic evaluation. Arthritis Rheum 1993; 36:1164–1174.
4. Xiu RJ, Jun C, Berglund O. Microcirculatory disturbances in AIDS patients—a first report. Microvasc Res 1991; 42:151–159.
5. Newsome DA, Green WR, Miller ED, Kiessling LA, Morgan B, Jabs DA, Polk BF. Microvascular aspects of acquired immune deficiency syndrome retinopathy. Am J Ophthalmol 1984; 98:590–601.
6. Geier SA, Klauss V, Goebel FD. Ocular microangiopathic syndrome in patients with acquired immunodeficiency syndrome and its relationship to alterations in cell adhesion and in blood flow. German J Ophthalmol 1994; 3:414–421.
7. Geier SA, Schielke E, Tatsch K, Sadri I, Bogner JR, Hammel G, Einhaupl KM, Goebel FD. Brain HMPAO-SPECT and ocular microangiopathic syndrome in HIV-1-infected patients. AIDS 1993; 7:1589–1594.
8. Glasgow BJ. Evidence for breaches of the retinal vasculature in acquired immune deficiency syndrome angiopathy. A fluorescent microsphere study. Ophthalmology 1997; 104:753–760.
9. Pomerantz RJ, Kuritzkes DR, de la Monte SM, Rota TR, Baker AS, Albert D, Bor DH, Feldman EL, Schooley RT, Hirsch MS. Infection of the retina by human immunode-ficiency virus type I. N Engl J Med 1987; 317:1643–1647.
10. Roh SS, Gertner E. Digital necrosis in acquired immune deficiency syndrome vasculopathy treated with recombinant tissue plasminogen activator. J Rheumatol 1997; 24:2258–2261.
11. Requena L, Farina C, Barat A. Degos disease in a patient with acquired immunodeficiency syndrome. J Am Acad Dermatol 1998; 38:852–856.
12. Eitner F, Cui Y, Hudkins KL, Schmidt A, Birkebak T, Agy MB, Hu SL, Morton WR, Anderson DM, Alpers CE. Thrombotic microangiopathy in the HIV-2-infected macaque. Am J Pathol 1999; 155:649–661.
13. Gadallah MF, el-Shahawy MA, Campese VM, Todd JR, King JW. Disparate prognosis of thrombotic microangiopathy in HIV-infected patients with and without AIDS. Am J Nephrol 1996; 16:446–450.
14. Sutor GC, Schmidt RE, Albrecht H. Thrombotic microangiopathies and HIV infection: report of two typical cases, features of HUS and TTP, and review of the literature. Infection 1999; 27:12–15.
15. Lee SD, Shroyer KR, Markham NE, Cool CD, Voelkel NF, Tuder RM. Monoclonal endothelial cell proliferation is present in primary but not secondary pulmonary hypertension. J Clin Invest 1998; 101:927–934.
16. Tabib A, Leroux C, Mornex JF, Loire R. Accelerated coronary atheroclerosis and

arteriosclerosis in young human-immunodeficiency-virus–positive patients. Coron Artery Dis 2000; 11:41–46.

17. Shannon RP, Simon MA, Mathier MA, Geng YJ, Mankad S, Lackner AA. Dilated cardiomyopathy associated with simian AIDS in nonhuman primates. Circulation 2000; 101:185–193.

18. Dubrovsky T, Curless R, Scott G, Chaneles M, Post MJ, Altman N, Petito CK, Start D, Wood C. Cerebral aneurysmal arteriopathy in childhood AIDS. Neurology 1998; 51:560–565.

19. Shah SS, Zimmerman RA, Rorke LB, Vezina LG. Cerebrovascular complications of HIV in children. Am J Neuroradiol 1996; 17:1913–1917.

20. Tinkle BT, Ngo L, Luciw PA, Maciag T, Jay G. Human immunodeficiency virus–associated vasculopathy in transgenic mice. J Virol 1997; 71:4809–4814.

21. Lebbe C, de Cremoux P, Millot G, Podgorniak MP, Verola O, Berger R, Morel P, Calvo F. Characterization of in vitro culture of HIV-negative Kaposi's sarcoma–derived cells. In vitro responses to alfa interferon. Arch Dermatol Res 1997; 289:421–428.

22. Ruszczak Z, Mayer-Da Silva A, Orfanos CE. Kaposi's sarcoma in AIDS. Multicentric angioneoplasia in early skin lesions. Am J Dermatopathol 1987; 9:388–398.

23. McNutt NS, Fletcher V, Conant MA. Early lesions of Kaposi's sarcoma in homosexual men. An ultrastructural comparison with other vascular proliferation in skin. Am J Pathol 1983; 111:62–77.

24. Delabesse E, Oksenhendler E, Lebbe C, Verola O, Varet B, Turhan AG. Molecular analysis of clonality in Kaposi's sarcoma. J Clin Pathol 1997; 50:664–668.

25. Rabkin CS, Janz S, Lash A, Coleman AE, Musaba E, Liotta L, Biggar RJ, Zhuang Z. Monoclonal origin of multicentric Kaposi's sarcoma lesions. N Engl J Med 1997; 336:988–993.

26. Wiley CA, Schrier RD, Nelson JA, Lampert PW, Oldstone MB. Cellular localization of human immunodeficiency virus infection within the brains of acquired immune deficiency syndrome patients. Proc Natl Acad Sci USA 1986; 83:7089–7093.

27. Ward JM, O'Leary TJ, Baskin GB, Benveniste R, Harris CA, Nara PL, Rhodes RH. Immunohistochemical localization of human and simian immunodeficiency viral antigens in fixed tissue sections. Am J Pathol 1987; 127:199–205.

28. Korber BT, Kunstman KJ, Patterson BK, Furtado M, McEvilly MM, Levy R, Wolinsky SM. Genetic differences between blood- and brain-derived viral sequences from human immunodeficiency virus type 1-infected patients: evidence of conserved elements in the V3 region of the envelope protein of brain-derived sequences. J Virol 1994; 68:7467–7481.

29. Moses AV, Bloom FE, Pauza CD, Nelson JA. Human immunodeficiency virus infection of human brain capillary endothelial cells occurs via a CD4/galactosylceramide-independent mechanism. Proc Natl Acad Sci USA 1993; 90:10474–10478.

30. Moses AV, Williams SE, Strussenberg JG, Heneveld ML, Ruhl RA, Bakke AC, Bagby GC, Nelson JA. HIV-1 induction of CD40 on endothelial cells promotes the outgrowth of AIDS-associated B-cell lymphomas. Nature Med 1997; 3:1242–1249.

31. Moses AV, Williams S, Heneveld ML, Strussenberg J, Rarick M, Loveless M, Bagby G, Nelson JA. Human immunodeficiency virus infection of bone marrow endothelium reduces induction of stromal hematopoietic growth factors. Blood 1996; 87:919–925.

32. Marciniak RA, Garcia-Blanco MA, Sharp PA. Identification and characterization of a HeLa nuclear protein that specifically binds to the trans-activation-response (TAR) element of human immunodeficiency virus. Proc Natl Acad Sci USA 1990; 87:3624–3628.

33. Jeang KT, Xiao H, Rich EA. Multifaceted activities of the HIV-1 transactivator of transcription. Tat J Biol Chem 1999; 274:28837–28840.

34. Westendorp MO, Frank R, Ochsenbauer C, Stricker K, Dhein J, Walczak H, Debatin KM, Krammer PH. Sensitization of T cells to CD95-mediated apoptosis by HIV-1 Tat and gp 120. Nature 1995; 375:497–500.

35. Frankel AD, Pabo CO. Cellular uptake of the tat protein from human immunodeficiency virus. Cell 1988; 55:1189–1193.
36. Albini A, Soldi R, Giunciuglio D, Giraudo E, Benelli R, Primo L, Noonan D, Salio M, Camussi G, Rockl W, Bussolino F. The angiogenesis induced by HIV-1 tat protein is mediated by the Flk-1/KDR receptor on vascular endothelial cells. Nature Med 1996; 2:1371–1375.
37. Seve M, Favier A, Osman M, Hernandez D, Vaitaitis G, Flores NC, McCord JM, Flores SC. The human immunodeficiency virus-1 Tat protein increases cell proliferation, alters sensitivity to zinc chelator-induced apoptosis, and changes Sp1 DNA binding in HeLa cells. Arch Biochem Biophys 1999; 361:165–172.
38. Ensoli B, Barillari G, Salahuddin SZ, Gallo RC, Wong-Staal F. Tat protein of HIV-1 stimulates growth of cells derived from Kaposi's sarcoma lesions of AIDS patients. Nature 1990; 345:84–85.
39. Albini A, Barillari G, Benelli R, Gallo RC, Ensoli B. Angiogenic properties of human immunodeficiency virus type 1 Tat protein. Proc Natl Acad Sci USA 1995; 92:4838–4842.
40. Albini A, Benelli R, Presta M, Rusnati M, Ziche M, Rubartelli A, Paglialunga G, Bussolino F, Noonan D. HIV-tat protein is a heparin-binding angiogenic growth factor. Oncogene 1996; 12:289–297.
41. Barillari G, Gendelman R, Gallo RC, Ensoli B. The Tat protein of human immuno-deficiency virus type 1, a growth factor for AIDS Kaposi sarcoma and cytokine-activated vascular cells, induces adhesion of the same cell types by using integrin receptors recog-nizing the RGD amino acid sequence. Proc Natl Acad Sci USA 1993; 90:7941–7945.
42. Barillari G, Sgadari C, Palladino C, Gendelman R, Caputo A, Morris CB, Nair BC, Markham P, Nel A, Sturzl M, Ensoli B. Inflammatory cytokines synergize with the HIV-1 Tat protein to promote angiogenesis and Kaposi's sarcoma via induction of basic fibroblast growth factor and the alpha v beta 3 integrin. J Immunol 1999; 163:1929–1935.
43. Ariyoshi K, Schim van der Loeff M, Cook P, Whitby D, Corrah T, Jaffar S, Cham F, Sabally S, O'Donovan D, Weiss RA, Schulz TF, Whittle H. Kaposi's sarcoma in the Gambia, West Africa is less frequent in human immunodeficiency virus type 2 than in human immunodeficiency virus type 1 infection despite a high prevalence of human herpesvirus 8. J Hum Virol 1998; 1:193–199.
44. Vogel J, Hinrichs SH, Reynolds RK, Luciw PA, Jay G. The HIV tat gene induces dermal lesions resembling Kaposi's sarcoma in transgenic mice. Nature 1988; 335:606–611.
45. Munshi N, Ganju RK, Avraham S, Mesri EA, Groopman JE. Kaposi's sarcoma-associated herpesvirus-encoded G protein-coupled receptor activation of c-jun amino-terminal kinase/stress-activated protein kinase and lyn kinase is mediated by related adhesion focal tyrosine kinase/proline-rich tyrosine kinase 2. J Biol Chem 1999; 274:31863–31867.
46. Dhawan S, Puri RK, Kumar A, Duplan H, Masson JM, Aggarwal BB. Human immu-nodeficiency virus-1-tat protein induces the cell surface expression of endothelial leuko-cyte adhesion molecule-1, vascular cell adhesion molecule-1, and intercellular adhesion molecule-1 in human endothelial cells. Blood 1997; 90:1535–1544.
47. Hofman FM, Wright AD, Dohadwala MM, Wong-Staal F, Walker SM. Exogenous tat protein activates human endothelial cells. Blood 1993; 82:2774–2780.
48. Cota-Gomez A, Flores NC, Cruz C, Casullo A, Aw TY, Ichikawa H, Schaack J, Schein-man R, Flores SC. The human immunodeficiency virus-1 Tat protein activates human umbilical vein endothelial cell E-selectin expression via an NF-kB-dependent mechanism. J Biol Chem 2002; 277:14390–14399.
49. Conant K, Ma M, Nath A, Major EO. Extracellular human immunodeficiency virus type 1 Tat protein is associated with an increase in both NF-kappa B binding and protein kinase C activity in primary human astrocytes. J Virol 1996; 70:1384–1389.
50. Demarchi F, d'Adda di Fagagna F, Falaschi A, Giacca M. Activation of transcription

factor NF-kappaB by the Tat protein of human immunodeficiency virus type 1. J Virol 1996; 70:4427–4437.

51. Park IW, Wang JF, Groopman JE. HIV-1 Tat promotes monocyte chemoattractant protein-1 secretion followed by transmigration of monocytes. Blood 2001; 97:352–358.

52. Oshima T, Flores SC, Vaitaitis G, Coe LL, Joh T, Park JH, Zhu Y, Alexander B, Alexander JS. HIV-1 Tat increases endothelial solute permeability through tyrosine kinase and mitogen-activated protein kinase-dependent pathways. AIDS 2000; 14:475–482.

53. Ganju RK, Munshi N, Nair BC, Liu ZY, Gill P, Groopman JE. Human immunodeficiency virus tat modulates the Flk-1/KDR receptor, mitogen-activated protein kinases, and components of focal adhesion in Kaposi's sarcoma cells. J Virol 1998; 72:6131–6137.

54. Gu Y, Wu RF, Xu YC, Flores SC, Terada LS. HIV Tat activates c-Jun amino-terminal kinase through an oxidant-dependent mechanism. Virology 2001; 286:62–71.

55. Park IW, Ullrich CK, Shoenberger E, Ganju RK, Groopman JE. HIV-1 tat induces microvascular endothelial apoptosis through caspase activation. J Immunol 2001; 167:2766–2771.

56. Flores SC, Marecki JC, Harper KP, Bose SK, Nelson SK, McCord JM. Tat protein of human immunodeficiency virus type 1 represses expression of manganese superoxide dismutase in HeLa cells. Proc Natl Acad Sci USA 1993; 90:7632–7636.

57. Westendorp MO, Shatrov VA, Schulze-Osthoff K, Frank R, Kraft M, Los M, Krammer PH, Droge W, Lehmann V. HIV-1 Tat potentiates TNF-induced NF-kappa B activation and cytotoxicity by altering the cellular redox state. EMBO J 1995; 14:546–554.

58. Eck HP, Gmunder H, Hartmann M, Petzoldt D, Daniel V, Droge W. Low concentrations of acid-soluble thiol (cysteine) in the blood plasma of HIV-1-infected patients. Biol Chem Hoppe Seyler 1989; 370:101–108.

59. Buhl R, Jaffe HA, Holroyd KJ, Wells FB, Mastrangeli A, Saltini C, Cantin AM, Crystal RG. Systemic glutathione deficiency in symptom-free HIV-seropositive individuals. Lancet 1989; 2:1294–1298.

60. Wang Y, Watson RR. Potential therapeutics of vitamin E (tocopherol) in AIDS and HIV. Drugs 1994; 48:327–338.

61. Revillard JP, Vincent CM, Favier AE, Richard MJ, Zittoun M, Kazatchkine MD. Lipid peroxidation in human immunodeficiency virus infection. J AIDS 1992; 5:637–638.

62. Staal FJ, Roederer M, Israelski DM, Bubp J, Mole LA, McShane D, Deresinski SC, Ross W, Sussman H, Raju PA, et al. Intracellular glutathione levels in T cell subsets decrease in HIV-infected individuals. AIDS Res Hum Retrovir 1992; 8:305–311.

63. Gu Y, Xu YC, Wu RF, Souza RF, Nwariaku FE, Terada LS. TNF alpha activates c-jun amino terminal kinase through p47phox. Exp Cell Res 2002; 272:62–74.

64. Sundaresan M, Yu ZX, Ferrans VJ, Irani K, Finkel T. Requirement for generation of H2O2 for platelet-derived growth factor signal transduction. Science 1995; 270:296–299.

65. Natoli G, Costanzo A, Ianni A, Templeton DJ, Woodgett JR, Balsano C, Levrero M. Activation of SAPK/JNK by TNF receptor 1 through a noncytotoxic TRAF2-dependent pathway. Science 1997; 275:200–203.

66. Lo YYC, Wong JMS, Cruz TF. Reactive oxygen species mediate cytokine activation of c-Jun NH2-terminal kinases. J Biol Chem 1996; 271:15703–15707.

67. Marumo T, Schini-Kerth VB, Fisslthaler B, Busse R. Platelet-derived growth factor-stimulated superoxide anion production modulates activation of transcription factor NF-kappaB and expression of monocyte chemoattractant protein 1 in human aortic smooth muscle cells. Circulation 1997; 96:2361–2367.

68. Sulciner DJ, Irani K, Yu ZX, Ferrans VJ, Goldschmidt-Clermont P, Finkel T. rac1 regulates a cytokine-stimulated, redox-dependent pathway necessary for NF-kappaB activation. Molec Cell Biol 1996; 16:7115–7121.

69. Shatrov VA, Boelaert JR, Chouaib S, Droge W, Lehmann V. Iron chelation decreases

human immunodeficiency virus-1 Tat potentiated tumor necrosis factor-induced NF-kappa B activation in Jurkat cells. Eur Cytokine Netw 1997; 8:37–43.

70. Barrett WC, DeGnore JP, Keng YF, Zhang ZY, Yim MB, Chock PB. Roles of superoxide radical anion in signal transduction mediated by reversible regulation of protein-tyrosine phosphatase 1B. J Biol Chem 1999; 274:34543–34546.

71. Ushio-Fukai M, Zafari AM, Fukui T, Ishizaka N, Griendling KK. p22phox is a critical component of the superoxide-generating NADH/NADPH oxidase system and regulates angiotensin II-induced hypertrophy in vascular smooth muscle cells. J Biol Chem 1996; 271:23317–23321.

72. Fukui T, Ishizaka N, Rajagopalan S, Laursen JB, Capers Qt, Taylor WR, Harrison DG, de Leon H, Wilcox JN, Griendling KK. p22phox mRna expression and NADPH oxidase activity are increased in aortas from hypertensive rats. Circ Res 1997; 80:45–51.

73. Cheng G, Cao Z, Xu X, van Meir EG, Lambeth JD. Homologs of gp91phox: cloning and tissue expression of Nox3. Nox4, and Nox5 Gene 2001; 269:131–140.

74. Jones SA, VB OD, Wood JD, Broughton JP, Hughes EJ, Jones OT. Expression of phagocyte NADPH oxidase components in human endothelial cells. Am J Physiol 1996; 271:H1626–H1634.

75. Hohler B, Holzapfel B, Kummer W. NADPH oxidase subunits and superoxide production in porcine pulmonary artery endothelial cells. Histochem Cell Biol 2000; 114:29–37.

76. Wang HD, Xu S, Johns DG, Du Y, Quinn MT, Cayatte AJ, Cohen RA. Role of NADPH oxidase in the vascular hypertrophic and oxidative stress response to angiotensin II in mice. Circ Res 2001; 88:947–953.

77. Gorlach A, Brandes RP, Nguyen K, Amidi M, Dehghani F, Busse R. A gp91phox containing NADPH oxidase selectivity expressed in endothelial cells is a major source of oxygen radical generation in the arterial wall. Circ Res 2000; 87:26–32.

78. Bayraktutan U, Blayney L, Shah AM. Molecular characterization and localization of the NAD(P)H oxidase components gp91-phox and p22-phox in endothelial cells. Arterioscler Thromb Vasc Biol 2000; 20:1903–1911.

79. Al-Mehdi AB, Zhao G, Dodia C, Tozawa K, Costa K, Muzykantov V, Ross C, Blecha F, Dinauer M, Fisher AB. Endothelial NADPH oxidase as the source of oxidants in lungs exposed to ischemia or high K+. Circ Res 1998; 83:730–737.

80. Lassegue B, Sorescu D, Szocs K, Yin Q, Akers M, Zhang Y, Grant SL, Lambeth JD, Griendling KK. Novel gp91 (phox) homologues in vascular smooth muscle cells: nox1 mediates angiotensin II-induced superoxide formation and redox-sensitive signaling pathways. Circ Res 2001; 88:888–894.

81. Archer SL, Reeve HL, Michelakis E, Puttagunta L, Waite R, Nelson DP, Dinauer MC, Weir EK. O2 sensing is preserved in mice lacking the gp91 phox subunit of NADPH oxidase. Proc Natl Acad Sci USA 1999; 96:7944–7949.

82. Pagano PJ, Clark JK, Cifuentes-Pagano ME, Clark SM, Callis GM, Quinn MT. Localization of a constitutively active, phagocyte-like NADPH oxidase in rabbit aortic adventitia: enhancement by angiotensin II. Proc Natl Acad Sci USA 1997; 94:14483–14488.

83. Patterson C, Ruef J, Madamanchi NR, Barry-Lane P, Hu Z, Horaist C, Ballinger CA, Brasier AR, Bode C, Runge MS. Stimulation of a vascular smooth muscle cell NAD(P)H oxidase by thrombin. Evidence that p47(phox) may participate in forming this oxidase in vitro and in vivo. J Biol Chem 1999; 274:19814–19822.

84. Lavigne MC, Malech HL, Holland SM, Leto TL. Genetic demonstration of p47phox-dependent superoxide anion production in murine vascular smooth muscle cells. Circulation 2001; 104:79–84.

85. Hsich E, Segal BH, Pagano PJ, Rey FE, Paigen B, Deleonardis J, Hoyt RF, Holland SM, Finkel T. Vascular effects following homozygous disruption of p47(phox): an essential component of NADPH oxidase. Circulation 2000; 101:1234–1236.

86. Schieffer B, Luchtefeld M, Braun S, Hilfiker A, Hilfiker-Kleiner D, Drexler H. Role of NAD(P)H oxidase in angiotensin II-induced JAK/STAT signaling and cytokine induction. Circ Res 2000; 87:1195–1201.

87. Xu YC, Wu RF, Gu Y, Yang YS, Yang MC, Nwariaku FE, Terada LS. Involvement of TRAF4 in oxidative activation of c-jun amino terminal kinase. J Biol Chem 2002; 277:28051–28057.

88. El Benna J, Ruedi JM, Babior BM. Cytosolic guanine nucleotide-binding protein Rac2 operates in vivo as a component of the neutrophil respiratory burst oxidase. Transfer of Rac2 and the cytosolic oxidase components p47phox and p67phox to the submembranous actin cytoskeleton during oxidase activation. J Biol Chem 1994; 269:6729–6734.

89. Nauseef WM, Volpp BD, McCormick S, Leidal KG, Clark RA. Assembly of the neutrophil respiratory burst oxidase. Protein kinase C promotes cytoskeletal and membrane association of cytosolic oxidase components. J Biol Chem 1991; 266:5911–5917.

90. Heyworth PG, Robinson JM, Ding J, Ellis BA, Badwey JA. Cofilin undergoes rapid dephosphorylation in stimulated neutrophils and translocates to ruffled membranes enriched in products of the NADPH oxidase complex. Evidence for a novel cycle of phosphorylation and dephosphorylation. Histochem Cell Biol 1997; 108:221–233.

91. Grogan A, Reeves E, Keep N, Wientjes F, Totty NF, Burlingame AL, Hsuan JJ, Segal AW. Cytosolic phox proteins interact with and regulate the assembly of coronin in neutrophils. J Cell Sci 1997; 110:3071–3081.

92. Kevil CG, Ohno N, Gute DC, Okayama N, Robinson SA, Chaney E, Alexander JS. Role of cadherin internalization in hydrogen peroxide-mediated endothelial permeability. Free Radic Biol Med 1998; 24:1015–1022.

93. Wojciak-Stothard B, Entwistle A, Garg R, Ridley AJ. Regulation of TNF-alpha–induced reorganization of the actin cytoskeleton and cell-cell junctions by Rho, Rac, and Cdc42 in human endothelial cells. J Cell Physiol 1998; 176:150–165.

94. Bradley JR, Thiru S, Pober JS. Hydrogen peroxide-induced endothelial retraction is accompanied by a loss of the normal spatial organization of endothelial cell adhesion molecules. Am J Pathol 1995; 147:627–641.

95. Plopper GE, McNamee HP, Dike LE, Bojanowski K, Ingber DE. Convergence of integrin and growth factor receptor signaling pathways within the focal adhesion complex. Mol Biol Cell 1995; 6:1349–1365.

96. Dadgostar H, Cheng G. Membrane localization of TRAF 3 enables JNK activation. J Biol Chem 2000; 275:2539–2544.

8

Causative Factors of Cardiovascular Complications in AIDS

Yinhong Chen
University of California, La Jolla, California, U.S.A.

Ronald Ross Watson
University of Arizona, Tucson, Arizona, U.S.A.

Acquired immunodeficiency syndrome (AIDS) is a health crisis; approximately 60 million people are affected worldwide (1). World Health Organization estimates that as many as 110 million people worldwide may be HIV-positive before the end of this century (2). One estimate of the prevalence of cardiac involvement in patients with HIV is from 28 to 73% (3). Cardiomyopathy and myocarditis now appear to be the most important cardiac complications of AIDS in the western world (4,5). Indeed, HIV cardiomyopathy was reported as being the fourth leading cause of dilated cardiomyopathy in the United States (2). Congestive heart failure has become the leading cause of death in pediatric patients with AIDS, half of whom die of within 6 to 12 months of diagnosis (6). Cardiac syndromes described in AIDS patients include myocarditis, myocardial necrosis, cardiomyopathy, arteriopathy, endocarditis, pericardial effusion, and cardiac neoplasm. The causative factors remain unknown. But these conditions suggest that the causative factors might be 1) HIV itself, 2) cocaine abuse, 3) multiple opportunistic infections, 4) nonspecific and specific inflammatory responses, 5) autoimmune reactions, 6) catecholamine excess, 7) drug-induced cardiotoxicity, and/or 8) nutritional deficiencies.

RETROVIRUS ATTACKS CARDIOVASCULAR TISSUE DIRECTLY

Retrovirus is capable of infecting various cell types, including monocytes, peripheral lymphocytes, corneal epithelial cells, glial cells, and myocytes (7). The direct effect of retrovirus on the cardiovascular system is not universally accepted. But much evidence supports that the retrovirus is a causative agent in AIDS with cardiovascular involvement. Researchers found the presence of an in situ hybridization signal for HIV-1 in the AIDS patient's myocardium (8–10). Other evidence of cardiac HIV-1 infection was based on isolation and the cultivation of HIV-1 from the patients' endomyocardial biopsies (11) by detection of nucleic acid sequences of extracted DNA (10–12). Barbaro et al. (13) found that cardiac myocytes were infected with

HIV-1 in 58 patients, and nearly two-thirds of those samples showed myocarditis. These findings suggested that the myocarditis was related to direct action of HIV-1. Cardiovascular endothelial cells infected by retrovirus are possibly related to endothelial cell dysfunction in AIDS. Altered function of vascular endothelial cells is associated with hyperactivity of the microcirculation and with coronary vasospasm, resembling the changes seen in cocaine abuse. Coronary artery spasm may lead to myocellular necrosis and subsequently cause hypertrophy (14). Recent studies (15) of the hypertensive rat demonstrated an increase of two orders of magnitude in the expression of endogenous retrovirus. Retroviruses infect the germlines of their hosts at the same time in the course of evolution and have persisted as stably integrated proviruses that are vertically transmitted. Retroviruses may integrate near or within host genes, occasionally upregulating or inactivating the host gene. Thus, consequences of integration may alter gene regulation and change phenotype.

COCAINE ABUSE

Cocaine abuse is the leading risk factor for the acquisition of AIDS (16). Cocaine itself has been associated with myocarditis, dilated cardiomyopathy, endocarditis, and arrhythmias. Onset of cocaine-associated angina pectoris or myocardial infarction was reported several hours after drug administration. The basic cellular mechanisms (17) of cocaine consist of (1) a catecholamine effect by inhibition of the presynaptic uptake carrier, (2) local anesthetic effect by the blockage of sodium channels, (3) procoagulant effect by combining with protein C or antithrombin (17,18) and cocaine-induced thrombosis by platelet activation and aggregation, (4) inflammatory alterations, and (5) intravenous cocaine abuse, impairing vascular endothelial cells and giving pathogens more chances of entry. Overall, it is possible that cocaine-abusing AIDS patients develop exaggerated cardiovascular manifestations. Indeed, Cho et al. (19), observed that the prevalence of idiopathic myocarditis and dilated cardiomyopathy was significantly greater in a group of HIV-infected patients addicted to cocaine than in homosexual patients.

AUTOIMMUNE REACTION

HIV-infected patients show high concentrations of immune complexes in serum. A murine AIDS model, induced by LP-BM5 murine leukemia virus, characteristically develops hypergammaglobulinemia, T-cell functional deficiency, and B-cell dysfunction. Acierno (20) suggested that myocardial damage could relate to hypersensitivity resulting from uncontrolled hypergammaglobulinemia. Many researchers (21–28) have proposed an autoimmune mechanism for HIV-related myocardial disease, similar to mechanisms described with antimyosin antibodies. They postulate that the viral gene alters the cell surface of the muscle fiber. Some of these cell surface proteins become immunogenic and elicit a progressive autoimmune reaction. A series of experiments revealed the presence of circulating cardiac autoantibodies to heavy-chain myosin in AIDS patients having cardiovascular complications. A large amount of class 1 and 2 histocompatibility marker, IL-1, and other cytokines may also contribute to the induction of heart-specific autoimmunity in AIDS.

NONSPECIFIC INFLAMMATORY INFILTRATION

In AIDS patients with cardiomyopathy, pathological findings show focal areas of inflammatory infiltrate containing lymphocytes, neutrophils, macrophages, histiocytes, and occasional plasma cells in the myocardial interstitium (29,30). Inflammatory infiltration is composed predominantly of CD3 and CD8 lymphocytes in over 80% of AIDS patients with myocarditis. An investigator foun a 74% prevalence of lymphocytic infiltrates of the myocardium. In another retrospective study, more than 500 histological sections of myocardium were reviewed; focal microscopic interstitial mononuclear infiltrates occurred in 16% of samples (31). Roldan and Baroldi (32,33) found higher lymphocytic infiltrates: 32 and 34%, respectively. In another autopsy series, the prevalence of myocardial inflammation was 52% (34). In animal experiments, we found that neutrophils were highly activated in murine AIDS (MAIDS). Myeloperoxidase (MPO) activity as a neutrophil infiltration marker is higher in MAIDS hearts than in control hearts (unpublished data). Reactive oxygen species (ROS) released from activated neutrophils and myocytes are toxic to heart tissue. The oxidative stress associated with HIV infection may be important for the progression of the heart disease because ROS activate the nuclear transcription factor NF-κB, which is obligatory for HIV replication (35). Overall, the prevalence of interstitial inflammation in AIDS was high, and the histological findings seen with myocarditis are often nonspecific inflammatory infiltrates without apparent myocyte damage.

PATHOGENIC AND OPPORTUNISTIC INFECTION

A number of opportunistic infections in AIDS involving the heart have been reported. Multiple infections are also frequent. Common pathogens include *Toxoplasma gondii*, *Myocobacterium tuberculosis*, *Cryptococcus neoformans*, *Pneumocystis carinii*, *Histoplasma capsulatum*, and *Cryptococcus neoformans*. More common is the finding of pericardial involvement as part of widely disseminated tuberculosis. Disseminated cytomegalovirus (CMV) infection also occurs frequently in HIV-infected patients. CMV antigen and CMV-mediated early gene expression were found in myocytes from HIV-infected patients. Because it is well known that CMV infections can cause tissue necrosis, it is possible that CMV-infected myocytes trigger cellular and humoral-mediated cardiac injury (36–38). Coxsackivirus B has also been associated with myocarditis in AIDS (39). Epstein-Barr virus is another opportunistic pathogen involved in the etiology of cardiac lymphomas (40).

CYTOKINES

Immunohistochemical, immunopathological and serological studies in animals and humans with AIDS and cardiovascular involvement have shown that the majority of inflamed cells express abnormally large amounts of class 1 and 2 histocompatibility markers, interleukin-1 (IL-1). Levy and Herskowitz (41,42) demonstrated that the degree of immunosupression, as evidenced by decreased CD4 lymphocyte counts, correlated strongly with echocardiographic evidence of myocardial dysfunction. It is reasonable to consider that circulating or local cytokines may be involved in cardio-vascular implications in AIDS (Fig. 1).

The cytokine IL-1 has a suppressive effect on adrenergic agonist–mediated increase in cAMP in neonatal rat cardiomyocytes. IL-2 and IL-6 have reversible myocardial depressant effect in vivo (43,44). IL-6 was identified as a mediator of myocardial injury (45,46). These effects might appear to be regulated by nitric oxide (NO). Increased expression of inducible nitric oxide syntheses (iNOS) was shown in vitro in cardiac myocyte treated with TNF-α, IL-1, and interferon (IFN-γ) (47). Myocyte death in culture paralleled increased NO and ROS. Long-term treatment of cardiomyocytes with IL-1 and TNF-α reduced contractility and cyclic adenosine monophosphate (cAMP) accumulation by inhibition of adrenergic responsiveness. Myocardial depression effects of TNF-α infusion in dogs resulted in LV dysfunction (48). Anti-TNF-α antibodies reduced cardiac dysfunction during sepsis (49). A study (50) demonstrated that TNF-α and iNOS immunohistochemical stains of endomyo-cardial biopsies had greater intensity in cardiomyopathy patiens with AIDS than those without AIDS.

Endothelin (ET) is a potent vasoconstrictor peptide that has long-term effects on cellular growth and phenotype (51,52). It is synthesized in vasculature and myocar-dium by various cell types, including vascular endothelial cells, ventricular myocytes, and fibroblasts. In vitro, ET stimulates myocyte hypertrophy and expression of a fetal phenotype (52,53). Plasma ET-1 level is elevated in patients with heart failure (54). On this basis, ET could be another marker of myocardial injury in AIDS.

Tat, a structural protein, is secreted by infected cells and contributes to the activation of endothelial cells (55), functional programs for angiogenesis, and in-

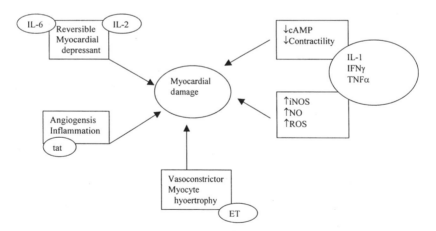

Figure 1 Cytokine dysregulation is a hallmark in AIDS individuals. IL-2 and IL-6 have reversible myocardial depressant effects in vivo (33,34). Tat is a structural protein secreted by HIV-infected cells. It contributes to the activation of endothelial cells, functional programs for angiogenesis, and inflammation (55). ET is a potent vasoconstrictor peptide that has long-term effects on cellular growth and phenotype (51,52). In vitro, ET stimulates myocyte hypertrophy and expression of a fetal phenotype (52,53). Increased expression of iNOS was shown in vitro in cardiac myocytes treated with TNF-α, IL-1, and IFN-γ (47). Myocyte death in culture paralleled increased NO and ROS. Long-term treatment of cardiomyocytes with IL-1 and TNF-α reduced contractility and cAMP accumulation by inhibition of adrenergic responsiveness. Therefore cytokine dysreguation in AIDS may be involved in cardiovascular implications.

flammation. Together, these observations support the suggestion that retrovirus-infected cells may release mitogenic tat to initiate a localized cascade of molecular events. The cascade could then result in the production of growth factors and cytokines relevant to the initiation and perpetuation of vascular cells.

DRUG-INDUCED CARDIOVASCULAR PROBLEMS

A variety of medications can be administered to HIV-infected patients, and many of these medications are associated with cardiovascular complications (Table 1). Pharmacologically induced cardiomyopathy occurs with AZT treatment of rats and mice (56–58,62,63) when AZT is administered for relatively long duration. Therefore, AZT may have negative clinical impacts in patients with AIDS. Altered mitochondrial deoxyribonucleic acid (mtDNA) replication is a hallmark of AZT. Some reporters (59,60) demonstrated that AZT therapy causes mitochondrial degeneration, swelling, enlargement, vacuolization, fragmentation, and lost cristae in myocytes. In one case, reversal of cardiac dysfunction followed the discontinuation of AZT therapy (60). AZT and dideoxyinosine, two other reverse transcriptase inhibitors used to inhibit replication of HIV, have been proposed as both deterrents to and inducers of cardiomyopathy in humans (61). AZT could inhibit mitochondrial DNA replication. There is also evidence that AZT is associated with myocardial dysfunction in children (61). Other therapeutic agents also have been related to cardiovascular complications in AIDS (62,63). For instance, the chemotherapy currently used for treatment of Kaposi's sarcoma in patients with AIDS includes vincristine, vinblastine, doxorubicin, and alpha interferon. Cardomyopathy is a well-recognized complication of doxorubicin. Alpha interferon has adverse cardiovascular effects, such as hypertension and tachycardia. AIDS patients with multiple infections have to use multiple antibiotics, such as trimethoprim/sulfamethoxazole (TMP/SMX), pentamidine, and amphotericin B. All of these drugs have been associated with cardiac arrest.

Table 1 Cardiotoxicity of Medications Used in the Treatment of AIDS

Drug	Treatment	Adverse effect on the cardiovascular system
AZT	Antiretroviral	Myocarditis and dilated cardiomyopathy
TMP/SMX	Antibacterial	QT prolongation and torsades de pointes
Pentammidine	Antibacterial	QT prolongation and torsades de pointes
Alpha interferon	Antiviral immunomodulator	Arrhythmia, myocardial infarction, cardiomyopathy, sudden death AV block and congestive heart failure
Doxorubicin	Kaposi's sarcoma	Cardiomyopathy
Amphotericin B	Antifungal	Dilated cardiomyopathy, hypertension, and bradycardia
Foscarnet sodium	CMV	Cardiomyopathy
Ganciclovir	CMV	Ventricular tachycardia

Source: Refs. 62 and 63.

NUTRITIONAL DEFICIENCY

The terminal stage of AIDS often involves significant nutritional problems. Selenium and carinitine deficiencies have been noted in malnourished HIV-infected patients and are potentially reversible causes of cardiomyopathy in other settings (64). Vitamin B deficiency can also cause myocardial dysfunction. Kavanaugh-Mchugh found that selenium deficiency is common in pediatric AIDS patients (64), and reversal of cardiomyopathy occurred after selenium supplementation. Multivitamin deficiencies can occur in the terminal stages of AIDS. Indeed, Allard et al. found that vitamin C, alpha-tocopherol, beta-carotene, and selenium concentrations were significantly lower in HIV-positive patients (65). Although there is no evidence to prove malnutrition as a direct factor of cardiomyopathy, decreases in left ventricular volume, ventricular function, and blood pressure have been associated with malnutrition (66).

CONCLUSION

As patient survival increases with more effective antiretroviral therapy, an increasingly prevalent cardiovascular involvement in AIDS has been shown by pathogenesis, pathophysiology, and epidemiology. These conditions may be progressive and disabling or fatal. Therefore cardiovascular dysfunction appears to be an important complication of AIDS. A number of causative factors may involve in cardiovascular complications. These factors may play important roles in cardiovascular involvement in AIDS, but the significant mechanisms are still unclear. Further animal experiments and clinical studies are necessary to clarify the causative factors on cardiovascular complications in AIDS.

ACKNOWLEDGMENT

This work was supported by grants HL 63667 and HL 59794.

REFERENCES

1. www.unaids.org/epidmic update/report dec01/index.html#full. AIDS epidemic update. December 2001
2. Epstein JE, Eichbaum QG, Lipshultz SE. Cardiovascular manifestations of HIV infection. Comp Ther 1996; 22:485–491.
3. Akhras F, Dubrey S, Gazzard B, Noble MI. Emerging patterns of heart disease in HIV infected homosexual subjects with and without opportunistic infections; a prospective colour flow Doppler echocardiographic study. Eur Heart J 1994; 15:68–75.
4. Currie PF, Boon NA. Cardiac involvement in human immunodeficiency virus infection. Q J Med 1993; 86:751–753.
5. Hsia JA, McQuinn LB. AIDS cardiomyopathy. Res Staff Phys 1993; 39:21–24.
6. Johann-Liang R, Cervia JS, Noel GJ. Characteristics of human immunodeficiency virus-infected children at the time of death: an experience in the 1990s. Pediatr Infect Dis J 1997; 16:1145–1150.

7. Bing OH, Sirokman G, Humphries DE. Hypothesis: link between endogenous retroviruses and cardiovascular disease. J Mol Cell Cardiol 1998; 30:1257–1262.

8. Grody WW, Cheng L, Lewis W. Infection of the heart by the human immunodeficiency virus. Am J Cardiol 1990; 66:203–206.

9. Lipshultz SE, Fox CH, Perez-Atayde AR, Sanders SP, Colan SD, McIntosh K, Winter HS. Identification of human immunodeficiency virus-1 RNA and DNA in the heart of a child with cardiovascular abnormalities and congenital acquired immune deficiency syndrome. Am J Cardiol 1990; 66:246–250.

10. Flomenbaum M, Soeiro R, Udem SA, Kress Y, Factor SM. Proliferative membranopathy and human immunodeficiency virus in AIDS hearts. J AIDS 1989; 2:129–135.

11. Calabrese LH, Proffitt MR, Yen-Lieberman B, Hobbs RE, Ratliff N.B. Congestive cardiomyopathy and illness related to the acquired immunodeficiency syndrome (AIDS) associated with isolation of retrovirus from myocardium. Ann Intern Med 1987; 107:691–692.

12. Wu AY, Forouhar F, Cartun RW, Berman MM, Shiue ST, Louie AT, Grunnet M. Identification of human immunodeficiency virus in the heart of a patient with acquired immunodeficiency syndrome. Mod Pathol 1990; 3:625–630.

13. Barbaro G, Di Lorenzo G, Grisorio B, Barbarini G. Incidence of dilated cardiomyopathy and detection of HIV in myocardial cells of HIV-positive patients. N Engl J Med 1998; 339:1093–1099.

14. Mohan P, Sys SU, Brutsaert DL. Mechanisms of endocardial endothelium modulation of myocardial performance. Adv Exp Med Biol 1995; 382:249–260.

15. Bing OH, Sirokman G, Humphries DE. Hypothesis: link between endogenous retroviruses and cardiovascular disease. J Mol Cell Cardiol 1998; 30:1257–1262.

16. National Institute on Drug Abuse. Research Report: Cocaine Abuse and Addiction. Bethesda, MD: NIDA, 1999:4.

17. Mouhaffel AH, Madu EC, Satmary WA, Fraker TD Jr. Cardiovascular complications of cocaine. Chest 1995; 107:1426–1434.

18. Rump AF, Theisohn M, Klaus W. The pathophysiology of cocaine cardiotoxicity. Forensic Sci Int 1995; 71:103–115.

19. Cho S, Matano S, Factor SM. Cardiac lesions in 118 autopsied acquired immune deficiency syndrome patients: intravenous drug abuser vs homosexual. Lab Inves 1989; 60:17.

20. Acierno LJ. Cardiac complications in acquired immunodeficiency syndrome (AIDS). J Am Coll Cardiol 1989; 13:1144–1154.

21. Herskowitz A, Neumann DA, Ansari AA. Concepts of autoimmunity applied to idiopathic dilated cardiomyopathy. J Am Coll Cardiol 1993; 22:1385–1388.

22. Hatillo A, Willis HE, Hess ML. The heart as a target organ of immune injury. Curr Probl Cardiol 1991; 16:377–442.

23. Herskowitz A, Willoughby S, Wu TC, Beschorner WE, Neumann DA, Rose NR, Baughman KL, Ansari AA. Immunopathogenesis of HIV-1-associated cardiomyopathy. Clin Immunol Immunopathol 1993; 68:234–246.

24. Kennedy JR. Does HIV disrupt a naturally occurring immune modulation system? Med Hypoth 1993; 41:445–449.

25. Lieberman EB, Herskowitz A, Rose NR, Baughman KL. A clinicopathologic description of myocarditis. Clin Immunol Immunopathol 1993; 68:191–196.

26. Neumann DA, Lane JR, Allen GS, Herskowitz A, Rose NR. Viral myocarditis leading to cardiomyopathy: do cytokines contribute to pathogenesis? Clin Immunol Immunopathol 1993; 68:181–190.

27. Neumann DA, Rose NR, Ansari AA, Herskowitz A. Induction of multiple heart autoantibodies in mice with coxsackievirus B3– and cardiac myosin–induced autoimmune myocarditis. J Immunol 1994; 152:343–350.

28. Rose NR, Herskowitz A, Neumann DA. Autoimmunity in myocarditis: models and mechanisms. Clin Immunol Immunopathol 1993; 68:95–99.

29. Blanchard DG, Hagenhoff C, Chow LC, McCann HA, Dittrich HC. Reversibility of cardiac abnormalities in human immunodeficiency virus (HIV)-infected individuals: a serial echocardiographic study. J Am Coll Cardiol 1991; 17:1270–1276.

30. Ensoli B, Markham P, Kao V, Barillari G, Fiorelli V, Gendelman R, Raffeld M, Zon G, Gallo RC. Block of AIDS-Kaposi's sarcoma (KS) cell growth, angiogenesis, and lesion formation in nude mice by antisense oligonucleotide targeting basic fibroblast growth factor. A novel strategy for the therapy of KS. J Clin Invest 1994; 94:1736–1746.

31. Lewis W, Grody WW. AIDS and the heart: review and consideration of pathogenetic mechanisms. Cardiovasc Pathol 1992; 1:53–64.

32. Baroldi G, Corallo S, Moroni M, Repossini A, Mutinelli MR, Lazzarin A, Antonacci CM, Cristina S, Negri C. Focal lymphocytic myocarditis in acquired immunodeficiency syndrome (AIDS): a correlative morphologic and clinical study in 26 consecutive fatal cases. J Am Coll Cardiol 1988; 12:463–469.

33. Roldan EO, Moskowitz L, Hensley GT. Pathology of the heart in acquired immunodeficiency syndrome. Arch Pathol Lab Med 1987; 111:943–946.

34. Anderson DW, Virmani R, Reilly JM, O'Leary T, Cunnion RE, Robinowitz M, Macher AM, Punja U, Villaflor ST, Parrillo JE, et al. Prevalent myocarditis at necropsy in the acquired immunodeficiency syndrome. J Am Coll Cardiol 1988; 11:792–799.

35. Treitinger A, Spada C, Verdi JC, Miranda AF, Oliveira OV, Silveira MV, Moriel P, Abdalla DS. Decreased antioxidant defence in individuals infected by the human immunodeficiency virus. Eur J Clin Invest 2000; 30:454–459.

36. Parravicini C, Baroldi G, Gaiera G, Lazzarin A. Phenotype of intramyocardial leukocytic infiltrates in acquired immunodeficiency syndrome (AIDS): a postmortem immunohistochemical study in 34 consecutive cases. Mod Pathol 1991; 4:559–565.

37. Wu TC, Pizzorno MC, Hayward GS, Willoughby S, Neumann DA, Rose NR, Ansari AA, Beschorner WE, Baughman KL, Herskowitz A. In situ detection of human cytomegalovirus immediate-early gene transcripts within cardiac myocytes of patients with HIV-associated cardiomyopathy. AIDS 1992; 6:777–785.

38. Kostianovsky M, Orenstein JM, Schaff Z, Grimley PM. Cytomembranous inclusions observed in acquired immunodeficiency syndrome. Clinical and experimental review. [review]. Arch Pathol Lab Med 1987; 111:218–223.

39. Schimmbeck PL, Schultheiss P, Strauer BE. Identification of a main autoimmunogenic epitope of adenosine nucleotide translocator which cross-reacts with coxsackie B3 virus: use in diagnosis of myocarditis and dilated cardiomyopathy. Circulation 1989; 80(suppl 2):II-665.

40. Gill PS, Chandraratna PA, Meyer PR, Levine AM. Malignant lymphoma: cardiac involvement at initial presentation. J Clin Oncol 1987; 5:216–224.

41. Herskowitz A, Vlahov D, Willoughby S, Chaisson RE, Schulman SP, Neumann DA, Baughman KL. Prevalence and incidence of left ventricular dysfunction in patients with human immunodeficiency virus infection. Am J Cardiol 1993; 71:955–958.

42. Levy WS, Simon GL, Rios JC, Ross AM. Prevalence of cardiac abnormalities in human immunodeficiency virus infection. Am J Cardiol 1989; 63:86–89.

43. Finkel MS, Oddis CV, Jacob TD, Watkins SC, Hattler BG, Simmons RL. Negative inotropic effects of cytokines on the heart mediated by nitric oxide. Science 1992; 257:387–389.

44. Barry WH. Mechanisms of immune-mediated myocyte injury. Circulation 1994; 89:2421–2432.

45. Finkel MS, Hoffman RA, Shen L, Oddis CV, Simmons RL, Hattler BG. Interleukin-6 (IL-6) as a mediator of stunned myocardium. Am J Cardiol 1993; 71:1231–1232.

46. Kawamura T, Inada K, Okada H, Okada K, Wakusawa R. Methylprednisolone inhibits increase of interleukin 8 and 6 during open heart surgery. Can J Anaesth 1995; 42:399–403.

47. Pinsky DJ, Cai B, Yang X, Rodriguez C, Sciacca RR, Cannon PJ. The lethal effects of cytokine-induced nitric oxide on cardiac myocytes are blocked by nitric oxide synthase antagonism or transforming growth factor beta. J Clin Invest 1995; 95:677–685.

48. Pagani FD, Baker LS, Hsi C, Knox M, Fink MP, Visner MS. Left ventricular systolic and diastolic dysfunction after infusion of tumor necrosis factor-alpha in conscious dogs. J Clin Invest 1992; 90:389–398.

49. Vincent JL, Bakker J, Marecaux G, Schandene L, Kahn RJ, Dupont E. Administration of anti-TNF antibody improves left ventricular function in septic shock patients. Results of a pilot study. Chest 1992; 101:810–815.

50. Barbaro G, Di Lorenzo G, Soldini M, Giancaspro G, Grisorio B, Pellicelli A, Barbarini G. Intensity of myocardial expression of inducible nitric oxide synthase influences the clinical course of human immunodeficiency virus–associated cardiomyopathy. Circulation 1999; 100:933–939.

51. Shubeita HE, McDonough PM, Harris AN, Knowlton KU, Glembotski CC, Brown JH, Chien KR. Endothelin induction of inositol phospholipid hydrolysis, sarcomere assembly, and cardiac gene expression in ventricular myocytes. A paracrine mechanism for myocardial cell hypertrophy. J Biol Chem 1990; 265:20555–20562.

52. Colucci WS. Molecular and cellular mechanisms of myocardial failure. Am J Cardiol 1997; 80:15L–25L.

53. Hunter JJ, Chien KR. Signaling pathways for cardiac hypertrophy and failure. N Engl J Med 1999; 341:1276–1283.

54. Wei CM, Lerman A, Rodeheffer RJ, McGregor CG, Brandt RR, Wright S, Heublein DM, Kao PC, Edwards WD, Burnett JC Jr. Endothelin in human congestive heart failure. Circulation 1994; 89:1580–1586.

55. Ensoli B, Buonaguro L, Barillari G, Fiorelli V, Gendelman R, Morgan RA, Wingfield P, Gallo RC. Release, uptake, and effects of extracellular human immunodeficiency virus type 1 Tat protein on cell growth and viral transactivation. J Virol 1993; 67:277–287.

56. Lewis W, Gonzalez B, Chomyn A, Papoian T. Zidovudine induces molecular, biochemical, and ultrastructural changes in rat skeletal muscle mitochondria. J Clin Invest 1992; 89:1354–1360.

57. Lewis W, Papoian T, Gonzalez B, Louie H, Kelly DP, Payne RM, Grody WW. Mitochondrial ultrastructural and molecular changes induced by zidovudine in rat hearts. Lab Invest 1991; 65:228–236.

58. Lewis W, Grupp IL, Grupp G, Hoit B, Morris R, Samarel AM, Bruggeman L, Klotman P. Cardiac dysfunction occurs in the HIV-1 transgenic mouse treated with zidovudine. Lab Invest 2000; 80:187–197.

59. Herskowitz A, Willoughby SB, Baughman KL, Schulman SP, Bartlett JD. Cardiomyopathy associated with antiretroviral therapy in patients with HIV infection: a report of six cases. An Intern Med 1992; 116:311–313.

60. Lewis W, Dalakas MC. Mitochondrial toxicity of antiviral drugs. Nat Med 1995; 1:417–422.

61. Leidig GA Jr. Clinical, echocardiographic, and electrocardiographic resolution of HIV-related cardiomyopathy. Mil Med 1991; 156:260–261.

62. Barbaro G, Lipshultz SE. Pathogenesis of HIV-associated cardiomyopathy. Ann NY Acad Sci 2001; 946:57–81.

63. Fantoni M, Autore C. Drugs and cardiotoxicity in HIV and AIDS. Ann NY Acad Sci 2001; 946:179–199.

64. Kavanaugh-McHugh AL, Ruff A, Perlman E, Hutton N, Modlin J, Rowe S. Selenium deficiency and cardiomyopathy in acquired immunodeficiency syndrome. JPEN 1991; 15:347–349.

65. Allard JP, Aghdassi E, Chau J, Salit I, Walmsley S. Oxidative stress and plasma antioxidant micronutrients in humans with HIV infection. Am J Clin Nutr 1998; 67:143–147.

66. Alden PB, Madoff RD, Dtahl TJ, Ring WS, Cerra FB. Cardiac function in malnutrition. In: Watson RR, ed. Nutrition and Heart Disease. Boca Raton, FL: CRC Press, 1987:71–81.

9

HIV-Associated Vascular Disease and Endothelial Injury

Changyi (Johnny) Chen, Peter H. Lin, Alan B. Lumsden, and Qizhi (Cathy) Yao
Baylor College of Medicine, Houston, Texas, U.S.A.

INTRODUCTION

With the advent of more effective therapies for human immunodeficiency virus (HIV) infection, HIV-infected patients are living longer; therefore HIV-associated disease and complications of antiviral therapy are becoming a significant concern in this population. HIV infection has been associated with the development of endocarditis, myocarditis, pericardial effusions, and dilated cardiomyopathy. Clinical use of HIV protease inhibitors has been associated with metabolic alteration and increased risk for cardiovascular disease. This chapter focuses on HIV-associated vascular disease and endothelial injury. Clinical investigations and possible mechanisms of atherosclerosis, pulmonary hypertension, and thrombosis in HIV-infected patients are discussed. Recent advances in molecular understandings of HIV-associated endothelial injury—including direct HIV infection, expression of cytokines and adhesion molecules, apoptosis, and endothelial permeability—are also discussed. Endothelial injury or dysfunction may contribute significantly to the pathogenesis of vascular disease in HIV-infected patients.

ATHEROSCLEROSIS

Clinical studies have indicated that atherosclerosis may be accelerated following HIV infection. These vascular lesions may involve coronary, peripheral, and cerebral arteries. Accelerated coronary atherosclerosis and arteriosclerosis have been observed in young HIV-positive patients. Autopsy reports were the first to describe an association between coronary artery disease and HIV infection (1,2). Joshi et al. (1) reported coronary artery pathology in an autopsy series of six children infected with HIV. Examination of their coronary arteries revealed inflammation of the endothelium—with lymphocytes and mononuclear giant cells, fragmentation of the elastin fibers, and intimal fibrosis—as well as luminal narrowing. Paton et al. (2) subsequently described a postmortem pathological examination of heart and lung specimens obtained from 8 HIV-seropositive patients. Major eccentric atherosclerotic lesions involving the proximal coronary vessels were discovered in 6 of these patients, who had a mean age of 27 years. The coronary arteries of 4 patients had 80 to 90% obstruction of the arterial lumen. Sclerohyalinosis and interstitial fibrosis of the smaller arteries were also demonstrated. This degree of coronary pathology occurred in the absence of traditionally associated coronary artery disease risk factors, which suggested an association between HIV and coronary artery pathology. Recently, Tabib et al. studied the coronary arteries of 13 men and 2 women who had died at ages ranging from 23 to 32 years after having been infected with HIV-1 virus for 2 to 5 years (3). In all 15 cases, thickening of the intima at least as great as that of the media was observed in the proximal coronary network. Proliferating intimal cells were phenotypically identified as smooth muscle cells, with exaggerated production of elastic fibers and in association with an increase in the expression of tumor necrosis factor alpha (TNF-α) and interleukin-1 (IL-1). In 9 cases, atherosclerosis had developed from this proliferation and on its surface, and in 4 cases arteriosclerosis had an unusual appearance, in the form of mamillated vegetations with endoluminal protrusions. A similar proliferation was found in the distal network in 4 cases, but with a significantly smaller proportion of elastic fibers. A case-control ultrasound study in 30 HIV-positive subjects indicated that atherosclerotic plaques in cervical arteries, the abdominal aorta, and femoral arteries occurred more often than in controls (36.7 versus 11.1%) (4). Nair et al. reported that 21 HIV-positive patients with mean age of 37 years had occlusive arterial disease. All patients had critical ischemia, involving the upper limbs in 4 and the lower limbs in 16 (5). In addition, many clinical and autopsy studies have suggested an increased incidence of strokes in HIV-infected patients, including children and young adults. Cerebral infarction in AIDS patients has been reported from as ranging 4 to 29% (6–10). These lesions may result from cerebral artery aneurysm formation and arteriosclerosis with occlusion. HIV infection may also cause endothelial damage and predispose to atherosclerotic disease through its effect on triglyceride levels. Hypertriglyceridemia was well described in AIDS patients before the introduction of protease inhibitor therapy and has been associated with elevations of circulating interferon gamma (IFN-γ) (11). Bobryshev et al. reported that there were significantly more HIV-1–infected dentritic cells in the atherosclerotic arteries than in the nondiseased segments by immunohistochemical staining and indicated that the accumulation of HIV-1 in dendritic cells in the arterial wall may influence the progression of atherosclerosis (12). HIV viral proteins may be able to affect smooth muscle cell proliferation, which is a major event of vascular lesion formation. HIV gp120 was a potent mitogen for rat smooth muscle cells (SMCs) in vitro (13). This effect seems to be mediated via gp120 sequences related to neuropeptide Y (13). Several mechanisms of HIV-induced endothelial injury or dysfunction described below may contribute to the formation of atherosclerosis and its exacerbation in HIV infected patients.

THROMBOSIS

HIV-associated deep venous thrombosis (DVT) in the lower extremities has been reported (14–16). Its incidence is about 1%, which is approximately 10 times greater than in the general population (16,17). Saber et al. reported 45 cases in patients with a mean age of 43 years (16). The distribution of the thromboses involved the femoral vein in 23 patients, the popliteal vein in 20 patients, and the iliofemoral system in 2 patients. Twelve patients had recurrent DVT and 3 developed a pulmonary embolism. Thrombosis in a retinal vein (18–20), cerebral vein (21), portal vein (21,22), brachial artery (23), and celiac artery (24) has also been reported. There is a significant correlation between thrombotic disease and CD4 cell counts ($<200/mm^3$) as well as the presence of opportunistic infections, AIDS-related neoplasms, or autoimmune disorders associated with HIV, such as autoimmue hemolytic anemia (25–27). In addition, widespread digital ischemia, with gangrene and malignant atrophic papulosis, which causes infarctive thrombosis of the skin and viscera, has been reported in HIV infection (28,29). Thrombotic microangiopathy, perhaps the second most common renal lesion seen in AIDS, causes intra- and extraglomerular arteriolar thrombus formation and is the hallmark histological lesion of hemolytic uremic syndrome and thrombotic thrombocytopenic purpura (TTP) (30–32), two AIDS-associated syndromes. TTP is a disorder characterized by intravascular platelet aggregates with abundant von Willebrand factor (vWF) in the thrombotic lesions (33). A recent study has demonstrated complete deficiency of vWF-cleaving protease and the presence of a concentration-dependent IgG1 inhibitor in the plasma of a patient with AIDS (34).

The pathogenesis of the increased risk of thrombosis in HIV-infected patients is not completely understood but is probably of a multifactorial nature. The prevalence of lupus anticoagulant in HIV infection has ranged as high as 70% (35). Anticardiolipin antibodies have been reported in 46 to 90% of HIV-infected patients (36). Sugerman et al. have reported that acquired protein-S deficiency is common in HIV-infected children (75%) and significantly more prevalent in those with a CD4 count $<200/cm^3$ (37). Another physiological coagulation inhibitor, heparin cofactor II, has also been reported to be deficient in HIV infection. Other possible contributing factors are hypoalbuminemia-related fibrin polymerization defects, endothelial dysfunction, and abnormalities of the fibrinolytic system (35). Various markers of endothelial cell damage—such as vWF, soluble thrombomodulin (sTM), adhesion molecule E-selectin, tissue-type plasminogen activator (t-PA), plasminogen activator inhibitor (PA-I), fibronectin, angiotensin-converting enzyme (ACE), and endothelin—have been shown to be increased in the course of HIV-1 infection (38–42). The secretion of t-PA, PA-I, sTM, and vWF creates alterations in the coagulation cascade and could predispose to thrombosis. Furthermore, HIV gp120 could induce tissue factor expression of vascular SMCs, which may have potential effects on the arterial wall's thrombogenicity (43).

PULMONARY HYPERTENSION

Pulmonary hypertension in an HIV-infected patient with hemophilia and membranoproliferative glomerulonephritis was first reported in 1987 (44). Subsequently, in 1988, 5 cases of classical hemophilia with HIV infection and pulmonary hypertension were reported (45). Initially, pulmonary hypertension in these cases was considered to be secondary to hemophilia or to the use of the therapeutically lyophilized factor VII concentrate. Thereafter, many cases of HIV-related pulmonary hypertension have been described in patients for whom no factor other than the HIV infection could explain the presence of pulmonary hypertension (46). The incidence of HIV-associated pulmonary hypertension is estimated to be 1 in 200, much higher than the 1 in 200,000 found in the general population (47). In a large series of case reports, pulmonary hypertension in HIV infection showed plexogenic pulmonary arteriopathy in 95% cases. Intimal fibrosis was revealed in the remaining 5% of patients (48). The plexiform lesion is a complex multichannel lesion of proliferative vascular endothelium with proximal luminal narrowing that is produced by a dysregulation of endothelial cell growth. Similarly, in an animal study of monkeys infected with simian immunodeficiency virus (SIV), 22% of monkeys developed an arteriopathy similar to that seen in HIV-related pulmonary hypertension (49). The exact mechanism of the development of pulmonary hypertension in HIV infection is not clear, although several hypotheses have been proposed (50). Increased expression of intrapulmonary platelet-derived growth factor (PDGF) has been demonstrated in cases of HIV-associated pulmonary vasculopathy (51). Exogenous Tat protein, an HIV gene product that functions as a transcription activator for HIV replication, has been shown to have synergy with TNF-α to activate endothelial cells, a process that directly results in the release of epidermal growth factor (EGF), transforming growth factor beta (TGF-β), platelet-derived growth factor (PDGF), and IL-6 (52,53). Increased expression of VEGF-A in T cells has been demonstrated in cases of HIV infection (54). VEGF-A increases vascular permeability and is a potent mitogen of endothelial cells. HIV may cause endothelial damage and mediator-related vasoconstriction through stimulation by the envelope gp 120, including direct release and effects of endothelin-1 (vasoconstrictor), IL-6, and TNF-α in the pulmonary arteries (55,56). HIV gp120 stimulates the production of endothelin-1 in a concentration-dependent manner (57). Chronically increased expression of endothelin-1 has been found in patients with HIV infection (58). Endothelin-1 acts as a vasoconstrictor and mitogen and thus may contribute to the proliferation of endothelia and SMCs in the pulmonary vascular bed. A decrease in the expression of prostacyclin synthase (the enzyme that produces prostacyclin) has also been demonstrated in HIV-infected patients (59). These elevated levels of endothelin-1 and decreased levels of prostacyclin, combined with abnormal regulation of the vasodilation/vasoconstriction balance and the endothelial cell and SMC proliferation, contribute to elevated pulmonary arterial pressure.

HIV INFECTION

The ability of HIV to infect endothelial cells is controversial. In certain types of endothelial cells or under certain conditions, actual infection of endothelial cells by HIV has been reported. In tissue obtained from HIV-infected patients, bone marrow microvascular endothelial cells (MEC) (60) as well as placental (61–63), retinal (64), and brain microvascular endothelial cells (MEC) (65–67) have shown staining for HIV antigens. In human brain MEC, HIV infection occurred in a CD4- and galactosyl ceramide–independent manner and suggested the presence of a unique cell surface receptor for HIV (68). The V3 loop of gp120 was important in the human brain MEC tropism of HIV. T cell–tropic, not macrophage–tropic, strains of HIV were capable of selectively infecting endothelium (69). In monkey models, SIV was able to infect brain MEC in a CD4-independent pathway involving CCR5 (70,71). Hepatic sinusoid endothelial cells have been found to express the CD4 cell marker (72), which is a pivotal cellular receptor required for the invasion of HIV. Indeed, Steffan et al. reported that the human liver sinusoid endothelial cell is permissive for HIV infection (73). In vitro study showed that 30 to 50% hepatic sinusoidal endothelial cells were infected by HIV (74). However, human umbilical vein endothelial cells (HUVEC) were less permissive for HIV. HIV particles could enter cells in a CD4-independent fashion and showed low level viral replication (0.02% of infected cells) (74). HIV was able to bind to HUVEC, but the virus was incapable of replicating in nonproliferating cultures. However, when endothelial cells were stimulated with IL-1 and TNF-α, viral adsorption and release were observed (75). In untreated cultures, the *gag* gene was expressed for a mean of 15 days, whereas stimulated endothelial cells continued to express the gag gene for over 20 days. Infection of proliferating HUVEC cultures released both p24 antigen and infectious virus (75). Furthermore, HUVEC infection with HIV probably occurs through a galactosyl ceramide receptor, as the CD4 receptor is not expressed on these cells (74–76). In another study, HIV infection of HUVEC and colon carcinoma cell lines was detected by the presence of p24 antigen in culture supernatants and HIV spliced RNA in cells (77). Again, this infection could not be blocked by an anti-CD4 antibody (18,76). Coculture of HIV-infected HUVEC with T cells allowed transfer of virus from HUVEC to T cells in an adhesion-dependent manner (78). This process was significantly enhanced by treatment with IFN-γ, which increased ICAM-1 expression and endothelium and T-cell interaction (78). Endothelial cells obtained from adipose tissue also showed susceptibility to HIV infection in vitro (79,80). Following infection of HIV, the presence of p24 and reverse transcriptase activity was detected in supernatants of endothelial cell cultures. Treatment with cyclohexamide decreased viral rescue, implying de novo synthesis of viral particles. Glomerular endothelial cells isolated from kidney were also permissive to HIV infection. When glomerular endothelial cells were cocultured with mononuclear cells, expression of p24 antigen was detected intra- and extracellularly, syncytia formation was observed, and HIV DNA was detected by PCR (81). HIV-1 does not possess the ability to infect certain types of endothelial cells. For example, Ades et al. demonstrated a lack of permissiveness of a line of immortalized human microvascular endothelial cells (HMEC-1) for HIV infection (82). In addition, two dual-tropic HIV-1 isolates failed to infect human lung microvascular endothelial cells (HLMEC) (83).

CYTOKINES AND ADHESION MOLECULES

Many clinical studies have demonstrated that endothelial injury and/or activation occurs in AIDS patients. Correlations have been discovered between levels of circulating VCAM-1 and decreased CD4 counts and increases in levels of TNF-α and neopterin (84). Nordoy et al. found higher levels of the soluble adhesion molecule sICAM-1 and sVCAM-1 in sera of HIV-infected patients compared to uninfected controls (84), while both sICAM-1 and sVCAM-1 correlated with TNF-α and neopterin levels. Aortic endothelial injury was manifested as enhanced cell surface expression of cell adhesion molecules, enhanced leukocyte adherence, and disturbed arrangement of cells compared to uninfected control individuals (85). In the brain tissue of patients with AIDS suffering from encephalitis, infiltration of macrophages was associated with increased levels of endothelial adhesion molecules. Expression of

E-selectin and VCAM-1 on endothelial cells paralleled expression of HIV gene products (86). Birdsall et al. found that transendothelial migration of CD4+ T cells in HIV-infected individuals was greatly enhanced (87). TNF-α is an inflammatory cytokine that has been shown to be secreted in large amounts by HIV-infected macrophages; it can activate endothelial function as well as enhance adhesion (88,89). The degree of lymphocyte migration was shown to correlate directly with expression of TNF-α. In in vitro cell culture, HIV particles could increase ICAM-1 expression of brain microvascular endothelial cells (BMECS) (90). HIV Tat activates mononuclear cells to secrete cytokines. Tat has also been shown to activate endothelial cells to express inflammatory cytokines and adhesion molecules and contribute to angiogenesis and the development of Kaposi's sarcoma (KS) (91,92). The endothelial receptor for Tat that binds and mediates angiogenesis appears to be Flk-1/KDR, which is a VEGF-A tyrosine kinase receptor (93). Tat protein can stimulate brain-derived endothelial cells to rapidly express IL-6 mRNA (94). This pathway appears to be dependent on activation of protein kinase A (PKA) and C (PKC), which occurred even at very low doses of Tat (10 ng/mL). Hofman et al. activated endothelial cells with Tat protein and showed that these cells expressed E-selectin, IL-6, and IL-8 (53,95). IL-6 is considered an acute-phase cytokine and can increase endothelial cell permeability, while IL-8 is chemotactic to leukocytes and assists in inflammatory cell recruitment. Dhawan et al. showed upregulation of adhesion molecules in HUVEC activated by Tat protein (96). Following exposure of HUVEC to Tat protein, surface expression of the adhesion molecules, ICAM-1, VCAM-1, and E-selectin were shown to increase rapidly, a process blocked by anti-Tat antibody. Tat contributes to endothelial cell activation by activating nuclear factor-κB (NF-κB) (97). Since NF-κB is essential for the activation of inflammatory cytokine and adhesion molecule genes, this has relevance to endothelial activation, because disorders such as atherosclerosis are characterized by endothelial activity of NF-κB (98). Tat protein also induced monocyte chemoattractant protein-1 (MCP-1) expression in brain astrocytes (99) and human lung microvascular endothelial cells (100). Increased MCP-1 expression resulted in the monocyte transmigration across the endothelial cells. PKC was involved in the signal transduction pathway of Tat-induced MCP-1 expression. In addition, Tat upregulated expression of the chemokine receptor CCR5 on monocytes in a time-dependent manner. HIV gp120 has several effects relevant to endothelial cell function. HIV gp120 has been shown to induce monocyte expression of proinflammatory cytokines, which could activate endothelial cells. HIV gp120 protein was able to activate monocytes and to increase expression of prostaglandin E2 and IL-1 in a dose-dependent manner (101). Both IL-1 and prostanoids can have profound effects on endothelial function with adhesive processes (102,103). Bragardo et al. studied two types of events mediating T cell–endothelial adhesion: dynamic adhesion mediated by selectins and static adhesion mediated by integrins; they showed that gp120 enhanced dynamic adhesion involving CD31, CD38, and CD49d (104). Gp120 alone could also quickly cause monocytes to adhere to endothelial cells (105). Soluble gp120 activated human brain microvascular endothelial cells (HBMEC) derived from children in upregulating ICAM-1 and VCAM-1 expression, IL-6 secretion and increased monocyte transmigration across monolayer in vitro. This study also demonstrated that the endothelial cells expressed CD4, which seemed to mediate gp120 effect (106). In a HIV-1 gp120 transgenic mouse model, ICAM-1, VCAM-1, and substance P were highly expressed in brain vessel endothelial cells, and there was a significant correlation between substance P and ICAM-1 expression (107). Furthermore, gp120 was able to enhance the TNF-α–mediated activation of NF-κB in Jurkat cells accompanied by increased formation of reactive intermediates such as H_2O_2 (108). Recently, we demonstrated that both soluble gp120 and membrane-associated gp120 on virus-like particles could induce ICAM-1 expression on several types of human endothelial cells in vitro and then increase monocyte adhesion on the gp120-treated endothelial monolayers. VCAM-1 and E-selectin were not affected by gp120 treatment (109).

APOPTOSIS

HIV-1–induced CD4+ T-cell apoptosis is a major mechanism of HIV pathogenesis. HIV-1 is also able to induce apoptosis in other types of cells, including endothelial cells. Endothelial apoptosis can impair endothelial integrity and function, thereby contributing to vascular lesion formation. In brain tissue obtained from AIDS patients, apoptosis of microvascular endothelial cells from small and medium-sized blood vessels was oberved using terminal deoxynucleotidyl transferase–mediated dUTP nick end-labeling (TUNEL), propiodium iodide staining, and electron microscopy (110). The occurrence of this apoptosis is distant from HIV-infected cells, suggesting the existence of soluble factors rather than direct viral infection for endothelial apoptosis. Apoptosis was also seen in astrocytes in brain tissue from AIDS patients (110). In brain tissue obtained from macaque monkeys infected with SIV, the occurrence of apoptosis in endothelial cells as well as neurons was demonstrated (111). There was an association between apoptotic endothelial and neural cells and perivascular inflammatory infiltrates of infected macrophages and giant cells. In an HIV-1 transgenic rat model, expression of the transgene, consisting of an HIV-1 provirus with a functional deletion of *gag* and *pol*, is regulated by the viral long-terminal repeat. Capillaries and endothelial cells in the brain tissue presented with atypical changes such as microscopic hemorrhages and endothelial cell apoptosis in a multifocal distribution (112). HIV proteins such as Tat and gp120 may be able to induce endothelial apoptosis. Park et al. reported that Tat caused apoptosis of primary microvascular endothelial cells of lung origin by a mechanism distinct from TNF secretion or the Fas pathway (113). This apoptosis occurred without induction of either Fas or TNF. Tat treatment increased the activity of caspase 3 but not caspase 9. Tat-induced apoptosis did not involve changes in bcl-2, Bax, and Bad regulatory proteins. Tat-derived peptides were also able to induce endothelial apoptosis (114). Treatment with Tat 21–40 or 23–34 peptides increased the percentage of apoptotic cells in HUVEC and also blocked the antiapoptotic effect of VEGF. Tat 27–38 peptide produced a similar striking apoptotic effect. Tat 46–57 peptide alone caused a modest increase in annexin V staining but completely blocked VEGF-induced antiapoptosis. Several studies have demonstrated the effect of HIV gp120 on endothelial apoptosis. Huang et al. reported that short exposure of HUVEC cultures to soluble gp120 caused significant levels of apoptosis with the biphasic nature of gp120 titration curves, suggesting that multiple cellular factors might be involved in the effect (115). The apoptotic effect was mediated through two cell surface receptors (CCR5 and CXCR4) on HUVECs and protein kinase C activation (115,116). Further studies revealed that gp120 on cell membranes or on virion particles was even more potent inducer of endothelial apoptosis than soluble gp120 (117). Caspases played an important role in this process, because the pretreatment of cells with a general caspase enzyme inhibitor decreased the extent of HUVEC apoptosis induced by gp120/160 (118). In fact, caspase 3 was activated and proapoptotic molecule Bax was increased by HUVECs following gp120/160 treatment (118). In addition, recombinant gp120 was able to induce apoptosis in human lung microvascular endothelial cells (HLMEC) (119).

ENDOTHELIAL PERMEABILITY

HIV-associated dementia occurs in about one-third of HIV-1 infected individuals (120,121). HIV-1 affects the central nervous system (CNS) early in almost every infected individual, and the subsequent decline of CNS function can affect quality of life and prognosis negatively. Several pathologic studies on brain tissues of HIV-positive autopsy cases have provided evidence of possible impairment of the blood-brain barrier (BBB) in the early stages of HIV infection occurring without neurological signs (122,123). Rhodes reported that the brain tissues obtained from AIDS patients with CNS lesions had serum protein immunoreactivity in some neurons, glial cells, gliomesenchymal cells, nodules, vascular endothelial cells, inflammatory cells, or microvascular walls (122). Petito and Cash demonstrated abnormalities of the BBB in the brain tissue of AIDS patients by immunohistochemical detection of fibrinogen and immunoglobulin G as the markers of vascular permeability (123). HIV antigen and specific antibody were also detected within the BBB in patients with AIDS as well as in the experimentally infected chimpanzees (124). In addition, an HIV-associated ocular microangiopathic syndrome is well documented (125). Clinical and morphological studies of ocular tissue from HIV-1–infected patients revealed endothelial permeability and vascular leakage (126). Alteration of endothelial barrier function in HIV-infected patients may also contribute to atherosclerosis and other vascular complications. The mechanisms of HIV-associated endothelial permeability are currently under active investigation. HIV gp120 has been shown to alter endothelial cell permeability. In a rat brain endothelial cell culture model, HIV-1 gp120 increased the permeability of the endothelium to albumin in a dose-dependent manner (127). Scanning electron microscopy revealed gp120-induced alterations in cell morphology, accounting for the increased permeability to macromolecules. The effect was blocked by anti-gp120 antibody, antisubstance P antibody, and spantide (a substance P antagonist). Following exposure to gp120, endothelial cells showed surface immunoreactivity for substance P, a molecule commonly associated with pain fiber transmission and inflammation-like responses. The investigators concluded that substance P was induced in brain endothelium by gp120 and bound to endothelial cells through a receptor-mediated mechanism, leading to some of the observed changes in function (127). In HIV-1 gp120 transgenic mice, the number of vessels with albumin extravasation in the brain was significantly higher than in the brains of nontransgenic mice (128). Substance P staining on endothelium and enhanced endothelial expression of ICAM-1 and VCAM-1 were also observed. More interestingly, a significant correlation was found between the number of vessels that were ICAM-1 positive and those positive for substance-P staining. These studies suggest that substance P plays a role in the gp120-mediated stimulation of rat brain endothelial cultures (128). HIV-1 gp120 was able to cross mice brain endothelial cells with a possible mechanism of lectin-like adsorptive endocytosis after intravenous injection of gp120 into mice (129). Wheat-germ agglutinin significantly increased the uptake of gp120 (129,130). Glycosylation of gp120 was critical for its uptake by adsorptive endocytosis, since the nonglycosylated form of gp120 was unaffected by wheat-germ agglutinin (131). This uptake of gp120 was significantly enhanced by lipopolysaccharide (131). Injection with HIV pseudoviruses also showed the uptake of brain tissue with gp120-dependent manner because viruses with mutant gp120 were not able to cross the BBB in mice (132). Recent studies indicate that HIV-1 entered brain microvascular endothelial cells in ICAM-1–lined macropinosomes by a mechanism involving lipid rafts, MAPK signaling, and glycosylaminoglycans, while CD4 and chemokine receptors played limited roles in this process (90). Tat may also have the ability to affect endothelial permeability. HUVEC monolayers treated with Tat showed a significant increase of albumin permeability in a dose-dependent manner (133,134). The blocker experiments suggested that tyrosine kinase and MAP kinase pathways, but not protein kinase G pathways, may mediated Tat-induced endothelial permeability (134). Tat was able to increase endothelial permeability in animal models (133,135). Tat synergized with bFGF in inducing vascular permeability and edema in guinea pigs and nude mice after systemic or local injection of Tat and bFGF (135).

SUMMARY

HIV-associated vascular disease and endothelial injury have become a significant clinical problem in HIV infection since, due to current advances in antiviral therapy, the mortality has decreased. There is strong evidence indicating the higher incidence of atherosclerosis, thrombosis, and pulmonary hypertension in HIV-infected patients. HIV is able to infect some types of endothelial cells under certain conditions. HIV and its viral proteins, Tat and gp120, are able to induce expression of several adhesion molecules and cytokines, such as ICAM-1, VCAM-1, E-selectin, TNF-α, and IL-6. This effect promotes the infiltration of inflammatory cells into tissues and causes tissue damage. In addition, HIV and its viral proteins can also induce endothelial apoptosis and increase endothelial permeability. These effects could significantly contribute to the formation of vascular disease. However, the molecular mechanisms of HIV-associated vascular disease and endothelial injury are not clear, although some direct and indirect effects of HIV infection on vascular systems are being studied. Recently, active investigations have been undertaken to elucidate HIV pathogenesis in vascular systems and develop new strategies to treat and prevent HIV-associated cardiovascular disease.

ACKNOWLEDGMENTS

This work was supported by NIH HL61943, HL65916, and HL72716 (C. Chen) and NIH AI49116 and DE15543 (Q. Yao).

REFERENCES

1. Joshi VV, Pawel B, Conner E, et al. Arteriopathy in children with AIDS. Pediatr Pathol 1987; 7:261–275.

2. Paton P, Tabib A, Loire R, Tete R. Coronary artery lesions and human immunodeficiency virus infection. Res Virol 1993; 144:225–231.

3. Tabib A, Leroux C, Mornex JF, Loire R. Accelerated coronary atherosclerosis and arteriosclerosis in young human immunodeficiency virus–positive patients [pathophysiology and natural history]. Coron Artery Dis 2000; 11:41–46.

4. Constants J, Marchand JM, Conri C, Peuchant E, Seigneur M, Rispal P, Lasseur C, Pellegrin JL, Leng B. Asymptomatic atherosclerosis in HIV-positive patients: a case-control ultrasound study. Ann Med 1995; 27:683–685.

5. Nair R, Robbs JV, Chetty R, Naidoo NG, Woolgar J. Occlusive arterial disease in HIV-infected patients: a preliminary report. Eur J Vasc Endovasc Surg 2000; 20:353–357.

6. Pinto AN. AIDS and cerebrovascular disease. Stroke 1996; 27:538–543.

7. Berger JR, Harris JO, Gregorios J, Norenberg M. Cerebrovascular disease in AIDS: a case-control study. AIDS 1990; 4:239–244.

8. Mizusawa H, Hirano A, Llena JF, Shintaku M. Cerebrovascular lesions in acquired immune deficiency syndrome (AIDS). Acta Neuropathol 1988; 76:451–457.

9. Rhodes RH. Histopathologic features in the central nervous system of 400 acquired immunodeficiency syndrome cases: implications of rates of occurrence. Hum Pathol 1993; 24:1189–1198.

10. Connor MD, Lammie GA, Bell JE, Warlow CP, Simmonds P, Brettle RD. Cerebral infarction in adult AIDS patients. Stroke 2002; 31:2117–2126.

11. Grunfeld C, Kotler DP, Hamadeh R, Tierney A, Wang J, Pierson RN. Hypertriglyceridemia in the acquired immunodeficiency syndrome. Am J Med 1989; 86:27–31.

12. Bobryshev YV, Cherian SM, Tran D. Identification of HIV-1 in the aortic wall of AIDS patients. Atherosclerosis 2000; 152:529–530.

13. Kim J, Ruff M, Karwatowska-Prokopczuk E, Hunt L, Ji H, Pert CB, Zukowska-Grojec Z. HIV envelope protein gp120 induces neuropeptide Y receptor-mediated proliferation of vascular smooth muscle cells: relevance to AIDS cardiovascular pathogenesis. Regul Pept 1998; 75–76:201–205.

14. Cohen JR, Lackner R, Wenig P, Pillari G. Deep venous thrombosis in patients with AIDS. NY State J Med 1990; 90:159–161.

15. Becker DM, Saunders TJ, Wispelwey B, et al. Case report: Venous thromboembolism in AIDS. Am J Med Sci 1992; 303:395–397.

16. Saber AA, Aboolian A, LaRaja RD, Baron H, Hanna K. HIV/AIDS and the risk of deep vein thrombosis: a study of 45 patients with lower extremity involvment. Am Surg 2001; 67:645–647.

17. Nordstrom M, Lindblad B, Bergquist D, et al. A prospective study of the incidence of deep-vein thrombosis within a defined urban population. J Intern Med 1992; 232:155–160.

18. Roberts SP, Haefs TMP. Central retinal vein occlusion in middle-aged adults with HIV infection. Optom Vis Sci 1992; 69:567–569.

19. Park KL, Marx JL, Lopez PF, Rao NA. Noninfectious branch retinal vein occlusion in HIV-positive patients. Retina 1997; 17:162–164.

20. Freidman SM, Margo CE. Bilateral central retinal vein occlusions in a patient with acquired immunodeficiency syndrome. Res Opthalmol 1995; 113:1184–1188.

21. Carr A, Brown D, Cooper DA. Portal vein thrombosis in patients reveiving indiavir, an HIV protease inhibitor. AIDS 1997; 11:1657–1658.

22. Narayanan TS, Narawane NM, Phadke AY, Abraham P. Multiple abdominal venous thrombosis in HIV-seropositive patient. Indian J Gastroenterol 1998; 17:105–106.

23. Witz M, Lehmann J, Korzets Z. Acute brachial artery thrombosis as the initial manifestation of human immunodeficiency virus infection. Am J Hematol 2000; 64:137–139.

24. Aouad K, Bouillot JL, Piketty C, et al. Splenic infarction in a HIV infected patient. Apropos of a case report and review of the literature. J Chir (Paris) 1996; 133:392–395 (French).

25. Saif MW, Bona R, Greenberg B. AIDS and thrombosis: retrospective study of 131 HIV-infected patients. AIDS Patient Care STDS 2001; 15:311–320.

26. Saif MW, Greenberg B. HIV and thrombosis: a review. AIDS Patient Care STDS 2001; 15:15–24.

27. Copur AS, Smith PR, Gomez V, Bergman M, Homel P. HIV infection is a risk factor for venous thromboembolism. AIDS Patient Care STDS 2002; 16:205–209.

28. Roh SS, Gertner E. Digital necrosis in acquired immune deficiency syndrome vasculopathy treated with recombinant tissue plasminogen activator. J Rheumatol 1997; 24:2258–2261.

29. Requena L, Farina C, Barat A. Degos disease in a patient with acquired immunodeficiency syndrome. J Am Acad Dermatol 1998; 38:852–856.

30. Eitner F, Cui Y, Hudkins KL, et al. Thrombotic microangiopathy in the HIV-2-infected macaque. Am J Pathol 1999; 155:649–661.

31. Gadallah MF, el-Shahawy MA, Campese VM, et al. Disparate prognosis of thrombotic microangiopathy in HIV-infected patients with and without AIDS. Am J Nephrol 1996; 16:446–450.

32. Sutor GC, Schmidt RE, Albrecht H. Thrombotic microangiopathies and HIV infection: report of two typical cases, features of HUS and TTP, and review of the literature. Infection 1999; 27:12–15.

33. Asada Y, Sumiyoshi A, Hayashi T, Suzumiya J, Kaketani K. Immunohistochemistry of vasculae lesion in thrombotic thrombocytopenic purpura, with special reference to factor VIII antigen. Thromb Res 1985; 38:469–479.

34. Sahud MA, Claster S, Liu L, Ero M, Harris K, Furlan M. von Willebrand factor–cleaving protease inhibitor in a patient with human immunodeficiency syndrome–associated thrombotic thrombocytopenic purpura. Br J Haematol 2002; 16:909–911.

35. Toulon P. Hemostasis and human immunodeficiency virus (HIV) infection. Ann Biol Clin (Paris) 1998; 56:153–160 (French).

36. Coyle TE. Hematologic complications of human immunodeficiency virus infection and the acquired immunodeficiency syndrome. Med Clin North Am 1997; 81:449–470.

37. Sugerman RW, Church JA, Goldsmith JC, et al. Acquired protein S deficiency in children infected with human immunodeficiency virus. Pediatr Infect Dis J 1996; 15:106–111.

38. Schved JF, Gris JC, Arnaud A, Martinez P, Sanchez N, Wautier JL, Sarlat C. von Willebrand factor agntigen, tissue-type plasminogen activator antigen, and reisk of death in human immunodeficiency virus 1-related clinical disease: independent prognostic relevance of tissue-type plasminogen activator. J Lab Clin Med 1992; 120:411–419.

39. Lafeuillade A, Alessi MC, Poizot-Martin I, Boyer-Neumann C, Zandotti C, Quilichini R, Aubert L, Tamalet C, Juhan-Vague I, Gastaut JA. Endothelial cell dysfunction in HIV infection. J AIDS 1992; 5:127–131.

40. Rolinsky B, Geier SA, Sadri I, Klauss V, Bogner JR, Ehrenreich H, Goebel FD. Endothelin-1 immunoreactivity in plasma is elevated in HIV-1 infected patients with retinal microangiopathic syndrome. Clin Invest 1994; 72:288–293.

41. Seigneur M, Constans J, Blann A, Renard M, Pellegrin JL, Amiral J, Boisseau M, Conri C. Soluble adhesion molecules and endothelial cell damage in HIV infected patients. Thromb Haemost 1997; 77:646–649.

42. Hadigan C, Meigs JB, Rabe J, D'Agostino RB, Wilson PW, Lipinska I, Tofler GH, Grinspoon SS. Increased PAI-1 and tPA antigen levels are reduced with metformin therapy in HIV-infected patients with fat redistribution and insulin resistance. J Clin Endocrinol Metab 2001; 86:939–943.

43. Schecter AD, Berman AB, Yi Lin A, Mosoian CM, McManus JW, Berman ME, Klotman MB. HIV envelope gp120 activates human arterial smooth muscle cells. PNAS 2001; 98:10142–10147.

44. Kim KK, Factor SM. Membranoproliferative glomerulonephritis and plexogenic pulmonary arteriopathy in a homosexual man with acquired immunodeficiency syndrome. Hum Pathol 1987; 18:1293–1296.

45. Goldsmith GH Jr, Baily RG, Brettler DB, et al. Primary pulmonary hypertension in patients with classic hemophilia. Ann Intern Med 1988; 108:797–799.

46. Mehta NJ, Khan IA, Mehta RN, Sepkowitz DA. HIV-related pulmonary hypertension. Analytic review of 131 cases. Chest 2000; 118:1133–1141.

47. Cool CD, Stewart JS, Werahera P, et al. Three-dimensional reconstruction of pulmonary arteries in plexiform pulmonary hypertension using cell-specific markers: evidence for a dynamic and heterogeneous process of pulmonary endothelial cell growth. Am J Pathol 1999; 155:411–419.

48. Rerkpattanapipat P, Wongpraparut N, Jacobs LE, Kotler MN. Cardiac manifestations of acquired immunodeficiency syndrome. Arch Intern Med 2000; 60:602–608.

49. Chalifoux LV, Simon MA, Pauley DR, et al. Arteriopathy in macaques infected with simian immunodeficiency virus. Lab Invest 1992; 67:338–349.

50. Mette SA, Palevsky HI, Pietra GG, et al. Primary pulmonary hypertension in association with human immunodeficiency virus infection: a possible viral etiology for some forms of hypertensive pulmonary arteriopathy. Am Rev Respir Dis 1992; 145:1196–1200.

51. Humbert M, Monti G, Fartoukh M, et al. Platelet-derived growth factor expression in primary pulmonary hypertension: comparison of HIV seropositive and HIV seronegative patients. Eur Respir J 1998; 11:554–559.

52. Voelkel NF, Tuder RM. Cellular and molecular mechanisms in pathogenesis of severe pulmonary hypertension. Eur Respir J 1995; 8:2129–2138.

53. Hofman FM, Wright AD, Dohadwala MM, et al. Exogenous tat protein activates human endothelial cells. Blood 1993; 82:2774–2780.

54. Ascheri G, Hohendl C, Schatz O, et al. Infection with human immunodeficiency virus-1 increases expression of vascular endothelial cell growth factor in T cells: implications for acquired immunodeficiency syndrome-associated vasculopathy. Blood 1999; 93: 4232–4241.

55. Pellicelli AM, Barbaro G, Palmieri F, et al. Primary pulmonary hypertension in HIV disease: a systematic review. Angiology 2001; 52:31–41.

56. Pellicelli AM, Palmieri F, D'Ambrosio C, et al. Role of human immunodeficiency virus in primary pulmonary hypertension: case reports. Angiology 1998; 49:1005–1011.

57. Ehrenreich H, Rieckmann P, Sinowatz F, et al. Potent stimulation of monocytic endothelin-1 production by HIV-1 glycoprotein 120. J Immunol 1993; 150:4601–4609.

58. Mesa RA, Edell ES, Dunn WF, Edwards WD. Human immunodeficiency virus infection and pulmonary hypertension. Mayo Clin Proc 1998; 73:37–44.

59. Nichols WC, Koller DL, Slovis B, et al. Localization of the gene for familial primary pulmonary hypertension to chromosome 2q31-32. Nat Genet 1997; 15:277–280.

60. Moses AV, Williams S, Heneveld ML, Strussenberg J, Rarick M, Loveless M, Bagby G, Nelson JA. Human immunodeficiency virus infection of bone marrow endothelium reduces induction of stromal hematopoietic growth factors. Blood 1996; 87:919–925.

61. Martin AW, Brady K, Smith SI, DeCoste D, Page DV, Malpica A, Wolf B, Neiman RS. Immunohistochemical localization of human immunodeficiency virus p24 antigen in placental tissue. Hum Pathol 1992; 23:411–414.

62. Villegas-Castrejon H, Paredes-Vivas Y, Flores-Rivera E, Gorbea-Robles MC, Arredondo-Garcia JL. Comparative study of the placenta from HIV + mothers. Ultrastructural analysis. Ginecol Obstet Mex 1996; 64:167–176.

63. Faulk WP, Labarrere CA. HIV proteins in normal human placentae. Am J Reprod Immunol 1991; 25:99–104.

64. Skolnik PR, Pomerantz RJ, de ja Monte SM, Lee SF, Hsiung GD, Foos RY, Cowan GM, Kosloff BR, Hirsch MS, Pepose JS. Dual infection of retina with human immunodeficiency virus type 1 and cytomegalovirus. Am J Ophthalmol 1989; 107:361–372.

65. Bagasra O, Lavi E, Bobroski L, Khalili K, Pestaner JP, Tawadros R, Pomerantz RJ. Cellular reservoirs of HIV-1 in the central nervous system of infected individuals: identification by the combination of in situ polymerase chain reaction and immunohistochemistry. AIDS 1996; 10:573–585.

66. Wiley CA, Schrier RD, Nelson JA, Lampert PW, Oldstone MB. Cellular localization of human immunodeficiency virus infection within the brains of acquired immune deficiency syndrome patients. Proc Natl Acad Sci USA 1986; 83:7089–7093.

67. Pumarola-Sune T, Navia BA, Cordon-Cardo C, Cho ES, Price RW. HIV antigen in the brains of patients with the AIDS dementia complex. Ann Neurol 1987; 21:490–496.

68. Moses AV, Bloom FE, Pauza CD, Nelson JA. Human immunodeficiency virus infection of human brain capillary endothelial cells occurs via a CD4/galactosyl-ceramide-independent mechanism. Proc Natl Acad Sci USA 1993; 90:10474–10478.

69. Moses AV, Nelson JA. HIV infection of human brain capillary endothelial cells: implications for AIDS dementia. Adv Neuroimmunol 1994; 4:239–247.

70. Strelow LI, Watry DD, Fox HS, Nelson JA. Efficient infection of brain microvascular endothelial cells by an in vivo-selected neuroinvasive SIVmac variant. J Neurovirol 1998; 4:269–280.

71. Edinger AL, Mankowski JL, Doranz BJ, Margulies BJ, Lee B, Rucker J, Sharron M, Hoffman TL, Berson JF, Zink MC, Hirsch VM, Clements JE, Doms RW. CD4-independent, CCR5-dependent infection of brain capillary endothelial cells by a neurovirulent simian immunodeficiency virus strain. Proc Natl Acad Sci USA 1997; 94:14742–14747.

72. Scoazec JY, Feldmann G. Both macrophages and endothelial cells of the human hapatic sinusoid express the CD4 molecule, a receptor for the human immunodeficiency virus. Hepatology 1990; 12:505–510.

73. Steffan AM, Lafon ME, Gendrault JL, Schweitzer C, Royer C, Jaeck D, Arnaud JP, Schmitt MP, Aubertin AM, Kim A. Primary cultures of endothelial cells from the human liver sinusoid are permissive for human immunodeficiency virus type 1. Proc Natl Acad Sci USA 1992; 89:1582–1586.

74. Lefon ME, Gendrault JL, Royer C, Jaeck D, Kirn A, Steffan AM. Human endothelial cells isolated from the hepatic sinusoids and the umbilical vein display a different permissiveness for HIV-1. Res Virol 1993; 144:99–104.

75. Conaldi PG, Srra C, Dolei A, Basolo F, Falcone V, Mariani G, Speziale P, Toniolo A. Productive HIV-1 infection of human vascular endothelial cells requires cell proferation and is stimulated by combined treatment with interleukin-1 beta plus tumor necrosis factor-alpha. J Med Virol 1995; 47:355–363.

76. Scheglovitova O, Capobianchi MR, Antonelli G, Guanmu D, Fais S, Dianzani F. CD4 positive lymphoid cells rescue HIV-1 replication from abortively infected human primary endothelial cells. Int Conf AIDS 1993; 9:142.

77. Corbeil J, Evans LA, McQueen PW, Wasak E, Edward PD, Richman DD, Penny R, Cooper DA. Productive in vitro infection of human umbilical vein endothelial cells and three colon carcinoma cell lines with HIV-1. Immunol Cell Biol 1995; 73:140–145.

78. Dianzani F, Scheglovitova O, Gentile M, Scanio V, Barresi C, Ficociello B, Bianchi F, Fiumara D, Capobianchi MR. Interferon gamma stimulates cell-mediated transmission of HIV type 1 from abortively infected endothelial cells. AIDS Res Hum Retrovir 1996; 12:621–627.

79. Cenacchi G, Re MC, Preda P, Pasquinelli G, Furlini G, Apkarian RP, La Placa M, Martinelli GN. Human immunodeficiency virus type-1 (HIV-1) infection of endothelial cells in vitro: a vriological, ultrastructural and immuno-cytochemical approach. J Submicrosc Cytol Pathol 1992; 24:155–161.

80. Re MC, Furlini G, Cenacchi G, Preda P, La Placa M. Human immunodeficiency virus type 1 infection of endothelial cells in vitro. Microbiologica 1991; 14:149–152.

81. Green DF, Resnick L, Bourgoignie JJ. HIV infects glomerular endothelial and mesangial but not epithelial cells in vitro. Kidney Int 1992; 41:956–960.

82. Ades EW, Hierholzer JC, George V, Black J, Candal F. Viral susceptibility of an immortalized human microvascular endothelial cell line. J Virol Methods 1992; 39:83–90.

83. Kanmogne GD, Kennedy RC, Grammas P. Analysis of human lung endothelial cells for susceptibility to HIV type 1 infection, coreceptor expression, and cytotoxicity of gp120 protein. AIDS Res Hum Retrovir 2001; 17:45–53.

84. Nordoy I, Aukrust P, Muller F, Froland S. Abnormal levels of circulating adhesion molecules in HIV-1 infection with characteristic alterations in opportunistic infections. Clin Immunol Immunopathol 1996; 81:16–21.

85. Zietz C, Hotz B, Sturzl M, Rauch E, Penning R, Lohrs U. Aortic endothelium in HIV-1 infection: chronic injury, activation, and increased leukocyte adherence. Am J Pathol 1996; 149:1887–1898.

86. Nottet HS, Persidsky Y, Sasseville VG, Nukuna AN, Bock P, Zhai QH, Sharer LR, McComb RD, Swindells S, Soderland C, Gendelman HE. Mechanisms for the trans-endothelial migration of HIV-1-infected monocytes into brain. J Immunol 1996; 156:1284–1295.

87. Bridsall HH, Trial J, Lin HJ, Green DM, Sorrentino GW, Siwak EB, de Jong AL, Rossen RG. Transendothelial migration of lymphocytes from HIV-1 infected donors: a mechanisms for extravascular dissemination of HIV-1. J Immunol 1997; 158:5968–5977.

88. Krishnaswamy G, Smith JK, Mukkamala R, Hall K, Joyner WLY, Chi DS. Multi-functional cytokine expression by human coronary endothelium and regulation by monokines and glucocorticoids. Microvasc Res 1998; 55:189–200.

89. Herbein G, Keshav S, Collin M, Montaner LJ, Gordon S. HIV-induces tumor necrosis factor and IL-1 gene expression in primary human macrophages independent of productive infection. Clin Exp Immunol 1994; 95:442–449.

90. Liu NQ, Lossinsky AS, Popik W, Li X, Gujuluva C, Kriederman B, Roberts J, Push-karsky M, Witte M, Weinand M, Fiala M. Human immunodeficiency virus type 1 enters brain microvascular endothelia by macropinocytosis dependent on lipid rafts and the mitogen-activated protein kinase signaling pathway. J Virol 2002; 76:6689–6700.

91. Mitola S, Soldi R, Zanon I, Barra L, Gutierrez MI, Berkhout B, Giacca M, Busso-linl F. Identification of specific molecular structures of human immunodeficiency virus type 1 Tat relevant for its biological effects on vascular endothelial cells. J Virol 2000; 74:344–353.

92. Albini A, Soldi R, Benelli R, Gallo RC, Ensoli B. Angiogenic properties of human immunodeficiency virus type 1 Tat protein. Proc Natl Acad Sci USA 1995; 92:4838–4842.

93. Albini A, Soldi R, Giunciuglio D, Giraudo E, Benelli R, Primo L, Noonan D, Salio M, Camussi G, Rockl W, Bussolino F. The angiogenesis induced by HIV-1 tat protein is mediated the Flk-1/KDR receptor on vascular endothelial cells. Nat Med 1996; 2:1371–1375.

94. Zidovetzki R, Wang JL, Chen P, Jeyaseekab R, Hofman F. Human immunodeficiency virus Tat protein induces interleukin 6 mRNA expression in human brain endothelial cells via protein kinase C- and cAMP-dependent protein kinase pathways. AIDS Res Hum Retrovir 1998; 14:825–833.

95. Hofman FM, Chen P, Incardona F, Zidovetzki R, Hinton DR. HIV-1 Tat protein induces the production of interleukin-8 by human brain-derived endothelial cells. J Neuroimmunol 1999; 94:28–39.

96. Dhawan S, Puri RK, Kumar A, Duplan H, Masson JM, Aggarwal BB. Human immunodeficiency virus-1-tat protein induces the cell surface expression of endothelial leukocyte adhesion molecule-1, vascular cell adhesion molecule-1, and intercellular adhesion molecule-1 in human endothelial cells. Blood 1997; 90:1535–1544.

97. Cota-Gomez A, Flores NA, Cruz C, Casullo A, Aw TY, Ichikawa H, Schaack J, Scheinman R, Flores SC. The human immunodeficiency virus-1 Tat protein activates human umbilical vein endothelial cell E-selectin expression via an NF-κB-dependent mechanism. J Biol Chem 2002; 277(17):14390–14399.

98. Brand K, Page S, Walli AK, Neumeier D, Bauerle PA. Role of nuclear factor-kappa B in atherogenesis. Exp Physiol 1997; 82:297–304.

99. Weiss JM, Nath A, Major EO, Berman JW. HIV-1 Tat induces monocyte chemo-attractant protein-1-mediated monocyte transmigration across a model of the human blood-brain barrier and up-regulates CCR5 expression on human monocytes. J Immunol 1999; 163:2953–2959.

100. Park IW, Wang JF, Groopman JE. HIV-1 Tat promotes monocyte chemoattractant protein-1 secretion followed by transmigration on monocytes. Blood 2001; 97:352–358.

101. Wahl LM, Corcoran ML, Pyle SW, Arthur LO, Harel-Bellan A, Farrar WL. Human immunodeficiency virus glycoprotein (gp120) induction of monocyte arachidonic acid metabolites and interleukin-1. Proc Natl Acad Sci USA 1989; 86:621–625.

102. Frenette PS, Wagner DD. Adhesion molecules. Part 1. N Engl J Med 1996; 334:1526–1529.

103. Frenette PS, Wagner DD. Adhesion molecules. Part II: Blood vessels and blood cells. N Engl J Med 1996; 335:43–45.

104. Bragardo M, Buonfiglio D, Feito MJ, Bonissoni S, Redoglia V, Rojo JM, Ballester S, Portoles P, Garbarino G, Malavasi F, Dianzani U. Modulation of lymphocyte interaction with endothelium and homing by HIV-1 gp120. J Immunol 1997; 159:1619–1627.

105. Stefano GB, Salzet M, Bilfinger TV. Long-term exposure of humao blood vessels to HIV gp120. morphine, and anandamide increases endothelial adhesion of monocytes: uncoupling of nitric oxide release. J Cardiovasc Pharmacol 1998; 31:862–868.

106. Stins MF, Shen Y, Huang SH, Gilles F, Kalra VK, Kim KS. Gp120 activates children's brain endothelial cells via CD4. J Neurovirol 2001; 7:125–134.

107. Toneatto S, Finco O, van der PH, Abrignani S, Annunziata P. Evidence of blood-brain barrier alteration and activation in HIV-1 gp120 transgenic mice. AIDS 1999; 13:2343–2348.

108. Shatrov VA, Ratter F, Gruber A, Droge W, Lehmann V. HIV type 1 glycoprotein 120 amplifies tumor necosis factor-induced NF-kappa B activation in Jurkat cells. AIDS Res Hum Retrovir 1996; 12:1209–1216.

109. Ren Z, Yao Q, Chen C. HIV-1 envelope glycoprotein 120 increases intercellular adhesion molecule-1 expression by human endothelial cells. Lab Invest 2002; 82:245–255.

110. Shi B, De Girolami U, He J, Wang S, Lorenzo A, Busciglion J, Gabuzda D. Apoptosis induced by HIV-1 infection of the central nervous system. J Clin Invest 1996; 98:1979–1990.

111. Adamson DC, Dawson TM, Zink MC, Clements JE, Dawson VL. Neurovirulent simian immunodeficiency virus infection induces neuronal, endothelial, and glial apoptposis. Mol Med 1996; 2:417–428.

112. Reid W, Sadwska M, Denaro F, Rao S, Foulke J, Hayes N, Jones O, Doodnauth D, Davis H, Sill A, O'Driscoll P, Huso D, Lewis G, Hill M, Kamin-Lewis R, Wei C,

Ray P, Gallo RC. An HIV-1 transgenic rat that develops HIV-related pathology and immunologic dyfunction. Proc Natl Acad Sci USA 2001; 98:9271–9276.

113. Park IW, Ullrich CK, Schoenberger E, Gasnju RK. HIV-1 Tat induces microvascular endothelial apoptosis through caspase activation. J Immunol 2001; 167:2766–2771.

114. Jia H, Lohr M, Jezequel S, Davis D, Shaikh S, Selwood D, Zachary I. Cysteine-rich and basic domain HIV-1 Tat peptides inhibit angiogenesis and induce endothelial cell apoptosis. Biochem Biophy Res Commun 2001; 283:469–479.

115. Huang MB, Hunter M, Bond VC. Effect of extracellular human immunodeficiency virus type-1 glycoprotein 120 on primary vascular endothelial cell cultures. AIDS Res Hum Retrovir, 1999; 1265–1277.

116. Huang MB, Bond VC. Involvement of protein kinase C in HIV-1 gp120-induced apoptosis in primary endothelium. J AIDS 2000; 25:375–389.

117. Huang MB, Khan M, Garcia-Barrio M, Powell M, Bond VC. Apoptotic effects in primary human umblical vein endothelial cell cultures caused by exposure to virion-associated and cell membrane–associated HIV-1 gp120. J AIDS 2001; 27:213–221.

118. Ullrich CK, Groopman JE, Ganju RK. HIV-1 gp120- and gp160-induced apoptosis in cultured endothelial cells is mediated by caspases. Blood 2000; 96:1438–1442.

119. Kanmogne GD, Kennedy RC, Grammas P. Analysis of human lung endothelial cells for susceptibility to HIV type 1 infection, coreceptor expression, and cytotoxicity of gp120 protein. AIDS Res Hum Retrovir 2001; 17:45–53.

120. Lipton SA. HIV-related neurotoxivity. Brian Pathol 1991; 1:193–199.

121. Vitkovix L, da Cunha A, Tyor WR. Cytokine expression and pathogenesis in AIDS brain. In: Price R, Perry SW, eds. HIV, AIDS and the Brain. New York: Raven Press, 1994; 203-221.

122. Rhodes RH. Evidence of serum-protein leakage across the blood-brain barrier in the acquired immunodeficiency syndrome. J Neuropathol Exp Neurol 1991; 50:171–183.

123. Petito CK, Cash KS. Blood-brain barrier abnormalities in the axquired immunodeficiency syndrome: immunohistochemical localization of serum protein in post-mortem brain. Ann Neurol 1992; 32:658–666.

124. Goudsmit J, Epstein LG, Paul DA, van der Helm HJ, Dawson GJ, Asher DM, Yanagihara R, Wolff AV, Gibbs CJ Jr, Gajdusek DC. Intra-blood-brain barrier synthesis of human immunodeficiency virus antigen and antibody in humans and chimpanzees. Proc Natl Acad Sci USA 1987; 84:3876–3880.

125. Pepose JS, Holland GN, Nestor MS, Cochran AJ, Foos RY. Acquired immune deficiency syndrome. Pathogenic mechanisms of ocular disease. Ophthalmology 1985; 92:472–484.

126. Gariano RF, Rickman LS, Freeman WR. Ocular examination and diagnosis in patients with the acquired immunodeficiency syndrome. West J Med 1993; 158:254–262.

127. Annunziata P, Cioni C, Toneatto S, Paccagnini E. HIV-1 gp120 increases the permeability of rat brain endothelium cultures by a mechanism involving substance P. AIDS 1998; 12:2377–2385.

128. Toneatto S, Finco O, van der PH, Abrignani S, Annunziata P. Evidence of blood-brain barrier alteration and activation in HIV-1 gp120 transgenic mince. AIDS 1999; 13:2343–2348.

129. Bank WA, Kastin AJ. Characterization of lectin-mediated brain uptake of HIV-1 gp120. J Neurosci Res 1998; 54:522–529.

130. Bank WA, Akerstrom V, Kastin AJ. Adsortive endocytosis mediates the passage of HIV-1 across the blood-brain barrier: evidence for a post-internalization coreceptor. J Cell Sci 1998; 111:533–540.

131. Bank WA, Kastin AJ, Brennan JM, Vallance KL. Adsorptive endocytosis of HIV-1 gp1120 by blood-brain barrier is enhanced by lipopolysaccharide. Exp Neurol 1999; 156:165–171.

132. Bank WA, Freed EO, Wolf KM, Robison SM, Franko M, Kumar VB. Transport of human immunodeficiency virus type 1 pseudoviruses across the blood-brain barrier: role of envelope proteins and adsorptive endocytosis. J Virol 2001; 75:4681–4691.

133. Arese M, Ferrandi C, Primo L, Camussi G, Bussolino F. HIV-1 Tat protein stimulates in vivo vascular permeability and lymphomonuclear cell recruitment. J Immunol 2001; 166:1380–1388.

134. Oshima T, Flores SC, Vaitaitis G, Coe LL, Joh T, Park JK, Zhu Y, Alexander B, Alexander JS. HIV-1 Tat increases endothelial solute permeability through tyrosine kinase and mitogen-activated protein kinase–dependent pathways. AIDS 2000; 14:475–482.

135. Toschi E, Barillari G, Sgadari C, Bacigalupo I, Cereseto A, Carlei D, Palladino C, Zietz C, Leone P, Sturzl M, Butto S, Cafaro A, Monini P. Activation of matrix-metalloproteinase-2 and membrane-type-1-matrix metalloproteinase in endothelial cells and induction of vascular permeability in vivo by human immunodeficiency virus-1 Tat protein and basic fibroblast growth factor. Mol Biol Cell 2001; 12:2934–2946.

10

Tat-Induced Angiogenesis

Harris E. McFerrin, Deborah E. Sullivan, Anne B. Nelson, Heather L. LaMarca, Bryan D. Shelby, and Cindy A. Morris
Tulane University Health Sciences Center, New Orleans, Louisiana, U.S.A.

Angiogenesis is the formation of new blood vessels from preexisting vessels by degradation of vessel basement membrane, endothelial cell sprouting, bridging, and intussusception. Normally, in a healthy adult, angiogenesis is limited to sites of vessel injury and to the female reproductive tract; however, pathological angiogenesis occurs in several disease processes including degenerative eye disease, atherosclerosis, and malignancies including Kaposi's sarcoma (KS) (1–4).

KS is a highly vascularized hyperplastic lesion characterized by proliferation of spindle-shaped cells of endothelial origin, unabated neoangiogenesis, and persistent inflammatory infiltration of T cells, B cells, and monocytes (5). KS has three forms, including (1) classical KS, which is seen sporatically in older men of Mediterranean–Eastern European descent or in immunosuppressed posttransplant patients; (2) endemic KS, which is prevalent in subequatorial Africa; and (3) acquired immunodeficiency disease syndrome–associated KS (AIDS-KS), which is commonly seen in human immunodeficiency virus type 1 (HIV-1)–infected individuals. As compared to classical KS, which is both rare and relatively indolent, AIDS-KS occurs more frequently and is more aggressive (6,7). Although KS is associated with the immunodeficiency that characterizes AIDS, Th1 immune activation, including influx of CD8 + T cells and monocytes, rather than immunodeficiency, may participate in the development of AIDS-KS (8,9) (For in-depth review, see Ref. 6).

Numerous studies suggest that KS pathogenesis requires reciprocal communication between spindle cells that produce proinflammatory cytokines and potent angiogenic growth factors and inflammatory infiltrates that produce additional factors that promote KS growth (5). The factors that collectively contribute to the increased aggressiveness of AIDS-KS are not fully known; however, specific viral gene products encoded by both human herpesvirus-8 (HHV-8/KSV) and HIV-1 appear to be involved (5,6).

Three key findings suggest that Tat, a small HIV-1 regulatory protein, may contribute to the pathogenesis of AIDS-KS (5). These include the demonstrations that (1) mice expressing *tat* as a transgene develop "KS-like" dermal lesions, (2) Tat is present in AIDS-KS lesions, and (3) Tat has angiogenic properties. Collectively, these findings support the hypothesis that Tat affects AIDS-KS pathogenesis, at least in part, by a mechanism that involves Tat-induced angiogenesis. This chapter focuses on the angiogenic effects of Tat that are known to date, with special emphasis on the molecular mechanisms by which Tat mediates these effects. The first part of this chapter introduces angiogenesis as a dynamic process that involves a complex interplay between soluble mediators, the extracellular matrix (ECM) and endothelial cell surface receptors. The subsequent section discusses the functional domains of Tat relevant to its role as a potent transcriptional transactivator and as an angiogenic factor. The chapter concludes with a discussion of future research directions that may further elucidate how Tat regulates angiogenesis and how these effects may contribute to the pathogenesis of AIDS-KS.

THE DYNAMIC PROCESS OF ANGIOGENESIS

Vascular Endothelial Cell Activation by Growth Factors

Angiogenesis is a multistep process requiring vascular endothelial cell adhesion, migration, invasion, proliferation, differentiation (formation of a new lumen) and survival (10). The initial step towards initiating this dynamic process involves the activation of vascular endothelial cells (EC) that are normally in a quiescent or "resting" state. Vascular endothelial cell growth factor (VEGF) and basic fibroblast growth factor (bFGF) belong to two different families of angiogenic growth factors (11). Both bFGF and VEGF activate the initiating steps toward new blood vessel formation, and together they act in synergy to induce angiogenesis. VEGF-A, that was initially identified based on its ability to stimulate EC proliferation and vascular permeability, induces angiogenesis in response to hypoxia and, therefore, is predictably important during embryonic development and tumor progression. The four isoforms of VEGF-A, generated through differential splicing, bind to two endothelial cell surface receptor tyrosine kinases, VEGF receptor-1 (VEGFR-1/Flt-1), and VEGFR-2 (Flk-1/KDR). The VEGFR-2 is the major receptor that mediates angiogenesis induced by VEGF-A. In contrast, the FGF family of angiogenic growth factors is much larger than the VEGF family and signals through four different receptors. Relative to either family, binding of specific angiogenic growth factors to their respective receptors on the surface of EC induces receptor tyrosine phosphorylation that subsequently activates a multitude of downstream signaling cascades within the cells, ultimately leading to angiogenesis. VEGF-A binding to VEGFR-2 induces dimerization and tyrosine phosphorylation of the receptor activating several intracellular signaling pathways. PLCγ, Sck, and VRAP are activated by direct interaction of VEGF-A with tyrosine phosphorylated VEGFR-2; whereas the mechanism(s) by which other signaling molecules, such as focal adhesion kinase (FAK), Src, mitogen activated protein kinase (MAPK), phosphatidylinositol-3-kinase (PI3K), and Akt are activated by VEGFR-2 are not completely clear (Fig. 1) (11–16).

Integrin Involvement in Growth Factor–Induced Vascular Endothelial Cell Adhesion, Migration, Proliferation, Extracellular Matrix Assembly, and Morphogenesis

Integrins belong to a family of heterodimeric transmembrane receptors composed of single α- and β-subunits that mediate both cell-ECM and cell-cell interactions, influencing endothelial cell behavior during angiogenesis (17–19). At least 18 α and 8 β subunits combine to generate more than 24 different αβ integrins, 7 of which are

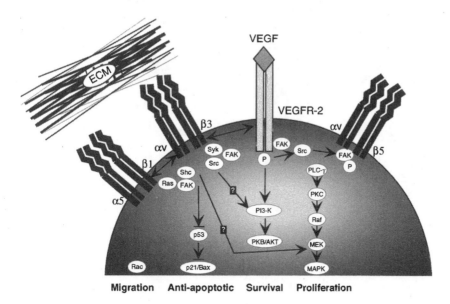

Figure 1 Cross talk between integrins and VEGF receptors in angiogenesis. Numerous signaling cascades, not all of which are depicted here, are activated by binding of specific ligands to the VEGFR-2 and to integrin receptors during angiogenesis, leading to migration, suppression of apoptosis, survival, and proliferation of endothelial cells. Solid lines indicate known pathways. Question marks indicate less well understood pathways. (Adapted from Ref. 12.)

expressed on EC and include $\alpha v\beta3$, $\alpha v\beta5$, $\alpha1\beta1$, $\alpha2\beta1$, $\alpha3\beta1$, $\alpha5\beta1$, and $\alpha6\beta1$ (10,20). Each integrin has its own binding specificity and signaling properties. Many of these adhesion receptors, although distinct, have overlapping specificities for ECM proteins [e.g., fibronectin (FN), vitronectin (VN), laminins, collagens, fibrinogen]. The biological significance of this is not clear. Conversely, the majority of ECM proteins are capable of binding more than one integrin. Of note, the intracellular signals and effectors induced by integrin-ECM interactions (such as, Ras, FAK, MAPK, Src, PI3K, PKC, Rac/Rho/cdc42 GTPases) are similar to those that are activated by growth factors (Fig. 1) (18,21). Cell proliferation, adhesion, and migration induced by growth factors in vitro often require specific integrin-ECM interactions. Accordingly, integrin-mediated endothelial cell adhesion to specific ECM molecules is required for optimal stimulation by growth factors such as VEGF, epidermal growth factor (EGF), insulin, or platelet-derived growth factor (PDGF) (18,21,22).

Growth factor signaling regulates endothelial cell expression of integrins. Different growth factors activate the expression of specific integrins. Specifically, VEGF stimulation of human microvascular endothelial cells (HMVEC) upregulates $\alpha v\beta3$, $\alpha2\beta1$, and $\alpha1\beta1$ integrins (23,24). VEGF has also been shown to upregulate the expression of integrins $\alpha v\beta5$ and $\alpha5\beta1$ and to enhance adhesion and migration mediated by $\alpha v\beta3$ integrin (Fig. 2) (25). The cellular microenvironment, as well as other growth factors, such as bFGF, can stimulate integrin expression in vascular EC. Hypoxia, for example, stimulates VEGF expression and nitric oxide synthesis in EC, both of which trigger integrin expression. Accordingly, bFGF, but not transforming growth factor beta (TGF-β), upregulates the normally low endothelial expression of

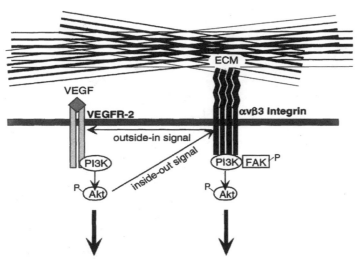

Figure 2 Inside-out and outside-in signaling. Integrins and VEGFR-2 bind their respective ligands and activate the PI3K/Akt signaling cascade, which induces endothelial cell survival, migration, invasion, tube formation, and proliferation. Angiogenesis induced by growth factors such as VEGF is dependent upon ECM-endothelial cell interactions ("outside-in signaling"). Growth factor receptor activation stimulates intracellular signaling that enhances integrin-mediated endothelial cell adhesion to ECM molecules ("inside-out signaling"). (Adapted from Ref. 13.)

αvβ3 integrin, whereas TGF-β increases the more abundantly expressed β1 integrins, which further demonstrates integrin-specific effects on growth factors (26–28).

Although integrins are most known for their ability to mediate cell adhesion and migration, they also function in the binding and assembly of the ECM as has been demonstrated by αvβ3- and α5β1- mediated assembly of FN matrices (29,30). Integrins are also involved in endothelial cell morphogenesis which is important for vascular lumen formation. In vitro, the specific integrins involved in this process are dictated by the specific matrix on which EC are cultured. For example, formation of endothelial luminal structures on fibrin matrices is arginine-glycine-aspartic acid (RGD)-dependent and involves integrins αvβ3 and α5β1 (31), as lumen formation is blocked by addition of anti-αvβ3 and anti-α5 antibodies or by expression of antisense β3 mRNA. In contrast, lumen formation in a three-dimensional collagen matrix is dependent upon α2β1 (32). The mechanisms involved in vascular lumen formation in vivo are not known, but are predictably more complex as both the composition and conformation of the ECM at any given time and in any given space may vary in response to environmental cues. However, the in vitro studies suggest the importance of integrin involvement during vascular endothelial cell morphogenesis (31,33).

Integrin Signaling and Downstream Effects on Vascular Endothelial Cells

Integrin signaling across the cellular membrane is bidirectional. "Outside-in" signaling as a result of extracellular ligand binding to integrins controls many processes important for endothelial cell migration, invasion, proliferation, differentiation, and survival (18,21,34). Integrin ligation induces integrin receptors to cluster in foci within the plasma membrane and signal through their interaction with adaptor proteins, such as Shc and CAS/Crk, that associate the integrins with cytoplasmic kinases, growth factor receptors, and the cytoskeleton (35,36). Some intracellular signaling events that occur upon integrin ligation have been demonstrated and include the activation of FAK, Src, MAPK, Ras, Rac, Rho, PI3K, integrin-linked kinase (ILK), cdc42 GTPases, and Abl (37–40). Other cellular effects of integrin signaling include stimulation of gene expression, cyclin synthesis, matrix degrading metalloproteinases, intracellular Ca2+ and pH, and inositol phosphate synthesis (41). Integrins mediate "inside-out" signaling upon growth factor-receptor binding that either alters integrin conformation to increase its binding affinity for ligand or enhances focal clustering of integrins on the plasma membrane to increase the strength of ligand binding. Of note, integrin ligation and growth factor receptor–ligand binding activate common intracellular effectors and signal transduction pathways, suggesting that integrins and growth factor receptors may work co-ordinately or in synergy to affect cell type–specific responses (Fig. 2) (18,21).

Cross Talk Between Integrins and Growth Factor Receptors During Angiogenesis

Induction of angiogenesis in vascular endothelial cells requires at least two signals, one from angiogenic growth factors that induce integrin receptor expression and one from the ECM (i.e., via FN or VN) (42,43). FN, through binding of its RGD sequence to the $\alpha5\beta1$ receptor, regulates both basal and growth factor-induced endothelial cell growth by modulating cell shape and by stimulating specific intracellular signaling pathways (43). Previous in vivo and in vitro studies demonstrate that FN can support primary human umbilical vein endothelial cell (HUVEC) adhesion, spread, and growth and can stimulate cell proliferation in response to bFGF (44). FN inoculated alone into athymic nude mice does not induce angiogenesis, possibly due to occupancy of its receptors by endogenous ECM proteins. However, FN acts synergistically with bFGF to induce both integrin expression and in vivo angiogenesis (42), thereby increasing the availability of and binding to integrin receptors by their specific ligands. Furthermore, injection of bFGF before FN injection in nude mice increases lesion development even beyond that seen as a result of their simultaneous inoculation (42).

Distinct angiogenic pathways may be defined by functional coupling of specific growth factors with distinct αv integrins (42,43). Recent in vivo studies indicate that angiogenesis induced by bFGF or by tumor necrosis factor alpha (TNF-α) is mediated by $\alpha v\beta3$; whereas angiogenesis induced by VEGF, TGF-α, or phorbol ester is more dependent upon $\alpha v\beta5$. Specifically, these studies demonstrate that antibody antagonists of $\alpha v\beta3$ completely block bFGF- or TNF-α–induced angiogenesis but only partially inhibit angiogenesis stimulated by VEGF. In contrast, antibody antagonists of $\alpha v\beta5$ specifically abrogate angiogenesis induced by VEGF, TGF-α, or phorbol ester. The idea of distinct angiogenic pathways is further substantiated by the ability of PKC and Src inhibitors to inhibit VEGF- but not bFGF-induced angiogenesis (10,17,45).

Cooperative effects of angiogenic growth factors and integrins promote the survival of vascular EC during angiogenesis. The importance of vascular cell interactions with the ECM during angiogenesis is well established. Disruption of cellular interactions with the ECM is associated with induction of apoptosis (10,17,45). Specifically, binding of integrin $\alpha_v\beta_3$ to its extracellular matrix substrate is necessary for both the survival and maturation of new blood vessels required for tumor progression as shown by perturbation of angiogenesis initiated on chick chorioallantoic membranes (CAMs) by intravenous inoculation of antibody and peptide antagonists of $\alpha_v\beta_3$ (42). These antagonists specifically promote apoptosis in vascular cells of these lesions, suggesting that $\alpha_v\beta_3$ mediates selective survival of these cells and thus contributes to vascular cell differentiation during angiogenesis (42). Antibody agonists of $\alpha_v\beta_3$ promote a critical and specific adhesion-dependent cell survival signal during angiogenesis leading to inhibition of p53 activity, decreased expression of p21$^{\text{WAF1/CIP1}}$, and suppression of the Bax cell death pathway, suggesting a mechanistic link between ligation of integrin $\alpha_v\beta_3$ and vascular cell survival during angiogenesis (46). Another study demonstrates that the $\alpha5\beta1$ integrin supports survival of serum-starved nonvascular cells (Chinese hamster ovary cells) on FN in association with upregulation of the protooncogene, *bcl-2* (47). The ability of integrins to mediate cell survival is not universal to all integrins as ligation of $\alpha_v\beta_1$ to its ECM substrate fails to suppress apoptotic cell death (47). Subsequent studies demonstrate that *bcl-2* transcription and cell survival is elevated in cells that attach to FN or VN through $\alpha5\beta1$ and $\alpha v\beta3$, respectively. The signaling pathway that leads to enhanced *bcl-2* transcription initiates with the integrin-mediated activation of Shc and FAK followed by a cascade of FAK activation of Ras, then activation of PI3K/Akt. Although this survival pathway is not delineated in vascular EC, VEGF has been shown to activate both a PI3K/Akt survival pathway and Bcl-2 expression in EC (48,49). A direct linkage of Bcl-2 as a downstream effector of the PI3K/Akt signaling pathway, however, has not yet been shown in vascular EC.

These studies collectively suggest that vascular endothelial cell survival during angiogenesis may be mediated by convergence of integrin and growth factor signaling at integrin-proximal locations that involve PI3K. In support of the model that direct communication between angiogenic growth factors and integrins during angiogenesis reflects convergence of their downstream intracellular signaling pathways, recent studies demonstrate that VEGF—through a signaling axis involving PI3K, PKB/Akt and PTEN (a lipid phosphatase that can dephosphoryate phophatidylinositol 3,4,5-triphosphate and thus negatively regulates PI3K signaling)—activates specific integrins through the VEGFR-2 effectively enhancing integrin-mediated adhesion and migration (25). Furthermore, by regulating cell adhesion to matrix, $\alpha v\beta3$ participates in the full activation of VEGFR-2 triggered by VEGF (50). Specifically, VEGF activates VEGFR-2 tyrosine kinase phosphorylation and PI3K in a $\beta3$-dependent manner (50). In these same studies, the mitogenic and motogenic effects of VEGF are enhanced by $\alpha v\beta3$ ligand binding and inhibited by wortmannin, a PI3K-specific inhibitor, by anti-$\beta3$ and anti-VEGFR-2 antibodies. Further, the VEGFR-2 immunoprecipitates, in a phosphorylated form, with $\beta3$ in VEGF-stimulated EC (50). These studies suggest a similarity or overlap in the functional responses of cells to engagement of growth factor receptors and integrins during angiogenesis. Mechanisms for direct communication between angiogenic factors and key integrins involved in angiogencsis remain relatively undefined; however, the ability of angiogenic factors to activate specific integrins and the requirement of specific integrins for growth factor receptor activation and effector function suggest a convergence of downstream intracellular signaling pathways. Accordingly, many of the signaling molecules and events induced by VEGFR-2 ligation and associated with integrin activation are shared. PKB/Akt, a downstream effector of PI3K and PTEN, has been directly implicated in the pathway from VEGF to integrin activation (Fig. 2) (25).

Many of the signaling pathways and effectors (e.g., Src, FAK, PI3K and Akt) that promote survival, migration and proliferation of vascular EC also promote cellular invasiveness. Angiogenesis requires vascular EC invasion into tissues, a process that involves coordinated interactions of matrix remodeling proteases and specific integrins. The 72-kDa matrix metalloproteinase (MMP)-2 plays a key role in vascular development and angiogenesis. The coordinated expression of MMP-2 and its activator, membrane-type metalloproteinase-1 (MT1-MMP) is limited to areas of neovascularization or cellular invasion during processes such as embryonic development and tumor growth and metastasis (51–53). In support of this, experiments show that angiogenesis and tumor growth is reduced in MMP-2 knockout mice (52). Additionally, concomitant reduction of vascular invasion and tumor growth in knockout mice defective in expression of Id, a transcriptional regulator of cell cycle progression and differentiation, correlates with absence of MMP-2 and αvβ3 in tumor-invading vascular EC, suggesting that vascular invasion may be mediated by coordinate regulation of MMP-2 and αvβ3 (54). In support of this, ligation of αvβ3 induces MMP-2 production. Additionally, the PEX domain of MMP-2, which is required for MMP-2 activation at the surface of invasive cells, interacts with αvβ3 (53,55). The PEX domain is also important for MMP-2 binding to tissue inhibitor of matrix metalloproteinase-2 (TIMP-2) that localizes MMP-2 to membrane type-1-matrix metalloproteinase (MT1-MMP), thus initiating the cascade of events leading to MMP-2 activation (53,56). Administration of recombinant MMP-2 PEX domain inhibits MMP-2 activation, tumor growth and angiogenesis by a mechanism that may involve both blocking initial MMP-2 binding to cell surface TIMP-2/MT1-MMP complexes and preventing binding of active MMP-2 to αvβ3 on the surface of invasive cells (53,57). The ability of αvβ3 to facilitate activation of MMP-2 by recruiting MT1-MMP in its active form to the surface of melanoma cells suggests that specific inhibition of MMP-2-αvβ3 binding may block angiogenesis and cellular invasion. In support, a recent study demonstrates the ability of an organic molecule to block angiogenesis and tumor growth in vivo by inhibiting MMP-2-αvβ3 binding without disrupting binding of the integrin to its natural ligand or affecting MMP-2 activation or catalytic function directly (58). This study suggests that the activated MMP-2 must be in a complex with αvβ3 to facilitate angiogenesis and tumor growth and invasion.

HIV-1 TAT

Tat as a Transcriptional Transactivator

Tat is best known as a regulatory protein encoded by HIV-1 that is essential for viral gene expression and replication (59). Anti-Tat antibodies inhibit HIV replication in culture and elevated titers of anti-Tat antibodies correlate with increased survival in HIV-infected individuals (60–62). The predominant and most potent functional role of Tat is as a transcriptional transactivator (59). Tat, representing a unique family of lentiviral transactivators, stimulates transcriptional activation through an RNA response element (TAR), to which it binds, located within the 5′-untranslated leader sequences of all HIV-1 mRNAs (59). Tat transactivates transcription in a TAR-dependent manner at the levels of initiation and elongation from the HIV-1 promoter (long terminal repeat, or LTR). HIV-1 LTR-directed viral gene expression occurs following differential processing of full-length viral transcripts generated from the proviral DNA template (for a review, see Refs. 63 and 64). In the absence of Tat, the process of generating full-length transcripts that serve as templates for expression of all HIV-1 genes is inefficient and results in the generation of abundant short nascent transcripts that contain TAR (63,64). These short transcripts are generated by promoter-proximal pausing of RNA polymerase II (RNAP II) elongation complexes. Promoter-proximal pausing is abolished in the presence of Tat, that either recruits and/or activates positive-acting transcription elongation factors.

Tat is a small protein consisting of 86 to 101 amino acids (aa) dependent upon the viral strain. The *tat* gene consists of 2 exons, the first of which is sufficient for mediating Tat-induced transcriptional transactivation (65). Exon 1 encodes a cysteine-rich or transactivation domain (7 cysteines within aa 22–37) that is important for formation of metal-linked dimers and is required for transactivation (66). Also encoded within exon 1 is a basic domain (2 lysines and 6 arginines within aa 48–57) responsible for Tat-TAR RNA binding and for nuclear localization of Tat (67,68). Although the second exon of Tat is dispensable for Tat-induced transactivation, it encodes an RGD domain that mediates the biological effects of extracellular Tat. All three domains contribute to the angiogenic effects of Tat.

One of the most significant and recent breakthroughs toward elucidating the molecular mechanism by which Tat affects transcription elongation is the discovery of an important host cell transcriptional coactivator for Tat that is a nuclear Tat-associated kinase, TAK (69,70). TAK is identical to the kinase subunit of P-TEFb (71,72), a positive-acting early elongation factor complex that mediates transcription elongation of many genes (73,74). A major substrate for TAK/P-TEFb activity is the carboxyl-terminal domain (CTD) of the RPB1 subunit of RNAP II that consists of 52 tandem repeats of the heptapeptide YSPTSPS, a region of the polymerase that plays a critical role in the control of transcription elongation (75). Hyperphosphorylation of the RNAP II CTD correlates with the transition of elongation-competent complexes to fully processive elongation complexes during transcription (75–77). TAR-dependent HIV-1 transactivation by Tat requires the RNAP II CTD and is sensitive to inhibition by specific protein kinase inhibitors, such as 5,6-dichloro-1-β-ribofuranosylbenzimidizole (DRB) (75). The transactivation domain of Tat (aa 1-48) interacts specifically and strongly with TAK/P-TEFb and in vivo and in vitro data suggest that Tat targets TAK/P-TEFb to TAR to enhance RNAP II processivity at an early step of elongation (75). The 42-kDa catalytic subunit of TAK/P-TEFb is a CDC2-related kinase, PITALRE, now designated cyclin-dependent kinase 9 (CDK9) (75). A dominant-negative mutant of CDK9 and CDK9 inhibitors block Tat trans-activation in vivo and in vitro, suggesting that CDK9 kinase activity is essential for Tat function (71,72,78). Moreover, Tat stimulates the high-affinity loop-specific binding of CDK9-containing TAK/P-TEFb complexes to TAR in HeLa nuclear extracts (79). The observation that TAK/P-TEFb contains a cell cycle regulatory protein suggests a link between activation of transcription and control of cell growth or differentiation.

A cyclin partner for CDK9, cyclin T, which is a component of the Tat-TAK/p-TEF-b complex in HeLa nuclear extracts, has recently been identified and cloned (79). Cyclin T is a novel cyclin C–related 87-kDa protein that interacts specifically with the activation domain of Tat and enhances its specific association with TAR (79). In this respect, the cyclin component of the Tat-TAK/P-TEFb complex serves as a cofactor for Tat-TAR binding (79). Recent studies have shown that P-TEFb associates with HIV-1 transcription preinitiation complexes and remains associated throughout elongation (76,80,81). Autophosphorylation of CDK9 regulates high-affinity binding of the Tat-P-TEFb complex to TAR RNA and Tat-induced HIV-1 transcriptional elongation (82–84). TFIIH, a general transcription factor with CTD kinase activity (CDK7) that is also present in HIV-1 transcriptional preinitiation complexes, inhibits autophosphorylation of CDK9 and hence the activity of CDK9 until the transcription complex has cleared the promoter and has synthesized between 14 and 36 nucleotides in the nascent RNA. At this time, TFIIH dissociates from the elongating complex, allowing autophosphorylation of CDK9 and subsequent binding of Tat-P-TEFb to the newly formed TAR element, facilitating transcription elongation (82–84). DRB-sensitivity inducing factor (DSIF) and negative elongation factor (NELF) are two negative elongation factors also present in the preinitiation complex that block productive elongation until they are released from the complex by hyperphosphorylation of the CTD by P-TEFb (Fig. 3) (85).

Unlike other cyclins, levels of C-type cyclins, such as cyclin T, do not change during the cell cycle (86). Some studies suggest that these cyclins are functional targets for environmental signaling pathways within cells (87). As a relevant example, TAK activity is elevated upon activation of peripheral blood mononuclear cells and peripheral blood lymphocytes (PBLs) by phytohaemagglutinin (PHA) or phorbol myristate acetate (PMA) and upon differentiation of promonocytic cell lines to macrophages by PMA (78). Activation of PBLs increases the expression of CDK9 and cyclin T at both the mRNA and the proteins levels. In contrast, phorbol ester–induced differentiation of promonocytic cells induces a dramatic induction of cyclin T protein expression from barely detectable levels but does not affect the constitutively high protein expression levels of CDK9. Therefore, TAK activity is regulated by distinct mechanisms in a cell type-specific manner. More recent studies demonstrate that treatment of purified resting CD4 + T lymphocytes with a combination of cytokines, including interleukin (IL)-2, IL-6, and TNF-α, increases expression of CDK9 and cyclin T protein levels that correlate with an increase in TAK activity (88). The increase in TAK activity does not require cell proliferation. As PMA, PHA and inflammatory cytokines stimulate HIV-1 transcription as well as cell growth and/or differentiation, it is likely that TAK, with other transcription factors, is a key regulator of HIV-1 transcription in HIV-1 infected cells (78).

From these studies, a plausible link between transcriptional regulation and cell growth and differentiation may be envisioned. CDK9/cyclin T likely stimulates transcription from numerous cellular genes that regulate growth and/or differentiation, yet is specifically targeted to certain genes by viral and/or cellular transcriptional activators. In support of this, a recent study demonstrates that NF-κB associates with P-TEFb to stimulate IL-8 transcription elongation by RNA polymerase II (89). Treatment of cells with TNF-α, a well-characterized inducer of NF-κB activity, results in the recruitment of P-TEFb to the NF-κB–regulated IL-8 gene. Additionally,

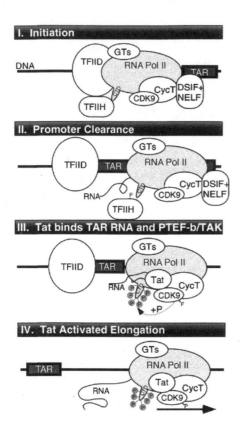

Figure 3 A model of Tat-induced elongation through activation of CDK9/cyclin T. I. During HIV-1 transcription, RNA polymerase II (RNAP II) binds to the HIV-1 LTR with TFIID, TFIIH, and other general transcription factors (GTs), p-TEFb/TAK composed of cyclin T/ CDK9, and negative elongation factors including DSIF and NELF. II. The CTD of RNAP II is partially phosphorylated by the CDK7 kinase subunit of TFIIH, which initiates promoter clearance of the HIV-1 transcription initiation complex. DSIF and NELF block elongation of the transcription complex by a mechanism intricately associated with the phosphorylation state of RNAP II. DSIF and NELF associate with only the hypophosphorylated form of RNAP II. TFIIH also prevents phosphorylation of CDK9. III. Once transcription proceeds past +36 relative to the transcription initiation start site at +1, TFIIH, DSIF, and NELF dissociate from the transcription elongation complex, which results in autophosphorylation and activation of CDK9. Once the nascent TAR RNA element is synthesized, Tat associates with P-TEFb and TAR (IV), enhancing the processivity of transcription elongation complexes.

inhibition of P-TEFb kinase activity by DRB in TNF-α-treated cells induces apoptosis, suggesting that P-TEFb is an essential cofactor of NF-κB, possibly stimulating the transcriptional elongation of anti-apoptotic genes (Fig. 4). These studies, as well as the established ability of TNF-α to support HIV replication in the absence of TAR in an NF-κB–dependent manner, provide a plausible explanation as to how the first rounds of HIV-1 transcription occur during viral replication at a time when Tat has yet to be expressed. In this scenario, NF-κB binds the two κB sites in the HIV LTR and recruits P-TEFb to stimulate transcription elongation.

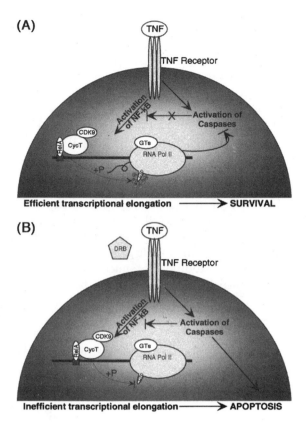

Figure 4 The role of CDK9/cyclin T in NF-κB transcription and apoptosis. (A) TNF-α induces translocation of NF-κB to the nucleus where it binds κB response elements and stimulates transcription. NF-κB recruits P-TEFb (cyclin T/CDK9) to the complex, leading to hyperphosphorylation of the RNAP II CTD and to efficient elongation of antiapoptotic genes that provide survival signals to cells and inhibit proapoptotic signaling through caspases. (B) When DRB is present upon TNF-α stimulation, phosphorylation of the CTD by CDK9 is inhibited and efficient elongation of antiapoptotic genes that inhibit caspases does not occur, leading to apoptosis. (Adapted from Ref. 89.)

Release and Uptake of Biologically Active Tat

During acute infection, HIV-1-infected cells can release significant amounts of Tat that is biologically active. Tat circulates in the blood of HIV-1-infected individuals (0.1–1 ng/mL 0.01–0.1 n*M*) (90) and exerts its effects on both infected and uninfected cells. Release of Tat from HIV-1-infected cells occurs without induction of cell death or alterations in cell permeability (91–93). Since Tat lacks a secretory signal, its release occurs through a specific leaderless secretory pathway that does not involve the endoplasmic reticulum or the Golgi apparatus, as has been shown for fibroblast growth factors and IL-1 (94). Release of Tat correlates with the extent of Tat expression such that maximal Tat release occurs at an early phase postinfection when Tat expression is high. Although Tat is known to localize to the nucleus (specifically the nucleolus) of cells via its basic rich domain, cytoplasmic localization of Tat appears to be important for its release, as mutation of the nuclear localization sequence of Tat results in an increase in both cytoplasmic concentrations and release of Tat (93).

The basic domain of Tat also allows a portion of released Tat to bind to cell membrane or ECM heparan sulfate proteoglycans, protecting Tat from degradation by proteases similar to the sequestration of growth factors such as bFGF (91,95). The ability of Tat to bind heparin through a functional domain that additionally mediates its nuclear localization, its interaction with TAR, and its cellular uptake suggests several mechanisms by which heparin blocks both transcriptional transactivation by Tat and the effects of extracellular (91,96,97).

Extracellular Tat may affect cells from the outside or inside, dependent upon its concentration (5). Tat must be present in nanomolar to micromolar concentrations to enter cells, a process that, for the most part, appears to be mediated by the basic region of the protein (98,99). Once inside an infected or uninfected cell, Tat has the capacity to transactivate cellular genes encoding various cytokines, chemokines and their receptors, integrins, and ECM proteins. Aberrant expression of these genes may contribute to viral spreading and the progression of AIDS. Additionally, micromolar concentrations of Tat induce apoptosis in T cells, which may contribute to the decline in CD4 + cells associated with AIDS (100). In contrast to these effects, picomolar concentrations of extracellular Tat modulate the expression of genes—such as *bcl-2*, *p53*, and that of CD95 ligand—to promote cell survival (101–106). Based on experimental evidence, the biological effects of picomolar concentrations of Tat are thought to be mediated through the interaction of Tat with specific cell surface receptors and the subsequent engagement of certain signal transduction pathways.

Angiogenic Properties of Tat

In addition to the discovery that *tat*-transgenic mice develop KS-like lesions, studies on the effects of Tat on cells derived from KS lesions (KSC) have provided the initial basis for investigating the role of Tat during angiogenesis (107,108). These studies have demonstrated that Tat-containing conditioned medium (CM) from *tat*-transfected or HIV-1 acutely infected cells stimulate KSC proliferation that can be inhibited by anti-Tat antibodies (92,93). Additionally, biologically active, recombinant Tat induces KSC proliferation to levels comparable to that observed upon mitogen (e.g., bFGF) stimulation (92,93). The concentration of Tat that mediates KSC proliferation ranges from 0.05 to 50 ng/mL; whereas concentrations of Tat greater than 100 ng/mL inhibit KSC growth (92,93). This suggests that Tat is mediating its KSC growth promoting effects by a mechanism that does not involve the transactivation function of Tat, the latter of which requires micromolar concentrations of extracellular Tat (93,109). Extracellular Tat, at picomolar concentrations, also induces KSC chemotaxis and invasion that likely involves the production and the activation of MMP-2 induced by Tat (110–112).

Although Tat stimulates the growth, migration and invasion of KSC, Tat alone does not induce KS-like, angiogenic lesions in nude mice (112). The ability of Tat to act in synergy with bFGF to induce these lesions in nude mice suggests that Tat may increase the aggressiveness of KS and that Tat has angiogenic properties (112).

Tat acts as an angiogenic factor in that it promotes endothelial cell adhesion, migration, differentiation, and growth and induces EC to organize into interconnecting tubular structures or new capillaries (Fig. 5) (5). Furthermore, Tat promotes

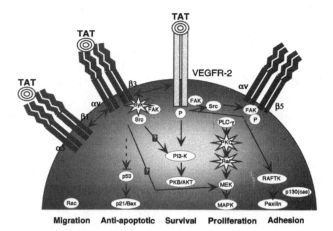

Figure 5 Cross-talk between integrins and VEGF receptors during Tat-induced angiogenesis. Tat-induced angiogenesis, like that induced by other angiogenic factors, requires at least two signals: one from integrin-ECM interaction and one from growth factor receptor activation. The signaling pathways stimulated by integrin and growth factor receptor interactions are only partially known but are essential for the angiogenic effects of Tat (see Fig. 1). Solid lines indicate known pathways. Dashed lines indicate less well understood pathways. Stars represent pathway members that are assumed but not known to be involved. (Adapted from Ref. 12.)

angiogenesis in vivo in CAM and nude mouse models (96,113–116). Other similarities between Tat and angiogenic factors include the ability of Tat to (1) bind heparin and to exist in soluble and extracellularly bound forms; (2) engage specific signal transduction pathways such as phosphorylation of FAK and induction of PI3K/Akt signaling; and (3) induce the release of active matrix metalloproteinases, such as MMP-2, to stimulate endothelial cell invasion (Table 1) (5,111,112,116–118). The role of HIV-1 in the angiogenic process must be indirect, because HIV damages or kills EC (119–125). Therefore HIV-1, through induction of inflammatory cytokines and Tat, may indirectly affect new blood vessel formation (5).

Table 1 Functional Mimicry of Angiogenic Growth Factors and ECM by Tat

Similarities between Tat and angiogenic factors	Similarities between Tat and ECM
Can be soluble or bound to ECM	Contains an RGD sequence
Binds heparin	Binds heparin
Binds VEGFR-2	Binds integrins
Phosphorylates FAK	Phosphorylates FAK
Activates PI3K	Promotes cellular adhesion
Promotes cell growth	Modulates cellular response to mitogens
Induces cellular migration	Induces cellular migration
Promotes vascular cell invasion	Induces and activates MMPs
Induces and activates MMPs	Binds heparan sulfate proteoglycans and
Promotes endothelial cell differentiation	release bFGF in soluble and biologically
Promotes angiogenesis in vivo	active form

Although Tat is considered to be an angiogenic factor due to the properties enumerated above, Tat differs from true angiogenic factors like VEGF and bFGF in that it promotes these angiogenic effects only on EC that are activated by inflammatory cytokines, including IFN-γ, IL-1β, and TNF-α, or by bFGF that is induced by cytokines (5,67,110–112,114,126–128). Although only IFN-γ is required for endothelial cell responsiveness to Tat, IL-1β, and TNF-α act in synergy with IFN-γ to augment the angiogenic effects of Tat (129). Factors that contribute to this synergy include the ability of IFN-γ to increase expression of the TNF receptor and the upregulation of the IFN-γ receptor by TNF-α and IL-1 (130). The levels of these inflammatory cytokines are elevated in blood and lesions of AIDS-KS patients as well as in the blood of HIV-1-infected individuals at risk of acquiring KS. These same inflammatory cytokines stimulate HIV-1 replication increasing the production of Tat. The increased growth rate of KS that is associated both with increased levels of circulating Tat and with localization of inflammatory cytokines and Tat in the microenvironment of the lesions support the notion that Tat plays a role in AIDS-KS progression that is dependent upon the expression of specific inflammatory cytokines. Of note, these same cytokines induce the expression of angiogenic growth factors also found within KS lesions, such as bFGF and VEGF. The development of KS-like lesions in *tat*-transgenic mice may be explained by Tat-mediated transactivation of inflammatory cytokine expression in cells expressing high levels of Tat (5).

Tat Interaction with Vascular Endothelial Cell Receptors

Tat, in picomolar concentrations, binds multiple endothelial cell surface receptors and thereby activates downstream signaling cascades and induces the expression of proteins necessary for angiogenesis. Importantly, Tat binds the α5β1, αvβ3 and αvβ5 integrins and the VEGFR-2 (50,67,111,112,114,116,128,131–133). Tat induces phosphorylation of tyrosine kinase receptors localized at cellular focal adhesion plaques including adhesion focal tyrosine kinase, p130^{cas}, c-Jun amino terminal kinase, Src kinase, and paxillin (116–118).

Many similarities are shared between Tat and extracellular matrix proteins, such as FN and VN. For example, Tat (1) has a heparin-binding domain and an RGD sequence (67,96,111,114,134); (2) binds specific integrins, including αvβ3, αvβ5, and α5β1 (50,67,111,112,114,116,128,131,133); (3) induces cellular migration and modulates cellular responses to angiogenic growth factors (96,110,111,113,114,116,135–138); (4) activates FAK (116–118,139); (5) stimulates cellular migration and invasion (96,110,111,113,114,116,128,135–138); (6) promotes the synthesis of specific matrix remodeling proteases (e.g., MMP-2) (111,112); and (7) affects the balance of soluble versus extracellularly sequestered angiogenic growth factors (Table 1) (5,111).

Vascular cell adhesion, migration, and invasion are mediated through the interaction of the RGD motif of Tat with the specific integrins αvβ3 and α5β1 that serve as the main receptors for FN and VN, respectively (67,140). Adhesion inhibition studies have demonstrated that KSC and endothelial cell adherence to FN or VN is abrogated by wild-type Tat and, conversely, that a peptide containing the RGD of FN blocks adhesion of KSC and endothelial cell to Tat (67). Anti-αvβ3 and α5β1 antibodies inhibit, though not completely, KSC and endothelial cell adhesion to Tat, suggesting the binding of Tat to these integrins is specific (67). These same integrins are expressed in KSC, in activated vascular EC lining the blood vessels of KS lesions and in cytokine-(IFN-γ, IL-1β, and TNF-α) or growth factor–(bFGF or VEGF) stimulated vascular EC grown in culture (112,127,128,141). Extracellular Tat is localized to regions of integrin staining within AIDS-KS lesion, suggesting functional relevance to Tat-integrin interaction in AIDS-KS pathogenesis and angiogenesis. The inability of integrin-specific antibodies to completely block adhesion to immobilized Tat is suggestive of the involvement of both the RGD motif and basic domains in cellular adhesion to Tat (116). Mutations in either the basic region or the RGD motif reduce the adhesive response to Tat. Also, these results are consistent with both regions of Tat being involved in FAK activation (116–118,139).

Angiogenic Effects Mediated by the Tat RGD Motif

Binding of Tat to αvβ3 and α5β1 specifically promotes KSC and EC migration, and antibodies against α5β1 and αvβ3 inhibit KSC and EC migration in response to Tat or to an RGD-containing Tat peptide (111). Using peptides spanning the entire length of Tat, only a peptide containing the RGD motif of Tat is capable of inducing endothelial cell locomotion (111). Interestingly, the basic domain of Tat has been implicated in the induction of migration of monocytes through a mechanism that is mediated through its interaction with VEGFR-1 (136,142); however, this does not occur in EC, as Tat fails to bind VEGFR-1 in these cells (113,142). Although Tat basic domain peptides fail to induce migration in EC, suggesting the exclusion of this domain in this angiogenic effect of Tat, studies employing basic domain mutants of Tat demonstrate that the basic region of Tat, indeed, may play a role in the migratory process (116). The effects of the basic region may be attributable to enhanced Tat–integrin interactions associated with the heparin-binding capacity of the Tat basic domain (91). However, the possibility that introduction of mutations in the basic domain of Tat may have altered the conformation and/or the spatial configuration of the RGD motif thus affecting RGD functionality cannot be excluded; therefore, the role of the basic region of Tat during endothelial cell migration is still unclear (5).

Earlier studies demonstrate that bFGF coordinately expresses MMP-2 and the αvβ3 and α5β1 integrins (111). Ligation of these integrins promotes the synthesis and release of the matrix remodeling protease, MMP-2. Since Tat synergizes with bFGF but not with VEGF in inducing vascular endothelial cell growth and in vivo angiogenesis, the angiogenic affects of Tat correlate with the expression of αvβ3 induced by bFGF and not with αvβ5 that is stimulated by VEGF (111,112). In support RGD-containing peptides, but not peptides in which the RGD is mutated to KGE, block the in vitro and in vivo angiogenic effects of Tat, suggesting again, that Tat RGD–integrin interactions are key mediators of Tat-induced angiogenesis (111). Further, antibodies against αvβ3 and α5β1 inhibit Tat-induced vascular endothelial cell invasion and Tat RGD-containing peptides induce MMP-2 expression to the same levels as does full-length Tat (111,112), indicating the importance of the RGD domain in this angiogenic process. More recent studies demonstrate that Tat cooperates with bFGF but not VEGF in the synthesis and release of activated MMP-2 in EC (143). These effects are apparently due to co-ordinate expression and activation of MT1-MMP and upregulation of cell membrane-bound TIMP-2 by bFGF and Tat as well as to inhibition of basal and bFGF-induced TIMP-1 and -2 secretion by Tat. Tat alone induces the expression of the proenzyme form of MMP-9 in both EC and monocytes (137, 138,143). The combination of Tat and bFGF further increases MMP-9 expression and release in EC in which MMP-9 expression is generally undetectable. However, increased MMP-9 expression induced by Tat and bFGF does not correlate with activation of MMP-9 (143). Tat and bFGF combined, but neither alone, induces vascular permeability and edema in both nude mouse and guinea pig models, although the edematous response is greater in the latter model (143). A synthetic cyclic peptide inhibitor of the gelatinases MMP-2 and -9 reduces the vascular permeability induced by bFGF and Tat in nude mice by 60%, suggesting that this in vivo effect of Tat and bFGF is due at least in part to MMP-2 and -9 induction (143). The biological relevance to this is suggested by the notably high MMP-2 expression in AIDS-KS lesions and in plasma from AIDS-KS patients compared with that observed in individuals with classical KS who are not infected with HIV-1 (143). The high expression of MMP-2, bFGF, Tat, $\alpha v \beta 3$, and $\alpha 5 \beta 1$ in AIDS-KS supports the in vivo involvement of these factors in mediating angiogenesis and edema that characterize KS lesion and may account for the increased aggressiveness of these lesions.

Endothelial cell function depends upon the interactions between growth factors and integrins (10,12,17,45). The signaling pathways induced by integrins and growth factors are convergent, and this "cross talk" between growth factor receptors and integrins is critical to angiogenesis. Since cell adhesion increases responsiveness to angiogenic growth factors, the RGD region of Tat additionally provides vascular EC with the adhesion signals required for their proliferation (5). Consequently, the association of the Tat RGD motif with $\alpha v \beta 3$ and $\alpha 5 \beta 1$ is additionally involved in vascular endothelial cell proliferation induced by Tat, as bFGF-induced growth of EC is elevated upon their adherence to immobilized Tat (111,112). Further, mutations in the RGD motif of Tat decrease the vascular endothelial cell proliferative response (116). Antibody antagonists of $\alpha v \beta 3$ and $\alpha 5 \beta 1$ or cyclic RGD peptides specifically impair bFGF-induced proliferation of EC bound to Tat (111). From these studies, Tat appears to be functioning analogously to FN or VN that likewise provide adhesion signals necessary for growth factor–induced proliferation of EC. The ability of Tat to modulate VEGFR-2, MAPK, and components of focal adhesion in KSC further supports this (5).

These studies suggest a role for Tat in angiogenesis as well as in KS progression that involves, in large part, its functional RGD motif. Studies on *tat*-transgenic mice support this in that KS develops in a milder form in transgenic animals expressing an RGD deletion mutant of Tat as compared to those expressing wild-type Tat (144). The mechanism(s) by which the RGD domain of Tat mediates angiogenesis appears to be one of extracellular matrix mimicry.

Angiogenic Effects Mediated by the Tat Basic Region

Vascular endothelial cell adhesion alone does not stimulate proliferation, but instead requires soluble angiogenic growth factors (10,12,17,42,45,146,147). Like other angiogenic growth factors, Tat has a highly basic domain (aa 48-57) that facilitates its binding to a number of cell surface molecules, presumably through nonspecific ionic interactions (140). The basic region of Tat mediates binding of Tat to $\alpha v \beta 5$ that interacts with the basic region of VN (131), heparan sulfate proteoglycans associated with the cell membrane or extracellular matrix (91,96,111,134), and VEGFR-1 and -2 (7,113,116,117,142,148). Tat peptides that contain the basic rich domain induce proliferation of EC and KSC (111). Additionally, Tat mutants that have disrupted basic domains have impaired ability to stimulate proliferation, suggesting that this region of Tat mediates endothelial cell proliferative responses to Tat (116).

The interaction of Tat with heparan sulfate proteoglycans greatly enhances its angiogenic effects. With respect to RGD-integrin interactions, binding of proteoglycans by Tat enhances the ligation of Tat-RGD to its specific integrin receptors (5,111). Additionally, both Tat and bFGF bind heparan sulfate proteoglycans on the ECM and cell surface, and Tat and bFGF compete for essentially the same heparin binding sites (111). Bound and soluble bFGF are both biologically active (149,150); however, the fraction of bFGF that is associated with the cell surface or extracellular matrix proteoglycans is protected from proteolysis and provides a localized storage of the active protein for rapid access (149,150). Thus, when Tat or the Tat basic peptide binds heparan sulfate proteoglycans, bFGF is released into the soluble fraction where it can more effectively promote angiogenesis (91,111,149–151). The ability of heparin to likewise retrieve sequestered extracellularly bound bFGF into a soluble form suggests a possible explanation for how Tat and heparin, combined, may induce in vivo angiogenesis. Neutralization of bFGF by anti-bFGF antibodies or blocking of bFGF synthesis and release using specific antisense oligonucleotides results in inhibition of endothelial cell and KSC proliferation induced by Tat (111,112).

VEGF-A binds both VEGFR-1 and 2 in EC, although the latter is the main mediator of VEGF-induced angiogenesis. This is due to the fact that VEGF binding to the VEGFR-2 activates signal transduction pathways, such as mitogen-activated protein kinases that are not induced by VEGF–VEGFR-1 interaction, stimulating endothelial cell migration and proliferation. In contrast, VEGF–VEGFR-1 binding induces endothelial cell migration but not proliferation. However, VEGFR1 and VEGFR-2 can homodimerize or heterodimerize following VEGF-A binding, and dimers containing VEGFR-2 can autophosphorylate and thus mediate angiogenesis (152).

Tat binds the VEGFR-2 through its basic domain, although this region of Tat contains an RKK sequence, as opposed to the RKH sequence that mediates the binding of VEGF-A to this receptor (153). Binding of Tat to VEGFR-2 stimulates the phosphorylation of this receptor in EC and KSC, and activates the same signal transduction pathways that are invoked by VEGF-A–VEGFR-2 interaction (50,113, 116,117). Tat basic region–containing peptides have the same effect as Tat in activating signal transduction pathways from the VEGFR-2 (116). However, Tat proteins bearing mutations in the basic domain are still competent in stimulating these pathways and in inducing EC proliferation (116). Since the signaling pathways activated by both Tat and VEGF are the same as those engaged upon integrin (αvβ3 and α5β1) ligation by VN, FN, or Tat, the RGD domain of this mutant Tat is likely providing the necessary adhesion signal to stimulate proliferation induced by growth factors (118,154–156). Although Tat binds VEGFR-1 in monocytes, it does not do so in EC, even though the receptors in both cell types are identical (113,142). This may help to explain the different effects that Tat and VEGF-A have on EC. For example, (1) VEGF-A induces both migration and growth in EC expressing VEGFR-1 and -2, whereas Tat can only do so if EC are prestimulated with cytokines (110,126–128,152); (2) VEGF-A induces angiogenesis in nude mice whose tissues express VEGFR-1 and-2, whereas Tat, alone, cannot (112,114); (3) Tat promotes KSC growth, whereas exogenous VEGF-A does not (151); and (4) αvβ5 integrin is required for VEGF-A– but not Tat-induced angiogenesis (43,111,131).

Tat mediates its angiogenic effects, including adhesion, migration, proliferation, invasion, and in vivo blood vessel formation in synergy with bFGF, that is induced by cytokine (IL-1β, TNF-α, and IFN-α) prestimulation of EC (5). Similarly, Tat induces in vivo angiogenesis in synergy with these same inflammatory cytokines. Although these inflammatory cytokines induce the expression of both bFGF and VEGF, Tat acts in synergy with only bFGF to exert its angiogenic effects. Tat enhances the proliferative response of EC induced by exogenous bFGF by effectively maintaining the growth factor in a soluble active state (5). Basic FGF but not VEGF induces the adhesion of EC to Tat via αvβ3 and α5β1, suggesting that Tat exerts its angiogenic effects through a distinct integrin-mediated pathway. Although the basic domain of Tat mediates the binding of Tat to αvβ5, anti-αvβ5 antibodies fail to inhibit the angiogenic effects of Tat, suggesting that Tat-αvβ5 does not have a functional role in Tat-induced angiogenesis (111,131). In vivo studies in support of this demonstrate that the angiogenic effects of Tat correlate with expression of β3 and β1 that are stimulated by either bFGF or inflammatory cytokines but not with β5 expression induced by VEGF (114). Therefore exogenous bFGF, or that which is induced by inflammatory cytokines, stimulates the expression of αvβ3 and α5β1, which mediate Tat-induced angiogenesis (67). Blocking of Tat-RGD binding to these receptors by antibodies specific to these integrins or with cyclic RGD–containing peptides abrogates the angiogenic effects of Tat (Fig. 6) (67,111,112,114,116–118,136,139,140). Although

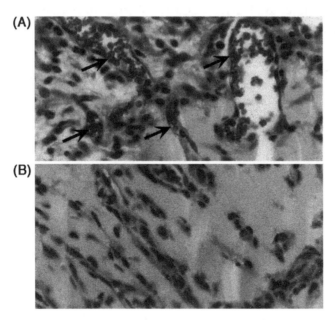

Figure 6 Inhibition of growth factor–induced angiogenesis by cyclic RGD peptides. Angiogenic lesions were induced in Balb/c (nu/nu) athymic mice by subcutaneous inoculation of equal amounts of bFGF dispersed in Matrigel (4 mice/group). After 72 hr, mice were inoculated intraperitoneally with cyclic peptides containing either KGE (A) or RGD (B). Seventy-two hours later, mice were sacrificed and tissues at the initial injection sites (including the Matrigel "plug") were retrieved and subjected to hematoxylin-eosin staining (×400 magnification). (A) KGE peptides fail to inhibit blood vessel formation (depicted by arrows). (B) RGD peptides efficiently block blood vessel formation. Accordingly, published studies (see text) have shown that these cyclic peptides inhibit angiogenesis induced by the combination of bFGF and Tat as well.

integrin antagonists do not block the binding of EC by bFGF or VEGF, they potently inhibit angiogenesis induced by these angiogenic growth factors, particularly those that target $\alpha v\beta 3$ (42,50,111,116,145). A mechanism for this has been suggested by a recent study in which VN binding to $\alpha v\beta 3$ in EC induces activation/phosphorylation of VEGFR-2, which correlates with VEGF-A–stimulated complex formation between VEGFR-2 and the integrin receptor (50). The net result of this receptor "cross talk" is full activation of the VEGFR-2 and consequent induction of EC proliferation. Although much remains to be learned about the molecular mechanism(s) that mediate Tat-induced angiogenesis, it is certain that the angiogenic effects of Tat involve the convergence of signaling pathways invoked by integrins and growth factor receptors.

Platelet-Activating Factor as a Mediator of Tat-Induced Angiogenesis

A potentially important secondary mediator of Tat-induced angiogenesis is platelet-activating factor (PAF), which is a phospholipid mediator of inflammation and of angiogenesis induced by certain cytokines and growth factors, including TNF, hepatocyte growth factor (HGF), and VEGF (157–160). PAF directly stimulates endothelial cell migration by these agonists in vitro and promotes in vivo angiogenesis (161). Although bFGF is able to induce PAF synthesis, bFGF-induced angiogenesis is not dependent upon synthesis of PAF (161).

A recent study demonstrates that Tat stimulates synthesis of PAF in HUVEC in a time- and dose-dependent manner. Doses of Tat as low as 0.1 ng/mL activate PAF and PAF levels plateau at concentrations of Tat from 10 to 20 ng/mL. Thus, PAF synthesis by Tat may have some biological relevance as the PAF stimulating doses of Tat are observed in the serum of HIV-1–infected patients (up to 1 ng/mL). In tissues where HIV-1 replication occurs, the levels of Tat may exceed that which is seen in the serum (103).

A specific PAF receptor antagonist, WEB 2170, inhibits both the in vitro migration of EC and the in vivo angiogenesis induced by Tat. Additionally, Tat-induced motility of KSC requires PAF synthesis (162). These studies suggest that PAF may be a critical mediator of the angiogenic effects of Tat.

THE MORE AND LESS KNOWN ABOUT TAT-INDUCED ANGIOGENESIS

The Role of the Transactivation Domain of Tat During Angiogenesis

Tat, acting in synergy with bFGF or combined inflammatory cytokines (IC), stimulates angiogenesis. Studies to date suggest a model in which the proangiogenic effects of Tat are mediated through the RGD and basic region domains of Tat that function by a molecular mimicry of extracellular matrix proteins. Only a few studies have addressed the potential proangiogenic effects mediated by the transcriptional activation function of Tat. Tat is known to be secreted from HIV-1-infected cells in circulation and in AIDS-KS lesions, and Tat is taken up efficiently by most cell types, including endothelial cells (5). Tat is present in KS lesions, mostly within uninfected EC, suggesting preferential uptake of Tat by the endothelium (163). In fact, the efficiency of Tat uptake has perpetuated its use as a vehicle to introduce heterologous recombinant proteins into a wide variety of cells (164,165). After entry into endothelial cells, Tat mediates similar transcriptional functions as have been observed in other cell types. Evidence for this includes the ability of endothelial cells, cultured in the presence of recombinant Tat, to support Tat transactivation of TAR-dependent transactivation from the HIV-1 LTR (166). Other evidence includes the ability of Tat to activate the expression of E-selectin and IL-8 in EC, both of which likely play a role in angiogenesis induced by Tat (167,168).

Recently, a short peptide of Tat (aa 21-40) that spans the cysteine-rich trans-activation domain has been shown to induce angiogenesis in chicken chorioallantoic membranes (115). The mechanism(s) by which this domain of Tat stimulates angio-genesis is not known. However, the cysteine-rich domain binds unstimulated EC (116) and similar cysteine-rich sequences occur in a number of angiogenic growth factors including VEGF, platelet-derived growth factor (PDGF), and placental growth factor (P1GF) (169). Although mutations in the cysteine-rich region of Tat do not affect Tat binding to EC through low-affinity binding sites of VEGFR-2 or Tat-mediated adhesion of EC, they reduce EC proliferation and fail to induce in vivo angiogenesis (116). Additionally, Tat variants with mutations in the cysteine-rich domain fail to induce tyrosine phosphorylation of VEGFR-2 and consequent endothelial cell signal-ing, such as PI3K, that is stimulated by wild-type Tat (116). These studies collectively suggest that the cysteine-rich region of Tat plays a role in Tat-induced angiogenesis. However, the Tat RGD motif that engages specific integrins and regulates VEGFR-2 activation is possibly indispensable for full activation of the angiogenic process in EC. The ability of anti-αvβ3 and anti-VEGFR-2 neutralizing antibodies to abrogate Tat-induced angiogenesis further suggests that Tat is able to bind to and activate both integrin and growth factor receptors to induce angiogenesis.

The Inability of Tat to Act in Synergy with VEGF

Since the cysteine-region mediates dimerization of Tat, the possibility exists that Tat activation of VEGFR-2 may require Tat to be in a dimeric form. Tat may conceivably regulate VEGFR-2 by heterodimerizing with VEGF-A through bridging of cysteine-rich regions, thus decreasing the levels of active VEGF-A, which is most active in signaling when homodimerized (5). A similar scenario has been shown for placental growth factor (P1GF) and VEGF-A (170). Alternatively, Tat may inhibit VEGF-A binding to VEGFR-2 by blocking the interaction of VEGF-A with cell surface heparan sulfate proteoglycans. This competitive inhibition by Tat may provide a possible explanation as to why Tat does not act in synergy to induce angiogenesis with VEGF, while bFGF does. Another possibility is that Tat, through its RGD, may compete with vitronectin for αvβ3 binding that is necessary for complete VEGFR-2 activation (50,67). The fact that VEGF can inhibit endothelial cell migration by Tat and can inhibit Tat binding to EC implies that perhaps Tat and VEGF reciprocally interfere with each other (113,142). Yet another possibility to explain the lack of synergy between Tat and VEGF is the fact that VEGF induces the expression of αvβ5 in particular, which does not mediate the angiogenic properties of Tat.

Tat-Induced Endothelial Cell Survival and Apoptosis

A recent study demonstrates that the interaction of Tat with VEGFR-2 activates PI3K/Akt-dependent survival pathways in KSC that correlate with enhanced phosphorylation and thus inhibition of the proapoptotic factor Bad (171). Vincristine treatment of KSC and serum withdrawal from HUVECs results in apoptosis (172). Tat protects KSC and EC from apoptosis in a dose-dependent manner through a mechanism that is independent of modulation of Fas, Bax, or Bcl-2 expression. However, in vincristine-treated KSC, Tat-induced survival correlates with increased expression of Bcl-X(L) and decreased caspase-3 activity (172). Tat activation of Akt is biphasic, with activation occurring early within 15 min (protein synthesis–independent) and delayed at 24 hr (protein synthesis–dependent) (171). Early activation of Akt implies direct stimulation of PI3K/Akt by Tat. Early activation of Akt is efficiently blocked by anti–VEGFR-2 antibodies suggesting that this survival pathway is stimulated through interaction of Tat with VEGFR-2. The delayed response suggests that Tat may induce the production of secondary mediators [e.g., VEGF, IL-3, insulin-like growth factor 1 (IGF-1)] that further activate Akt (171). The fact that anti-VEGFR-2 antibodies only partially block delayed Akt activation suggests that Tat-mediated synthesis of mediators in addition to increased VEGF are important. These studies suggest a putative functional role for the transactivation function of Tat in mediating survival during angiogenesis (171).

Other studies support a role for Tat in inducing the expression of anti-apoptotic genes that correlate with cellular survival. Specifically, Tat upregulates *bcl-2* expression in Jurkat cells and in peripheral blood mononuclear cells (102). This presumably occurs through a mechanism that involves both exons of Tat (173). Although the precise mechanisms mediating Tat-induced activation of Bcl-2 are not known, studies suggest that transcriptional, posttranslational and signaling effects may be involved. Specifically, it is feasible that Tat, through RGD-dependent adhesion, through growth factor receptor binding, or through transactivation of the *bcl-2* gene, may stimulate the expression of Bcl-2. The biphasic, Tat-induced activation of Akt, a second messenger that invokes numerous parallel survival pathways in vascular endothelial cells including Bcl-2 (13,174), does not correlate with changes in Bcl-2 expression in KSC; however, KSC express abundant amounts of Bcl-2 and induction above already high levels of expression may not be detectable in these cells in response to Tat (175). In contrast, resting vascular EC that are unstimulated express minimal, if any, Bcl-2. Consequently, during Tat-induced angiogenesis, Bcl-2 levels may likely increase in ECs, along with increased levels of Akt phosphorylation. Akt is a critical regulator of EC survival that is activated by a number of endothelial cell stimuli, including VEGF, angiopoetin-1, IGF-1, insulin, HGF, sphingosine-1-phosphate, decorin, estrogen, shear stress, corticosteroids, and reactive oxygen species (13). Predictably, Tat may play a role in activating some of the numerous downstream effectors of Akt signaling in EC, including Bcl-2 activation (13,174). Other mediators of Akt signaling may also be induced by Tat during angiogenesis, although currently little is known.

Recently, a study using Tat-expressing cells (T53) derived from an adenocarcinoma of a *tat*-transgenic mouse has demonstrated that blocking of both intracellular and extracellular Tat results in a decrease in *bcl-2* gene expression, proliferation, tumorigenesis, and angiogenesis. Collectively, these studies suggest that Tat provides a survival signal for EC and KSC (176).

In sharp contrast to the notion that Tat acts as a survival factor for EC, a recent study demonstrates in primary lung microvascular endothelial cells (HMVEC-L) that Tat induces apoptosis occurring without induction of Fas or TNF(177). Additionally, Tat promotes the cleavage of a caspase substrate, poly(A/DP)-ribose polymerase.

Anti-Tat antibodies inhibit caspase-3 activity, markedly reducing apoptosis in these cells that does not correlate with modulated expression of Bcl-2, Bax, or Bad (177).

The disparity among these studies may be due to experimental design and cell type–specific differences in which Tat may be invoking different signaling pathways. Investigators have speculated that the ability of Tat to activate several cellular receptors, including VEGFR-2, VEGFR-1, $\alpha v\beta 3$, and $\alpha 5\beta 1$ may confuse cells due to induction of multiple signaling pathways simultaneously (113,117,131,136,177,178). Such confused signaling can result from changes in normal adhesion and growth factor signaling that results in apoptosis (179). Interestingly, high concentrations of Tat RGD–containing peptides induce apoptosis in HMVEC-L; whereas, equimolar amounts of Tat (picomolar range) do not (177). These results suggest that the role of the RGD motif in Tat-mediated apoptosis in EC is nominal, at best, and that the signaling pathways that lead to Tat-induced angiogenesis (a survival pathway) and to Tat-induced apoptosis (a death pathway) are distinct (177). In support, RGD peptides, in general induce apoptosis directly, requiring no integrin-mediated clustering or signaling (180). They enter cells and induce conformational alterations leading to autoprocessing and activation of procaspase 3 (180).

This same sort of rationale may help explain the ability of cysteine-rich and basic domain Tat peptides to induce apoptosis in HUVEC and to inhibit angiogenesis (181). These peptides inhibit VEGF-induced binding of VEGFR-2 and its putative coreceptor, neuropilin-1 (NP-1) and abrogate VEGF- and bFGF-mediated ERK activation, blocking EC proliferation. Importantly, the ability of these peptides to induce an apoptotic response in EC is independent of their effects on VEGF and bFGF activity, suggesting involvement of different signaling pathways and downstream effectors (181).

A Role for Transactivation Function of Tat During Angiogenesis

Although immediate-early effects of Tat on EC during angiogenesis appear to be mediated by the ability of Tat to activate adhesion and GFR signaling, the delayed effects of Tat may feasibly involve the transcriptional transactivation function of Tat, particularly mediating EC survival, and possibly differentiation. Tat is well known to transcriptionally activate a number of genes that likely play a role during angiogenesis. For example, Tat activates transcription of IGF-1 and IL-3 in KSC that correlates with both a delayed Tat-induced Akt activation response and protection from apoptosis (171). Additionally, Tat induces the expression of antiapoptotic genes, such as Bcl-2 (173). These studies, as well as others not discussed here, suggest that Tat-induced survival during angiogenesis may be mediated, in part, through the transactivation function of Tat. The ability of Tat to upregulate expressin of MT1-MMP in the activation and release of MMP-2 in EC suggests that the transactivation function of Tat may additionally have a role in differentiation of EC that ensues upon switching from a proliferative to an invasive state to initiate the process of vessel formation. Identifying the downstream targets of Tat transactivation that are involved in these processes is critical to understanding how Tat induces angiogenesis.

One intriguing aim toward studying the transactivation function of Tat during angiogenesis would be to determine whether the cellular cofactor complex that is critical for Tat transactivation of the HIV-1 LTR is likewise important for transactivation of cellular genes in EC that contain no TAR response element. Recently, studies have demonstrated that P-TEF-b, the catalytic subunit of TAK (cyclin T/

CDK9) mediates NF-κB (specifically Rel A)–activated transcription elongation of the chemokine/angiogenic factor IL-8 (89,182). These studies suggest a role for cyclin T/P-TEFb in human cells beyond activation of genes involved in heat-shock response and antigen processing and presentation (183). Since many of the TAR-independent transactivation effects of Tat are mediated through NF-κB, it is feasible to propose that cyclin T/CDK9 may mediate Tat transactivation of specific cellular genes such as IL-8 or Bcl-2. Alternatively, induction of angiogenesis by angiogenic growth factors with or without Tat may trigger increases in CDK9 activity that correlate with endothelial cell survival and/or differentiation. Studies testing this have yet to be published. However, preliminary data from ongoing studies demonstrate that stimulation of serum-starved, primary HUVEC with bFGF and VEGF increases expression of cyclin T but not CDK9 and correlates with stimulation of CDK9 activity (A.B. Nelson, unpublished). Increases in CDK9 activity and cyclin-T expression are coincident with upregulation of Bcl-2 and endothelial cell survival induced by bFGF. These studies suggest a putative, novel role for cyclin T/CDK9 in vascular endothelial cell survival, although additional experiments are required for confirmation of this. In support of this hypothesis, recent studies have attributed a functional role for CDK9 activity induced during monocyte differentiation. Specifically, these studies show that PMA-induced differentiation of pro-monocytic cell lines induces a significant increase in cyclin T1 protein; whereas, CDK9 protein levels remain constitutively high. Overexpression of a dominant-negative mutant of CDK9 in the promonocytic cell line U937 sensitizes the cells to apoptosis, particularly after PMA treatment, to induce differentiation, suggesting that CDK9 may have an anti-apoptotic function during monocyte differentiation (184). A similar scenario may be occurring in EC induced to form new blood vessels, and the presence of Tat may enhance the angiogenic process.

Potential Cooperative Effects of Tat and HHV-8 During Angiogenesis and Kaposi's Sarcoma

A recent study demonstrates that the HHV-8 G protein-coupled receptor (HHV-8 ORF74) promotes NF-κB–dependent endothelial cell survival through Akt signaling (185,186). HHV-8 is present in EC of KS lesions and is able to infect EC in vitro (186). Although only a small portion of cultured cells are infected, the cells as a whole adopt a spindle-shaped morphology and have an increased proliferative life span, suggesting that HHV-8 infection induces paracrine and phenotypically altering effects on neighboring, uninfected cells (186). In HIV-1 infected individuals, Tat may contribute to HHV-8 infection and KS pathogenesis by activating the P13K/Akt signaling survival pathway and possibly by cooperating with HHV-8 ORF74 in the induction of angiogenesis. Studies designed to test these hypotheses and to determine the molecular mechanisms involved may elucidate novel targets for therapeutic intervention of KS as well as for other pathologies that are dependent upon angiogenesis.

REFERENCES

1. Ferrara N, Chen F, Davis ST, Gerber HP, Nguyen TN, Peers D, Chisolm V, Hillan KJ, Schwall RH. Vascular endothelial growth factor is essential for corpus luteum angiogenesis. Nat Med 1998; 4:336–340.

2. Aiello LP. Vascular endothelial growth factor and the eye: biochemical mechanisms of actin and implication for novel therapies. Opthal Res 1997; 29:354–362.
3. Sueishi K, Yonemitsu Y, Nakagawa K, Kaneda Y, Kumamoto M, Nakashima Y. Atherosclerosis and angiogenesis: its pathophysiological significance in humans as well as in an animal model induced by the gene transfer of vascular endothelial growth factor. Ann N Y Acad Sci 1997; 811:311–322.
4. Zetter BR. Angiogenesis and tumor metastasis. Annu Rev Med 1998; 49:407–424.
5. Barillari G, Ensoli B. Angiogenic effects of extracellular human immunodeficiency virus type 1 Tat protein and its role in the pathogenesis of AIDS-associated Kaposi's sarcoma. Clin Microbiol Rev 2002; 15(2):310–326.
6. Reitz M, Nerurkar L, Gallo RC. Perspective on Kaposi's sarcoma: facts, concepts, and conjectures. J Natl Cancer Inst 1999; 91(17):1453–1458.
7. Morini M, Benelli R, Giunciuglio D, Carlone S, Arena G, Noonan DM, Albini A. Kaposi's sarcoma cells of different etiologic origins respond to HIV-Tat through the Flk-1/KD (VEGFR-2): relevance in AIDS-KS pathology. Biochem Biophys Res Commun 2000; 273(1):267–271.
8. Beckstead JH. Oral presentation of Kaposi's sarcoma in a patient without severe immunodeficiency. Arch Pathol Lab Med 1992; 116:543–545.
9. Kestens L, Melbye M, Biggar RJ, Stevens WJ, Piot P, De Muynck A, Taelman H, De Feyter M, Paluku L, Gigase PL. Endemic African KS is not associated with immuno-deficiency. Int J Cancer 1985; 36:49–54.
10. Rupp P, Little C. Integrins in vascular development. Circ Res 2001; 89:566–572.
11. Cross MJ, Cclaesson-Welsh L. FGF and VEGF function in angiogenesis: signaling pathways, biological responses and therapeutic inhibition. Trends Pharmacol Sci 2001; 22:201–207.
12. Smyth SS, Patterson C. Tiny dancers: the integrin-growth factor nexus in angiogenic signaling. J Cell Biol 2002; 158:17–21.
13. Shiojima I, Walsh K. Role of Akt signaling in vascular homeostasis and angiogenesis. Circ Res 2002; 90(12):1243–1250.
14. Post MJ. Angiogenesis: initiation and maintenance. Ann N Y Acad Sci 2002; 961:249–250.
15. Hlatky L, Hahnfeldt P, Folkman J. Clinical application of antiangiogenic therapy: microvessel density, what it does and doesn't tell us. J Natl Cancer Inst 2002; 94(12):883–893.
16. Chavakis E, Dimmeler S. Regulation of endothelial cell survival and apoptosis during angiogenesis. Arterioscler Thromb Vasc Biol 2002; 22(6):887–893.
17. Eliceiri B. Integrin and growth factor receptor crosstalk. Circ Res 2001; 89:1104–1110.
18. Giancotti FG, Ruoslahti E. Integrin signaling. Science 1999; 285(5430):1028–1032.
19. Hynes RO. Integrins: versatility, modulation and signaling in cell adhesion. Cell 1992; 69:11–24.
20. Drake CJ, Little CD. The morphogenesis of primary vascular networks. In: Little C, Mironov V, Sage EH, eds. Vascular Morphogenesis: In vivo, in Vitro, in Mente. Boston, MA: Birkhauser, 1998:3–21.
21. Shattil SJ, Ginsberg MH. Integrin signaling in vascular biology. J Clin Invest 1997; 100(suppl 11):S91–S95.
22. Schwartz MA, Baron V. Interactions between mitogenic stimuli, or, a thousand and one connections. Curr Opin Cell Biol 1999; 11:197–202.
23. Senger DR, Claffey KP, Benes JE, Perruzzi CA, Sergiou AP, Detmar M. Angiogenesis promoted by vascular endothelial growth factor: regulation through alpha1beta1 and alpha2beta1 integrins. Proc Natl Acad Sci USA 1997; 94(25):13612–13617.
24. Senger DR, Ledbetter SR, Claffey KP, Papadopoulos-Sergiou A, Peruzzi CA, Detmar M. Stimulation of endothelial cell migration by vascular permeability factor/vascular

endothelial growth factor through cooperative mechanisms involving the alphavbeta3 integrin, osteopontin, and thrombin. Am J Pathol 1996; 149(1):293–305.

25. Byzova VT, Goldman KC, Pampori N, Thomas AK, Bett A, Shattil JS, Plow FE. A mechanism for modulation of cellular responses to VEGF activation of integrins. Mol Cell 2000; 6:851–860.

26. Senger DR, Ledbetter SR, Claffey KP, Papadopoulos-Sergiou A, Peruzzi CA, Detmar M. Stimulation of endothelial cell migration by vascular permeability factor/vascular endothelial growth factor through cooperative mechanisms involving alphavbeta3 integrin, osteopontin, and thrombin. Am J Pathol 1996; 149:293–305.

27. Enenstein J, Waleh NS, Kramer RH. Basic FGF and TGF-beta differentially modulate integrin expression of human microvascular endothelial cells. Exp Cell Res 1992; 203(2):499–503.

28. Sepp NT, Li LJ, Lee KH, Brown EJ, Caughman SW, Lawley TJ, Swerlick RA. Basic fibroblast growth factor increases expression of the alpha v beta 3 integrin complex on human microvascular endothelial cells. J Invest Dermatol 1994; 103(3):295–299.

29. Wennerberg K, Lohikangas L, Gullberg D, Pfaff M, Johansson S, Fassler R. Beta 1 integrin-dependent and -independent polymerization of fibronectin. J Cell Biol 1996; 132(1–2):227–238.

30. Fogerty FJ, Akiyama SK, Yamada KM, Mosher DF. Inhibition of binding of fibronectin to matrix assembly sites by anti-integrin (alpha 5 beta 1) antibodies. J Cell Biol 1990; 111(2):699–708.

31. Bayless KJ, Salazar R, Davis GE. RGD-dependent vacuolation and lumen formation observed during endothelial cell morphogenesis in three-dimensional fibrin matrices involves the alpha(v)beta(3) and alpha(5)beta(1) integrins. Am J Pathol 2000; 156(5):1673–1683.

32. Davis GE, Camarillo CW. An alpha 2 beta 1 integrin-dependent pinocytic mechanism involving intracellular vacuole formation and coalescence regulates capillary lumen and tube formation in three-dimensional collagen matrix. Exp Cell Res 1996; 224(1):39–51.

33. Dallabrida SM, De Sousa MA, Farrell DH. Expression of antisense to integrin subunit beta 3 inhibits microvascular endothelial cell capillary tube formation in fibrin. J Biol Chem 2000; 275(41):32281–32288.

34. Shattil SJ, Ginsberg MH. Perspectives series: cell adhesion in vascular biology. Integrin signaling in vascular biology. J Clin Invest 1997; 100(1):1–5.

35. Klemke RL, Leng J, Molander R, Brooks PC, Vuori K, Cheresh DA. CAS/Crk coupling serves as a "molecular switch" for induction of cell migration. J Cell Biol 1998; 140(4):961–972.

36. Collins LR, Ricketts WA, Yeh L, Cheresh D. Bifurcation of cell migratory and proliferative signaling by the adaptor protein Shc. J Cell Biol 1999; 147(7):1561–1568.

37. Aplin AE, Howe A, Alahari SK, Juliano RL. Signal transduction and signal modulation by cell adhesion receptors: the role of integrins, cadherins, immunoglobulin-cell adhesion molecules, and selectins. Pharmacol Rev 1998; 50(2):197–263.

38. Schwartz MA, Shattil SJ. Signaling networks linking integrins and rho family GTPases. Trends Biochem Sci 2000; 25(8):388–391.

39. Miyamoto S, Teramoto H, Gutkind JS, Yamada KM. Integrins can collaborate with growth factors for phosphorylation of receptor tyrosine kinases and MAP kinase activation: roles of integrin aggregation and occupancy of receptors. J Cell Biol 1996; 135 (6 Pt 1):1633–1642.

40. Ridley A. Rho GTPases. Integrating integrin signaling. J Cell Biol 2000; 150(4):F107–F109.

41. Schwartz MA, Schaller MD, Ginsberg MH. Integrins: emerging paradigms of signal transduction. Annu Rev Cell Dev Biol 1995; 11:549–599.

42. Brooks PC, Clark RA, Cheresh DA. Requirement of vascular integrin avB3 for angiogenesis. Science 1994; 264:569–571.

43. Friedlander MP, Brooks C, Shaffer RW, Kincaid CM, Varner JA, Cheresh DA. Definition of two angiogenic pathways by distinct av integrins. Science 1995; 270:1500–1502.

44. Ingberg D. Extracellular matrix and cell shape potential control points for inhibition of angiogenesis. Biochem 1991; 47:236–241.

45. Eliceiri B, Cheresh DA. Adhesion Events in angiogenesis. Curr Opin Cell Biol 2001; 13:563–568.

46. Stromblad S, Becker JC, Yebra M, Brooks PC, Cheresh DA. Suppression of p53 activity and p21waf/cp1 expression by vascular cell integrin avB3 during angiogenesis. J Clin Invest 1996; 98:426–433.

47. Zhang Z, Vuori K, Reed JC, Ruoslahti E. The alpha 5 beta 1 integrin supports survival of cells on fibronectin and up-regulates Bcl-2 expression. Proc Natl Acad Sci USA 1995; 92(13):6161–6165.

48. Gerber HP, McMurtrey A, Kowalski J, Yan M, Keyt BA, Dixit VM, Ferrara N. Vascular endothelial growth factor regulates endothelial cell survival through the phosphoinositol 3′-kinase/Akt signal transduction pathway. Requirement for Flk-1/KDR activation. J Biol Chem 1998; 273:30336–30343.

49. Gerber HP, Dixit VM, Ferrara N. Vascular endothelial growth factor induces expression of the antiapoptotic proteins Bcl-2 and A11 in vascular endothelial cells. J Biol Chem 1998; 273:13313–13316.

50. Soldi R, Mitola S, Strasly M, Defilippi P, Tarone G, Bussolino F. Role of alpha V beta 3 integrin in the activation of vascular endothelial growth factor receptor-2. EMBO J 1999; 18:882–892.

51. Kinoh H, Sato H, Tsunezuka Y, Takino T, Kawashima A, Okada Y, Seiki M. MT-MMP, the cell surface activator of proMMP-2 (pro-gelatinase A), is expressed with its substrate in mouse tissue during embryogenesis. J Cell Sci 1996; 109:953–959.

52. Itoh T, Tanioka M, Yoshida H, Yoshioka T, Nishimoto H, Itohara S. A novel phosphatidylinositol-5-phosphate 4-kinase (phosphatidylinositol-phosphate kinase llgamma) is phosphorylated in the endoplasmic reticulum in response to mitogenic signals. J Biol Chem 1998; 273:143–149.

53. Silletti S, Cheresh DA. Fibrinolysis proteinolysis 1999; 13:226–238.

54. Lyden D, Young AZ, Zagzag D, Yan W, Geerald W, O'Reilly R, Bader BL, Hynes RO, Zhuang Y, Manova K, Benezra R. Id1 and Id3 are required for neurogenesis, angiogenesis and vascularization of tumour xenografts. Nature (London) 1999; 401:670–677.

55. Brooks PC, Stromblad S, Sanders LC, von Schalscha TL, Aimes RT, Stetler-Stevenson WG, Quigley JP, Cheresh DA. Chemokines are the main proinflammatory mediators in human monocytes activated by *Staphylococcus aureus*, peptidoglycan, and endotoxin. Cell 1996; 85:683–693.

56. Wang Z, Juuterman R, Soloway PD. Specialized surface protrusions in invasive cells, invadopodia and lamellipodia, have differential MT1-MMP, MMP-2, and TIMP-2 localization. J Biol Chem 2000; 275:26411–26415.

57. Chen WT, Wang JY. Disruption of matrix metalloproteinase 2 binding to integrin alpha vbeta 3 by an organic molecule inhibits angiogenesis and tumor growth in vivo. Ann N Y Acad Sci 1999; 878:361–371.

58. Silletti S, Kessler T, Goldberg J, Boger D, Cheresh DA. Disruption of matrix metalloproteinase 2 binding to integrin alpha-v-beta-3 by an organic molecule inhibits angiogenesis and tumor growth in vivo. Proc Natl Acad Sci USA 2001; 98(1):119–124.

59. Arya SK, Guo C, JS F, Wong-Staal F. Transactivator gene of human T-lymphotropic virus type III (HTLV-III). Science 1985; 229:69–73.

60. Re M, Furlini G, Vignoli M, Ramazzotti E, Roderigo G, DeRosa V, Zauli G, Lolli S,

Capitani S, LaPlaca M. Effect of antibody to HIV-1 Tat protein on viral replication in vitro and progression of HIV-1 disease in vivo. J AIDS Hum Retrovir 1995; 10:408–416.

61. Re M, Furlini G, Vignoli M, Ramazzotti E, Zauli G, LaPlaca M. Antibody against human immunodeficiency virus type 1 (HIV-1) Tat protein may have influenced the progression of AIDS in HIV-1-infected hemophiliac patients. Clin Diagn Lab Immunol 1996; 3:230–232.

62. van Baalen C, Pontesilli O, Huisman RC, Geretti AM, Klein MR, De W, Miedema F, Fruters RA, Osterhaus AD. Human Immunodeficiency virus type I Rev- and Tat-specific cytotoxic T-lymphocyte frequencies inversely correlate with rapid progression to AIDS. J Gen Virol 1997; 78:1913–1918.

63. Cullen B. Does HIV-1 Tat induce a change in viral initiation rights? Cell 1993; 73:417–420.

64. Jones KA, Peterlin BM. Control of initiation and elongation at the HIV-1 promoter. Annu Rev Biochem 1994; 63:717–743.

65. Jeang KT, Xiao H, Rich EA. Multifaceted activities of the HIV-1 transactivator of transcription, Tat. J Biol Chem 1999; 274(41):28837–28840.

66. Frankel AD, Biancalana S, Hudson D. Activity of synthetic peptides from the Tat protein of human immunodeficiency virus type 1. Proc Natl Acad Sci USA 1989; 86:7397–7401.

67. Barillari G, Gendelman R, Gallo RC, Ensoli B. The Tat protein of human immunodeficiency virus type 1, a growth factor for AIDS Kaposi sarcoma and cytokine-activated vascular cells, induces adhesion of the same cell types by using integrin receptors recognizing the RGD amino acid sequence. Proc Natl Acad Sci USA 1993; 90(17):7941–7945.

68. Drake DA, Debouck C, Biesecker G. Identification of an Arg-Gly-Asp (RGD) cell adhesion site in human immunodeficiency virus type I transactivator protein. J Cell Biol 1990; 111:1275–1281.

69. Herrman C, Rice A. Specific interaction of the human immunodeficiency virus Tat proteins with a cellular protein kinase. J Virol 1993; 197:601–608.

70. Herrman C, Rice A. Lentivirus Tat proteins specifically associate with a cellular protein kinase, TAK, that phosphorylates the carboxyl-terminal domain of the large subunit of RNA polymerase II: candidate for a Tat cofactor. J Virol 1995; 69:1612–1620.

71. Mancebo H, Lee G, Flygare J, Tomassini J, Luu P, Zhu Y, Blau C, Hazuda D, Price D, Flores O. PTEF-b kinase is required for HIV Tat transcriptional activation in vivo and in vitro. Genes Dev 1997; 11:2633–2644.

72. Zhu Y, Pe'ery T, Peng T, Ramanathan Y, Marshall N, Marshall T, Amendt B, Matthews M, Price D. Transcriptional elongation factor PTEF-b is required for HIV-1 Tat transactivation in vitro. Genes Dev 1997; 11:2622–2632.

73. Marshall N, Price D. Control of formation of two distinct classes of RNA polymerase II elongation complexes. Mol Cell Biol 1992; 12:2078–2090.

74. Marshall N, Price D. Purification of PTEF-b, a transcription factor required for the transition into productive elongation. J Biol Chem 1995; 270:12335–12336.

75. Jones KA. Taking a new TAK on tat transactivation. Genes Dev 1997; 11(20):2593–2599.

76. Zhou M, Halanski MA, Radonovich MF, Kashanchi F, Peng J, Price DH, Brady JN. Tat modifies the activity of CDK9 to phosphorylate serine 5 of the RNA polymerase II carboxyl-terminal domain during human immunodeficiency virus type 1 transcription. Mol Cell Biol 2000; 20(14):5077–5086.

77. Wimmer J, Fujinaga K, Taube R, Cujec TP, Zhu Y, Peng J, Price DH, Peterlin BM. Interactions between Tat and TAR and human immunodeficiency virus replication are facilitated by human cyclin T1 but not cyclins T2a or T2b. Virology 1999; 255(1):182–189.

78. Yang X, Gold MO, Tang DN, Lewis DE, Aguilar-Cordova E, Rice AP, Herrmann CH. TAK, an HIV Tat-associated kinase, is a member of the cyclin-dependent family of

protein kinases and is induced by activation of peripheral blood lymphocytes and differentiation of promonocytic cell lines. Proc Natl Acad Sci USA 1997; 94(23):12331–12336.

79. Wei P, Garber ME, Fang SM, Fischer WH, Jones KA. A novel CDK9-associated C-type cyclin interacts directly with HIV-1 Tat and mediates its high-affinity, loop-specific binding to TAR RNA. Cell 1998; 92(4):451–462.

80. Garcia-Martinez LF, Ivanov D, Gaynor RB. Association of Tat with purified HIV-1 and HIV-2 transcription preinitiation complexes. J Biol Chem 1997; 272(11):6951–6958.

81. Ping YH, Rana TM. Tat-associated kinase (P-TEFb): a component of transcription preinitiation and elongation complexes. J Biol Chem 1999; 274(11):7399–7404.

82. Zhou M, Nekhai S, Bharucha DC, Kumar A, Ge H, Price DH, Egly JM, Brady JN. TFIIH inhibits CDK9 phosphorylation during human immunodeficiency virus type 1 transcription. J Biol Chem 2001; 276(48):44633–44640.

83. Garber ME, Mayall TP, Suess EM, Meisenhelder J, Thompson NE, Jones KA. CDK9 autophosphorylation regulates high-affinity binding of the human immunodeficiency virus type 1 tat-P-TEFb complex to TAR RNA. Mol Cell Biol 2000; 20(18):6958–6969.

84. Fong YW, Zhou Q. Relief of two built-in autoinhibitory mechanisms in P-TEFb is required for assembly of a multicomponent transcription elongation complex at the human immunodeficiency virus type 1 promoter. Mol Cell Biol 2000; 20(16):5897–5907.

85. Garber ME, Jones KA. HIV-1 Tat: coping with negative elongation factors. Curr Opin Immunol 1999; 11:480–485.

86. Li H, Lahti J, Kidd V. Alternately spliced cyclin C mRNA is widely expressed, cell cycle regulated, and encodes a truncated protein. Oncogene 1996; 13:705–712.

87. Cooper K, Mallory M, Smith J, Strich R. Stress and development regulation of the yeast type-C cyclin Ume3p. EMBO J 1997; 16:4665–4675.

88. Ghose R, Liou LY, Herrmann CH, Rice AP. Induction of TAK (cyclin T1/P-TEFb) in purified resting CD4(+) T lymphocytes by combination of cytokines. J Virol 2001; 75(23):11336–11343.

89. Barboric M, Nissen R, Kanazawa S, Jabrene-Ferrat N, Peterlin BM. NF-kappa-B binds P-TEFb to stimulate transcriptional elongation by RNA polymerase II. Mol Cell 2001; 8:327–337.

90. McKenzie SW, Dallialo G, North M, Frame P, Means RJ. Serum chemokine levels in patients with non-progressing HIV infection. AIDS 1996; 10:F29–F33.

91. Chang HC, Samaniego F, Nair BC, Buonaguro L, Ensoli B. HIV-1 Tat protein exits from cells via a leaderless secretory pathway and binds to extracellular matrix-associated heparan sulfate proteoglycans through its basic region. AIDS 1997; 11(12):1421–1431.

92. Ensoli B, Barillari G, Salahuddin SZ, Gallo RC, Wong-Staal F. Tat protein of HIV-1 stimulates growth of cells derived from Kaposi's sarcoma lesions of AIDS patients. Nature 1990; 345(6270):84–86.

93. Ensoli B, Buonaguro L, Barillari G, Fiorelli V, Gendelman R, Morgan RA, Wingfield P, Gallo RC. Release, uptake, and effects of extracellular human immunodeficiency virus type 1 Tat protein on cell growth and viral transactivation. J Virol 1993; 67(1):277–287.

94. Noonan D, Albini A. From the outside in: extracellular activities of HIV Tat. In: Jeang K-T, ed. HIV-1: Molecular Biology and Pathogenesis Viral Mechanisms: Advances in Pharmacology. San Diego, CA: Academic Press, 2000:229–250.

95. Raines EW, Ross R. Compartmentalization of PDGF on extracellular binding sites dependent on exon 6-encoded sequences. J Cell Biol 1992; 116:533–543.

96. Albini A, Benelli R, Presta M, Rusnati M, Ziche M, Rubartelli A, Paglialunga G, Bussolino F, Noonan D. HIV-tat protein is a heparin-binding angiogenic growth factor. Oncogene 1996; 12(2):289–297.

97. Rusnati M, Coltrini D, Oreste P, Zoppetti G, Albini A, Noonan D, d'Adda di Fagagna F,

Giacca M, Presta M. Interaction of HIV-1 Tat protein with heparin. Role of the backbone structure, sulfation, and size. J Biol Chem 1997; 272(17):11313–11320.

98. Green M, Loewenstein PM. Autonomous function domains of chemically synthesized human immunodeficiency virus tat transactivator protein. Cell 1988; 55:1179–1188.

99. Vives E, Brodin P, Lebleu B. A truncated HIV-1 Tat protein basic domain rapidly translocates through the plasma membrane and accumulates in the cell nucleus. J Biol Chem 1997; 272:16010–16017.

100. Li CJ, Friedman DJ, Pardee AB, Wang C, Metelev V, Pardee AB. Induction of apoptosis in uninfected lymphocytes by HIV-1 Tat protein. Science 1995; 268:429–431.

101. Li CJ, Wang C, Friedman DJ, Pardee AB. Reciprocal modulations between p53 and Tat of human immunodeficiency virus type 1. Proc Natl Acad Sci USA 1995; 92:5461–5464.

102. Zauli G, Gibellini D, Caputo A, Bassini A, Negrini M, Monne M, Mazzoni M, Capitani S. The human immunodeficiency virus type-1 Tat protein upregulates Bcl-2 gene expression in Jurkat T cel lines and primary peripheral blood mononuclear cells. Blood 1995; 86:3823–3834.

103. Westendorp MO, Frank R, Oschenbauer C, Stricker K, Dhein J, Walczak H, Debatin KM, Krammer PH. Sensitization of T cells to CD95-mediated apoptosis by HIV-1 Tat and gp120. Nature 1995; 375:497–500.

104. Ranki A, Lagerstedt A, Ovod V, Aavik A, Krohn K. Expression kinetics and subcellular localization of HIV-1 regulatory proteins Nef, Tat and Rev in acutely and chronically infected lymphoid cell lines. Arch Virol 1994; 139:365–378.

105. Zauli G, Gibellini D, Milani D, Mazzoni M, Borgatti P, La Placa M, Capitani S. Human immunodeficiency virus type-1 Tat protein protects lymphoid, epithelial and neuronal cell lines from death by apoptosis. Cancer Res 1993; 53:4481–4485.

106. Zauli G, La Placa M, Vignoli M, Re M, Gibellini D, Furlini G, Milani D, Marchisio M, Mazzoni M, Capitani S. An autocrine loop of HIV-1 Tat protein is responsible for the improved survival/proliferation capacity of permanently tat-transfected cells and required for optimal human immunodeficiency virus type-1 long terminal repeat trans-activating activity. J AIDS Hum Retrovir 1995; 10:306–316.

107. Corallini A, Altavilla G, Pozzi L, Bignozzi F, Negrini M, Rimessi P, Gualandi F, Barbanti-Brodano G. Systemic expression of HIV-1 tat gene in transgenic mice induces endothelial proliferation and tumors of different histotypes. Cancer Res 1993; 53(22):5569–5575.

108. Vogel J, Hinrichs SH, Reynolds RK, Luciw PA, Jay G. The HIV Tat gene induces dermal lesions resembling Kaposi's sarcoma in transgenic mice. Nature 1988; 335:606–611.

109. Frankel AD, Pabo CO. Cellular uptake of the tat protein from human immunodeficiency virus. Cell 1988; 55:1189–1193.

110. Albini A, Barillari G, Benelli R, Gallo RC, Ensoli B. Angiogenic properties of human immunodeficiency virus type 1 Tat protein. Proc Natl Acad Sci USA 1995; 92(11):4838–4842.

111. Barillari G, Sgadari C, Fiorelli V, Samaniego F, Colombini S, Manzari V, Modesti A, Nair BC, Cafaro A, Sturzl M, Ensoli B. The Tat protein of human immunodeficiency virus type-1 promotes vascular cell growth and locomotion by engaging the alpha5beta1 and alphavbeta3 integrins and by mobilizing sequestered basic fibroblast growth factor. Blood 1999; 94(2):663–672.

112. Ensoli B, Gendelman R, Markham P, Fiorelli V, Colombini S, Raffeld M, Cafaro A, Chang HK, Brady JN, Gallo RC. Synergy between basic fibroblast growth factor and HIV-1 Tat protein in induction of Kaposi's sarcoma. Nature 1994; 371(6499):674–680.

113. Albini A, Soldi R, Giunciuglio D, Giraudo E, Benelli R, Primo L, Noonan D, Salio M, Camussi G, Rockl W, Bussolino F. The angiogenesis induced by HIV-1 tat protein is mediated by the Flk- 1/KDR receptor on vascular endothelial cells. Nat Med 1996; 2(12):1371–1375.

114. Barillari G, Sgadari C, Palladino C, Gendelman R, Caputo A, Morris CB, Nair BC, Markham P, Nel A, Sturzl M, Ensoli B. Inflammatory cytokines synergize with the HIV-1 Tat protein to promote angiogenesis and Kaposi's sarcoma via induction of basic fibroblast growth factor and the alpha v beta 3 integrin. J Immunol 1999; 163(4):1929–1935.

115. Boykins RA, Mahieux R, Shankavaram UT, Gho YS, Lee SF, Hewlett IK, Wahl LM, Kleinman HK, Brady JN, Yamada KM, Dhawan S. Cutting edge: a short polypeptide domain of HIV-1-Tat protein mediates pathogenesis. J Immunol 1999; 163(1):15–20.

116. Mitola S, Soldi R, Zanon I, Barra L, Gutierrez MI, Berkhout B, Giacca M, Bussolino F. Identification of specific molecular structures of human immunodeficiency virus type 1 Tat relevant for its biological effects on vascular endothelial cells. J Virol 2000; 74(1):344–353.

117. Ganju RK, Munshi N, Nair BC, Liu ZY, Gill P, Groopman JE. Human immunodeficiency virus tat modulates the Flk-1/KDR receptor, mitogen-activated protein kinases, and components of focal adhesion in Kaposi's sarcoma cells. J Virol 1998; 72(7):6131–6137.

118. Milani D, Mazzoni M, Zauli G, Mischiati D, Gibellini M, Giacca M, Capitani S. HIV-1 Tat induces phosphorylation of p125fak and its association with phosphoinositide 3-kinase in PC12 cells. AIDS 1998; 12:1275–1284.

119. Annunziata P, Cioni C, Toneatto S, Paccagnini E. HIV-1 gp120 increases the permeability of rat brain endothelium cultures by a mechanism involving substance P. AIDS 1998; 12:2377–2385.

120. Conaldi PG, Serra C, Dolei A, Basolo F, Falcone V, Mariana G, Speziale P. Productive HIV-1 infection of human vascular endothelial cells requires cell proliferation and is stimulated by combined treatment with interleukin-1 beta plus tumor necrosis factor-alpha. J Med Virol 1995; 47:355–363.

121. Huang MB, Hunter M, Bond VC. Effect of extracellular human immunodeficiency virus type-1 glycoprotein 120 on primary human vascular endothelial cell cultures. AIDS Res Hum Retrovir 1999; 15:1265–1277.

122. Lafon ME, Gendrault JL, Royer C, Jaeck D, Kirn A. Human endothelial cells isolated from the hepatic sinusoids and the umbilical vein display a different permissiveness for HIV-1. Res Virol 1993; 144:99–104.

123. Lafon ME, Steffen AM, Royer C, Jaeck D, Beretz A, Kirn A, Gendrault JL. HIV-1 infection induces functional alterations in human liver endothelial cells in primary culture. AIDS 1994; 8:747–752.

124. Moses AV, Nelson JA. HIV infection of human brain capillary endothelial cells: implications for AIDS dementia. Adv Neuroimmunol 1994; 4:239–247.

125. B, De Girolami U, He J, Wang S, Lorenzo A, Busciglio J, Gabuzda D. Apoptosis induced by HIV-1 infection of the central nervous system. J Clin Invest 1996; 98:1979–1990.

126. Barillari G, Buonaguro L, Fiorelli V, Hoffman J, Michaels F, Gallo RC, Ensoli B. Effects of cytokines from activated immune cells on vascular cell growth and HIV-1 gene expression. Implications for AIDS-Kaposi's sarcoma pathogenesis. J Immunol 1992; 149(11):3727–3734.

127. Fiorelli V, Gendelman R, Samaniego F, Markham PD, Ensoli B. Cytokines from activated T cells induce normal endothelial cells to acquire the phenotypic and functional features of AIDS-Kaposi's sarcoma spindle cells. J Clin Invest 1995; 95(4):1723–1734.

128. Fiorelli V, Barillari G, Toschi E, Sgadari C, Monini P, Sturzl M, Ensoli B. IFN-gamma induces endothelial cells to proliferate and to invade the extracellular matrix in response to the HIV-1 Tat protein: implications for AIDS-Kaposi's sarcoma pathogenesis. J Immunol 1999; 162(2):1165–1170.

129. Albrecht H, Stellbrink HJ, Gross G, Berg B, Helmchen U, Mensing H. Treatment of atypical leishmaniasis with interferon-gamma resulting in progression of Kaposi's sarcoma in AIDS patients. Clin Invest 1994; 72:1041–1047.

130. Krakauer T, Oppennheim JJ. IL-1 and tumor necrosis factor-alpha each upregulate both the expression of IFN-gamma and enhance IFN-gamma-induced HLA-DR expression on human monocytes and on human monocytic cell line. J Immunol 1993; 150:1205–1211.

131. Vogel BE, Lee SJ, Hieldebrand A, Craig W, Pierschbacher MD, Wong-Staal F, Ruoslahti E. A novel integrin specificity exemplified by binding of the avb3 integrin to the basic domain of the HIV Tat protein and vitronectin. J Cell Biol 1993; 121:461–468.

132. Weeks BS, Deasai K, Lowenstein PM, Klotman ME, Klotman PE, Green M, Kleinman HK. Identification of a novel cell attachment domain in the HIV-1 Tat protein and its 90kDa cell surface binding protein. J Biol Chem 1993; 268:1167–1174.

133. Zauli G, Gibellini D, Caputo A, Bassini A, Negrini M, Monne M, Mazonni M, Capitani S. Pleiotropic effects of immobilized versus soluble recombinant HIV-1 Tat protein on CD3-mediated activation, induction of apoptosis, and HIV-1 long terminal repeat trans-activation in purified CD4+ T lymphocytes. J Immunol 1996; 2:850–856.

134. Rusnati M, Tulipano G, Urbinati C, Tanghetti E, Giuliani R, Giacca M, Ciomei M, Corallini A, Presta M. The basic domain in HIV-1 Tat protein as a target for poly-sulfonated heparin-mimicking extracellular Tat antagonists. J Biol Chem 1998; 273(26): 16027–16037.

135. Albini A, Benelli R, Giunciuglio D, Cai T, Mariani G, Ferrini S, Noonan DM. Identification of a novel domain of HIV tat involved in monocyte chemotaxis. J Biol Chem 1998; 273(26):15895–15900.

136. Benelli R, Mortarini R, Anichini A, Giunciuglio D, Noonan DM, Montalti S, Tacchetti C, Albini A. Monocyte-derived dendritic cells and monocytes migrate to HIV-Tat RGD and basic peptides. AIDS 1998; 12(3):261–268.

137. Lafrenie RM, Wahl LM, Epstein JS, Hewlett IK, Yamada KM, Dhawan S. HIV-1-Tat protein promotes chemotaxis and invasive behavior by monocytes. J Immunol 1996; 157(3):974–977.

138. Lafrenie RM, Wahl LM, Epstein JS, Hewlett IK, Yamada KM, Dhawan S. HIV-1-Tat modulates the function of monocytes and alters their interactions with microvessel endothelial cells. A mechanism of HIV pathogenesis. J Immunol 1996; 156(4):1638–1645.

139. Milani D, Mazzoni M, Borgatti P, Zauli G, Cantley L, Capitani S. Extracellular human immunodeficiency virus type-1 Tat protein activates phosphatidylinositol 3-kinase in PC12 neuronal cells. J Biol Chem 1996; 271(38):22961–22964.

140. Brake DA, Debouck C, Biesecker G. Identification of an Arg-Gly-Asp (RGD) cell adhesion site in human immunodeficiency virus type 1 transactivation protein, tat. J Cell Biol 1990; 111(3):1275–1281.

141. Fiorelli V, Gendelman R, Sirianni MC, Chang HK, Colombini S, Markham PD, Monini P, Sonnabend J, Pintus A, Gallo RC, Ensoli B. gamma-interferon produced by CD8+ T cells infiltrating Kaposi's sarcoma induces spindle cells with angiogenic phenotype and synergy with human immunodeficiency virus-1 Tat protein: an immune response to human herpesvirus-8 infection? Blood 1998; 91(3):956–967.

142. Mitola S, Sozzani S, Luini W, Primo L, Borsatti A, Weich H, Bussolino F. Tat-human immunodeficiency virus-1 induces human monocyte chemotaxis by activation of vascular endothelial growth factor receptor-1. Blood 1997; 90(4):1365–1372.

143. Toschi E, Barillari G, Sgadari C, Bacigalupo I, Cereseto A, Carlei D, Palladino C, Zietz C, Leone P, Sturzl M, Butto S, Cafaro A, Monini P, Ensoli B. Activation of matrix-metalloproteinase-2 and membrane-type-1-matrix-metalloproteinase in endothelial cells and induction of vascular permeability in vivo by human immunodeficiency virus-1 Tat protein and basic fibroblast growth factor. Mol Biol Cell 2001; 12(10):2934–2946.

144. Prakash O, Tang ZY, He E, Ali MS, Coleman R, Gill J, Farr G, Samaniego F. Human Kaposi's sarcoma cell-mediated tumorigenesis in human immunodeficiency type 1 tat-expressing transgenic mice. J Natl Cancer Inst 2000; 92:721–728.

145. Brooks PC, Montgomery AM, Rosenfeld M, Reisfeld RA, Hu T, Klier G, Cheresh DA. Integrin avB3 antagonists promote tumor regression by inducing apoptosis of angiogenic blood vessels. Cell 1994; 79:1157–1164.

146. Gospodarowitcz D, Greenburg G, Birdwell CR. Determination of cellular shape by the extracellular matrix and its correlation with the control of cellular growth. Cancer Res 1978; 38:4155–4171.

147. Ingber DE, Prusty D, Frangioni JV, Cragoe EJ Jr, Lechene C, Schwartz MA. Control of intracellular pH and growth by fibronectin in capillary endothelial cells. J Cell Biol 1990; 110(5):1803–1811.

148. Montaldo F, Maffe A, Morini M, Noonan D, Giordano S, Albini A, Prat M. Expression of functional tyrosine kinases on immortalized Kaposi's sarcoma cells. J Cell Physiol 2000; 184(2):246–254.

149. Baird A, Schubert D, Ling N, Guillemin R. Receptor- and heparin-binding domains of basic fibroblast growth factor. Proc Natl Acad Sci USA 1988; 85:2324–2328.

150. Folkman J, Klagsbrun M, Sasse J, Wadzinski M, Ingberg D, Vlodavsky I. A heparin-binding angiogenic protein—basic fibroblast growth factor—is stored within the basement membrane. Am J Pathol 1988; 130:393–400.

151. Samaniego F, Markham P, Gendelman R, Watanabe T, Kao V, Kowalski K, Ferrara N, Sonnabend J, Pintus A, Zon G, Gallo RC, Ensoli B. Vacular endothelial growth factor and basic fibroblast growth factor present in Kaposi's sarcoma (KS) are induced by inflammatory cytokines and synergize to promoter vascular permeability and KS lesion development. Am J Pathol 1998; 152:433–443.

152. Neufeld G, Cohen T, Gengrinovitch S, Poltorak Z. Vascular endothelial growth factor (VEGF) and its receptors. FASEB J 1999; 13:9–22.

153. Keyt BA, Berleau LT, Nguuyen HU, Chen H, Heinsohn H, Vandlen R, Ferrara N. The carboxyl-terminal domain (111-165) of vascular endothelial growth factor is critical for its mitogenic potential. J Biol Chem 1996; 271:7788–7795.

154. Clark EA, Brugge JS. Integrins and signal transduction pathways: the road taken. Science 1995; 268(5208):233–239.

155. Zietz C, Hotz B, Sturzl M, Rauch E, Penning R, Lohrs U. Aortic endothelium in HIV-1 infection: chronic injury, activation, and increased leukocyte adherence. Am J Pathol 1996; 149(6):1887–1898.

156. Touloumi G, Hatzakis A, Potouridou I, Milona I, Strarigos J, Katsambas A, Giraldo G, Beth-Giraldo E, Biggar RJ, Mueller N, Trichopoulos D. The role of immunosuppression and immune-activation in classic Kaposi's sarcoma. Int J Cancer 1999; 82(6): 817–821.

157. Del Sorbo L, Arese M, Giraudo E, Tizzani M, Biancone L, Bussolino F, Camussi G. Tat-induced platelet-activating factor synthesis contributes to the angiogenic effect of HIV-1 Tat. Eur J Immunol 2001; 31(2):376–383.

158. Montrucchio G, Lupia E, Battaglia E, Del Sorbo L, Boccellino M, Biancone L, Emanuelli G, Camussi G. Platelet-activating factor enhances vascular endothelial growth factor-induced endothelial cell motility and neoangiogenesis in a murine matrigel model. Arterioscler Thromb Vasc Biol 2000; 20(1):80–88.

159. Montrucchio G, Lupia E, Battaglia E, Passerini G, Bussolino F, Emanuelli G, Camussi G. Tumor necrosis factor alpha-induced angiogenesis depends on in situ platelet-activating factor biosynthesis. J Exp Med 1994; 180(1):377–382.

160. Camussi G, Montrucchio G, Lupia E, Soldi R, Comoglio PM, Bussolino F. Angiogenesis induced in vivo by hepatocyte growth factor is mediated by platelet-activating factor synthesis from macrophages. J Immunol 1997; 158(3):1302–1309.

161. Camussi G, Montrucchio G, Lupia E, De Martino A, Perona L, Arese M, Vercellone A, Toniolo A, Bussolino F. Platelet-activating factor directly stimulates in vitro migration of endothelial cells and promotes in vivo angiogenesis by a heparin-dependent mechanism. J Immunol 1995; 154(12):6492–6501.

162. Biancone L, Cantaluppi V, Boccellino M, Bussolati B, Del Sorbo L, Conaldi PG, Albini A, Toniolo A, Camussi G. Motility induced by human immunodeficiency virus-1 Tat on Kaposi's sarcoma cells requires platelet-activating factor synthesis. Am J Pathol 1999; 155(5):1731–1739.

163. Kelly GD, Ensoli B, Gunthel CJ, Offermann MK. Purified Tat induces inflammatory response genes in Kaposi's sarcoma cells. Aids 1998; 12(14):1753–1761.

164. Schwartz HA, Mermelstein SJ, Waksman G, Dowdy SF. Synthetic protein transduction domains: enhanced transduction potential in vitro and in vivo. Cancer Res 2001; 61:474–477.

165. Fawell S, Seery J, Daikh Y, Moore C, Chen LL, Pepinsky B, Barsoum J. Tat-mediated delivery of heterologous proteins into cells. Proc Natl Acad Sci USA 1994; 91(2):664–668.

166. Cooper JT, Stroka DM, Brostjan C, Palmetshofer A, Bach FH, Ferran C. A20 blocks endothelial cell activation through a NF-kappaB-dependent mechanism. J Biol Chem 1996; 271(30):18068–18073.

167. Hofman FM, Chen P, Incardona F, Zidovetzki R, Hinton DR. HIV-1 tat protein induces the production of interleukin-8 by human brain-derived endothelial cells. J Neuroimmunol 1999; 94(1–2):28–39.

168. Cota-Gomez A, Flores NC, Cruz C, Casullo A, Aw TY, Ichikawa H, Schaack J, Scheinman R, Flores SC. The human immunodeficiency virus-1 Tat protein activates human umbilical vein endothelial cell E-selectin expression via an NF-kappa B–dependent mechanism. J Biol Chem 2002; 277(17):14390–14399.

169. Thomas KA. Vascular endothelial growth factor, a potet and selective angiogenic agent. J Biol Chem 1996; 271(2):603–606.

170. Nicosia RF. What is the role of vascular endothelial growth factor-related molecules in tumor angiogenesis? Am J Pathol 1998; 153:11–16.

171. Deregibus MC, Cantaluppi V, Doublier S, Brizzi MF, Deambrosis I, Albini A, Camussi G. HIV-1-Tat protein activates phosphatidylinositol 3-kinase/AKT- dependent survival pathways in Kaposi's sarcoma cells. J Biol Chem 2002; 277(28):25195–25202.

172. Cantaluppi V, Biancone L, Boccellino M, Doublier S, Benelli R, Carlone S, Albini A, Camussi G. HIV type 1 Tat protein is a survival factor for Kaposi's sarcoma and endothelial cells. AIDS Res Hum Retrovir 2001; 17(10):965–976.

173. Wang Z, Morris GF, Rice AP, Xiong W, Morris CB. Wild-type and transactivation-defective mutants of human immunodeficiency virus type 1 Tat protein bind human TATA-binding protein in vitro. J AIDS 1996; 12(2):128–138.

174. Matter M, Ruoslahti E. A signaling pathway from the alpha-5-beta-1 and alpha-v-beta-3 integrins that elevates bcl-2 transcription. J Biol Chem 2001; 276(30):27757–27763.

175. Bohan Morris CA, Gendelman R, Marrogi AJ, Lu M, Lockyer JM, Alperin-Lea W, Ensoli B. Immunohistochemical detection of Bcl-2 in AIDS-associated and classical Kaposi's sarcoma. Am J Pathol 1996; 148:1055–1063.

176. Corallini A, Sampaolesi R, Possati L, Merlin M, Bagnarelli P, Piola C, Fabris M, Menegatti M, Talevi S, Gibellini D, Rocchetti R, Caputo A, Barbanti-Brodano G. Inhibition of HIV-1 tat activity correlates with down-regulation of bcl- 2 and results in reduction of angiogenesis and oncogenicity. Virology 2002; 299(1):1.

177. Park IW, Ullrich CK, Schoenberger E, Ganju RK, Groopman JE. HIV-1 Tat induces microvascular endothelial apoptosis through caspase activation. J Immunol 2001; 167(5):2766–2771.

178. Kaaya EE, Castanos-Velez E, Amir H, Lema L, Luande J, Kitinya J, Patarroyo M, Biberfeld P. Expression of adhesion molecules in endemic and epidemic Kaposi's sarcoma. Histopathology 1996; 29(4):337–346.

179. Murphy PM. Pirated genes in Kaposi's sarcoma. Nature 1997; 385(6614):296–297, 299.

180. Buckley CD, Pilling D, Henriquez NV, Parsonage G, Threlfall K, Scheel-Toellner D, Simmons DL, Akbar AN, Lord JM, Salmon M. RGD peptides induce apoptosis by direct caspase-3 activation. Nature 1999; 397(6719):534–539.

181. Jia H, Lohr M, Jezequel S, Davis D, Shaikh S, Selwood D, Zachary I. Cysteine-rich and basic domain HIV-1 Tat peptides inhibit angiogenesis and induce endothelial cell apoptosis. Biochem Biophys Res Commun 2001; 283(2):469–479.

182. Lis JT, Mason P, Peng J, Price DH, Werner J. P-TEFb kinase recruitment and function at heat shock loci. Genes Dev 2000; 14(7):792–803.

183. Kanazawa S, Okamoto T, Peterlin BM. Tat competes with CIITA for the binding to P-TEFb and blocks the expression of MHC class II genes in HIV infection. Immunity 2000; 12(1):61–70.

184. Foskett SM, Ghose R, Tang DN, Lewis DE, Rice AP. Antiapoptotic function of Cdk9 (TAK/P-TEFb) in U937 promonocytic cells. J Virol 2001; 75(3):1220–1228.

185. Montaner S, Sodhi A, Pece S, Mesri EA, Gutkind JS. The Kaposi's sarcoma-associated herpesvirus G protein-coupled receptor promotes endothelial cell survival through the activation of Akt/protein kinase B. Cancer Res 2001; 61(6):2641–2648.

186. Cesarman E, Mesri EA, Gershengorn MC. Viral G protein-coupled receptor and Kaposi's sarcoma: a model of paracrine neoplasia? J Exp Med 2000; 191(3):417–417.

11

Nutrients as Modulators of Immune Dysfunction and Dyslipidemia in AIDS

Raxit J. Jariwalla
California Institute for Medical Research, San Jose, California, U.S.A.

INTRODUCTION

Acquired immunodeficiency syndrome (AIDS) is characterized by infection with human immunodeficiency virus (HIV) and progressive depletion of CD4+ (helper) T cells, leading to opportunistic infections and malignancies (1). In addition to CD4+ cell loss, HIV-infected patients manifest impairment of immune response, affecting both CD4+ and CD8+ T-cell subsets, that resembles an anergic state of immune dysfunction (2). These defective immunological responses include decreased interleukin-2 (IL-2) secretion and unresponsiveness to recall antigens or stimulation through the CD3/TCR complex (3).

HIV infection is also associated with lipid abnormalities (dyslipidemia), which can be potentiated by antitetroviral treatment (see below). Since dyslipidemia is linked to cardiovascular disease, HIV infection and its current treatment pose an increased risk for coronary artery disease.

It has also been reported that both asymptomatic and symptomatic HIV-infected persons manifest imbalance of key antioxidant micronutrients, such that specific nutrient deficiencies may contribute to loss of cell-mediated immune responses (4–6). Supplementation with specific micronutrients has been correlated to a reduced hazard of AIDS development (4–6). Some of the nutrients lowered in HIV infection can suppress virus expression in infected cell lines (reviewed in Ref. 6). Other nutrients have been demonstrated to manifest lipid-lowering properties (see below). Accordingly, nutrients are potential candidates for the treatment of immune dysfunction and dyslipidemia underlying HIV/AIDS.

NEED FOR ALTERNATIVE/COMPLEMENTARY THERAPY IN AIDS

Since the advent of highly active antiretroviral therapy (HAART), which includes HIV protease inhibitors in combination with nucleoside analogues, reports have appeared suggesting increased survival of HIV-infected patients. Whereas HAART can suppress HIV replication and reduce viral burden, latent virus persists in a dormant state and patients undergo only partial immune recovery. Furthermore, prolonged antiretroviral treatment is often accompanied by severe side effects, and a fraction of patients develop resistance to HAART, indicating limitations to this regimen.

Recent analysis of T-cell dynamics has unraveled the limited efficacy of these newer drug cocktails in restoring the immune system (7–9). Thus, the increase in CD4+ cell counts associated with HAART is primarily due to the redistribution of memory cells and only slow repopulation with newly produced naive T cells (9). Consequently subsets of naive T cells may not attain normal levels and the functionality of the immune response is not restored, posing a risk for recurrence of opportunistic infection. Hence there is a need for alternative and/or complementary treatment that can restore the immune system that has been ravaged by HIV infection.

Additionally, HAART is associated with the development of lipodystrophy, a syndrome characterized by body fat redistribution and metabolic abnormalities that may pose a risk for cardiovascular disease (10). The body fat changes include peripheral fat wasting and abdominal adiposity, which may affect patients psychologically and contribute to a negative impact on their quality of life. Metabolic changes involve lipid abnormalities (dyslipidemia) and insulin resistance, which occur in over 50% of patients receiving HAART. Both parameters have been recognized as risk factors for cardiovascular disease and may affect long-term morbidity. The dyslipidemia associated with HAART is characterized by elevated serum total and low-density lipoprotein (LDL) cholesterol and elevated serum triglycerides.

Although the etiology of lipodystrophy remains unknown, specific guideline have been proposed to treat HIV-associated dyslipidemia (11). However, current lipid-lowering drugs are linked to adverse side effects (myopathy, liver damage) and a major class, the statins, can interact negatively with protease inhibitors in HAART due to metabolism by a common pathway (cytochrome CYP34A). Hence, the use of conventional lipid-lowering agents is limited in HIV patients. Since dyslipidemia is a major risk factor for cardiac disease, there is, in addition to the need for immune-reconstituting agents, a real need for a less toxic, complementary therapy that will keep lipid abnormalities in check.

NUTRIENTS AND AIDS

Several lines of evidence suggest that nutrient supplementation may be a desirable therapeutic strategy for improving immune responses and managing dyslipidemia in AIDS. First, nutrition and immunity are interrelated and intertwined with one another (reviewed in Ref. 12). It is well established that nutritional deficiencies can lower immunity and increase susceptibility to infection. Conversely, viral infection is known to alter nutritional status and reduce immunity.

Second, the immunological abnormalities seen in AIDS resemble those associated with protein calorie malnutrition (PCM), a wasting disease characterized by loss of lean body mass and imbalance of amino-acid levels in blood plasma (13). PCM has been linked to T-cell anergy, a state of immunological unresponsiveness that leads to a breakdown in resistance to infectious agents. Third, prospective studies (4,5) have shown that micronutrient consumption in asymptomatic HIV-seropositive persons is associated with reduced risk of AIDS development. Micronutrients deficient in HIV infection and those reported to correlate with reduced AIDS risk are known to affect humoral and/or cell-mediated responses (6,12). Finally, specific nutrients, especially plant-based phytonutrients, manifest lipid-lowering properties that may be of value in treating HIV-associated dyslipidemia (see "Phytonutrients," below). Hence, nutrients may positively impact AIDS treatment by improving immunological and lipid parameters that respond poorly to antiretroviral drugs. This article reviews specific micronutrients and phytonutrients with reference to their known effects on the immune and lipid parameters respectively and the potential significance of these actions in the treatment of AIDS.

VITAMINS

Vitamin A and Beta-Carotene

These fat-soluble vitamins are closely related, with beta-carotene serving as a precursor of vitamin A. In animal studies, supplementation with retinol (vitamin A) and beta-carotene was shown to improve antibody response and resistance to infection (14). Vitamin A deficiency has been reported in AIDS patients. It is not clear whether supplementation can reverse this deficiency. In one study (5), supplementation with less than 9000 IU or more than 20,000 IU/day was linked to increased risk of AIDS development in HIV-positive persons. Therefore supplementation with vitamin A must be approached with caution.

Beta-carotene, a carotenoid, occurs as provitamin A in vegetables containing yellow or orange pigment. Unlike vitamin A, it is a strong antioxidant and can be taken in larger doses without attendant toxicity. Consumption of beta-carotene at 60 to 180 mg/day was reported to stabilize CD4 cell counts and elevate CD4/CD8 ratios in HIV-infected patients (15).

Vitamin C (Ascorbate)

Vitamin C (ascorbic acid, or ascorbate) is an essential vitamin and a primary water-soluble antioxidant that the body needs to prevent scurvy, fight infection, and maintain optimal health. It participates in maintenance, reparative, and restorative reactions, including collagen formation, tissue repair, immune function, and metabolism. It is vital for the infection-fighting activity of white blood cells, which accumulate ascorbate to 10 to 150 times higher levels than blood plasma. Foods rich in vitamin C include citrus fruits, potatoes, strawberries, broccoli, and green leafy vegetables. Ascorbate deficiency has been linked to HIV infection in nonsupplementing subjects (16).

A role for vitamin C in influencing the course of HIV infection is suggested by the following lines of evidence.

First, in vivo, vitamin C has been shown to modulate cell-mediated immune responses, which include activation of phagocytic activity, stimulation of production/function of B and T lymphocytes, and enhancement of natural-killer (NK) cell activity (reviewed in Refs. 17 and 18). The immunodeficiency disease–related conditions ameliorated by vitamin C supplementation include restoration of (1) impaired phagocytic function in Chediak-Higashi disease, (2) abnormal helper/suppressor T-cell ratios in childhood measles, and (3) cell-mediated immune responses in the elderly. More recently, vitamin C was identified as one among several micronutrients whose consumption correlated positively with a reduced risk of AIDS development in asymptomatic HIV-infected persons (4).

Second, in vitro, ascorbate has been demonstrated to inhibit the activity of a wide spectrum of viruses, including human retroviruses (18). Most importantly, the addition of ascorbate to growing cultures of acutely, chronically, or latently infectd cells resulted in suppression of HIV expression without adverse effects on host cells (17,18). The mechanism of HIV suppression by ascorbate differs from that of nucleoside analogues as well as other antioxidants, suggesting a unique mode of action of the vitamin on HIV (19).

Third, HIV-infected patients exhibit widespread glutathione (GSH) deficiency. Vitamin C supplementation has been shown to elevate GSH levels in healthy adults (20). Similarly, reduced levels of plasma GSH associated with human diets low in vitamin C were restored with an ascorbate-supplemented diet (21). Additionally, in animal models of drug-induced GSH deficiency, vitamin C acts as an essential antioxidant by sparing GSH, protecting against oxidant-induced organ damage, and lowering mortality in a dose-dependent fashion (22).

A significant proportion of men and women in the United States practice regular vitamin supplementation (23). Large doses of vitamin C are believed by some clinicians and their patients to ameliorate the common cold, cardiovascular disease, and cancer. Many HIV-infected persons believe that the ingestion of large doses may positively influence the clinical course of their disease (24). Although large clinical trials have not been conducted, amelioration of opportunistic infection and stabilization of helper CD4 cell counts was seen in patients ingesting doses of vitamin C large enough to approach the bowel tolerance level (25,26).

The recommended daily allowance for vitamin C was recently revised to 90 mg/ day for nonsmokers and additional 35 mg/day for smokers. These guidelines also set, for the first time, the upper limits for vitamin C to 2000 mg/day. Although these recommendations assert that dosages exceeding the upper limit may not confer any benefit due to preferential excretion of the vitamin by the body, they are based on pharmacokinetic data from healthy human volunteers (27). The bowel tolerance level (i.e., the dose at which ascorbate produces a laxative effect) in persons with disease may be much higher. Thus, it has been reported that the bowel tolerance dose increases with severity of illness/infection, with HIV-positive individuals capable of tolerating up to 40 g/day and persons with AIDS tolerating up to 200 g/day without exhibiting diarrhea (26,27). Furthermore, the minimal dose of vitamin C found to suppress HIV in vitro was 25 µg/mL, with higher levels up to 150 µg/mL conferring dose-dependent suppression of virus production (28). Based on pharmacokinetics of vitamin C up to 12 g/day (29), an oral dose of at least 6 to 7 (and up to 12) g/day would be needed to achieve the ascorbate level in blood plasma equivalent to that required for minimal HIV suppression in vitro. Much higher levels of ascorbate in plasma (up to 40 mg/dL or 400 µg/mL) can be attained by intravenous infusion (30). As the influence of ascorbate on viral load and immune function in AIDS patients is not known and given the frequent failure of antiretroviral therapy, it is important to evaluate the efficacy of high-dose ascorbate in this patient population.

Vitamin E

Vitamin E or d-alpha tocopherol is an important fat-soluble antioxidant that protects cell membranes from oxidative damage. HIV-infected patients have been reported to have reduced vitamin E levels compared to normal controls (31). In experimental studies, vitamin E enhanced immune function in various species of mamals (32). The natural form of the vitamin (d-alpha tocopherol) is more readily absorbed than the synthetic form (dl-alpha-tocopherol). Food sources of d-alpha tocopherol include nuts, seeds, liver, whole grains, and leafy vegetables. The natural form is relatively nontoxic in doses up to 1500 IU/day, which correspond to the upper limit set recently by the NAS. The upper limit for the synthetic form was set at 1100 IU/day. Since vitamin E can act as an anticoagulant at high levels, it is contraindicated with other anticoagulants, with which it may interact adversely. In addition to its antioxidant and immune-stimulating activities, a role for vitamin E in AIDS has been suggested based on:

1. The ability of alpha-tocopheryl succinate to suppress NF-κB, the key cellular transcription factor required for expression of HIV provirus (33)
2. Enhancement of antiviral activity of AZT when used in combination on HIV-infected cells (34)
3. The identification of vitamin E as a micronutrient correlating positively with a reduced hazard of AIDS development in asymptomatic HIV-infected men consuming micronutrients at baseline (4,5)

B Vitamins

HIV infection has been linked to deficiencies in three members of the vitamin B complex family. These include vitamins B_6 (pyridoxine), B_{12} (cyanocobalamin), and folic acid. Pyridoxine plays an important role as an apoenzyme in the conversion of methionine to cysteine. B_{12} is involved in the formation of red blood cells and plays a role in mental functioning and cognitive awareness. Folic acid is required for DNA and RNA synthesis. Adequate amounts of B_{12} are required for folic acid metabolism. When supplementation is considered, both B_{12} and folic acid should be taken together, since a deficiency in either vitamin results in anaemia. In addition to these B-complex vitamins, consumption of vitamins B_1 and niacin at baseline in a prospective study was linked to reduced risk of AIDS progression in HIV-positive men (5). The relationship of these B vitamins to immune function has been reviewed by other authors (35).

TRACE MINERALS

Selenium

Selenium is an important trace element which, as a cofactor of GSH peroxidase (along with vitamin E), is involved in the reduction of lipid peroxides and prevention of damage to cellular membranes. Selenium is also involved in the recycling of oxidized GSH back to its reduced form. Studies carried out by Taylor and colleagues have shown that HIV and other RNA-containing viruses encode a selenium-dependent GSH peroxidase gene that may allow the virus to monitor intracellular selenium levels

(36). HIV-infected persons have been reported to have a selenium deficiency, which may favor virus proliferation (37). Selenium is required for the proper functioning of T lymphocytes and has been shown to potentiate the action of IL-2 (37). Selenium supplementation has been shown to increase T-cell proliferation and cytotoxicity in response to mitogens and antigens (37). Selenium deficiency in HIV infection is associated with reduced NK cell activity (38). Treatment of HIV-infected cells with selenium selenite was demonstrated to reduce HIV activation following cell stimulation with cytokine or exposure to oxidative stress (39). Selenium supplementation has been reported to stabilize AIDS patients in a University of Miami study (cited in Ref. 36). Rich food sources of selenium include seafood, meat, and grains. The upper limit for selenium supplements was recently set by NAS at 400 µg/mL/day. Larger amounts may cause selenosis, a toxic reaction marked by hair loss and nail damage.

Zinc

Zinc together with copper is an integral component of the antioxidant enzyme superoxide dismutase, which neutralizes peroxides. Zinc deficiency in blood plasma is common in HIV infection. This plasma deficiency may arise from the acute-phase response to viral infection, which results in the concentration of zinc by the liver (40). This trace element is important for the proper development of lymphocytes in the thymus gland (41). Excessive zinc can be immunosuppressive and can interfere with copper absorption. To prevent the latter effect, zinc and copper supplements should be taken at different times of the day. Intake of zinc in excess of 10 to 15 mg/day was reported in one study to increase the risk of disease progression in HIV-positive persons (5).

AMINO ACID/PEPTIDE THIOLS

Glutathione

In recent years, several reports have suggested that impaired antioxidant defenses, in particular glutathione (GSH) deficiency, may play a role in the immunopathogenesis of HIV infection (12,42–44). HIV-infected and AIDS patients manifest decreased GSH levels in plasma, lung epithelial lining fluid, and in CD4+/CD8+ lymphocyte subsets (44,45).

GSH, a cysteine-containing tripeptide (glutamyl-L-cysteinyl-glycine, or GSH) is the major redox buffering thiol within cells and a central molecule for lymphocytic function. Depletion of intracellular GSH inhibits IL-2–dependent lymphocyte proliferation and cell-mediated cytotoxicity (45). In a recent study in HIV-infected patients, oxidized GSH was strongly correlated with low numbers of CD4+ lymphocytes and impaired IL-2 production and proliferation in peripheral blood mononuclear cells (44). Furthermore, GSH redox disturbances induced by the generation of reactive oxygen species (ROS) were associated with an increased rate of cellular apoptosis (46).

Since several immunological functions related to HIV infection are dependent on adequate intracellular GSH balance, GSH restoration may have value in the treatment of HIV infection. Although both GSH and its monoester have been shown to suppress cytokine-stimulated HIV expression in latently infected cell lines (47), these compounds have found limited use in HIV treatment on account of the poor bioavailability of GSH and limited tolerance of its monoester (22). Accordingly, an alternative strategy for GSH restoration has focused on utilizing precursors of GSH (see below).

Cysteine and N-acetyl Cysteine (NAC)

As cysteine, a monothiol, is a rate-limiting precursor in GSH synthesis and its blood levels are lowered in HIV infection (48), cysteine and its derivatives have been considered for GSH replenishment. Cysteine is crucial for lymphocyte activation, and it can suppress HIV production in chronically infected cells (45,49). However, the use of cysteine supplementation in vivo is limited by its conversion to toxic by-products in the gut (32).

N-acetyl cysteine (NAC) has been suggested as an alternative to cysteine supplementation. NAC can act as a precursor of GSH and also as an antioxidant. It is commonly indicated as an antidote for acetaminophen overdose. It has been reported to inhibit apoptosis and HIV-1 production in infected cells (50,51) and to stimulate colonial growth of T cells derived from ARC/AIDS patients (6). Recently, NAC treatment in vitro was also reported to enhance CD3-mediated proliferative responses in freshly prepared peripheral blood mononuclear cells from AIDS patients (3). However, early data on use of NAC in AIDS patients were ambiguous (reviewed in Ref. 6). Although intravenous NAC was reported to lower viral p24 antigen levels (52), it did not improve surrogate immune parameters such as CD4 cell number and beta$_2$-microglobulin level. In another study, NAC was reported to enhance HIV-1 replication in monocyte-derived macrophages (53). More recently, helper T cell–associated GSH deficiency in HIV-infected patients was associated with decreased survival, and oral administration of NAC was correlated to increased survival (54). It is important to note that although NAC increases intracellular GSH during in vitro treatment, oral administration of NAC or OTC (procysteine), in another study, did not result in increase in plasma or lymphocyte levels in HIV-infected patients (55). Accordingly, the use of these monothiols for effecting GSH augmentation and immune restoration is rather limited.

ALPHA-LIPOIC ACID (THIOCTIC ACID)

In contrast to monothiols, dithiols such as alpha-lipoic acid (ALA) have been demonstrated to efficiently enhance intracellular GSH levels in models of oxidative stress (56,57) and to augment GSH levels in human blood plasma (57). ALA, which is readily converted intracellularly to its reduced form, dihydrolipoate (DHLA), functions as a universal antioxidant neutralizing reactive oxygen and nitrogen radicals in both aqueous and lipid-soluble compartments of the cell (57). ALA also functions as a redox regulator of proteins such as thioredoxin and NF-κB, which in turn regulate transcription of proinflammatory genes and latent HIV in immune cells (57). In cultured T cells, ALA and DHLA have been shown to prevent HIV replication (58) as well as cytokine-stimulated activation of NF-κB in T cells (59), which are regulated by oxidative stress.

ALA appears to be safe in the dosages prescribed clinically. The LD$_{50}$ was 400 to 500 mg/kg after oral dosing in dogs (57). It is recommended that it should not be given in high doses to patients suspected of having a thiamine deficiency unless the thiamine deficiency is also corrected (60). There have not been sufficient studies to guarantee safety for its use in pregnancy. In humans, reported side effects include allergic skin conditions and possible hypoglycemia in diabetic patients as a consequence of improved glucose utilization (57).

To date, limited data exist on the effects of ALA in HIV-infected patients. In a small study of ALA on AIDS patients utilizing oral doses of 450 mg/day for 14 days, plasma glutathione levels increased in 100% of participants, vitamin C levels increased in 90% of participants, T4 cells increased in 66%, and other markers of oxidative stress (lipid peroxidation) decreased in 90% of participants (61). However, no in vivo measurements of viral load were made and the effects of ALA supplementation on lymphocyte function were not determined. In mice, ALA increases immunity by specificaly enhancing helper T cells (62). In vitro, ALA inhibits the growth of HIV and blocks the activation of the NF-κB transcription factor more effectively than NAC. Thus, preincubation of T cells with ALA prior to cell stimulation completely inhibited NF-κB activation with only a small amount (2 to 4 mM) compared to the 20 mM needed for complete inhibition by NAC (62). ALA was recently shown in a triple antioxidant formulation with silymarin (from milk thistle) and selenium to regenerate the liver in a small number of patients with hepatitis C (63). These results suggest that further research is warranted on the immunomodulatory and antiviral effects of ALA in HIV infection. Elucidation of these effects is important, as this approach could identify novel complementary compounds for reconstituting immune function and controlling viral infection.

PHYTONUTRIENTS

Many plant-derived nutrients are antioxidants that manifest synergistic activity. The role of phytonutrients and their metabolites as synergistic antioxidants in HIV/AIDS has been reviewed by Greenspan and Aruoma (43). This review focuses on key phytonutrients with relevance to AIDS and heart disease.

Bioflavonoids

These are phenolic antioxidants that can scavenge peroxy radicals and chelate metal ions involved in redox reactions, which generate highly reactive hydroxyl radicals. Members of this group include quercetin, hesperidin, and catechin, which also have strong antiviral activity. Quercetin and catechin have been shown to inhibit viral reverse transcriptase activity (64). Certain catechin derivatives (flavans) were shown to inhibit HIV and SIV infection of target cells through interaction with the surface glycoprotein on the viral envelope (65). Clinical trails evaluating the usefulness of these compounds in HIV/AIDS patients are needed.

Coenzyme Q-10 and L-Carnitine

Coenzyme Q-10 (CoQ-10) is a lipid-soluble antioxidant that is abundant in beets and salmon. It plays an important role in cellular respiration and energy generation in the mitochondria and synergizes with vitamin E in the neutralization of peroxy radicals. CoQ-10 deficiency has been reported in HIV/AIDS patients (66). In a small study in healthy volunteers, ingestion of CoQ-10 (100 mg/day) for 2 months was reported to improve the CD4/CD8 ratio (67).

L-Carnitine facilitates transport of long-chain fatty acid into mitochondria. In concert with CoQ-10, it may increase efficiency of energy production in the mitochondria. An altered electrochemical potential across the mitochondrial membrane has been detected in peripheral blood lymphocytes (PBL) from AIDS patients (68). Treatment of patient-derived PBL in vitro with NAC, L-acetyl carnitine, or nicotinamide was shown to modify the electrochemical gradient and reduce the rate of spontaneous apoptosis (68).

Inositol and Inositol Hexaphosphate

Inositol, a major component of rice bran, is a B vitamin–like sugar alcohol. Inositol deficiency has been linked to hair loss (alopecia) and abnormal vertebrate development. The biologically active form is myoinositol which occurs abundantly in skeletal muscle (69). Myoinositol can exist in a free or bound form. In its bound form, myoinositol occurs as a constituent of phospholipids in biological membranes and as inositol hexaphosphate (IP6 or phytate) in plant seeds, whole grains, and cereals. IP6 is the major dietary or food source of phosphatidyl inositol, which serves as a lipid precursor to intracellular molecules (second messengers) involved in cell signaling. Experimental studies have demonstrated that both inositol and IP6 have lipid-lowering effects (reviewed in Ref. 70). Specifically, IP6 was shown to lower elevated serum total cholesterol and triglycerides in hyperlipemic animals (71). In another study, myoinositol and IP6 prevented the development of fatty liver by inhibiting sucrose-induced elevation in hepatic total lipids and trigycerides (72). In addition, IP6 has also been shown to have other beneficial effects relevant to heart disease, namely antiplatelet activity (73) and inhibition of aortic calcification and lipid peroxidation in ischemic kidneys (cited in Ref. 70).

Other Rice Bran–Derived Products

Aside from inositol and IP6, which are derived primarily from the defatted fraction of rice bran, the fraction containing rice oil is rich in antioxidant polyphenols, which include plant sterol, its ester (γ-oryzanol) and tocotrienol. These polyphenolic compounds have been shown in experimental studies to have significant lipid-lowering properties relevant to the treatment of hyperlipidemia. These studies have recently been reviewed (74).

Another important group of plant-based alcohols are policosanols, which are derived from waxes extracted primarily from sugar cane, beeswax, or rice bran wax. In human studies conducted in Latin America, policosanol (from sugar cane wax) was found to have significant cholesterol-lowering properties. It is a new lipid-lowering agent with potential for the treatment of dyslipidemia that may offer advantages over conventional cholesterol-lowering drugs (75).

CONCLUSION

Immune system restoration and management of metabolic abnormalities associated with antiretroviral treatment is highly desired in persons afflicted with HIV infection.

In addition to a decrease in immune function, HIV/AIDS patients manifest deficiencies in specific micronutrients including vitamins A, B complex (B_6, B_{12}, folic acid), C and E, trace minerals selenium and zinc, and amino acid/peptide thiols—namely, cysteine and glutathione. The affected micronutrients and thiols have been shown in experimental animal and human studies to influence humoral/cell-mediated immune responses. In addition, other nutrients, specifically phytonutrients, manifest lipid-lowering effects relevant to the treatment of dyslipidemia linked to HIV infection. Further studies in human subjects are urgently needed to determine the impact of micronutrient and phytonutrient supplementation on immune function and dyslipidemia in HIV/AIDS patients currently on antiretroviral therapy as well as in those who fail such treatment.

REFERENCES

1. Lane HC, Fauci A. Immunologic abnormalities in the acquired immunodeficiency syndrome. Annu Rev Immunol 1985; 3:477.
2. Clerici M, et al. Detection of three distinct patterns of T-helper cell dysfunction in asymptomatic, human immunodeficiency virus–seropositive patients. Independence of CD4+ cell numbers and clinical staging. J Clin Invest 1989; 84:1892.
3. Alfonso C, et al. In vitro antioxidant treatment recovers proliferative response of anergic CD4+ lymphocytes from human immunodeficiency virus-infected individuals. Blood 1996; 87(11):4746–4753.
4. Abrams B, et al. A prospective study of dietary intake and acquired human deficiency syndrome in HIV-seropositive homosexual men. J AIDS 1993; 6:949.
5. Tang AM, et al. Dietary micronutrient intake and risk of progression to AIDS in human immunodeficiency virus type 1 (HIV-1)-infected homosexual men. Am J Epidemiol 1993; 138:937.
6. Jariwalla RI. Experimental studies with antioxidants. In: Watson R, ed. Nutrients and Foods in AIDS. Boca Raton, FL: CRC Press, 1998:99–115.
7. Roederer M. Getting to the HAART of T cell dynamics. Nat Med 1998; 4(2):145–146.
8. Autran B, et al. Positive effects of combined antiretroviral therapy on CD4+ T cell homeostasis and function in advanced HIV disease. Science 1997; 277:112–116.
9. Pakker NG, et al. Biphasic kinetics of peripheral blood T cells after triple combination therapy in HIV-1 infection: a composite of redistribution and proliferation. Nat Med 1998; 4:208–214.
10. Behrens GMN, Stoll M, Schmidt RE. Lipodystrophy syndrome in HIV infection. What is it, what causes it and how it can be managed? Drug Saf 2000; 23:57–76.
11. Dube MP, et al. Preliminary guidelines for the evaluation and management of dyslipidemia in adults infected with human immunodeficiency virus and receiving antiretroviral therapy: recommendations of the adult AIDS Clinical Trial Group Cardiovascular Disease Focus Group. Clin Infect Dis 2000; 31:1216–1224.
12. Jariwalla RJ. Micronutrient imbalance in HIV infection and AIDS: relevance to pathogenesis and therapy. J Nutr Environ Med 1995; 5:297.
13. Gray RH. Similarities between AIDS and PCM [letter]. Am J Public Health 1983; 73:1332.
14. Bendich A. Antioxidant vitamins and their functions in immune responses. Adv Exp Mol Biol 1990; 262:35–55.
15. Coodley GO. Vitamins in HIV infection. In: Watson RR, ed. Nutrition and AIDS. Boca Raton. FL: CRC Press, 1994:89–103.
16. Bodgen JD, Baker H, Frank O, Perez G, Kemp F, Breuning K, Louria D. Micronutrient

status and human immunodeficiency virus (HIV) infection. Ann N Y Acad Sci USA 1990; 587:189.

17. Jariwalla RJ, Harakeh S. Mechanisms underlying the action of vitamin C in viral and immunodeficiency disease. In: Packer L, Fuchs J, eds. Vitamin C in Health and Disease. New York: Marcel Dekker, 1997:309–322.

18. Jariwalla RJ, Harakeh S. Antiviral and immunomodulatory activities of ascorbic acid. In: Harris JR, ed. Subcellular Biochemistry: Vol 25. Ascorbic Acid: Biochemistry and Biomedical Cell Biology. New York: Plenum Press, 1995:215–231.

19. Harakeh S, Jariwalla RJ. NF-κB independent suppression of HIV expression by ascorbic acid. AIDS Res Hum Retrovir 1997; 13:3.

20. Johnston CS, Meyer CG, Srilakshmi JC. Vitamin C elevates red blood cell glutathione in healthy adults. Am J Clin Nutr 1993; 58:103–105.

21. Henning SM, et al. Glutathione blood levels and other oxidant defense indices in men fed diets low in vitamin C. J Nutr 1991; 121:1969–1975.

22. Martensson J, Han J, Griffith OW, Meister A. Glutathione ester delays the onset of scurvy in ascorbate-deficient guinea pigs. Proc Natl Acad Sci USA 1993; 90:317.

23. Kim I. et al. Vitamin and mineral supplement use and mortality in a US cohort. Am J Public Health 1993; 83(4):546–550.

24. Martin JB, Easley-Shaw T, Collins C. Use of selected vitamin and mineral supplements among individuals infected with human immunodeficiency virus. J Am Diet Assoc 1991; 91(4):476–478.

25. Cathcart RF. Vitamin C in the treatment of acquired immune deficiency syndrome (AIDS). Med Hypoth 1984; 14:423.

26. Cathcart RF. Glutathione and HIV infection [letter]. Lancet 1990; 335(8683):234–236.

27. Levine M, et al. Vitamin C pharmacokinetics in healthy volunteers: evidence for a recommended dietary allowance. Proc Natl Acad Sci USA 1996; 93:3704–3709.

28. Harakeh S, Jariwalla RJ, Pauling L. Suppression of human immunodeficiency virus replication by ascorbate in chronically and acutely infected cells. Proc Natl Acad Sci USA 1990; 87:7245–7249.

29. Harris A, Robinson AB, Pauling L. Blood plasma L-ascorbic acid concentration for oral L-ascorbic acid dosage up to 12 grams a day. IRCS J Med Sci 1973; 10:19.

30. Riordan NH, Riordan HD, Meng X, et al. Intravenous ascorbate as a tumor cytotoxic chemotherapeutic agent. Med Hypoth 1995; 44:207–213.

31. Picardo M, et al. Vitamin E, polyunsaturated fatty acids of phospholipids, lipoperoxides and glutathione peroxidase status in HIV sero-positive patients. VIIth International Conference on AIDS. Florence, Italy, 1991.

32. Waterson SK. Glutathione deficiency: therapeutic target in human immunodeficiency virus infection. J Orthomol Med 1992; 7:104–110.

33. Suzuki YJ, Packer L. Inhibition of NF- kappaB DNA binding activity by alpha-tocopheryl succinate. Biochem Mol Biol Int 1993; 31:693–700.

34. Matthes E, Langen P, Brachwitz H. Alteration of DNA topoisomerase II activity during infection of H9 cells by human immunodeficiency virus type 1 in vitro: a target for potential therapeutic agents. Antivir Res 1990; 13:273.

35. Baum M, et al. Association of vitamin B status with parameters of immune function in early HIV-1 infection. J AIDS 1991; 4:1122–1132.

36. Taylor EW. Selenium and viral diseases: facts and hypotheses. In: Proceedings of the American College of Advanced Medicine. Tampa, FL: Spring Conference, April 1997.

37. Dworkin B, et al. Selenium deficiency in the acquired immune deficiency syndrome. J Parenteral Enteral Nutr 1986; 10:405–407.

38. Mantero-Atienza E, et al. Selenium status and immune function in early HIV infection VIIth International Conference on AIDS. Florence, Italy, 1991.

39. Sappey C, Legrand-Poels S, Best-Belpomme M, Favier A, Rentier B, Piette J. Stimulation

of glutathione peroxidase activity decreases HIV type 1 activation after oxidative stress. AIDS Res Hum Retrovir 1994; 10(11):1451–1461.

40. Graham NMH. On specific nutrient abnormalities in asymptomatic HIV infection. AIDS 1992; 6:1552–1553.

41. Fraker PJ, King LE, Gravy B, et al. Immunopathology of zinc deficiency: a role for apoptosis. In: Klurfeld DM, ed. Human Nutrition: A Comprehensive Treatise. Vol 8. New York: Plenum Press, 1993:267–283.

42. Baruchel S, Wainberg MA. The role of oxidative stress in disease progression in individuals infected by the human immunodeficiency virus. J Leuk Biol 1992; 52:111.

43. Greenspan HC, Arouma O. Could oxidative stress initiate programmed cell death in HIV infection? A role for plant derived metabolites having synergistic antioxidant activity. Chem Biol Interact 1994; 91:187.

44. Aukrust P, et al. Increased levels of oxidized glutathione in CD4 + lymphocytes associated with disturbed intracellular redox balance in human immunodeficiency virus type 1 infection. Blood 1995; 86(1):258–267.

45. Droge W, Eck HP, Mihm S. HIV-induced cysteine deficiency and T-cell dysfunction—a rationale for treatment with N-acetylcysteine. Immunol Today 1992; 13(6):211.

46. Sato J, et al. Thiol-mediated redox regulation of apoptosis. J Immunol 1995; 154:3194.

47. Kalebic T, Kinter A, Guide P, Anderson ME, Fauci AS. Suppression of human immuno-deficiency virus expression in chronically infected monocytic cells by glutathione ester and N-acetyl cysteine. Proc Natl Acad Sci USA 1991; 88:986.

48. Eck H-P, et al. Low concentration of acid-soluble thiol (cysteine) in the blood plasma of HIV-infected patients. Biol Chem Hoppe Seyler 1989; 370:101–108.

49. Mihm S, Ennen J, Pessara U, Kurth R, Dröge W. Inhibition of HIV-1 replication and NF-κB by cysteine and cysteine derivatives. AIDS 1991; 497:503.

50. Malorni W, Rivabene R, Santini MT, Donelli G. N-Acetylcysteine inhibits apoptosis and decreases viral particles in HIV-chronically infected U937 cells. FEBS Lett 1993; 327(1): 75–78.

51. Roederer M, et al. Cytokine-stimulated human immunodeficiency virus replication is inhibited by N-acetyl-L-cysteine. Proc Natl Acad Sci USA 1990; 87:4884.

52. Clotet B, et al. Effects on surrogate markers of intravenous N-acetylcysteine in AIDS patients. VIIIth International Conference on AIDS. Amsterdam, 1992.

53. Nottet HSLM, et al. Role for oxygen radicals in the self-sustained HIV-1 replication in monocyte-derived macrophages: enhanced HIV-1 replication by N-acetylcyteine. IXth International Conference on AIDS. Berlin, 1992.

54. Herzenberg LA, et al. Glutathione deficiency is associated with impaired survival in HIV disease. Proc Natl Acad Sci USA 1997; 94:1967–1972.

55. Witschi A, et al. Supplementation of N-acetylcysteine fails to increase glutathione in lymphocyte and plasma of patients with AIDS. AIDS Res Hum Retrovir 1995; 11:141.

56. Busse E, et al. Influence of alpha-lipoic acid on intracellular glutathione in vitro and in vivo. Arzneimittel Forsch 1992; 42:829–831.

57. Packer L, et al. Alpha-lipoic acid as a biological antioxidant. Free Radic Biol Med 1995; 19:227–250.

58. Baur A, et al. Alpha-lipoic acid is an effective inhibitor of human immuno-deficiency virus (HIV-1) replication. Klin Wochensch 1991; 69:722–724.

59. Suzuki YJ, Aggarwal BB, Packer L. Alpha-lipoic acid is a potent inhibitor of NF-κB activation in human T cells. Biochem Biophys Res Commun 1992; 189:1709–1715.

60. Gal EM. Reversal of selective toxicity of alpha-lipoic acid by thiamine in thiamine-deficient rats. Nature 1965; 205:535.

61. Lands S. NAC, glutamine and alpha lipoic acid. In: James J, ed. AIDS Treatment News. no. 268, April 4, 1997.

62. Sosin A, Jacobs BL. Alpha lipoic acid and HIV. In: Alpha Lipoic Acid: Nature's Ultimate Antioxidant. New York: Kensington, 1998:154–161.

63. Berkson BM. A triple antioxidant approach to the treatment of hepatitis C using alpha-lipoic acid, silymarin, selenium and other fundamental nutraceuticals. Clin Pract Alt Med 2000; 1:27–33.

64. Nakaul H, et al. Differential inhibition of HIV-reverse transcriptase and various DNA and RNA polymerase by some catechin derivatives. Nucleic Acid Res Symp Series 21, 1989.

65. Mahmood N, et al. Inhibition of HIV infection by caffeoyl-quinic acid derivatives. Antivir Chem Chemother 1993; 4(4):235–240.

66. Biochemical deficiencies of coenzyme Q10 in HIV infection and exploratory treatment. Biochem Biophys Res Commun 1988; 153:188.

67. Folkers K, et al. Coenzyme Q 10 increases T4/T8 ratio of lymphocytes in ordinary subjects and relevance to patients having the AIDS-related complex. Biochem Biophys Res Commun 1991; 176:786–791.

68. Cossarizza A, et al. Mitochondrial alterations and dramatic tendency to undergo apoptosis in peripheral blood lymphocytes during acute HIV syndrome. AIDS 1997; 11:19–26.

69. Ogawa S. Chemical components of rice bran: myo-inositol and related compounds. Anticancer Res 1999; 19:3635–3644.

70. Jariwalla RJ. Inositol hexaphosphate (IP6) as an anti-neoplastic and lipid-lowering agent. Anticancer Res 1999; 19:3699–3702.

71. Jariwalla RJ, et al. Lowering of serum cholesterol and triglycerides and modulation of divalent cations by dietary phytate. J Applied Nutr 1990; 42:18–28.

72. Katayama T. Hypolipidemic action of phytic acid (IP6): prevention of fatty liver. Anticancer Res 1999; 19:3695–3698.

73. Vucenik JJ, et al. Anti-platelet activity of inositol hexaphosphate (IP6). Anticancer Res 1999; 19:3689–3693.

74. Jariwalla RJ. Rice-bran products: phytonutrients with potential applications in preventive and clinical medicine. Drugs Exp Clin Res 2001; 27:17–26.

75. Gouini-Berthold I, Berthold HK. Policosanol: clinical pharmacology and therapeutic significance of a new lipid-lowering agent. Am Heart J 2002; 143:356–365.

12

Antioxidant Vitamins and Heart Disease Prevention

Jin Zhang

Brigham and Women's Hospital and Harvard Medical School, Boston, Massachusetts, U.S.A.

Ronald Ross Watson

University of Arizona, Tucson, Arizona, U.S.A.

INTRODUCTION

Coronary heart disease (CHD) is a major cause of mortality and morbidity worldwide. About 13 million Americans have CHD, 1.5 million have a myocardial infarction (MI) each year, and about 450,000 die of CHD each year (1). It is of great public health benefit to find simple, feasible, and cost-effective preventive therapies that decrease the incidence of CHD. Research on the cause of CHD has been ongoing for approximately a century (2). It is known that CHD is caused by atherosclerosis, a process characterized by endothelial dysfunction in association with hypertension, diabetes, smoking, and elevated homocysteine concentrations and cholesterol deposition in macrophages and smooth muscle cells in the arterial wall as the result of elevated low-density lipoproteins (LDLs) and remnant lipoproteins as well as decreased high-density lipoproteins (HDLs). In addition, smooth muscle proliferation, inflammation, thrombosis, and calcification occur in this process. The basis of therapy for CHD is its prevention through the modification of risk factors (3).

Epidemiological studies find lower CHD morbidity and mortality in people who consume larger quantities of antioxidants in foods or supplements (4). Therefore, substantial interest has recently focused on the hypothesis that the naturally occurring antioxidant vitamins—such as vitamin E, vitamin C, and beta-carotene—may prevent the progression of CHD. This chapter provides a comprehensive review of antioxidant vitamins (vitamins E, and C, and beta-carotene) in CHD prevention in animal studies, human epidemiological studies, and randomized clinical trials.

PATHOPHYSIOLOGY OF ATHEROSCLEROSIS

Significant progress has been made in understanding the underlying atherosclerotic process during the last decades. Several hypotheses have been proposed to explain the initiating events in atherosclerosis—e.g., the response to injury, response to retention, and oxidation hypotheses (5–7). These hypotheses are not mutually exclusive and may even be compatible with each other. The oxidation hypothesis emphasizes the importance of oxidative modification in the atherosclerotic process, because compared with native LDL, oxidized LDL is preferentially taken up in the arterial wall (7). This hypothesis shows a role for diet and lifestyle in atherosclerosis; for example, LDL can be oxidized by smoking. Such oxidation can be prevented by dietary antioxidants, e.g., vitamins and polyphenols.

Atherosclerosis is the initial step in the development of CHD, which is a complex process involving the deposition of plasma lipoproteins and the proliferation of cellular elements in the artery wall (8). The key determinants of early lesion initiation are as follows:

1. Enhanced focal intimal influx and accumulation of plasma LDL, in which LDL crosses the endothelium in a concentration-dependent manner and can become trapped in the extracellular matrix.
2. Increased net intimal oxidative stress status. The subendothelium is an oxidizing environment, and if the LDL remains trapped for a sufficiently long period of time, it undergoes oxidative change.
3. Oxidative modifications of LDL components, which promote focal monocyte recruitment to the arterial intima. Mildly oxidized forms of LDL contain biologically active phospholipid oxidation products that affect the pattern of gene expression in endothelial cells via activation of the transcription factor NF-κB, leading to, among other things, changes in the expression of monocyte binding molecules, monocyte chemoattractant protein, and macrophage colony stimulating factors. These factors, in turn, promote the recruitment of monocytes.
4. Intimal monocyte/macrophage activation and their phenotypic differentiation to macrophages.
5. Foam cell formation. Further oxidation leads to alterations in apolipoprotein B such that LDL particles are recognized and internalized by macrophages, progenitors of the lipid-laden foam cells. Marked increases in lipid and cholesterol oxidation products render the LDL particles cytotoxic, leading to further endothelial injury and favoring further entry of LDLs and circulating monocytes, and thus a continuation of the disease process.

The occurrence of CHD depends not only on the rate at which atherosclerotic plaques grow but also on endothelial function, smooth muscle proliferation, thrombosis, and plaque rupture. It is gradually being recognized that reactive oxygen and nitrogen species directly interact with signaling mechanisms in the arterial wall to regulate vascular function (9,10). The activities of oxidant-generating enzymes in the arterial wall are regulated by both receptor activation and non-receptor-mediated pathways. The occurrence of CHD depends not only on endothelial function, smooth muscle cell proliferation, thrombosis, and plaque rupture. Such effects might also be influenced by antioxidant effects on the signaling processes in the arterial wall to regulate vascular funtion, thus providing alternative mechanisms by which antioxidant supplementation might ameliorate vascular pathology, as by improving endothelial function (10,11). Complex interactions between diet, lifestyle, and lipoprotein metabolism determine the development of atherosclerosis and its complications. Since oxidation is essential for the generation of atherosclerotic plaques, the prevention or reduction of lipid peroxidation is of significant medical importance.

ARE EXOGENOUS ANTIOXIDANTS EFFECTIVE?

As we know, the antioxidant defense system includes both endogenously and exogenously (diet) derived compounds: antioxidant enzymes, chain-breaking antioxidants, and transition metal-binding proteins. Major antioxidant enzymes include superoxide dismutase (SOD), catalase, and glutathione peroxidase (GPx). SOD was the first genuine ROS (reactive oxygen species)-metabolizing enzyme discovered and exists mainly in mitochondria (12). In the reaction catalyzed by SOD, two molecules of superoxide form hydrogen peroxide and molecular oxygen and are thereby a source of cellular hydrogen peroxide—Reaction (1). The reaction catalyzed by SOD is extremely efficient in eliminating superoxide.

$$O_2 + e^- + 2H^+ \rightarrow H_2O_2 \tag{1}$$

Another enzyme, catalase, is mainly a heme-containing enzyme (13). Its predominant subcellular localization in mammalian cells is in peroxisomes, where catalase catalyzes the dismutation of hydrogen peroxide to water and molecular oxygen—Reaction (2).

$$2H_2O_2 \rightarrow O_2 + 2H_2O \tag{2}$$

The third enzyme is GPx. There are at least four different GPx enzymes in mammals (GPx1 to 4), all containing selenocysteine (14). GPx1 and GPx4 (or phospholipid hydroperoxide GPx) are both cytosolic enzymes abundant in most tissues (15). All GPxs catalyze the reduction of H_2O_2 using glutathione as substrate. They can also reduce other peroxides (e.g., lipid peroxides in cell membranes) to alcohols—Reactions (3) and (4).

$$H_2O_2 + 2GSH \rightarrow GSSG + H_2O \tag{3}$$

$$ROOH + 2GSH \rightarrow ROH + GSSG + H_2O \tag{4}$$

The major chain-breaking antioxidants include the aqueous-phase chain-breaking antioxidant vitamin C (ascorbic acid), lipid-phase chain breaking-antioxidant vitamin E (α-tocopherol), and beta-carotene (provitamin A). Vitamin E prevents the peroxidation of polyunsaturated fatty acid in membranes. The most active and efficient form of vitamin E is alpha-tocopherol. Vitamin E is incorporated into lipoproteins and cell membranes, limiting LDL oxidation and scavenging lipid peroxyl radicals to yield lipid hydroperoxides and the tocopheroxyl radical. Vitamin E is the predominant antioxidant in LDL. It also inhibits platelet activation and monocyte adhesion. Vitamin C (ascorbic acid) is the predominant plasma antioxidant. This water-soluble vitamin scavenges plasma free radicals (e.g., superoxide anion, hydrogen peroxide, the hydroxyl radical, and singlet oxygen) and prevents their entry into LDL particles. Vitamin C also regenerates active vitamin E and increases cholesterol excretion. Vitamin C improves endothelium-dependent vasodilation and reduces monocyte adhesion as well. Beta-carotene (provitamin A) is a vitamin A precursor carried in plasma and LDL. It reduces oxidized LDL uptake but does not prevent LDL oxidation.

Additionally, emerging evidence also suggests an important role of antioxidants in modulating endothelial function, which is probably in part mediated by their antioxidant activity (10). In animal models, alpha-tocopherol was found to preserve nitric oxide–mediated vascular relaxation. In vitro studies showed a reduction in cell adhesion molecule expression and monocyte adhesion to the endothelium and improvement in endothelium-dependent vasodilation after incubation with antioxidants. In addition to the in vitro evidence, there is growing clinical evidence to support a favorable effect of antioxidants on endothelial function (11). Studies of the effect of antioxidant supplementation on endothelial function, ranging in duration from 1 week to 3 months, used either vitamin C or vitamin E supplementation and assessed soluble markers of endothelial activation or endothelium-dependent vasodilation in conduit arteries.

EVIDENCE SUPPORTING THE ROLE OF ANTIOXIDANT VITAMINS IN CHD PREVENTION

Dietary antioxidants—including vitamin C, vitamin E, and beta-carotene—have received the greatest attention with regard to cardiovascular disease prevention (4). Evidence that antioxidant vitamins potentially reduce the risk of CHD comes from animal studies, human studies, epidemiological studies, and randomized trials. Animal studies suggest that vitamin E can slow the development of atherosclerosis (16). Many studies have now shown that antioxidant supplementation in healthy subjects or patients with CHD can reduce free radical damage and protect LDLs against oxidation. Both beta-carotene and vitamin C have produced extensions in lag time to oxidation in only a few studies, although it remains possible that they might have a beneficial effect in individuals with poor baseline status (17,18).

Large-scale epidemiological studies generally show that a low intake of antioxidants is associated with increased cardiovascular risk after correcting for other risk factors. The epidemiological evidence is strongest in the case of vitamin E. Two particularly illustrative prospective cohort studies in the United States examined the association between antioxidant intake and the risk of CHD. In a group of 39,910 male health professionals, men who took a vitamin E supplement (≥60 IU/day) for 4 years had—after adjustment for age, coronary risk factors, and intake of vitamin C and beta-carotene—a 37% lower relative risk of CHD than those who did not take vitamin E supplements (19). In the nurses' health study of 87,245 female nurses, women who took vitamin E supplements (≥30 IU/day) for 8 years had a 41% lower relative risk of major coronary disease (20).

The evidence linking the water-soluble vitamin C with CHD is less strong than that for vitamin E. Only one prospective study involving 11,348 adults who took vitamin C for over 10 years demonstrated an inverse relation between vitamin C intake and overall cardiovascular mortality (21). Results were not adjusted for the intake of other antioxidants, however. This effect resulted largely from the use of vitamin C in supplements and might have been related to other antioxidant vitamins in multivitamin preparations.

There is also some indication that increased dietary intake of beta-carotene is associated with reduced risk of CHD, although again the evidence is less convincing than that for vitamin E. Tavani et al. found that the risk of acute myocardial infarction was inversely related to beta-carotene intake, with an OR of 0.5 (95% CI: 0.3 to 0.8) for the highest quintile of intake compared to the lowest ($p < 0.01$) (22). Rimm et al. also observed a lower risk of major coronary events in men reporting high versus those reporting low intakes of beta-carotene, but in subgroup analyses, this relationship was significant only in current and former smokers (19). These findings are consistent with several other studies indicating an inverse association between dietary intake of beta-carotene or provitamin A carotenoids and risk of cardiovascular disease, particularly among smokers (23,24).

In a study of the effect of antioxidant vitamins on death from cardiovascular disease in 34,486 postmenopausal women (25), Kushi et al. found that the intake of vitamin E from food is inversely associated with the risk of death from coronary heart disease and that such women can lower their risk without using vitamin supplements. By contrast, the intake of vitamins A and C was not associated with a lower risk of dying from coronary disease.

Although epidemological studies have provided support for the potential health benefits of antioxidants, there remains little direct experimental evidence from randomized trials. Currently, there is no strong evidence from primary prevention trials (8,26). However, results from secondary prevention trials have been more supportive of the potential health benefits of antioxidants. The Cambridge Heart Antioxidant Study tested the effects of high doses (400 or 800 IU/day) of alpha-tocopherol on subsequent cardiovascular events in patients with angiographic evidence of coronary atherosclerosis (27). On the basis of the combined results for the two dose levels, the risk of myocardial infarction and all cardiovascular events was reduced by 77 and 47%, respectively, in the treatment group, with a delay in the onset of treatment benefit of ≈ 200 days.

EVIDENCE OPPOSING THE ROLE OF ANTIOXIDANT VITAMINS IN CHD PREVENTION

DeMaio et al. investigated 100 patients who had undergone percutaneous transluminal coronary angioplasty with the treatment of 1200 IU/day of vitamin E supplementation for 4 months; no significant benefit was found (28). In a study conducted by Laura and coworkers, vitamin E from foods had a protective effect on death from stroke. However, intake of supplemental vitamin E (at 2053 IU/day) or other antioxidant vitamins (vitamin C, 9.7 mg/day; carotenoids, 678 µg/day; retinol equivalents, 2053 µg/day; and retinol 1178 µg/day) in 41,836 postmenopausal women (55 to 69 years of age) did not have a protective role (29). Another study investigated 1511 men and women who were at high risk for cardiovascular events for a mean of 4.5 years. Vitamin E supplementation of 400 IU/day had no significant effects on death due to cardiovascular disease (30).

In 1996, Omenn et al. reported that in 18,314 male smokers and asbestos workers who received the supplement beta-carotene (30 mg/day) and retinol (25,000 IU/day) for 4 years, the combination of beta-carotene and retinol had no benefit and may have increased the risk of cardiac death (31). In the same year, a study in 22,071 male physicians concluded that the combination of beta-carotene at 50 mg/day and aspirin 325 mg/day for 12 years showed no benefit on risk of cardiovascular disease (32). And later in 1999, Lee et al. found no statistically significant differences in the overall incidence of cardiovascular disease in 39,876 women (45 years or older) with a supplement of 50 mg of beta-carotene on alternate days (33).

In several studies, dietary vitamin C was found to reduce CHD. However, supplemental vitamin C had little effect (34–36). This suggests that the benefit attributed to dietary vitamin C may be due to other dietary and lifestyle factors among individuals consuming a diet high in vitamin C. Rimm et al. reported that in 39,910 male health professionals with an intake of 1162 mg/day, vitamin C supplementation did not show any benefit with regard to cardiovascular disease (34). In 1996, Azen et al. investigated 146 subjects with previous coronary artery bypass graft surgery with a drug plus vitamin C supplements of at least 250 mg/day. These supplements did not show any benefit for intimal-medial thickness (35). The Scottish Heart Health Study reported significant benefits from vitamin C but only in men, while no benefit was observed in women (36). The study of dietary antioxidant vitamins and death from CHD in postmenopausal women showed that the intake of vitamin C was not associated with a lower risk of dying from such disease (25).

When antioxidants were used in combination, the results were also inconclusive. The Alpha-Tocopherol, Beta-Carotene Cancer Prevention study group examined the effects of vitamin E and beta-carotene over a period of 5 to 8 years in 29,133 male smokers with supplement of beta-carotene (20 mg/day) and vitamin E (50 IU/day) in Finland. No reduction in heart disease or death was found. Moreover, an increase in mortality from hemorrhagic stroke was found with the use of vitamin E supplements. An increased incidence of cardiac death was also found in the group taking beta-carotene supplements (37). The Multivitamins and Probucol Study showed that the combination of vitamins C, E, and beta-carotene had no effect in reducing the rate of restenosis in patients after angioplasty (38).

DIETARY SOURCES AND SAFETY OF ANTIOXIDANT VITAMINS

Dietary sources of vitamin E include vegetable and seed oils, wheat germ, and, in smaller quantities, meats, fish, fruits, and vegetables. Sources of dietary vitamin C include citrus fruits, strawberries, cantaloupe, tomatoes, and vegetables. Beta-carotene can be found in fruits, yellow-orange vegetables (e.g., carrots, squash, and sweet potatoes) and deep-green vegetables (e.g., spinach and broccoli).

Vitamins C, E, and beta-carotene have few side effects. The current RDA for vitamin E is 15 mg/day of alpha-tocopherol for both men and women (39). No significant toxicity has been noted for vitamin E in dosages of 800 to 3,200 IU/day. Vitamin E has been found to prolong thrombin time in some animals, and it may increase vitamin K requirements. Therefore caution is recommended when vitamin E supplementation is used in patients receiving anticoagulant therapy. The RDA for vitamin C is 75 mg/day for females and 90 mg/day for males (39). Vitamin C supplementation is usually nontoxic, although diarrhea, bloating, and false-negative occult blood tests can occur at dosages greater than 2 g/day. The intestinal absorptive capacity for vitamin C is approximately 3 g/day. Excess vitamin C is excreted in the urine but does not increase urinary oxalic acid. However, confusion arises about excess vitamin C intake causing increased oxalic acid excretion (and thus a possibly an increased risk of oxalate kidney stones), as urinary vitamin C is converted to oxalate with air exposure. No RDA for beta-carotene is established in humans (39). Data about adverse effects of beta-carotene are very limited as well. However, this does not mean that there is no potential for adverse effects resulting from high intake. Recent studies have shown a potential risk of lung cancer with high-dose beta-carotene. Extra caution may be warranted.

CONCLUSIONS AND RECOMMENDATIONS

Oxidation of LDL plays an important role in the development of atherosclerosis, the disease process that leads to CHD. Increasing evidence suggests that using antioxidant vitamins, both in the diet and in supplements, can prevent LDL oxidation and its biological effects. These data are from various sources: basic science, epidemiology, experiments in animals, and limited clinical trials. However the beneficial effects are inconsistent, as reviewed above. There are many possible explanations for the differences in those studies. (1) Individual lifestyle can significantly affect the study results. The positive outcomes are not obvious in those samples that have a healthy lifestyle. (2) The synergistic effects between ingested nutrients will conceal the effect of antioxidant supplements. Therefore supplementation with antioxidants alone may not show significant effects on CHD. (3) The bioavailability of antioxidant vitamins may be responsible for the different results of the studies (26). (4) If the dose of antioxidant supplements is too high, it can lead to a toxic effect instead of beneficial one.

In conclusion, the benefits of antioxidant vitamins for the prevention of CHD have not been demonstrated consistently. A complex interplay exists between antioxidants, which makes it difficult to predict how antioxidants will function in vivo and to answer which antioxidant is most important. Standardization and optimization of antioxidant use based on pharmacokinetic considerations are warranted. Furthermore, additional randomized clinical trials are needed to define the role of antioxidant vitamins in the prevention and treatment of CHD. Generally, diets rich in antioxidants are also lower in saturated fat and cholesterol and higher in fiber. For example, foods rich in vitamins C, and E, and beta-carotene also contain minerals, flavonoids, and indoles as well as carotenoids other than beta-carotene (40). Considering these findings, the most practical and scientifically supportable recommendation for the general population is to consume a balanced diet with emphasis on antioxidant-rich fruits and vegetables and whole grains. This advice considers the role of the total diet in influencing disease risk, which is consistent with the current dietary guidelines of the American Heart Association (41). Healthy foods should always provide the foundation for a healthy diet, and supplements should be used to complement, not replace, healthy foods.

ACKNOWLEDGMENT

This work was supported by grants HL63667 and HL59794 and their NIDA supplements as well as the Wallace Genetics Foundation.

REFERENCES

1. American Heart Association. 2000 Heart and Stroke Statistical Update. Dallas: American Heart Association, 2000:1–10.
2. Connor WE. Diet-heart research in the first part of the 20th century. Acta Cardiol 1999; 54:135–139.
3. Schaefer EJ. Lipoproteins, nutrition, and heart disease. Am J Clin Nutr 2002; 75(2):191–212.
4. Adams AK, Wermuth EO, Mcbride PE. Antioxidant vitamins and the prevention of coronary heart disease. Am Fam Physician 1999; 60(3):895–904.
5. Ross R. The pathogenesis of atherosclerosis: a perspective for the 1990s. Nature 1993; 362:801–809.
6. Boren J, Gustafsson M, Skalen K, Flood C, Innerarity TL. Role of extracellular retention of low density lipoproteins in atherosclerosis. Curr Opin Lipidol 2000; 11:451–456.
7. Young IS, McEneny J. Lipoprotein oxidation and atherosclerosis. Biochem Soc Trans 2001; 29(Pt 2):358–362.
8. Tribble D. AHA Science Advisory. Antioxidant consumption and risk of coronary heart disease: emphasis on Vitamin C, Vitamin E, and β-carotene. Circulation 1999; 99:591–595.
9. Young IS, Woodside JV. Antioxidants in health and disease. J Clin Pathol 2001; 54(3):176–186.
10. Brown AA, Hu FB. Dietary modulation of endothelial function: implications for cardiovascular disease. Am J Clin Nutr 2001; 73(4):673–686.
11. Aminbakhsh A, Mancini J. Chronic antioxidant use and changes in endothelial dysfunction: a review of clinical investigations. Can J Cardiol 1999; 15:895–903.
12. McCord JM, Fridovich I. Superoxide dismutase: an enzymatic function for erythrocuprein (hemocuprein). J Biol Chem 1969; 244:6049–6055.
13. Aebi H. Catalase. In: Bergmeyer HU ed. Methods of Enzymatic Analyses. New York: Academic Press, 1974:673–683.
14. Ursini F, Maiorino M, Brigelius-Flohe R, Aumann KD, Roveri A, Schomburg D, Flohe L. Diversity of glutathione peroxidases. Methods Enzymol 1995; 252:38–53.
15. Mates JM, Perez-Gomez C, Nunez de Castro I. Antioxidant enzymes and human diseases. Clin Biochem 1999; 32:595–603.
16. Verlangieri AJ, Bush MJ. Effects of d-alpha-tocopherol supplementation on experimentally induced primate atherosclerosis. J Am Coll Nutr 1992; 11:131–138.
17. Stocker R, Bowry VW, Frei B. Ubiquinol-10 protect human low-density lipoprotein more efficiently against lipid peroxidation than does alpha-tocopherol. Proc Natl Acad Sci USA 1991; 88:1646–1650.
18. Esterbauer H, Puhl H, Dieber-Rotheneder M, Waeg G, Rabl H. Effect of antioxidants on oxidative modification of LDL. Ann Med 1991; 23:573–581.
19. Rimm EB, Stampfer MJ, Ascherio A, Giovannucci E, Colditz GA, Willett WC. Vitamin E consumption and the risk of coronary heart disease in men. N Engl J Med 1993; 328:1450–1456.
20. Stampfer MJ, Hennekens CH, Manson JE, Colditz GA, Willett WC. Vitamin E consumption and the risk of coronary heart disease in women. N Engl J Med 1993; 328:1444–1449.

21. Enstrom JE, Kanim LE, Klein MA. Vitamin C intake and mortality among a sample of the United States population. Epidemiology 1992; 3:194–202.
22. Tavani A, Negri E, D'Avanzo B, Vecchia CL. Beta-carotene intake and risk of nonfatal acute myocardial infarction in women. Eur J Epidemiol 1997; 13:631–637.
23. Gaziano JM, Manson JE, Branch LG, Colditz GA, Willett WC, Buring JE. A prospective study of consumption of carotenoids in fruits and vegetables and decreased cardiovascular mortality in the elderly. Ann Epidemiol 1995; 5:255–260.
24. Kritchevsky SB, Tell GS, Shimakawa T, Dennis B, Li R, Kohlmeier L, Steere E, Heiss G. Provitamin A carotenoid intake and carotid artery plaques: the atherosclerosis risk in communities study. Am J Clin Nutr 1998; 68:726–733.
25. Kushi LH, Folsom AR, Prineas RJ, Mink PJ, Wu Y, Bostick RM. Dietary antioxidant vitamins and death from coronary heart disease in postmenopausal women. N Engl J Med 1996; 334:1156–1162.
26. Wattanapitayakul SK, Bauer JA. Oxidative pathways in cardiovascular disease: roles, mechanisms, and therapeutic implications. Pharmacol Ther 2001; 89(2):187–206.
27. Stephens NG, Parsons A, Schofield PM, Kelly F, Cheeseman K, Mitchinson MJ. Randomised controlled trial of vitamin E in patients with coronary disease: Cambridge Heart Antioxidant Study (CHAOS). Lancet 1996; 347:781–786.
28. DeMaio SJ, King SB, Lembo NJ, Roubin GS, Hearn JA, Bhagavan HN, Sgoutas DS. Vitamin E supplementation, plasma lipids and incidence of restenosis after percutaneous transluminal coronary angioplasty (PTCA). J Am Coll Nutr 1992; 11:68–73.
29. Laura AY, Aaron RF, Lawrence HK. Intake of antioxidant vitamins and risk of death form stroke in postmenopausal women. Am J Clin Nutr 2000; 72:476–483.
30. Yusuf S, Sleight P, Pogue J, Bosch J, Davies R, Dagenials G. Effects of an angiotensin-converting-enzyme inhibitor, rampipril, on cardiovascular events in high-risk patients. The Heart Outcomes Prevention Evaluation Study Investigators. N Engl J Med 2000; 342:145–153.
31. Omenn GS, Goodman GE, Thornquist MD, Balmes J, Cullen MR, Blass A, Keogh JP, Meyskens FL, Valanis B, Williams JH, Barnhart S, Hammar S. Effects of a combination of beta carotene and vitamin A on lung cancer and cardiovascular disease. N Engl J Med 1996; 334:1150–1155.
32. Henneckens CH, Buring JE, Manson JE, Stampfer M, Rosner B, Cook NR, Belanger C, LaMotte F, Baziano JM, Ridker PM, Willett W, Peto R. Lack of effect of long-term supplementation with beta carotene on the incidence of malignant neoplasms and cardiovascular disease. N Engl J Med 1996; 334:1145–1149.
33. Lee IM, Cook NR, Manson JE, Buring JE, Hennekens CH. Beta-carotene supplementation and incidence of cancer and cardiovascular disease: the Women's Health Study. J Natl Cancer Inst 1999; 91:2102–2106.
34. Rimm EB, Stampfer MJ, Ascherio A. Vitamin E consumption and the risk of coronary heart disease in men. N Engl J Med 1993; 328:1450–1456.
35. Azen SP, Qian D, Mack WJ, Sevanian A, Selzer RH, Liu CR, Liu CH, Hodis HN. Effect of supplementary antioxidant vitamin intake on carotid arterial wall intima-media thickness in a controlled clinical trial of cholesterol lowering. Circulation 1996; 94:2369–2372.
36. Bolto-Smith C, Woodward M, Tunstall-Pedoe H. The Scottish Heart Health Study. Dietary intake by food frequency questionnaire and odds ratios for coronary heart disease risk. II. The antioxidant vitamins and fibre. Eur J Clin Nutr 1992; 46(2):85–93.
37. The Alpha-Tocopherol, Beta-Carotene Cancer Prevention Study Group. The effect of vitamin E and beta-carotene on the incidence of lung cancer and other cancers in male smokers. N Engl J Med 1994; 330:1029–1053.
38. Tardif JC, Cote G, Lesperance J, Bourassa M, Lambert J, Doucet S, Bilodeau L, Nattel S, de Guise P. Probucol and multivitamins in the prevention of restenosis after coronary angioplasty. Multivitamins and Probucol Study Group. N Engl J Med 1997; 337(6):365–372.

39. Brown ML. Present Knowledge in Nutrition. 7th ed. Washington DC: International Life Sciences Institute–Nutrition Foundation, 1996.
40. Weisburger JH. Nutritional approach to cancer prevention with emphasis on vitamins, antioxidants, and carotenoids. Am J Clin Nutr 1991; 53(1 suppl):226S–237S.
41. Krauss RM, Eckel RH, Howard B, Appel LJ, Daniels SR, Deckelbaum RJ, Erdman JW Jr, Kris-Etherton P, Goldberg IJ, Kotchen TA, Lichtenstein AH, Mitch WE, Mullis R, Robinson K, Wylie-Rosett J, St Jeor S, Suttie J, Tribble DL, Bazzarre TL. AHA Dietary Guidelines: revision 2000: A statement for healthcare professionals from the Nutrition Committee of the American Heart Association. Stroke 2000; 31(11):2751–2766.

13

Nutrients and Treatment of Heart Disease in AIDS

Ramón Tomás Sepulveda and Ronald Ross Watson
University of Arizona, Tucson, Arizona, U.S.A.

Human immunodeficiency virus (HIV) infections are a major health threat to populations worldwide. For those burdened with acquired immunodeficiency syndrome (AIDS) due to HIV infection, damage to many organs can occur, including the heart. Novel therapies available that combat the retroviral infection keep the disease at an apparent stalemate; however, malnutrition and wasting are becoming central factors in the care of long-term survivors. The function of the immune system is tightly related the nutritional status of the host and is of paramount importance in AIDS patients.

Micronutrient supplementation in conjunction with antiretroviral therapy can extend and improve the quality and quantity of life in patients infected with HIV as well as in those living with AIDS.

Malnutrition affects the status of the immune system and conditions the host to pathogenic diseases. For HIV-positive individuals, a well-balanced diet is essential. Nutritional supplementation is helpful in treating nutritional deficiencies and immunosuppression in AIDS (1). Its been shown that HIV-infected individuals present selenium and vitamin E deficiencies and that supplementation with both antioxidants retards the progression of the immunodeficiency (1–4). Preliminary data are encouraging and supplementation treatment of HIV/AIDS patients should be considered (5).

Our intent in this chapter is to present data from diverse areas of research that establish a link between the effects of alcohol consumption on heart function and micronutrient deficiencies and the effectiveness of antioxidant supplementation in ameliorating cardiovascular diseases in HIV/AIDS patients.

MICRONUTRIENT DEFICIENCY AND AIDS

Recent studies with HIV-infected patients indicate that micronutrients play a role in the progression of HIV disease. Some of the more promising nutrients are discussed here.

Vitamins

Vitamin A participates in many normal processes, including immunity, reproduction, growth, and vision (6–8).

In AIDS patients, mother-to-child transmissio of HIV is inversely correlated with vitamin A levels (9–11), and up to 50% of AIDS individuals are vitamin A–deficient before death (9). Although vitamin A treatment in AIDS patients improves the immune system, dietary supplementation is a better preventive measure (12).

Of importance is that mothers with low levels of the vitamin lost their infants within 1 year (13). Vitamin A deficiency seems to play a crucial role in vertical transmission of HIV, influencing several parameters: impairment of the immune response in both mother and child and increased HIV viral load in breast milk and blood (1,14). Possible causes of low serum vitamin A levels are (1) decreased dietary intake (15), (2) poor gastrointestinal absorption (16), (3) high urinary losses, (4) impaired hepatic protein synthesis (17,18), and (5) increased nutritional demands due to chronic infection.

Depending on the stage and chronicity of the disease, vitamin supplementation can be affected due to malabsorption related to mucosal gut damage (19–21).

Although there is evidence the vitamin A supplementation improves the performance of the immune system (22–25), some studies have concluded otherwise (26,27). Based on the experimental data of more then a decade of research, the effectiveness of vitamin A supplementation in AIDS seems to be determined by (1) treatment in the early stages of the diseases (2) absorption at the gut level, (3) dose of vitamin A, and (4) duration of treatment.

Another vitamin that has been used as a preventive treatment in individuals who might be infected with HIV is vitamin B_6. It has been shown that vitamin B_6 [as pyridoxal 5′-phosphtate (PLP)] binds to CD4 soluble and surface molecules and therefore prevents viral attachment to the cell (28).

Pyridoxine (vitamin B_6) is essential for the proper metabolism of various neurotransmitters (29–31). Shor-Posner et al. examined vitamin B_6 status and psychological distress in HIV-infected individuals. Vitamin B_6 levels were significantly lower in AIDS patients with symptoms of depression, and normalization of vitamin B_6 status ameliorated their psychological distress (32). In AIDS patients under antiretroviral therapy, a condition called serotinin syndrome develops, inducing a state of depression. It is possible that vitamin B_6 promotes the degradation of the excess of serotonin caused by the treatment.

Vitamin B_6 deficiency influences both the humoral immune response, specifically immunoglobulins G and E, as well as the cellular immune response diminishing lymphocyte proliferation, reduced CD4 cell counts, and lowered NK cell activity, although excess supplementation can have the same negative effects, suppressing not only antibody production but also interleukin-2 (IL-2) and lymphocyte proliferation (33).

Partial restoration of NK cell activity can be obtained by vitamin B_{12} supplementation after only 14 days of treatment in patients suffering from anemia due to its deficiency (34).

Baum et al. measured plasma levels of vitamin B_{12} and CD4+ T-cell counts in HIV patients; they observed that as the HIV infection progressed, the vitamin B_{12} levels diminished, correlating with the T-cell counts (35).

Although vitamin B_{12} supplementation in AIDS patients who develop neurological diseases does not improve their condition, supplementation should still be encouraged for HIV-infected pregnant women, since vitamin B_{12} deficiency as been related to abnormalities of fetal nervous system development (36,37).

Vitamin B_{12} deficiency can negatively influence NK cell activity as well as CD4/CD8 lymphocyte ratio, all essential in responding against secondary infections such as varicella, cytomegalovirus, tuberculosis, and syphilis, which affect the central nervous system (38).

There is a strong correlation between the degree of oxidative stress and the progression to AIDS once an individual has been diagnosed HIV-positive (33).

In part due to digestive complications as well as malnutrition, AIDS patients present lower levels of antioxidants. In general, one of the antioxidant deficiencies most studied in regard to these diseases has been vitamin E. Vitamin E deficiencies have been seen in patients that are susceptible to opportunistic infections and the development of tumors (39).

In both human and murine retroviral infections, the protective Th1 response changes to an aberrant Th2 response, promoting progression to AIDS (40). In a study by Wang et al., where vitamin E supplements of up to 15 times the normal levels were given to mice with AIDS, non-vitamin E–treated mice with AIDS presented an exacerbated Th2 response of IL-4, -5, and -6, which ranged from 50 to 100% above normal levels. Mice with murine AIDS (MAIDS) that were treated with vitamin E showed a reduced Th2 cytokine response, ranging between 40 and 60% higher when compared to uninfected, untreated controls. Total immunomodulation of the Th2 response in mice with MAIDS was achieved when the immunodeficient animals were treated with interferon gamma (IFN-γ) and vitamin E (41). Similar effects of vitamin E supplementation on the Th2 response have been seen in different human and animal conditions (42,43).

In AIDS, CD4+ T-cell apoptosis is accentuated due to increased oxidative stress and lower levels of bcl-2 protein, an antiapoptotic/antioxidative molecules (44–51). The use of antioxidant supplementation in combination with antiviral therapy should improve the prognosis of AIDS or HIV infected patients.

There are several nonantioxidant effects of alpha-tocopherol: lowering of pro-inflammatory cytokines (IL-1β) as well as tumor necrosis factor alpha (TNF-α) (52); reduction of superoxide and lipid oxidation, and inhibition of monocyte–endothelial cell interaction by way of lowering the expression of CD11b and VLA-4 (53).

Vitamin E deficiency has been associated with atherosclerosis, diabetes, and progression of some types of cancers (53). Recently, vitamin E succinate has been shown to induce human breast cancer dormancy via inhibition of vascular endothelial growth factor (VEGF) gene expression (54).

In a study done by Liang et al. of C57BL/6 mice infected with LP-BM5 retrovirus, treatment with human TCR V-β 8.1 peptide, a CDR1 16-mer peptide, largely prevented the retrovirus-induced reduction in B- and T-cell proliferation and Th1 cytokines, including IL-2 and IFN-γ secretion (55). It also suppressed the excessive production of Th2 cytokine IL-6 and IL-10 stimulated by retroviral-infection. Retroviral infection in mice promotes a lower Th1/Th2 cytokine ratio and induces hepatic and cardiac vitamin E deficiency. Treatment with TCR peptide 2 to 4 weeks after retroviral infection maintained production of IL-2 and prevented retrovirus-induced elevated production of IL-6 by splenocytes in vitro. It also maintained low levels of hepatic lipid peroxides and kept loss of hepatic vitamin E to a minimum (56). Treatment with TCR peptide could be important in the prevention of the T-cell immune dysfunction and vitamin E deficiency seen in HIV-infected individuals.

Minerals

In AIDS, the concentration of micronutrients like copper (Cu) and zinc (Zn) normalizes after supplementation, yet the amounts required to maintain normal serum concentrations suggest a persistent intracellular deficiency, possibly correlating to poor absorption, low intake, vomiting, diarrhea, or even sequestration by HIV. In the case of HIV disease, Cu can works as a passive inhibitor by blocking the intracellular activation HIV protease (57,58).

Zinc is associated with more than 200 enzymatic systems. It is involved in the synthesis of proteins, nucleic acids, hormone secretion, and brain function. Zn also protects against the formation of free radical reactive oxygen species (ROS) by Cu-Zn superoxide dismutases (59). Zn deficiency can promote an unbalanced Th1:Th2 response by favoring a humoral Th2-type response, which is less effective against viral infections (58,59).

Nitric oxide, one of the factors of oxidative stress, appears to be able to free Zn from metallothioneine, a molecule used by the cells to store metal ions such as Zn and Cu. Moreover, alcohol consumption, a common problem in HIV sufferers, seem to accentuate the loss of magnesium (Mg), which is essential for the conduction of nerve impulses and in muscle and heart contraction (61).

Another micronutrient that is being recognize as an essential component of the immune system is selenium (Se). Se deficiency is associated with glutathione peroxidase (GPX) activity, cardiomyopathy, carcinogeneis, and immune dysfunction, including impaired phagocytic function, decreased numbers of CD4-lymphocyte cells, and AIDS (62). Se deficiency affects both the cellular and antibody mediated immune responses (3,63–65). Therefore Se plays an important role both in Th1 and Th2 responses. HIV-infected individuals have shown low levels of Se; supplementation with the micronutrient enhances T-cell function while reducing apoptosis (2). Se deficiency has been found to be associated with a nearly threefold higher likelihood of genital mucosal shedding of HIV-1–infected cells, suggesting that deficiency may increase the infectiousness of women with HIV-1 as well as mother-to-child transmission (66). The enzyme GPX uses Se as a cofactor; its deficiency decreases the enzymatic activity considerably.

GPX, a major antioxidant system that reduces the levels of free radicals, will also create an unfavorable environment for HIV replication and CD4-lymphocyte cell apoptosis.

Thus, as Se concentration decreases, it gives rise to an increase in oxidative stress, HIV replication, and CD4-lymphocyte cell death (33). Also, Se has been shown to inhibit reverse transcriptase activity, suggesting that supplementation in the early stages of HIV infection may retard the development of AIDS. Furthermore, HIV may carry several genes to encode selenoproteins, and one of these proteins may bind with DNA, repressing HIV viral transcription. This mechanism results in turning off HIV expression and thus slowing the viral proliferation (67).

In terms of cytokine regulation, Se supplementation will increase IL-2 while decreasing IL-8; the former will induce T-cell activation while a decrease in the latter has been associated with a good prognosis (2). A major drawback of Se supplementation is the degree of toxicity seen in animal models even at low doses. A dose 100 µg/day Se, which is in the safe intake range, is sufficient to restore normal plasma concentrations, improve oxidative stress, and decrease $beta_2$ microglobulin, all markers of a good prognosis in HIV infection (68,69).

Micronutrient Deficiency and Heart Disease

Se is one of the micronutrients that as been widely studied in heart disease in both human and animal studies.

Two of the major contributors to this field have been Beck and Levander (63,70–73), who have done groundbreaking work in establishing the relationship between Se deficiency and increased viral pathogenicity. Based on the observation that Se supplementation prevented the development of cardiomyopathy (Keshan's disease) in people living in certain regions of China and that the peak of the condition coincided with the season for transmission of enteroviruses, Beck and Levander started a series of experiments using a mouse model, showing that mice, fed a diet deficient in Se were more susceptible to myocarditis due to coxsackievirus B3 (an enterovirus), while control mice fed a diet adequate in Se developed mild or no cardiopathology. Moreover, when an amyocarditic strain of coxsackievirus B3 was used to infect Se-deficient mice, it was found that an avirulent virus can acquire virulence as a result of passage through an Se-deficient host.

Patients with AIDS also show a marked deficiency in Se (74), which is also seen in MAIDS (75). Our studies have shown that Se supplementation of retrovirally induced immunodeficiency will promote a balanced Th1/Th2 response sufficient to protect the host against a secondary viral infection, thus providing a longer life span and better quality of life (76).

CONCLUSIONS

Oxidative stress is being recognized more and more as a key element in the pathogenesis of HIV disease. Both animal and human research support the important role that micronutrients play in establishing a more efficient and balanced immune system. Micronutrient deficiency influences the status of the immune system, accentuating and accelerating the immunodeficient conditions that HIV promotes and opens the window for secondary infections. Supplementation with antioxidants offers a safe and economic treatment to slow the progression of HIV infection.

Multimicronutrient supplementation together with antiretroviral therapy is expected to give better results. Caution must be exercised when antioxidant supplementation is considered because of the toxicity that some micronutrients will have at high levels. Consultation with a medical practitioner should always be considered when any other therapy is being taken (73) and becomes paramount when micronutrients are used in combination with allopathic medication (77). It is also important for physicians to acknowledge the importance of a basic balanced diet as the essential groundwork underlying any additional supplementation or drug treatment. We have come a long way in understanding how antioxidants are related to AIDS, but we still need to do more research to decipher the optimal conditions in which micronutrients can help modulate or immunopotentiate the body's defenses as well as how the host's nutritional status influences the virulence of some pathogens.

REFERENCES

1. Tang AM, Smit E. Selected vitamins in HIV infection: a review. AIDS Patient Care STDs 1998; 12:263–273.
2. Baum MK, Miguez-Burbano MJ, Campa A, Shor-Posner G. Selenium and interleukins in persons infected with human immunodeficiency virus type 1. J Infect Dis 2000; 182: S69–S73.
3. Swain BK, Johri TS, Majumdar S. Effect of supplementation of vitamin E, selenium and their different combinations on the performance and immune response of broilers. Br Poultry Sci 2000; 41:287–292.
4. Batterham M, Gold J, Naidoo D, Lux O, Sadler S, Bridle S, Ewing M, Oliver C. A preliminary open label dose comparison using an antioxidant regimen to determinine the effect on viral load and oxidative stress in men with HIV/AIDS. Eur J Clin Nutr 2001; 55:107–114.
5. Watson RR. Nutrients, Foods for AIDS. Boca Raton, FL: CRC Press, 1997.
6. Semba RD. Vitamin A, immunity, and infection. Clin Infect Dis 1994; 19:489–499.
7. Linney E. Retinoic acid receptors: transcription factors modulating gene regulation, development, and differentiation. Curr Top Dev Biol 1992; 27:309–350.
8. Maciaszek JW, Coniglio SJ, Talmage DD, Viglianti G. Retinoid-induced repression of human immunodeficiency virus type 1 core promoter activity inhibits virus replication. J Virol 1998; 72:5862–5869.
9. Semba RD, Caiaffa WT, Graham NM, Cohn S, Vlahov D. Vitamin A deficiency and wasting as predictors of mortality in human immunodeficiency virus-infected injection drug users. J Infect Dis 1995; 171:1196–1202.
10. Semba RD. Overview of the potential role of vitamin A in mother-to-child transmission of HIV-1. Acta Paediatr Suppl 1997; 421:107–112.
11. Greenberg BL, Semba Rd, Vink PE, et al. Vitamin A deficiency and maternal-infant transmissions of HIV in two metropolitan areas in the United States. AIDS 1997; 11:325–332.
12. Semba RD, Lyles CM, Margolick JB, Caiaffa WT, Farzadegan H, Cohn S, Vlahov D. Vitamin A supplementation and human immunodeficiency virus load in injection drug users. J Infect Dis 1998; 177:611–616.
13. Nduati RW, John GC, Richardson BA, et al. Human immunodeficiency virus type 1-infected cells in breast milk: association with immunosuppression and vitamin A deficiency. J Infect Dis 1995; 172:1461–1468.
14. Thorne C, Newell ML. Epidemiology of HIV infection in newborn. Early Hum Dev 2000; 58:1–16.
15. Silveira SA, Figueiredo JF, Jordao Junior A, de Unamuno MD, Rodrigues MdeL, Vannucchi H. Malnutrition and hypovitaminosis A in AIDS patients. Rev Soc Bras Med Trop 1999; 32:119–124.
16. Purvin V. Through a shade darkly. Surv Ophthalmol 1999; 43:335–340.
17. Ullrich R, Zeitz M, Heise W. Small intestinal structure and function in patients infected with HIV: evidence for HIV-induced enteropathy. Ann Intern Med 1989; 111:15–21.

18. Russell RM. The vitamin A spectrum: from deficiency to toxicity. Am J Clin Nutr 2000; 71:878–884.

19. Kelly P, Musonda R, Kafwembe E, Kaetano L, Keane E, Farthing M. Micronutritent supplementation in AIDS diarrhoea-wasting syndrome in Zambia: a randomized controlled trial. AIDS 1999; 13:495–500.

20. Kelly P, Musuku J, Kafwembe E, Libby G, Zulu I, Murphy J, Farthing MJ. Impaired bioavailability of vitamin A in adults and children with persistent diarrhoea in Zambia. Aliment Pharmacol Ther 2001; 15:973–979.

21. Jimenez-Exposito MJ, Garcia-Lorda P, Alonso-Villaverde C, de Virgala CM, Sola R, Masana L. Effect of malabsorption on nutritional status and resting energy expenditure in HIV-infected patients. AIDS 1998; 12:1965–1972.

22. Watson RR, Yahya MD, Darban HR, Prabhala RH. Enhanced survival by vitamin A supplementation during a retrovirus infection causing murine AIDS. Life Sci 1988; 43: 13–18.

23. Semba RD, Muhilal, Ward BJ, Friggin DE, Scott AL, Natadisastra G, West KP Jr, Sommer A. Abnormal T-cell subset proportions in vitamin A–deficient children. Lancet 1993; 341:5–8.

24. Rousseau E, Davison AJ, Dunn B. Protection by beta-carotene and related compounds against oxygen-mediated cytotoxicity and genotoxicity. Free Radic Biol Med 1992; 12: 407–433.

25. Fawzi WW, Mbsise RL, Hertzmark E, Fataki MR, Herrera MG, Ndossi G, Spiegelman D. A randomized trial of vitamin A supplements in relation to mortality among human immunodeficiency virus–infected and uninfected children in Tanzania. Pediatr Infect Dis J 1999; 18:127–133.

26. Pillay K, Coutsoudis A, York D, Kuhn L, Coovadia HM. Cell-free virus in breast milk of HIV-1-seropositive women. J AIDS 2000; 24(4):330–336.

27. Benn CS, Lisse IM, Bale C, Michaelsen KF, Olsen J, Hedegaard K, Aaby P. No strong long-term effect of vitamin A supplementation in infancy on CD4 and CD8 T-cell subsets. A community study from Guinea-Bissau, West Africa. Ann Trop Paediatr 2000; 20(4):259–264.

28. Salhany JM, Schopfer LM. Pyridoxal 5'-phosphate binds specifically to soluble CD4 protein, the HIV-1 receptor. Implications for AIDS therapy. J Biol Chem 1993; 268:7643–7645.

29. De Silva KE, Le Flore DB, Marston BJ, Rimland D. Serotonin syndrome in HIV-infected individuals receiving antiretroviral therapy and fluoxetine. AIDS 2001; 15:1281–1285.

30. Miodownik C, Lerner V, Cohen H, Kotler M. Serum vitamin B6 in schizophrenic and schizoaffective patients with and without tardive dyskinesia. Clin Neuropharmacol 2000; 23:212–215.

31. Shiloh R, Weizman A, Weizer N, Dorfman-Etrog P, Munitz H. Antidepressive effect of pyridoxine (vitamin B6) in neuroleptic-treated schizophrenic patients with co-morbid minor depression—preliminary open-label trial. Harefuah 2001; 140:369–373.

32. Shor-Posner G, Feaster D, Blaney NT, Rocca H, Mantero-Atienza E, Szapocznik J, Eisdorfer C, Goodkin K, Baum MK. Impact of vitamin B6 status on psychological distress in a longitudinal study of HIV infection. Int J Psychiatr Med 1994; 24:209–222.

33. Lee J, Yoshi K, Watson RR. Nutritional deficiencies in AIDS patients: a treatment opportunity. In: Standish LJ, Calabrese C, Galantino ML, eds. AIDS and Alternative Medicine. Kenmore, WA: Bastyr Research, 2001:56–70.

34. Tamura J, Kubota K, Murakami H, Sawamura M, Matsushima R, Tamura T, Saitoh T. Immunomodulation by vitamin B12: augmentation of CD8 + T lymphocytes and natural killer (NK) cell activity in vitamin B12–deficient patients by methyl-B12 treatment. Clin Exp Immunol 1999; 116:28–32.

35. Baum MK, Shor-Posner G, Lu Y, et al. Micronutrients and HIV-1 disease progression. AIDS 1995; 9:1051–1056.

36. Di Rocco A, Simpson DM. AIDS-associated vacuolar myelopathy. AIDS patient Care STDs 1998; 12:457–461.
37. Frenkel EP, Yardley DA. Clinical and laboratory features and sequelea of deficiency of folic acid (folate) and vitamin B12 (cobalamin) in pregnancy and gynecology. Hematol Oncol Clin North Am 2000; 14:1079–1100.
38. Brannagan TH. Retroviral-associated vasculitis of the nervous system. Neurol Clin 1997; 15:927–944.
39. Moriguchi S, Muraga M. Vitamin E and immunity. Vitam Horm 2000; 59:304–306.
40. Clerici M, Shearer GM. A Th1 → Th2 switch is a critical step in the etiology of HIV infection. Immunol Today 1993; 14:107–111.
41. Wang JY, Liang B, Watson RR. Vitamin E supplementation with interferon-γ administration retards immune dysfunction during murine retrovirus infection. J Leuk Biol 1995; 58:698–703.
42. Fogarty A, Lewis S, Weiss S, Briton J. Dietary vitamin E, IgE concentrations, and atopy. Lancet 2000; 356:1573–1574.
43. Hann SN, Wu D, Ha WK, Beharka A, Smith DE, Bender BS, Meydani SN. Vitamin E supplementation increases T helper 1 cytokine production in old mice infected with influenza virus. Immunology 2000; 100:487–493.
44. Elbim C, Pillet S, Prevost MH, Preira A, Girard PM, Rogine N, Hakim J, Israel N, Gougerot-Pocidalo MA. The role of phagocytes in HIV-related oxidative stress. J Clin Virol 2001; 20:99–109.
45. Vouldoukis I, Sivan V, Vozenin MC, Kamate C, Calenda A, Mazier D, Dugas B. Fc-receptor-mediated intracellular delivery of Cu/Zn-superoxide dismutase (SOD1) protects against redox-induced apoptosis through a nitric oxide dependent mechanism. Mol Med 2000; 6:1042–1053.
46. Aoki M, Nata T, Morishita R, Matsushita H, Nakagami H, Yamamoto K, Yamazaki K, Nakabayashi M, Ogihara T, Kaneda Y. Endothelial apoptosis induced by oxidative stress through activation of NF-kappaB: antiapoptotic effect of antioxidant agents on endothelial cells. Hypertension 2001; 38:48–55.
47. Torre D, ZeroliC C, Martegani R, Pugliese A, Basilico C, Speranza F. Levels of the bcl-2 protein, fibronectin and alpha(5)beta(1) fibronectin receptor in HIV-1–infected patients with Kaposi's sarcoma. Microbes Infect 2000; 2:1831–1833.
48. Airo P, Torti C, Uccelli MC, Malacarne F, Palvarini L, Carosi G, Castelli F. Naïve CD+ T lymphocytes express high levels of Bcl-2 after highly active antiretroviral therapy for HIV infection. AIDS Res Hum Retrovir 2000; 16:1805–1807.
49. Kline K, Yu W, Sanders BG. Vitamin E: mechanisms of action as tumor cell growth inhibitors. J Nutr 2001; 131:161S–163S.
50. Muller F, Svardal AM, Norday I, Berge RK, Aukrust P, Froland SS. Virological and immunological effects of antioxidant treatment in patients with HIV infection. Eur J Clin Invest 2000; 30:905–914.
51. Perl A, Banki K. Genetic metabolic control of the mitochondrial transmembrane potential and reactive oxygen intermediate production in HIV disease. Antioxid Redox Sign 2000; 2:551–573.
52. Devaraj S, Jiala I. Alpha-tocopherol decreases interleukin-1 beta release from activated human monocytes by inhibition of 5-lipoxygenase. Arterioscler Thromb Vasc Biol 1999; 19:1125–1133.
53. Azzi A, Stoker A. Vitamin E: non-antioxidant roles. Progr Lipid Res 2000; 39:231–255.
54. Malafa MP, Neitzel LT. Vitamin E succinate promotes breast cancer tumor dormancy. J Surg Res 2000; 93:163–170.
55. Liang B, Ardestani S, Watson RR, et al. T-cell receptor dose and the time of treatment during murine retrovirus infection for maintenance of immune function. Immunology 1996; 87:198–204.

56. Liang B, Eskelson C, Watson RR, et al. Vitamin E deficiency and immune dysfunction in retrovirus-infected C57BL/6 mice are prevented by T-cell receptor peptide treatment. J Nutr 1996; 126:1389–1397.

57. Sprietsma JE. Cysteine (GSH) and zinc and copper ions together are effective, natural intracellular inhibitors of (AIDS) viruses. Med Hypoth 1999; 6:529–538.

58. Sprietsma JE. Modern diets and diseases: NO-Zn balance. Under Th1, zinc and nitrogen monoxide (NO) collectively protect against viruses, AIDS, autoimmunity, diabetes, allergies, asthma, infectious diseases, atherosclerosis and cancer. Med Hypoth 1999; 53: 6–16.

59. Konin D, Keul J, Northoff H, Halle M, Berg A. Effect of 6-week nutritional intervention with enzymatic yeast cells and antioxidants on exercise stress and antioxidant status (German). Wien Med Wochenschr 1999; 149:13–18.

60. Lai H, Lai S, Shor-Posner G. Plasma zinc, copper, copper:zinc ratio, and survival in a cohort of HIV-1-infected homosexual men. J AIDS 2001; 27:56–62.

61. Bogden JD, Kemp FW, Han S, Li W, Bruening K, Denny T, Oleske JM, Lloyd J, Baker H, Perez G, Kloser P, Skurnick J, Louria DB. Status of selected nutrients and progression of human immunodeficiency virus type 1 infection. Am J Clin Nutr 2000; 72:809–815.

62. Badmaev V, Majeed M, Passwater RA. Selenium: a quest for better understanding. Alt Ther Health Med 1996; 2:59–62, 65–67.

63. Beck MA, Levander OA. Host nutritional status and its effect on a viral pathogen. J Infect Dis 2000; 182:S93–S96.

64. Forceville X, Vitoux D, Gauzit R, Combes A, Lahilaire P, Chappuis P. Selenium, systemic immune response syndrome, sepsis, and outcome in critically ill patients. Crit Care Med 1998; 26:1536–1544.

65. Hegazy SM, Adachi Y. Comparison of the effects of dietary selenium, zinc, and selenium and zinc supplementation on growth and immune response beween chick groups that were inoculated with *Salmonella* and aflatoxin or *Salmonella*. Poultry Sci 2000; 79:331–335.

66. Baeten JM, Mostad SB, Hughes MP. Selenium deficiency is associated with shedding of HIV-1-infected cells in the female genital tract. J AIDS 2001; 26:360–364.

67. Taylor EW, Ramanathan CS, Jalluri RK, et al. A basis for new approaches to the chemotherapy of AIDS: novel genes in HIV-1 potentially encode selenoproteins expressed by ribosomal frameshifting and termination suppression. J Med Chem 1994; 37:2637–2654.

68. Schrauzer GN, Sacher J. Selenium in the maintenance and therapy of HIV-infected patients. Chem Biol Interact 1994; 91:199–205.

69. Hori K, Hatfield D, Lee BJ, et al. Selenium supplementation suppresses tumor necrosis factor alpha-induced HIV-1 replication in vitro. AIDS Res Hum Retrovir 1997; 13:1325–1332.

70. Beck MA, Levander OA. Dietary oxidative stress and the potentiation of viral infection. Annu Rev Nutr 1998; 18:93–116.

71. Beck MA, Levander OA. Effects of nutritional antioxidants and other dietary constituents on coxsackievirus-induced myocarditis. Curr Top Microbiol Immunol 1997; 223:81–96.

72. Levander OA, Beck MA. Interacting nutritional and infectious etiologies of Keshan disease. Insights from coxsackie virus B–induced myocarditis in mice deficient in selenium or vitamin E. Biol Trace Elem Res 1997; 56(1):5–21.

73. Snodgrass E, Rumack BH, Sullivan JB Jr, Peterson RG, Chase HP, Cotton EK, Sokol R. Selenium: Childhood poisoning and cystic fibrosis. Clin Toxicol 1981; 18:211–220.

74. Constans J, Conri C, Sergeant C. Selenium and HIV infection. Nutrition 1999; 15:719–720.

75. Chen C, Zhou J, Xu H, Jiang Y, Zhu G. Effect of selenium supplementation on mice infected with LP-BM5 MuLV, a murine AIDS model. Biol Trace Elem Res 1997; 59:187–193.

76. Sepulveda RT, Watson RR. Selenium supplementation decreases coxsackievirus heart disease during murine AIDS. Cardiotoxicology 2002; 4:25–28.

77. Scevola D, Di Matteo A, Uberti F, Minoia G, Poletti F, Faga A. AIDS reader 2000; 10:365–369.

14

Will Soy Protein Help HIV Patients with Cardiovascular Risk?

Kelly J. Blackstock
Colorado State University, Fort Collins, Colorado, U.S.A.

CARDIOVASCULAR PATHOLOGY AND HIV

Recent developments in HIV treatments have allowed for decreased morbidity in infected patients. Because of these patients' longer survival, late-stage manifestations will be seen, including HIV-related cardiac diseases. This article postulates that the addition of soy protein to the diets of HIV-infected patients has cardioprotective effects. The most common pathology of infected individuals includes pericardial effusion, myocarditis, cardiomyopathy, and pulmonary hypertension (1). With the exception of the last, these conditions result from viral and bacterial infection and are not likely altered with dietary manipulation (2). For that reason the focus here remains on pulmonary hypertension along with other substantiated risk factors for cardiovascular disease (CVD).

Cardiopathology related to HIV infection is described in multiple autopsy and echocardiographic reports. Although the prevalence is uncertain, it was predicted as far back as 1990 that between 2800 to 5000 HIV patients would develop CVD per year (2). The most common and severe metabolic component is hyperlipidemia, most often associated with elevated total cholesterol and triglycerides (3). Another major pathophysiological component found at autopsy is premature coronary atherosclerosis (1,3). Nonbacterial thrombotic endocarditis has also been described in AIDS patients and has similar ischemic effects, causing coronary artery blockage by embolism. As noted earlier, pulmonary hypertension is a significant risk factor, affecting 1 of every 200 HIV patients, as opposed to 1 out of 200,000 in the general population (1). In a review article by Pantel et al. (2), several reports were cited suggesting a positive association between HIV infection and primary pulmonary hypertension. This evidence has raised concern that HIV patients may exhibit an increase in incidence of CVD similar to that of syndrome X (4). For that reason, strategies to prevent cardiac disease are warranted.

The pathogenesis of HIV-related CVD is unclear. Due to the lack of genetic evidence in pulmonary endothelial cells by immunochemistry, DNA hybridization, and polymerase chain reaction, it is thought that the condition is not a result of direct infection but rather due to an aspect of some autoimmune process (1,2). A recent focus for blame has been the new antiretroviral agents called protease inhibitors (PIs). These drugs act to inhibit the protease necessary for the formation and maturation of infectious HIV virons (3). Although PIs have had a positive impact on morbidity, significant adverse metabolic effects have been increasingly recognized, including exacerbation of hyperlipidemia, hyperglycemia, and lipidystrophy (3,5). The PI ritonavir has been found to increase total cholesterol 30 to 40% and triglycerides (TG) 200 to 300% from baseline (3). A case study released at the 38th Interscience Conference on Antimicrobial Agents and Chemotherapy showed TG levels at 40 times the upper limit of normal due to antiretroviral treatment (3). In a 5-year analysis of an HIV-infected population, PI use affected new-onset hyperglycemia, hypercholesterolemia, hypergriglyceridemia, and lipodystrophy positively by 5, 24, 19, and 13%, respectively. Atherosclerosis and atherothrombosis from PI-related dyslipidemia is also described (5). Whether these risk factors would directly translate into CVD is uncertain. Studies have been cited where PI use appeared to have no association with increased CVD rates when compared to controls (4). However, premature infarction has been noted (4).

BENEFITS OF SOY PROTEIN

The cardioprotective nature of soy protein was first hypothesized after cultural comparisons were made between rates of CVD and diet. Epidemiological data have shown that Asians, whose diets are primarily plant-based, have the lowest incidence of heart disease (6). On average, Asians consume 50 g of soy per day, as opposed to the 1 to 3 g in a typical American diet (7). It is argued that lower rates of CVD are indicative of improved lipid profiles. While the health advantages of a low intake of saturated fat are well documented (6,8), mounting evidence is proving that soy has benefits of its own.

Soybeans are the most common and significant source of isoflavones (6,7,9,10), containing between 0.2 and 4.2 mg/g dry weight (9). Isoflavones, along with lignans and coumestans, belong to a group of compounds called phytoestrogens (PEs). PEs are naturally occurring plant-based diphenolic compounds similar in structure to estradiol (6). It appears that they are the active cardioprotective components of soy. Meta-analysis has shown that isoflavone PEs have significant cholesterol-lowering effects (8). A study done by Anthony et al. reported that monkeys fed soy protein that included PEs (soy+) had lower total and low-density-lipoprotein (LDL) cholesterol and higher high-density-lipoprotein (HDL) cholesterol than monkeys fed either soy without PEs (soy-) or a casein/lactoalbumin mix. Atherosclerotic lesions were also less frequent in the soy+ group compared to the other two (7,9).

The effectiveness of PEs stems from their close structural similarity to endogenous estrogens, agents long known to decrease risk factors associated with CVD (6,9) (see Fig. 1). The aromatic ring and hydroxyl groups are key to binding to the estrogen receptor (ER) (6,10). Whether PEs would trigger identical responses is debatable, since binding affinity does not necessarily translate into biological action. It appears that PEs have both agonistic and antagonistic actions to estrogen. The antiestrogenic effects are perhaps due to competitive inhibition at the ER and the availability of natural circulating estrogens, but they are more likely explained by the recent discovery of a second subtype of ER, ER-β (6,10,11). The role of this

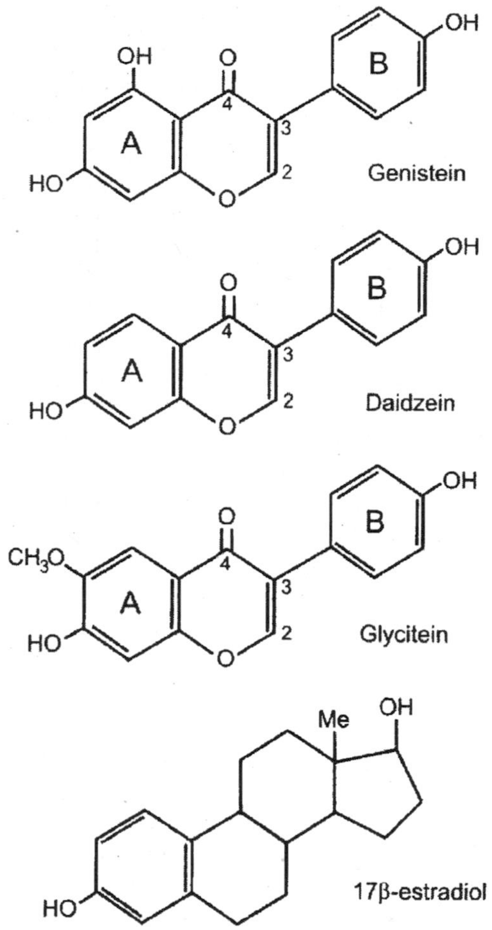

Figure 1 Chemical structural comparisons of estradiol-17β and genistein and daidzein, two prominent isoflavones.

receptor is still under investigation, though it is known to be expressed in non-reproductive tissues such as bone and vascular epithelium (11). Isoflavones are able to bind to both subtypes of receptors, but they have a 20-fold greater affinity for ER-β than for ER-α (11). The antiestrogenic effects of PEs allow for another potential benefit, given that endogenous estrogens have been known to induce endometrial hyperplasia and tumorigenesis (6,9,10,12). The ability of PEs to decrease the risk for CVD without increasing the risk for cancer could convince many that estrogen agonists such as PEs may be superior to conventional estrogens.

PLASMA LIPIDS

The majority of soy research is directed toward cholesterol modification, and the hypocholesterolemic effects of soy are well documented. Meta-analysis of 38 controlled trials concluded that soy protein rather than animal protein was responsible for decreasing total serum cholesterol, LDLs, and triglycerides, noting that 60 to 70% of the effects seen were accounted for by the PEs (8). Even when both animal and soy proteins were combined with a low intake of saturated fats, more potent cholesterol-lowering alterations were seen with soy (6). In a study comparing casein to soy with medium and high levels of isoflavones, only the soy groups displayed significant decreases in non-HDL cholesterol and increases in HDLs (6). The U.S. Food and Drug Administration (FDA) substantiated these health claims in 1999 and recommend that soy be added to a diet low in fat and cholesterol (13).

The extent that soy can reduce cholesterol is thought to be due to baseline concentrations (6,9,11). Moderately hypercholesterolemic individuals (259 to 333 mg/dL) and severely hypercholesterolemic (>335 mg/dL) who were ingesting soy protein are cited as having total cholesterol decreases of 7.4 and 19.6%, respectively (6). One study comparing a low-fat soy diet to a low-fat animal-protein diet showed no change in 24 normocholesterolemic men, while hyperlipoproteinemic subjects saw a 16% decrease of both total and LDL cholesterol (6). However, Wong et al. (14) found the hypocholesterolemic effects of soy protein to be independent of age, body weight, and pretreatment plasma lipid concentrations, noting significant differences in LDL levels in all groups. Discrepancies about whether or not benefits are universal might be due in part to dosage amounts. The FDA recommends 25 g of soy per day to attain desired lipid modifications (13). A study of hypercholester-olemic subjects ingesting 50 g of protein with different ratios of soy to casein found that 20 g of soy elicited lowering of LDLs, but only by 2.2% (15). Meta-analysis (8) claimed that 47 g of soy protein was necessary for a 12.9% drop in LDLs. This evidence suggests that individuals with a normal baseline cholesterol level would have to ingest greater amounts of soy to observe the same benefits seen in hyper-cholesterolemic individuals. Consideration must also be given to the type of soy protein utilized, since the isoflavone content of these products is highly variable (6,9,10). Research done strictly with isoflavones is as yet inconsistent, claiming significant reductions in cholesterol in subjects with normal cholesterol levels with dosages ranging from 45 to 129 mg of isoflavones per day.

The exact mechanisms behind soy's cholesterol-lowering effects have not been elucidated. Several hypotheses have been proposed; these include increased bile acid synthesis, increased apolipoprotein B, induction of a hypothyroid state, or increased estrogen receptor (ER) activity and suppressed hepatic metabolism—both known to clear cholesterol from the blood (6,9). Research suggests that PEs upregulate LDL receptors, thereby enhancing receptor activity and cholesterol clearance (16). Li-poprotein (a), an independent risk factor for CHD, is successfully depressed by estrogen treatment, so PEs could potentially have the same effect (10). Lignans may also alter cholesterol metabolism by inhibiting cholesterol-7α-hydroxylase, the rate-limiting enzyme in the formation of bile acids from cholesterol (10).

VASOREACTIVITY

Although research involving soy protein and vasoreactivity is scant, the initial assessment is that PEs have a direct effect on arterial walls (11). A study investigating renal transporters found isoflavones to induce considerable vasodilation (17). Honoré et al. (18) recently used female and male macaques with preexisting diet-induced atherosclerosis to examine vasodilatory effects. The monkeys were fed diets of either soy+ or soy− for 6 months. Acetylcholine was intravenously injected to test vascular reactivity. In females, constriction of coronary arteries was associated with the soy− group, while vasodilation was associated with the soy+ group. No statistically significant differences were observed in males. Another study isolated rabbit coronary artery rings and contracted them with potassium chloride. Tissue samples were induced to relax in PE baths. Results were dose-dependent, with the greatest effects seen at 40 μM genistein (isoflavonoid). No difference between males and females was observed. The concentrations of genistein utilized in the organ baths are equivalent to attainable human plasma levels, indicating the potential for effects in humans in vivo (19). The intake of soy has also been shown to improve systemic arterial compliance (11).

The mechanisms behind PE vasodilation are unclear. Similar relaxation effects are seen with ER-α inhibitors, excluding a mechanism by that receptor (19). However, since ER-β has been discovered in vascular tissue, it must still be considered. Gemma et al. (19) have suggested that the PEs act as Ca++ antagonists Ca++ is an important mediator of excitation-contraction coupling in smooth muscle cells. This is similar to the inhibitory mechanisms of estrogen and progesterone.

BLOOD PRESSURE

Claims that soy protein can lower blood pressure are largely based on renal studies. Within the thick ascending limb of the loop of Henle there is a Na+/K+/2Cl-cotransporter which is responsible for the majority of luminal NaCl reabsorption. Genistein and daidzein, two prominent isoflavones, are said to inhibit this cotransporter in vitro (17,20). Inhibition would result in stimulation of Na+ and H_2O excretion, followed concurrently by a loss of blood volume. This mechanism of *osmosalidiuretic* potency is plausible but not readily accepted. Another study reported genistein to stimulate the same cotransporter (21). Perhaps this explains the finding of Hodgson et al. (22), whose study comprised 59 subjects with high to normal systolic blood pressure who participated in an 8-week randomized, placebo-controlled trial. The experimental group took 55 mg of isoflavonoids (30 mg of which was genistein). No significant differences in blood pressure were seen after adjustment for baseline values.

ATHEROSCLEROSIS

Vascular endothelial injury due to hyperlipidemia or toxic or infectious agents is generally believed to be the cause of atherosclorotic lesions (11). Soy protein has been reported to inhibit the progression of atherosclorosis in the coronary, iliac, and common and internal carotid arteries of both males and females (23). Platelet aggregation induced by collagen and thromboxane A_2 was entirely prevented in human platelets preincubated for 5 min. in 10 $\mu g/mL$ genistein. Inhibition of tyrosine kinase appears to be the underlying reason for the antithrombolytic effect. Without tyrosine kinase, platelets will not be activated, thereby reducing their deposition and aggregation. The outcome will be a halt in the progression of atherosclerosis (10,16a).

SOY AND HIV

Current evidence indicates that there are many potential benefits from increasing intakes of soy protein. It has even been endorsed by the FDA for its ability to modify plasma lipids, provide antioxidant protection against LDLs, and affect vascular reactivity. Such effects suggest that soy is capable of decreasing CVD risk. Given the information provided, it would seem plausible to recommend a soy-based diet to HIV patients; however, on closer examination, a potential for adverse effects involving hyperkalemia becomes apparent.

Hyperkalemia is defined as a high serum potassium (K+) level (>5.5 mmol/L) (24). Blood measurements reflect only 2% of total body potassium. The remaining amount comprises intracellular stores. K+ is necessary for the activity of muscle tissue, enzyme reactions involving digestion and metabolism, and electrical and chemical homeostasis. Hyperkalemia stems from increases in total body K+ or excessive transfer of intracellular levels into the blood. Pathology is most often associated with kidney disease, but it can also be linked to aberrant aldosterone levels, tissue trauma, medications, or diet. Problems arising from this condition include arrthymias, bradycardia, ventricular fibrillation, respiratory arrest, paresthesias, and changes in neuromuscular control (14). Soy products contain high levels of potassium, ranging from 620 mg in soybeans to 2515 mg in soy flour (24). Normal healthy individuals can compensate for these levels; but if pathology exists, soy may exacerbate problems associated with a hyperkalemic condition.

A number of HIV-infected patients are reported to have hyperkalemia; however, this has been attributed to treatment with pentamidine or trimethoprim/sulfamethoxazole or to hyporeninemic hypoaldosteronism. It has recently been proposed that HIV infection alone is accompanied by a defect in transmembrane K+ equilibrium due to defective ionic transport mechanisms. Cited was a study by Lachaal and Venuto, who observed high serum K+ levels after the first day of pentamidine treatment—too soon for it to be a treatment effect (25). Caramelo et al. (25) assessed abnormalities in K+ equilibrium by intravenous injection of L-arginine into HIV-positive and HIV-negative subjects and the observation of changes in K+ concentrations. Two-fifths of the HIV patients were on trimethoprim/sulfamethoxazole. At baseline, no differences were noted between infected subjects and controls; however, 1 hr after L-arginine injection, a significant rise in plasma K+ was seen in HIV patients, and this was not related to renal factors. This finding raises the possibility that hyperkalemia can develop in HIV patients in previously unsuspected ways—for example, amino acid infusions or protein meals.

More disturbing than the threat of cytotoxicity is the finding that HIV thrives in hyperkalemic environments (26). HIV is capable of modifying intracellar ion concentrations, so that it might preferentially influence translation of viral mRNA or induce cytopathology (27). In an important study done by Choi et al. (26), CD4+ lymphoid cells infected with HIV-1 were incubated in graded levels of K+ concentrations. Cells incubated in K+-free mediums were discovered to have 40 to 50% lower levels of HIV-1 production than those in a control medium (5mM). Mediums of 25 to 50 mM K+ showed an approximately threefold elevation of viral production in a single round replication. From these data, it can be hypothesized that any factor, including diet, which increases K+ levels can have severe consequences for individuals infected with HIV.

SUMMARY

Advances in medicine have allowed patients suffering from HIV to extend their lives. Longer life has meant the introduction of new diseases, including CVD. Tremendous focus has been placed on dietary changes to decrease the risk of CVD. Epidemiological data and a variety of research studies have credited soy protein with cardioprotective effects. The FDA has acknowledged soy's ability to lower cholesterol. Blood pressure modification and vasoreactivity effects have also been attributed to soy. It would appear that HIV patients would benefit greatly from the addition of soy to their diets; however, problems may arise because of possible ionic disturbances in infected individuals. Hyperkalemia is increasingly being described in HIV patients. Choi et al. (26) have shown that the virus thrives in high-K+ environments, tripling virus production within a single round. Given the high levels of K+ found in soy products, it is suggested that HIV-infected patients avoid soy protein. This topic warrants further investigation, but until confounding factors can be ruled out, HIV patients will have to be exempt from the cardioprotective benefits of soy.

REFERENCES

1. Rerkpattanapipat P, Wongpraparut N, et al. Cardiac manifestations of acquired immunodeficiency syndrome. Arch Intern Med 2000; 160:602–608.
2. Panel RC, Frishman WH. Management of the HIV-infected patient: Part I. Cardiac involvement in HIV infection. Med Clin North Am 1996; 80(6):1493–1512.
3. Penzak SR, Chuck SK. Hyperlipidemia associated with HIV protease inhibitor use: pathophysiology, prevalence, risk factors and treatment. Scand J Infect Dis 2000; 32:111–123.
4. Tsiodras S, Mantzoros C, et al. Effects of protease inhibitors on hyperglycemia hyperlipidemia, and lipodystrophy. Arch Intern Med 2000; 160(13).
5. Carr A, Samaras K, et al. Pathogenesis of HIV-1-protease inhibitor-associated peripheral lipodystrophy, hyperlipidaemia, and insulin resistance. Lancet 1998; 351:1881–1883.
6. Lissin LW, Cooke JP. Phytoestrogens and cardiovascular health. J Am Coll Cardiol 2000; 35(6):1403–1410.
7. Davis SR, Dalais FS, et al. Phytoestrogens in Health and Disease. Recent Progr Hormone Res 1999; 54:185–210.
8. Anderson JW, Johnstone BM, et al. Meta-analysis of the effects of soy protein intake on serum lipids. N Engl J Med 1995; 333:276–282.
9. Kurzer MS, Xu X. Dietary phytoestrogens. Annu Rev Nutr 1997; 17:353–381.
10. Tham DM, Gardner CD, Haskell WL. Potential health benefits of dietary phytoestrogens: a review of the clinical, epidemiological and mechanistic evidence. J Clin Endocrinol Metab 1998; 83(7):2223–2235.
11. Tikkanen MJ, Adlercreutz H. Dietary soy-derived isoflavone phytoestrogens. Could they have a role in coronary heart disease prevention? Biochem Pharm 2000; 60(1):1–5.
12. Messina M, Messina V. Soyfoods, soybean isoflavones, and bone health: a brief overview. J Renal Nutr 2000; 10(2):63–68.
13. www.fda.gov
14. Wong WW, Smith EO. Cholesterol-lowering effect of soy protein in normocholesterolemic and hypercholesterolemic men. Am J Clin Nutr 1998; 68:1385S–1389S
15. Teixeira SR, Potter SM, et al. Effects of feeding 4 levels of soy protein for 3 and 6 wk on

blood lipids and apolipoproteins in moderately hypercholesterolemic men. Am J Clin Nutr 2000; 71(5):1077–1084.

16. Sirtori CR, Lovati MR. Soy and cholesterol reduction: clinical experience. J Nutr 1995; 125:5985–6055.

16a. Nakashima S, Koike T. Genistein, a protein kinase inhibitor, inhibits thromboxane A_2–mediated human platelet responses. Mol Pharm 1990; 39:475–480.

17. Martinez RM, Gimenez I. Soy isoflavonoids exhibit in vitro biological activities of loop diuretics. Am J Clin Nutr 1998; 68(suppl 6):1354S–1357S.

18. Honoré EK, Williams JK, et al. Soy isoflavones enhance coronary vascular reactivity in atherosclerotic female macaques. Fertil Steril 1997; 67:148–154.

19. Gemma A, Gigtree MB, et al. Plant-derived estrogens relax coronary arteries in vitro by a calcium antagonistic mechanism. J Am Coll Cardiol 2000; 35(7):1977–1985.

20. Garay RP, Alvarez-Guerra M, et al. Regulation of renal Na-K-Cl cotransporter NKCC2 by humoral natriuretic factors: relevance in hypertension. Clin Exp Hypertens 1998; 20(5–6):675–682.

21. Niisato N, Ito Y, Marunaka Y. Activation of Cl– channel and Na+/K+/2Cl– cotransporter in renal epithelial A6 cells by flavonoids: genistein, daidzein, and apigenin. Biochem Biophy Res Commun 1999; 254(2):368–371.

22. Hodgson JM, Puddey IB. Effects of isoflavonoids on blood pressure in subjects with high-normal ambulatory blood pressure levels: a randomized controlled trial. Am J Hypertens 1999; 12(1 pt 1):47–53.

23. Clarkson TB, Anthony MS. Phytoestrogens and coronary heart disease. Baillieres Clin Endocrinol Metab 1998; 12(4):589–604.

24. www.nal.usda.gov

25. Caramelo C, Bello E, et al. Hyperkalemia in patients infected with the human immuno-deficiency virus: involvement of a systemic mechanism. Kidney Int 1999; 56:198–205.

26. Choi B, Gatti PJ, et al. Role of potassium in human immunodeficiency virus production and cytopathic effects. Virology 1998; 247(2):189–199.

27. Voss TG, Fermin CD, et al. Alteration of intracellular sodium and potassium concentrations correlates with induction of cytopathic effects by human immunodeficiency virus. J Virol 1996; 70:5447–5454.

15

N-3 Fatty Acid Supplementation in AIDS Patients with Cardiac Complications

Zeina Makhoul
University of Arizona, Tucson, Arizona, U.S.A.

INTRODUCTION

Acquired immune deficiency syndrome (AIDS), first identified in 1981, is the final stage of a viral infection caused by the human immunodeficiency virus (HIV). AIDS is now the seventh leading cause of death in 1- to 4-year-olds, sixth among 15- to 24-year olds, and third among 25- to 44-year-olds in the United States. Cardiac involvement in AIDS, which was previously felt to be an unusual manifestation of the disease, appears to be an important complication of AIDS and is now being reported with increased frequency (1).

Because of the increased frequency of heart disease in AIDS patients and the correlation between consuming n-3 fatty acids and reduced incidence of cardiovascular disease (CVD), I hypothesize that supplementing AIDS patients' diets with n-3 fatty acids may reduce cardiac complications of AIDS.

AIDS AND IMMUNITY

HIV can infect several cell types in the human body, the most important of which belong to the immune system. The human immune system is able to mount a highly specific response against any foreign substances, even those never seen before. It is able to do so because of different kinds of cells called lymphocytes. Lymphocytes circulate in blood and lymph tissue and are present in large numbers in lymphoid organs such as bone marrow, thymus, lymph nodes, spleen, tonsils, adenoids, appendix, and the clumps of lymphoid tissue in the small intestine called Peyer's patches. The blood and lymphatic fluids transport lymphocytes to and from all the immune system organs (1).

Lymphocytes are divided into two classes: B cells, derived from and maturing in bone marrow, and T cells, which are derived from bone marrow but travel to the thymus gland and mature in it (2).

T cells make up the majority of circulating lymphocytes. They play a major role in the immune response by destroying infected cells, controlling inflamatory responses, and helping B cells to make antibodies. The three major kinds of T cells are cytotoxic (CD8) or killer T cells, helper T cells (T4 cells), and suppressor T cells (T8 cells).

Helper T cells carry the CD4 marker and are most often referred to as T4 cells. They alert the immune system to the presence of an antigen and activate other cells in the system. T4 cells have receptors that are specialized for the recognition of antigens found on the surface of viruses, fungi, and other parasites. When a T4 cell receptor binds to the antigen, the T4 cell becomes activated and secretes a variety of stimulatory factors called lymphokines. The T4 cell does little to repel the intruding substance on its own, but it is vital for activating the other lymphocytes—B cells, natural killer cells, and phagocytes—by secretion of lymphokines, interleukin-2 (IL-2), and interferon gamma (IFN-γ). As a result, B lymphocytes multiply and produce specific antibodies that attach to the antigen on infected cells, leading to their destruction.

Cytotoxic T cells, also known as killer T cells, express the CD8 molecule and are most often referred to as T8 cells. They are crucial for the immune response to viral infections. A T8 cell becomes activated when it recognizes an antigen and is assisted by an activated T4 cell. Activated T8 cells are largely responsible for recovery from a viral infection by eliminating virus-infected cells.

Suppressor T cells also carry the CD8 molecule. Suppressor T8 cells turn off antibody production and other immune responses after an invader has been destroyed. This allows the immune system to rest when its functions are not needed (2).

T4 CELL FUNCTION AND HIV DISEASE

In general, T-cell disorders are more severe than B-cell disorders. Individuals with defective T-cell function suffer from infections and clinical problems for which there is no treatment.

In the case of HIV disease, the T cells are deleted as a result of a series of events initiated by the binding of HIV to the CD4 molecule. Once HIV enters a T4 cell, it begins to lose its normal function. The takeover of HIV is a quiet event and not immediately apparent. Little or no viral replication takes place when the virus joins the host cell's DNA. When some antigen—not necessarily another HIV but some unrelated viral, fungal, or parasitic invader—activates the T4 cell, it manufactures the invader's viral RNA strands. Consequently, T4 cells are destroyed by HIV. The loss of T4 cells severely reduces cell-mediated immunity and eliminates the T4 cell–dependent production of antibodies by B cells. HIV-infected patients become more susceptible to opportunistic infection and subsequent death. AIDS is diagnosed when the T4 cell count drops to less than 200/μL, the normal level in adults being 600 to 1200/μL (1).

T8 CELL FUNCTION AND HIV DISEASE

Other lymphocyte functions are impaired as well. T8 cells help the immune system recognize the cells of its own body and thus avoid attacking them. In HIV-infected persons, some T8 cells are lost. Therefore the immune system may not be properly suppressed and it may attack the body's cells (autoimmune response).

Thus HIV specifically infects the T4 helper cell or CD4 + cell. Because of the T4 cell's destruction, the ratio of T4 to T8 cells changes. Normally, the number of T4 cells is greater than that of T8 cells. The impaired ratio signals the progress of the immune system's deterioration. The T4 cells become much less responsive to antigen deterioration, macrophages are not as responsive, and B cells produce fewer specific antibodies (1).

ANTIBODIES AND HIV DISEASE

B-cell function is almost normal in most HIV-infected persons. Small defects in B-cell function may occur because of disrupted communication with other cells, such as the T cell–independent B-cell response or the T4 cell–dependent B-cell response.

Antibodies secreted by B cells do not work effectively against HIV. They have difficulty in neutralizing the virus and therefore provide little protection.

Humans create antibodies against a number of HIV proteins, namely the envelope proteins (gp 120), the transmembrane protein (gp 41), and the protein of the HIV core (gp 24). The antibodies can attack HIV only in the plasma. Once inside a host cell, therefore, HIV is protected from antibodies.

The envelope of HIV is studded with proteins made by the virus. Gp 120 proteins protrude from the viral envelope. The gp 120 protein contains a CD4-binding domain (the area that binds to the T4 lymphocyte), which is believed to be the most important site responsible for HIV's infectivity. Once inside the body, because of its specific glycoprotein "spikes" (gp 120) that extend out from the viral envelope, HIV is attracted primarily to those cells that display the CD4 receptor-site antigen. All sites that carry a CD4 or T4 receptor antigen are susceptible to HIV infection (1).

Cell types other than T4 cells known to carry the CD4 or T4 receptor antigen are monocytes, macrophages, glial cells, chromaffin cells of the lower intestine and vaginal lining, and retinal cells in the eye. The viral protein gp 120 then binds specifically and tightly to the CD4 receptor site. Thus HIV suppresses the human immune defense by infecting the cells that govern the immune system—most importantly, the T4 lymphocytes and macrophages.

T4 CELL DEPLETION AND IMMUNE SUPPRESSION

Research using the polymerase chain reaction, a method of amplifying unmeasurable quantities of HIV DNA in T4 cells into measurable quantities, has revealed that about one in every 10 to 100 T4 cells is HIV-infected in an AIDS patient. Thus, T4 helper cells serve as reservoirs of HIV in the body.

In vitro studies show that HIV can attack CD4 receptor sites in two ways. First, it can attach via its gp 160 "spikes" to CD4 receptor sites. Second, it can release its exterior gp 120 envelope glycoprotein, thereby generating a molecule that can actively bind to CD4-containing cells. As a result, T4 cells lose their immune function after their receptor sites are filled with the virus. The T4 cells do not have to be infected to lose their function. Filled T4 cells become targets for immune attack. This would result in the destruction not only of infected but also of uninfected CD4 cells (1).

Infected macrophages, which normally interact with the T4 cells to stimulate the immune function, can transfer HIV into uninfected T4 lymphocytes. In any case, immediate viral or proviral replication kills the T4 cell.

It is believed that some cofactors may be responsible for activating or increasing HIV production. Agents such as nutrition, stress, and infections organisms may accelerate HIV expression after infection.

Another abnormality associated with HIV infection is the inability of the T4 cells to produce a variety of lymphokines such as interleukins. These chemical stimulants are necessary for the proper maturation of B-cells into plasma and the maturation and induction of the cytotoxic T-cell functions (3).

Thus, the critical basis for the immunopathogenesis of HIV infection is the depletion of the T4 helper cells, which results in profound immunosuppression.

CARDIAC INVOLVEMENT IN AIDS

More recently, however, the virus was found to infect other cell types as well, including monocytes/macrophages, endothelial cells, glial cells, bowel epithelium cells, and possibly neurons. These results suggest a broader host cell range for HIV than was previously suspected and may account for some of the clinical manifestations of AIDS (4).

Based on the involvement of the above-mentioned cell types, the brain is documented as a target organ of HIV infection, manifest by the encephalopathic syndrome that is emerging as a major clinical feature of AIDS. Although it has received less attention, heart muscle disease is another clinical manifestation. Cardiac involvement in AIDS, which was previously felt to be an unusual manifestation of the disease, is now being described with increasing frequency. Studies have suggested that HIV may exhibit a cardiac tropism. More commonly, the hearts of patients can be infected by other viruses, fungi, and protozoa that cause opportunistic infections in AIDS. Cardiac disease in AIDS patients may be caused by the infectious or neoplastic complication of AIDS and their therapies or perhaps by HIV infection of the myocardium itself (5).

Grody et al. (5) reported evidence for direct infection of the heart in AIDS, not by an opportunistic pathogen but by the AIDS virus itself, HIV. For this study the technique of in situ deoxyribonucleic acid (DNA) hybridization was applied to cardiac tissues obtained at autopsy from AIDS patients. Using sulfur 35–labeled ribonucleic acid (RNA) probes encompassing the entire HIV genome, HIV nucleic acid sequences were detected in cardiac tissue sections from 6 of 22 patients examined who had died of AIDS.

The mechanism by which HIV enters muscle cells is not clear. Studies done on normal human myocardium using an anti-CD4 antibody showed that no CD4 antigen was detected in this tissue. The cardiac conditions seen in patients with AIDS include myocardial, endocardial and pericardial disease.

Once myocardial failure develops in AIDS patients, it has a poor prognosis despite the observation that patients often respond to traditional heart failure therapies.

Pericardial involvement in AIDS is frequent, often asymptomatic, and usually manifest as a nonspecific pericardial effusion, although neoplasms and opportunistic infections may also be seen.

Endocardial involvement in AIDS is most likely related to marantic endocarditis; however, bacterial endocarditis may also complicate the course of AIDS patients who are intravenous drug abusers. Infection with HIV does not appear to make patients more susceptible to bacterial endocarditis (5).

Important clinical syndromes described in patients with HIV infection that involve the heart include cardiac tamponade resulting from pericardial effusion or hemorrhage, dilated cardiac myopathy, other forms of myocardial failure, refractory ventricular tachyarrythmias or sudden death, and systemic thromboembolic disease caused by infectious and noninfectious thrombotic endocarditis (4).

In another study by Valdes et al. (6), 50 patients of both sexes with severe immunosuppression were evaluated. All had severe HIV infection with a CD4 count of less than 200 μL. Diastolic ventricular dysfunction was present in 40% of the cases, even as systolic dysfunction occurred in 18%. Global hypokinesia was present in 12% of the cases. Clinically, 6 patients presented with left ventricular failure, 5 with pericarditis and effusion, 1 with severe arhythmia, and 1 with endocarditis. The pathophysiological interpretation of the observed findings is difficult in the light of the current knowledge. Ventricular dysfunction in AIDS has been associated with a specific or direct viral cytopathic action or nonspecific myocarditis of multifactorial physiopathology: myocardialcytopathic immune complexes, myocardiotoxic cytokines produced by macrophages stimulated by viral replication, other opportunistic viral infections, and nutritional deficiencies (selenium).

Some studies have suggested that immunosuppression may predispose patients with HIV to myocarditis. Some studies in which T4 helper lymphocytes were used as a marker of immunosuppression could not show any quantitative differences in numbers of T4 cells between HIV patients with and without cardiomyopathy. However, other studies showed a direct relationship between decreased CD4 lymphocyte counts and the presence of myocardial pathology in HIV patients (4).

Acierno (7) suggested that myocardial damage could relate to hypersensitivity resulting from uncontrolled hypergammaglobulinemia from altered T-cell function. HIV infected patients do show high concentrations of immunocomplexes in their serum, but the relationship between these findings and myocardial damage requires further study.

Another study, done by De Castro et al. (8), evaluated the incidence of cardiac involvement and its clinical correlates during the various phases of infection. The results demonstrated that cardiac involvement in present in 45% HIV-infected patients, but only in the end stage of the disease and presumably due to opportunistic infections and/or secondary malignancies.

The direct role of HIV in the genesis of cardiomyopathy remains uncertain and should be evaluated by further studies. Cardiac involvement can occur without any clinical manifestations, or it can complicate the course of the disease, thus causing death in some patients [5.5% in the study of De Castro et al. (8)].

Echocardiography appears to be the most appropriate way to detect heart involvement during HIV infection; it provides early diagnosis and time to find the most suitable way of treating cardiac abnormalities even when they occur during the early, asymptomatic phase of the disease (8).

Physicians should now be alert to the high frequency of cardiac involvement with AIDS, which might affect the treatment and supportive care that these individuals need.

FATTY ACIDS AND IMMUNITY

The successful initiation of an immune response to foreign antigens depends on lymphocytes, macrophages, and natural killer cells. Cooperation among these cell types is essential to the inflammatory response. This communication is through cytokines that serve as protein mediators between different cells. Another name used to describe most mediators is *interleukins*. Cytokines are produced mainly by cells of the immune system. The target for cytokines includes both immune and nonimmune cell types; therefore the physiological and pathological effects of cytokines extend beyond the immune system. Specific cytokines have been implicated in the pathogenesis of cardiovascular and other diseases (9). Thus dietary manipulation of these compounds will have important implications, as discussed below.

CYTOKINES

Cytokines are highly interdependent. They can act in an additive, synergistic, or suppressive fashion. Therefore dietary change in one cytokine may have a profound effect on other cytokines.

Important cytokines are interleukins: interleukin-1 (IL-1), IL-2, IL-6, and tumor necrosis factor (TNF). IL-1 is one of the key mediators in response to microbial invasion, immunological reactions, inflammatory response, and tissue injury. Macrophages are the major source of IL-1. IL-1 production is under negative control by prostaglandin E_2 (PGE_2).

IL-2 is produced by T cells, especially T-helper cells, and is essential for antigen-stimulated proliferation of T cells. In addition, IL-2 increases activity of natural killer cells and antibody production by B lymphocytes. A reduced ability to produce IL-2 or to respond to IL-2 has been implicated in acquired immunodeficiency and auto-immune diseases.

IL-6 is produced during the immune response and can influence the growth and differentiation of both T and B cells.

TNF includes TNF-α, which is macrophage-derived, and TNF-β, derived from lymphocytes. TNF induces synthesis of several proteins (including IL- 1) and alters homeostatic properties of the vascular endothelium. TNF also increases PGE_2 levels (9).

Lipid biology plays a significant role in the normal and pathological findings of cells of the immune system. In addition to these cells' physiological requirements for essential fatty acids, dietary fatty acid modulation of the membrane composition and functions of immune cells can affect both normal and pathological processes. Free fatty acids are produced and secreted during the activation of immune cells (10).

Studies in cultured cells, animal models, and human subjects have shown that both the amounts and types of fatty acids are important for growth and activity of immune cells.

IMMUNONUTRITION: THE ROLE OF N-3 FATTY ACIDS

Epidemiological and biochemical studies have suggested an anti-inflammatory effect of n-3 fatty acids. N-3 fatty acids are long chain polyunsaturated fatty acids (PUFA) with a double bond between carbon atoms 3 and 4 proximal to the methyl end of the fatty acids. Species of this lipid class that naturally occur in appreciable amounts are eicosapentaenoic acid (EPA; 20:5 w-3), docosahexaenoic acid (DHA; 22:6 w-3) and α-linoleic acid (ALA). Both EPA and DHA inhibited a number of immune cell functions when tested in vitro and in animal models, although stimulation was found in some animal studies (11).

Results from other studies have indicated that EPA and DHA may differ in their effects on the immune cells and act through different mechanisms. Thus recombinant IL-2 partly restored the inhibition of human lymphocyte proliferation caused by EPA but not by DHA.

A number of studies have examined the effect of n-3 PUFA on human immune status by supplementing diets with flax-seed oil rich in ALA, fish oil rich in EPA and DHA, and purified sources of EPA and DHA. All these diets inhibited the immune response regardless of the carbon-chain length and number of double bonds in the n-3 PUFA used.

Subtle changes in immune status are noted from the onset of HIV infection. These may be related to many factors, including nutritional deficiencies. Because supplementation with n-3 fatty acids (fish oil) correlates with improved immune function in various clinical conditions, Pichard et al. (12) hypothesized that long-term (6 months) oral nutritional supplementation enriched with n-3 fatty acids and arginine may contribute to preserving the immune status of HIV-infected patients. The experimental group received 1.7 g n-3 fatty acids. Changes between the two groups over the 6-month trial period were not statistically significant. The variations of lymphocytes, CD4, and CD8 cell counts were similar in experimental and control groups. Viremia and TNF-soluble receptors remained unchanged. Thus Pichard et al. (12) concluded from this trial that enrichment of diet with n-3 fatty acids (and arginine) did not improve immunological parameters.

Another study discussing dietary modulation and autoimmune disease was done by Fernandes et al. (13). Recently, a murine retrovirus (LpBM5 MuLV), which induces immunodeficiency syndrome in mice, termed MAIDS, has been found to have several features similar to those seen in human AIDS, such as B-cell lymphoma, altered B- and T-cell function, and dysregulation of cytokines such as IL-1, IL-2, an IL-6. It is interesting to note that altered immune dysfunction in MAIDS could be modulated by n-3 fatty acid supplementation. The work of Fernandes et al. (13) on mice showed that changes induced by dietary n-3 PUFA and/or energy restriction on the composition of lymphocytes can modulate the production and response of lymphokines, including immunosuppressive PGE_2, which appear to delay progression of retroviral infection. However, further nutritional studies are required to understand the role of n-3 fatty acids in delaying retroviral infection in humans.

Clearly, there is much evidence to show that under well-controlled dietary conditions, fatty acid intake can have profound effects on animal models of auto-immune disease. Studies in human autoimmune disease have been less dramatic. However, human trials have been subject to uncontrolled dietary and genetic back-grounds, infection, and other environmental influences. The impact of dietary fatty acids on animal models of autoimmune disease appears to depend on the animal model and the type and amount of fatty acids fed to the animal. Diets high in n-3 fatty acids from fish oils increase survival and reduce disease severity in spontaneous autoantibody-mediated disease. In experimentally induced T cell–mediated autoimmune disease, diets supplemented with n-3 fatty acids appear to augment disease.

Suppression of autoantibody and T-lymphocyte proliferation, apoptosis of autoreactive lymphocytes, and reduced proinflammatory cytokine production by high doses of fish oils are all likely mechanisms by which n-3 fatty acids ameliorate autoimmune disease. However, treatment with these substances could lead to an undesirable long-term effect of high-dose fish oil, which can compromise host immunity. In addition to the effects of dietary fatty acids on immunoregulation, inflammation as a consequence of immune activation in autoimmune disease may also be an important mechanism of action whereby dietary fatty acids modulate disease activity.

Meydani (14) found that fish oil supplementation for 24 weeks reduced the relative percentage of peripheral blood CD4 cells and increased the percentage of CD8 cells in humans. He also found that plasma vitamin E levels were maintained and suggested that, in the presence of adequate vitamin E concentrations, lymphocyte mitogenic proliferative responses are enhanced. This indicates that vitamin E may have an independent effect on immune function and that the balance of n-3 fatty acids and vitamin E is important, because the immunosuppression caused by n-3 PUFA may be in part attributed to increased lipid peroxidation and decreased levels of antioxidant, especially vitamin E.

From the above studies, one can say that n-3 fatty acids can have immunosuppressive and immunostimulatory effects. Examples of immunosuppressive effects are reduced lymphocyte proliferation, decreased expression of major histocompatibility complex class II and adhesion molecules, and reduced cytokine production and chemotaxis by monocytes and neutrophils, discussed below.

Whereas many of the studies in humans and rats point toward an inhibitory effect of an n-3 PUFA diet on proinflammatory cytokines such as TNF and IL-1, several if not most of the studies performed in mice show that n-3 PUFA have stimulatory effects on TNF and IL-1. Most human studies have shown that n-3 PUFA inhibit cytokine production. However, while these studies have investigated the effect of short-term n-3 PUFA diets, studies employing longer-term studies (4 to 12 months) failed to find any effect on cytokine production (15).

In conclusion, although there is evidence that diets rich in n-3 PUFA might be beneficial in the treatment of inflammatory conditions, their effects are complex—both immunosuppressive and immunostimulatory—and still not fully understood.

N-3 FATTY ACIDS AND CVD

N-3 PUFA have been shown to reduce the risk of cardiovascular and inflammatory diseases. However, they have also been shown to suppress T cell–mediated immune function, an undesirable effect, especially in immunosuppressed individuals.

The low incidence of mortality from CHD among the Eskimos was initially attributed to the relatively large proportion of n-3 fatty acids from fish in their diet. Human and animal experimental studies have also demonstrated the beneficial effects of n-3 fatty acids on cardiovascular health. Fish oils may improve cardiovascular health because they lower serum triglycerides and inhibit platelet aggregation (16).

In addition to modulation of blood lipids and platelet activity, the anti-inflammatory properties of n-3 PUFA have been suggested as a mechanism for modulation endothelial/immune interaction in the prevention of CVD.

In general, the n-3 fatty acids diminish inflammatory and vascular responses because of their effect on cytokines and eicosanoid production. Therefore they have been beneficial in the treatment of diseases associated with inflammation and vascular pathology. However, prospective, randomized, placebo-controlled clinical trials have not always been consistent and have not always shown the anticipated effect.

LONG-CHAIN FATTY ACIDS

When incorporated into the plasma membrane, long-chain fatty acids (LCFA) alter membrane fluidity, cell-to-cell signaling, interaction of receptors with their agonists, mobility of cells, membrane function such as capping, and the formation of secondary signals. When they are released from the cell membrane or when they gain entrance to the cell from an extracellular milieu, they may undergo degradation through the eicosanoid pathways and/or influence the production of eicosanoids by inhibiting or increasing the activity of the appropriate enzymes. The eicosanoids have significant effects on intracellular signaling as well as a variety of inflammatory and other biological processes. In addition, the LCFA themselves may act as secondary messengers within cytoplasm, particularly influencing the formation of protein kinase C and diacylglycerol, calcium flux, and the distal pathways that influence the formation of cytokines and other cellular proteins that may be involved in inflammatory processes. Therefore, the amount and type of LCFA in dietary sources may profoundly influence cell function and the alteration of inflammatory processes (17).

THE EFFECT OF N-3 FATTY ACIDS ON LEUKOCYTE FUNCTION

Atherosclerosis, the major cause of morbidity and mortality from CVD, is an inflammatory disease of the vascular system in the treatment of which dietary fish and fish oil are known to play important roles. Activation and expression of adhesion molecules and recruitment of immune cells by the vascular endothelium are now recognized as inflammatory processes in the development and progression of atherosclerosis.

Monocytes play a major role in the early stages of atherogenesis. A sequence of monocyte adhesion to vascular endothelium, migration of monocytes into arterial intima, uptake of cholesterol by monocytes evolving into foam cells and fatty streaks, preceding the development of more advanced atherosclerotic lesions as fibrous plaque, has been documented in experimental models (18).

Circulating neutrophils and monocytes/macrophages are involved in the formation of leukotrienes from fatty acids. Arachidonic acid yields the 4 series of leukotrienes (LT), including LTB4, which is strongly chemotactic, whereas EPA yields the 5 series of leukotrienes, which are only weakly chemotactic. A relative reduction in chemotaxis might be expected by an antiatherogenic diet therapy. The response of monocytes to recruiting signals (chemotaxis) is important for their participation in physiological and pathophysiological processes. That is why researchers studied the effect of dietary supplementation with n-3 PUFA on monocyte chemotaxis (19).

In one of the studies, monocyte chemotaxis was reduced in healthy men supplemented with 5.3 g n-3 PUFA/day for 6 weeks. Next, it was demonstrated that the effect of n-3 PUFA on monocyte chemotaxis was dose-related.

Other investigators have reported that n-3 PUFA reduce the generation of platelet activating factor, reduce thromboplastin synthesis, decrease formation of IL-1, IL-2, IL-6, and TNF, and inhibit superoxide production and chemiluminescence from activated monocytes, in addition to the reduced formation of LTB4 previously mentioned. Neutrophil chemotaxis in response to LTB4 was also shown to be reduced by n-3 PUFA in healthy humans (18). In conclusion, n-3 PUFA reduce monocyte and neutrophil reactivity, which may be important for their possible effect on the development of atherosclerosis and CHD.

In a recent study (14), supplementation of patients with fish oil following coronary angioplasty elevated levels of lipid peroxides and two adhesion molecules in plasma, suggesting a proinflammatory action of fish oil. However, decreases in several plasma markers of endothelial hemostatic activity have indicated a healthier and better vasculature associated with fish oil supplementation. The notion that n-3 PUFA from fish oil might be proinflammatory to the vascular system, based on the increase of soluble adhesion molecules, is not well founded and contradicts several studies in which n-3 PUFA treatment demonstrated anti-inflammatory effects.

N-3 FATTY ACIDS: SIDE EFFECTS AND CONCERNS

The n-3 PUFA improve cardiovascular health and are also used in the management of human autoimmune disorders. There is concern that these health benefits come at the cost of increased susceptibility to other infections. Animals fed diets containing fish oils have shown slower clearance of bacteria and a decreased survival rate compared with those fed diets devoid of n-3 PUFA. Even in healthy humans, fish oil consumption has been found to attenuate the maximal increase in oral temperature after typhoid vaccination. Because the normal ranges for most indices of human immune response are very wide, the values of these indices after n-3 PUFA supplementation are often within the normal range. Most studies conducted in healthy subjects have not found an increased incidence of infection after n-3 PUFA supplementation. This, however, does not rule out the increased susceptibility of these subjects, which is of special concern in subjects with a compromised immune system such as AIDS patients (20).

It remains to be determined whether there are separate requirements for EPA and DHA. Dose-response studies need to be conducted to establish the amounts of n-3 PUFA that will serve the need to improve cardiovascular health without impairing the immune response. The safe levels may differ with the total fat intake and its composition and in different population groups. Based on the existing knowledge, an ALA intake of 5 g/day or an EPA + DHA intake of 400 mg/day can be considered safe for adult humans (20).

CONCLUSION

Although all the studies of n-3 PUFA and heart disease were not AIDS studies, fish oil may or may not be appropriate in treating some HIV-infected patients with heart problems or lipid abnormalities due to the use of antiretroviral drugs. Therefore my hypothesis that n-3 fatty acid supplementation may be helpful to AIDS patients with cardiac complications should be supported by further studies. Future studies focused on elucidating the molecular mechanism(s) modified by dietary fish oil or n-3 PUFA will ultimately lead to improved dietary strategies to aid in the prevention of auto-immune disease and CVD. In the future, manipulation of the dietary LCFA, especially of the n-3 series, as part of multimodality pharmacology, will be increasingly important in therapeutic regimens.

REFERENCES

1. Stine GJ. Acquired Immune Deficiency Syndrome: Biological, Medical, Social, and Legal Issues. 2d ed. Saddle River, NJ: Prentice Hall, 1996.
2. Chandra RK. Nutrition and the immune system: an introduction. Am J Clin Nutr 1997; 66:460S–463S.
3. Kubena KS, McMurray DN. Nutrition and the immune system: a review of nutrient-nutrient interactions. J Am Diet Assoc 1996; 96:1156–1164.
4. Patel RC, Frishman WH. AIDS and the heart: clinicopathologic assessment. Cardiovasc Pathol 1995; 4(3):173–183.
5. Grody WW, Cheng L, Lewis W. Infection of the heart by the human immunodeficiency virus. Am J Cardiol 1990; 66:203–206.
6. Valdes EF. Cardiovascular involvement during HIV infection. Eur Heart J 1996; 17(10):1605.
7. Acierno LJ. Cardiac complication in acquired immunodeficiency syndrome (AIDS): review. J Am Coll Cardiol 1989; 13:1144–1154.
8. De Castro S, Migliau G, Silvestri A, D'Amati G, Giannantoni P, Cartoni D, Kol A, Vullo V, Cirelli A. Heart involvement in AIDS: a prospective study during various stages of the disease. Eur Soc Cardiol 1992; 13:1452–1459.
9. Meydani SN. Dietary modulation of cytokine production and biologic functions. Nutr Rev 1990; 48(10):361–369.
10. Harbige LS. Dietary n-6 and n-3 fatty acids in immunity and autoimmune disease. Proc Nutr Soc 1998; 57:555–562.
11. Endres S, De Caterina R, Schmidt EB, Kristensen SD. N-3 polyunsaturated fatty acids: update 1995. Eur J Clin Invest 1995; 25:629–638.
12. Pichard C, Surde P, Karsegard V, Yerly S, Slosman DO, Delly V, Perrin L. A randomized double-blind controlled study of 6 months of oral nutritional supplementation with arginine ad ω-3 fatty acids in HIV-infected patients. AIDS 1998; 12:53–63.
13. Fernandes G, Tomar V, Mohan N, Venkatraman JT. Potential of diet therapy on murine AIDS. J Nutr 1992; 122:716–722.
14. Meydani M. Omega-3 fatty acids alter soluble markers of endothelial function in coronary heart disease patients. Nutr Rev 2000; 58:56–59.
15. Grimble RF. Nutritional modulation of cytokine biology. Nutrition 1998; 14:634–640.
16. Kelly DS, Taylor PC, Nelson GJ, Schmidt PC, Ferretti A, Erickson KL, Yu R, Chandra RK, Mackey BE. Docosahexaenoic acid ingestion inhibits natural killer cell activity and production of inflammatory mediators in young healthy men. Lipids 1999; 34(4):317–324.

17. Alexander JW. Immunonutrition: the role of ω-3 fatty acids. Nutrition 1998; 14:627–633.
18. Schmidt EB. N-3 fatty acids and the risk of coronary heart disease. Danish Med Bull 1997; 44:1–17.
19. Singleton CB, Walker BD, Campbell TJ. N-3 polyunsaturated fatty acids and cardiac mortality. Aust N Z J Med 2000; 30:246–251.
20. Darshan SK, Ingrid LR. Effect of individual fatty acids of ω-6 and ω-3 type on human immune status and role of eicosanoids. Nutrition 2000; 16:143–145.

16

A Role for Dietary Protein in the AIDS Wasting Syndrome and Heart Disease?

Jaclyn Maurer
University of Arizona, Tucson, Arizona, U.S.A.

INTRODUCTION

The human immunodeficiency virus (HIV) that causes acquired immunodeficiency syndrome (AIDS) shook the American nation in the early 1980s. Since that time, extensive research has been devoted to understanding the disease and finding answers to the many questions that arise from it. With the "discovery" of AIDS, numerous other diseases associated with the virus have emerged. Along with cancers, lymphomas, and immune diseases, heart disease has emerged as a risk for those living with AIDS. The etiology of and risk factors for heart disease in AIDS patients need further clarification. While there is yet no cure for HIV, AIDS, or many of the complications that arise from these diseases, there are numerous therapies devoted to reducing the suffering associated with AIDS as well as helping to prolong life. With increasing knowledge of the AIDS disease itself and how it relates to the risk for other diseases, nutrition—specifically adequate protein intake—emerges as an essential factor in the treatment of the progression from HIV to AIDS. Protein also appears to have a role in the treatment of AIDS-related conditions like the AIDS wasting syndrome.

THE AIDS WASTING SYNDROME: WHAT AND WHY?

What?

Numerous AIDS-related conditions exist; the second most prevalent is the AIDS wasting syndrome (1). The Centers for Disease Control (CDC) define the AIDS wasting syndrome (AWS) as an involuntary loss of more than 10% of one's body weight coinciding with fever, diarrhea, or weakness for more than 30 days (1). This definition may be a bit loose, since additional research shows that weight loss of only 1 to 5% of total body weight, even without concurrent or prior complications from AIDS, can promote the development of opportunistic infections as well as threaten survival (2–4). Emerging evidence like this suggests that while the AWS is prevalent among 20 to 30% of those affected with AIDS (3), its prevalence may be even higher than is reported under the CDC's definition.

The AWS is characterized by disproportionate decreases in lean body tissue with relative sparing of fat mass (2,3,5,6). Since the loss of lean tissue is associated with an increased risk of mortality and morbidity, this syndrome is a major threat to the health and well-being of people living with AIDS (3,7).

Why?

The causes of AWS are presently not fully understood; however, several factors appear to contribute: inadequate food intake, malabsorption, metabolic dysregulation, and hypermetabolism (1,7,8). Inadequate food intake may result from decreased appetite due to medications, opportunistic infections, depression, anorexia, decreases in energy, and even lack of funds (1,7,8). Malabsorption often arises due to infections in the intestinal lining and other factors that disrupt normal digestive processes. Metabolic dysregulation or altered metabolism is impairment of the body's mechanisms to preserve lean body mass in states of nutrient insufficiency. Metabolic dysregulation appears to be prevalent in some AIDS patients (7).

A study by Faber and Mannix investigating the biochemical events in exercising skeletal muscle of AIDS patients found that patients with AIDS relied more on anaerobic metabolism and less on oxidative phosphorylation than did non-HIV-infected controls (7). This evidence suggests that the increased reliance on anaerobic energy metabolism seen in AIDS patients may be a result of metabolic dysregulation and contributes to the negative energy balance and weight loss typically seen in patients with AWS (7).

Hypermetabolism, or increased energy expenditure, due possibly to the increased activity of the immune system (especially increased cytokine activity), appears to be prevalent even in patients progressing through the early stages of HIV infection, before any symptoms arise (1,7,8). The evidence for altered fat oxidation and higher protein oxidation rates, along with enhanced de novo lipogenesis (which is associated with accelerated fat oxidation and loss of lean tissue mass) in HIV-infected patients, all constitute abnormalities of hypermetabolism and present themselves as possible reasons for the loss of lean tissue mass (7). While more evidence on metabolic dysregulation and hypermetabolism in HIV and AIDS is needed, both of these conditions are associated with the loss of lean body mass.

NUTRITIONAL NEEDS OF THE AIDS PATIENT WITH AWS—A LOOK AT PROTEIN REQUIREMENTS

Nutrition plays an all-important role in the treatment and prevention of the AWS. The inadequate food intake and malabsorption associated with AWS indicate nutritional intervention to correct such deficiencies may have positive effects on the health and well-being of the AIDS patient. People affected with HIV and AIDS appear to have altered levels of certain hormones important in metabolism (1,7,8). Of these, cytokines, which are proteins producing inflammation to help the body overcome infection, are highly elevated in people with HIV and AIDS (1,7). These high levels of cytokines cause the body to produce more sugars and fats but also, unfortunately, less protein (the macronutrient an AIDS patient with AWS desperately needs) (1,7,8).

The building blocks of protein, amino acids, are used to help build immune factors; therefore, protein follows energy in importance of maintaining optimal immune function (9). Two amino acids in particular, glutamine and arginine, have shown promise in the treatment of AIDS patients. Glutamine is associated with maintaining the function and structure of the intestinal mucosa, while arginine is a sole source of the antimicrobial agent nitric oxide (10). The maintenance of intestinal mucosal health may ward off malabsorption, and adequate amounts of nitrix oxide help to prevent microbiotic infections. Protein also plays an important role in preventing catabolism of lean body mass (11).

Clearly, the protein needs of an AIDS patient are elevated due to the multitude of factors listed above, especially the increased metabolic requirements associated with fighting infection. In terms of recommendations, protein intakes for people infected with HIV and AIDS range between 1.0 and 2.5 g/kg body weight, depending on the severity of lean body mass wasting (9,11,12). Protein intake should also comprise between 15 to 20% of total calories (12). Meeting increased protein requirements is particularly hard for patients infected with HIV and AIDS, since the disease itself perpetually stimulates immune responses that divert protein intake and stimulate depletion of body protein reserves (i.e., from the skeletal muscle) (9). Research shows that the mucosal barrier in AIDS patients is abnormal because of increases in enteric losses, which contribute to protein malnutrition (10). Further, the anorexia that many HIV and AIDS patients experience makes it difficult for them to reach even the RDA for protein (0.8 g/kg body weight) let alone the higher requirements associated with their disease. Thus arises a serious nutritional obstacle. The HIV or AIDS patient needs adequate and often additional protein; however, consuming it from diet alone may not be sufficient; this is where other means of adding protein come into play.

ALTERNATIVE MECHANISMS FOR INCREASING PROTEIN INTAKE

Anabolic agents like steroids and hormone treatments are emerging as potential mechanisms for increasing lean body mass and reversing the disproportionate loss of lean body mass and fat accumulation that is associated with AWS (1,2,5,6,13,15–17). Anabolic steroids stimulate increases in muscle tissue mass by enhancing the body's ability to utilize protein in the production of muscle (4,13). Since HIV infection can affect the means via which the body utilizes amino acids, anabolic steroids aid in returning amino acids to the muscles and ultimately support muscle repair and growth (13). In a study of Grinspoon et al., the androgen deficiency seen in 20 hypogonadal men with AWS demonstrated a significant ($p = 0.02$) association between hypogonadal function and decreased lean body mass (5). Grinspoon et al. concluded that androgen deficiency may contribute to this decrease in lean body mass; however, the exact mechanism by which this occurs remains unknown. Therefore Grinspoon et al. hypothesized that gonadal dysfunction contributes to the loss of lean body mass associated with AWS and that androgen replacement therapy would increase lean body mass in hypogonadal men with AWS (5). This hypothesis is promising, since testosterone (an androgen) has shown stimulatory effects on the secretion of growth hormone (GH), and it is possible that loss of growth hormone (GH) insulin-like growth factor I (GH-IGF-I) axis is a mechanism for the decreased lean body mass associated with AWS (5).

In a later study, Grinspoon et al. explored how testosterone administration may affect the GH-IGF-I axis in men with AWS. Results showed that administration of testosterone decreased the level of GH in hypogonadal men with AWS, and this decrease in GH was inversely associated with a gain in lean body mass as a result of testosterone administration ($p = 0.024$) (15). Further results showed that along with androgen deficiency in patients with AWS, undernutrition (as often occurs with the inadequate intake of dietary protein or the protein-energy malnutrition seen in AIDS patients) might contribute to the changes observed in the GH-IGF-I axis of men with AWS (15). Therefore, according to the results of this later study by Grinspoon et al., administration of testosterone to patients with AWS appears to be a beneficial means for increasing lean body mass. However, it should be noted that proper nutrition must accompany this testosterone dosage in order to maximize its effects. Sattler et al. explored the potential use of another anabolic steroid, nandrolone decanoate, for increasing lean tissue mass in HIV- and AIDS-infected men. Results showed that subjects taking nandrolone decanoate and those enriching nandrolone decanoate with progressive resistance training experienced significant increases in body weight (3.2 +/− 2.7 kg) and lean body mass (4.0 +/− 2.0 kg) (2).

Further studies have explore administering growth hormone and insulin-like growth factor I (IGF-I) therapy to patients with AWS (14,16,17). Results show that administration of GH in GH-deficient children and adults (without HIV or AIDS) has led to positive nitrogen balance and an increase in lean body mass; however, the results of a study by Lee et al. failed to show a significant effect on body composition, weight, or clinical status in patients with AWS administered recombinant GH and recombinant IGF-I for 12 weeks, despite increases in total body weight at weeks 3 and 6 (16). Conversly, evidence from a study by Mulligan et al. showed that 3-month administration of recombinant human GH in patients with AWS increased lean body mass (+ 3.2 kg +/− 0.6 kg), decreased fat (−1.0 kg +/− 0.5 kg), increased resting energy expenditure (REE), and increased lipid oxidation (14). These two studies present conflicting results and reveal the need for further studies (and perhaps longer test periods) to explore the potential use of GH in the treatment of AWS. While GH administration shows the potential to increase lean body mass, the increase in REE that was shown in the study of Lee et al. because of recombinant GH administration presents problems for the HIV and AIDS patient. The increase in REE is likely due to an increase in lean body mass, but in the study of Mulligan et al., even when adjusting for changes in lean body mass, the increases seen in REE were close to significant (14). Since HIV and AIDS patients already have elevated REE due to stress, those patients who are not clinically stable and capable of meeting their current caloric needs may not fully benefit from recombinant GH therapy and its subsequent added demand for calories. Also, since recombinant GH administration increases lipid oxidation, the existing body fat stores in the absence of adequate energy intake may limit the degree to which lean body mass can increase in conjunction with recombinant GH administration in patients with AIDS.

These studies suggest potential uses of anabolic agents in the treatment of AWS; however, their use does not negate the importance of optimal nutrition and protein intake. Anabolic steroids may help the HIV or AIDS patient gain weight;

however, in order to maintain this weight, the patient must consume foods rich in amino acids and high-quality protein (13). Without the building blocks for lean muscle mass—amino acids—the effects of anabolic steroids are reduced. This fact reinforces the increased need for protein in patients with HIV and AIDS. While the studies mentioned above mainly employed male subjects, Grinspoon et al. also found, in a study exploring the body composition and endocrine function of women with AWS, that women, too, demonstrate an androgen deficiency that may contribute to the syndrome of wasting (6).

COMPLICATIONS WITH HEART DISEASE AND HIV INFECTION

Although evidence is still emerging on its prevalence and magnitude, heart disease (or cardiovascular dysfunction) appears to be a serious complication of HIV infection (18). While some research suggests that abnormalities of the heart are seen frequently in patients infected with AIDS, clinical manifestations of such abnormalities remain uncommon (19). Still more evidence suggests that only 5 to 20% of AIDS patients appear to have clinically important cardiac lesions (19). Research has reported a prevalence of echocardiographic abnormalities in 15 to 60% of HIV-infected persons, with left ventricular dysfunction being the most commonly seen abnormality (19). These large variations in prevalence (15 to 45%) suggest that the exact extent to which AIDS patients are affected by heart diseases is debatable and requires additional research.

The mechanisms by which HIV infection may lead to heart disease are also still unclear. Some evidence proposes that the virus itself may invade the myocytes, while other evidence suggests that the bacterial, viral, mycotic, and protozoal infections to which AIDS patients are exposed and susceptible may be to blame for the myocarditis seen in some patients. Still more theories propose that humorally mediated autoimmune reactions employing antimyosin antibodies may lead to the development of cardiomyopathy (19). Despite these various theories, there is enough evidence to indicate heart disease as a serious complication of HIV infection (7,18,19). Additionally, the protease inhibitor therapy frequently employed in the treatment of HIV and AIDS is associated with increased amounts of intra-abdominal visceral fat, which is another factor associated with an increased risk of heart disease (2).

AIDS WASTING SYNDROME AND HEART DISEASE

The main function of the heart is to deliver oxygen and nutrient-rich blood to tissues and remove waste products and carbon dioxide (20). Certain heart diseases disrupt this function. Congestive heart failure is associated with chronic undernutrition (7); likewise, the AWS is characterized by undernutrition. Undernutrition or starvation will cause myocardial mass to decrease, followed by a proportionate decrease in stroke volume and cardiac output. The effects of this myocardial atrophy, however, are often masked by compensatory mechanisms. Conversely, HIV infection appears to modulate the normal response expected of malnutrition in relation to the heart. With HIV infection and malnutrition, there arises an increased heart rate that has effects opposite to those of other malnutritional states, and this may, in association with hypermetabolism, contribute to wasting (20). Moreover, cardiac cachexia (tissue wasting in congestive heart failure) is propagated via hypermetabolism, one of the causative factors of AWS. The similarities between congestive heart failure and AWS suggest a link between the two conditions; however, unclear associations require additional research to further define this link.

COMPLICATIONS OF PROTEIN INTAKE AND HEART DISEASE

As already addressed, adequate and even increased protein intakes are important for proper care and maintenance of the HIV infected patient. Recommended protein intakes for HIV-infected patients range between 1.0 and 2.5 g/kg of body weight and this high protein intake (11,12), potentially poses a threat to increasing heart disease risk. There is a well-established link between plasma cholesterol levels and heart disease as well as epidemiological evidence supporting a relationship between dietary saturated fat intake and plasma cholesterol levels (22). This is where the problem arises between increasing protein intake and potentially increasing the risk for cardiovascular disease. Animal protein sources, the typical protein sources in the American diet (21), are often rich sources of saturated fat and cholesterol. Therefore, if AIDS patients are meeting their increased protein requirements by consuming animal protein sources rich in saturated fat, they potentially exacerbate their risk for heart disease; whereas if AIDS patients are meeting their protein requirements with mainly plant protein sources, they may risk inadequate consumption of essential amino acids, since plant protein sources have lower biological value than animal protein sources and also do not contain all the essential amino acids all in one source (soy is the exception) (22). While these concerns are valid, ultimately the relationship between increased protein intake and risk for heart disease in AIDS patients is speculative. Any concrete associations cannot be made without supplementary research.

Inadequate protein intake can also have adverse affects on heart disease. Malnourishment is associated with primary congestive heart failure and has been seen in malnourished non-HIV-infected children (19). Protein-energy malnutrition (PEM) in human adults without HIV infection has led to reduced heart rate, stroke volume, cardiac output, and heart size. Patients with anorexia nervosa (suffering from PEM) have shown a reduced left ventricular mass, one-half to one-third the size of age and sex-matched controls (19). Furthermore, patients with anorexia nervosa may have periodic reductions in heart rate and systolic blood pressure (19). The undernourished AIDS patient does not express the same cardiac responses as the non-HIV-infected, individual with PEM (the heart rate increases in the AIDS patient); therefore PEM does not appear to affect the cardiovascular system of the AIDS patient in the same manner as it does the non-HIV-infected PEM patient.

COMPLICATIONS OF ANABOLIC AGENTS AND HEART DISEASE

There may be an association between anabolic agents and heart disease. Evidence associating anabolic androgenic steroids with sudden cardiac death, myocardial infarction, altered serum lipoproteins, altered hematocrit, clotting factors, hypertension, and cardiac hypertrophy exists; however, no research directly links anabolic androgenic steroids with cardiovascular diseases (23). Anabolic agents such as nandrolone and testosterone stimulate the enzyme hepatic triglyceride lipase that removes HDL from the circulation and thereby lowers the cholesterol/HDL ratio. This lowered ratio potentially puts the AIDS patient at risk for heart disease. Conversely, though, this hepatic triglyceride lipase enzyme removes trigylerides from the blood, and since high triglyceride levels may promote heart disease, the two functions of this enzyme may counterbalance each other and negate any additional risk for heart disease (4). Further, excess testosterone can be associated with polycythemia, abnormally high numbers of red blood cells (4). Polycythemia has been implicated in heart disease; therefore testosterone administration to the AWS patient should be monitored to avoid inflating the risk for heart disease. While associations between the use of anabolic agents and heart disease exist, the adverse cardiovascular effects of using anabolic agents are not completely understood.

CONCLUSION

There is much uncertainty arise among protein intake, use of anabolic agents, and risk for heart disease among patients with AWS. Perhaps, the only certainty is that AWS is a serious, common, and fatal condition of AIDS. Proper treatment of the factors involved in AWS (inadequate food intake, malabsorption, altered metabolism, and hypermetabolism) is necessary to reverse or slow the progression of the AWS. Nutrition, especially adequate protein intake, is an essential component of this treatment. However, along with dietary protein intake, anabolic agents such as testosterone and growth hormone emerge as potential aids in the treatment and prevention of the AWS. While there does appear to be a risk for heart disease as a complication of AIDS, the unclear effects that increased protein intake and use of anabolic agents may have on heart disease risk suggest that continued research into this area is needed. The associations between nutritional intake, anabolic agents, and heart disease in the AWS patient require further exploration in order to clearly define any existing relationships and help clarify therapeutic recommendations.

REFERENCES

1. AIDS InfoNet. Wasting syndrome. Available at http://www.aidsinfonet.org. Accessed October 23, 2000.
2. Sattler FR, Jaque SV, Schroeder ET, et al. Effects of pharmacological doses of nandrolone decanoate and progressive resistance training in immunodeficient patients with human immunodeficiency virus. J Clin Endocrinol Metab 1999; 84:1268–1276.
3. Cone LA. Wasting and AIDS in the era of highly active antiretroviral therapy. In: Watson RR, ed. Nutrition and AIDS. 2d ed. Boca Raton, FL: CRC Press, 2001:1–8.
4. Body Positive. Fighting Wasting. Available at http://www.thebody.com. Accessed October 23, 2000.
5. Grinspoon S, Corcoran C, Lee K, Burrows B, et al. Loss of lean body and muscle mass correlates with androgen levels in hypogonadal men with acquired immunodeficiency syndrome and wasting. J Clin Endocrinol Metab 1996; 81:4051–4058.
6. Grinspoon S, Corcoran C, Miller, Biller K, Askari H, et al. Body composition and

endocrine function in women with acquired immunodeficiency syndrome wasting. J Clin Endocrinol Metab 1997; 82:1332–1337.

7.   Faber MO, Mannix ET. Tissue wasting in patients with chronic obstructive pulmonary disease, the acquired immune deficiency syndrome, and congestive heart failure. Neurol Clin 2000; 18:245–262.

8.   Maddox TG. HIV/AIDS management in office practice. Primary Care 1997; 24:517–529.

9.   Bahl S. Body weight, illness, and death. In: Bahl SM, Hickson JF, eds. Nutritional Care for HIV-Positive Persons: A Manual for Individuals and Their Caregivers. Boca Raton, FL: CRC Press, 1995:37–49.

10. Beisel WR. AIDS. In: Gershwin ME, German JB, Keen CL, eds. Nutrition and Immunology: principles and practice. Totowa, NJ: Humana Press, 2000:389–401.

11. Gardner CF, Thompson CA, Rhodes RR. Oral nutrition interventions. A Clinician's Guide to Nutrition in HIV and AIDS. Chicago: American Dietetic Association, 1997:43–64.

12. Nutritional Management of Symptoms. In: Fahey JL, Flemming DS, eds. AIDS/HIV Reference Guide for Medical Professionals. 4th ed. Baltimore, MD: Williams & Wilkins, 1997:441–451.

13. The AIDS Treatment Data Network. Anabolic steroids. Available at http://www.aidstreatmentdatanetwork.com. Accessed October 23, 2000.

14. Mulligan K, Tai VW, Schambelan M. Effects of chronic growth hormone treatment on energy intake and resting energy metabolism in patients with human immunodeficiency virus-associated wasting—a clinical research center study. J Clin Endocrinol Metab 1998; 83:1542–1547.

15. Grinspoon S, Corcoran C, Stanley T, Katzenlson L, et al. Effects of androgen administration on the growth hormone-insulin-like growth factor I axis in men with acquired immunodeficiency syndrome wasting. J Clin Endocrinol Metab 1998; 83:4251–4256.

16. Lee PDK, Pivarnik JM, Bukar JG, Muurahainen N, et al. A randomized, placebo-controlled trial of combined insulin-like growth factor I and low dose growth hormone therapy for wasting associated with human immunodeficiency virus infection. J Clin Endocrinol Metab 1996; 81:2968–2975.

17. McNurlan MA, Garlick PJ, Frost RA, Decristofaro KA, et al. Albumin synthesis and bone collagen formation in human immunodeficiency virus-positive subjects: differential effects of growth hormone administration. J Clin Endocrinol Metab 1998; 83:3050–3055.

18. Patel RC, Frishman WH. Management of the HIV-infected patient, part I. Med Clin North Am 1996; 80:P1493–P1512.

19. Cheitlin MD. Aids and the cardiovascular system. In: Alexander RW, Schlant RC, Fuster V, O'Rouke RA, Roberts R, Sonnenblick, eds. Hurst's The Heart: Vol 2. 9th ed. New York: McGraw-Hill, 1998:2143–2149.

20. Lichtenstein AH. Atherosclerosis. In: Ziegler EE, Filer LJ, eds. Present Knowledge in Nutrition. 7th ed. Washington, DC: ISLI Press, 1996:430–437.

21. Zeman FJ, Ney DM. Cardiovascular disease. In: Davis KM, ed. Applications in Medical Nutrition Therapy. 2d ed. Englewood Cliffs, NJ: Prentice Hall, 1996:251–262.

22. Sizer F, Whitney E. The proteins and amino acids. In: Bass J, ed. Nutrition Concepts and Controversies. 7th ed. Belmont, CA: West/Wadsworth, 1997:206–210.

23. Blue JG. Steroids and steroid-like compounds. Clin Sports Med 1999; 18:667–689.

17

Role of Antioxidants in Reducing Heart Disease in HIV-Infected Patients

Yingying Liu and Ronald Ross Watson
University of Arizona, Tucson, Arizona, U.S.A.

INTRODUCTION

Cardiovascular disease (CVD) is an important complication of human immunodeficiency virus (HIV) infection. It is now being reported with greater frequency, since a necropsy study first described cardiac involvement in an acquired immune deficiency syndrome (AIDS) patient (1). So far, cardiac abnormalities are found at autopsy in two-thirds of patients with AIDS, but they are often not detected by clinical examination. Although the cause and pathogenesis of CVD remain unresolved in many situations, opportunistic infections, vasculitis, hypoxia, catecholamine excess, and nutritional deficiencies have been suggested (2).

Viruses can cause oxidative stress by disturbing cellular antioxidant systems or inducing oxidative reactions. There is evidence of the presence of oxidative stress in the early stage of HIV infection (3–5), including glutathione and other antioxidant loss in serum and decreased activity of antioxidant enzymes. This pro-oxidant state is a result of an imbalance between the generation of reactive oxygen and nitrogen species (RONS) and the antioxidant system. Excess production of RONS (superoxide anion radical, hydrogen peroxide, hydroxyl radical, and nitric oxide) may occur following activation of polymorphonuclear leukocytes and macrophages (6). Furthermore, over the past decade, experimental and epidemiological evidence has demonstrated that macrophage-mediated oxidation of low-density lipoprotein (LDL) has a central role in atherogenesis (7,8). This is the underlying cause of most of the morbidity and mortality associated with CVD. Therefore the metabolic oxidation disturbance in AIDS patients may be involved in the decline of cardiovascular function.

Conversely, antioxidant confer protection against oxidative damage. Vitamins E and C and the carotenoids have been investigated most extensively for their antioxidant activity and potential roles in disease prevention (9,10). Indeed, human, animal, and epidemiological studies have demonstrated that administration of various antioxidant compounds can reduce the susceptibility of LDL oxidation and retard the development of atherosclerosis (11–13). However, no attention was paid to the potential benefit of antioxidants to HIV patients with heart disease.

In this review, we propose the hypothesis that treatment of HIV-infected patients with dietary antioxidants would overcome antioxidant deficiencies and reduce the risk of cardiovascular disease. This hypothesis is developed from the following ideas: (1) oxidant stress and loss of antioxidants occur in HIV-infected populations; (2) inflammation and excessive production of RONS may be involved in cardiovascular disease (CVD) in AIDS; (3) both animal and in vitro experiments have shown that antioxidants reduce oxidative stress, improve immune function, and decrease HIV replication; and (4) certain benefits of supplemental intake of antioxidants to reduce the risk of CVD have been demonstrated in uninfected humans.

CVD IN HIV-INFECTED PATIENTS

HIV infection is characterized by an acquired, irreversible immunosuppression that predisposes the patient to multiple opportunistic infections and a progressive dysfunction of multiple organ systems. Cardiac involvement related to HIV infection has been described in many autopsy and echocardiographic series. In one large autopsy series from Europe (14), cardiac disease was the cause of death in 9.1% of HIV-infected patients. In an echocardiographic study, patients with CD4$^+$ cell counts <100/mm^3 displayed higher rates of left ventricular dysfunction (15). Furthermore, it was reported that large amounts of HIV proteins, rather than the whole virus, can be found bound to fibers in heart muscle (16). Other researchers also found the same results by using different methods (17). These studies suggested that the cardiac myocyte is a target for HIV.

The pathological conditions that occur in HIV patients have often been explained in terms of deficient immune surveillance stemming from cytolytic infection of T-helper lymphocytes by HIV. The degree of immunosuppression, as evidenced by decreased CD4 lymphocyte counts, is correlated strongly with myocardial dysfunction (15). On the other hand, based on measurements of lipid peroxidation indices in plasma and expired breath, several studies have now documented an excessive production of RONS during activation of polymorphonuclear leukocytes and macrophages in the HIV-infected population. An elevated concentration in plasma of free radicals means enhanced oxidative stress. Once oxidative stress occurs, accelerated atherosclerosis may be present (18). Furthermore, significant nutritional problems were found in patients in the terminal stages of HIV infection. Previous studies have shown that patients with HIV infection may be deficient in antioxidant micronutrients, including selenium, vitamins A, E, and C, and carotenoids (19,20).

With the rapidly escalating incidence of HIV infection and AIDS, it is anticipated that the incidence of cardiac complications will also increase. Although the traditional heart failure therapies may be effective, alternative approaches must be tried as well to reduce morbidity and mortality associated with CVD in HIV patients.

"OXIDATION THEORY" OF CVD

Atherosclerosis is the underlying cause of most of the morbidity and mortality associated with CVD. The "oxidation theory" of atherosclerosis proposes that oxidation of LDL contributes to atherogenesis. Although little direct evidence for a causative role of "oxidized LDL" in atherogenesis exists, oxidized LDL has exhibited potentially atherogenic activity in several vitro studies, and lipoproteins isolated from atherosclerotic lesions have been found to be oxidized (21).

Each LDL particle contains one apolipoprotein B-100 (apo B) molecule embedded in a mixture of various lipids, including free cholesterol, phospholipids, cholesterol esters (CE), and triglycerides. The modification of LDL to oxidative lipid is thought to be the primary oxidative event preceding and contributing to the modification of apo B and formation of high-uptake LDL. Circulating LDL filters through the arterial intima and into the subintimal space, where it initiates the atherosclerotic process. The immune and inflammatory cells interact with the en dothelium and then migrate into subendothelium, together with some of the modified LDL accumulated in the macrophages. The macrophages become engorged with cholesterol and are transformed into foam cells. In addition, oxidized LDL acts both as an injurious agent and as a chemoattractant that promotes cellular reactions leading to plaque development (22).

Although the development of this oxidation theory was based on studies of uninfected humans and animals, it is very possible that these events are also involved in the mechanisms of CVD in AIDS patients, due to their excessive production of RONS and oxidative stress.

ANTIOXIDANTS AND CVD IN UNINFECTED POPULATIONS

Numerous epidemiological and experimental studies have demonstrated a lower risk of CVD associated with an increased intake of fruits and vegetables. This is reportedly due to the ability of dietary antioxidants to prevent oxidative damage to DNA and lipoproteins. Large trials have focused on vitamin A and beta-carotene, vitamin E, and vitamin C; other dietary antioxidants, such as flavonoids and the trace mineral selenium, also received more attention for their potential health benefit in preventing CVD. Key points from these recent studies are presented here.

Beta-Carotene/Vitamin A

More than 600 carotenoid compounds have been identified; beta-carotene is only one with strong antioxidant properties. More detailed reviews of the epidemiological evidence supporting carotenoids in the prevention of CVD can be found elsewhere, although the evidence from clinical trials does not support a specific benefit from beta-carotene. In the 4-year follow-up of the Health Professional Follow-up Study, men consuming a diet high in total carotenoids had a significantly lower risk of developing coronary heart disease (23). This result was corroborated in the report of a large European collaborative case-control study of adipose carotenoid concentrations (24) and risk of nonfatal myocardial infarction and in a small nested case-control study in the United States (25). In all these studies, the lower risk of CVD was limited to current or former smokers with high levels of carotenoids in adipose tissue or serum. The inverse association between beta-carotene and CVD from observational studies is most plausibly explained by other dietary components found in fruits and vegetables with high carotene concentrations. Beta-carotene is probably important in human health, but not necessarily by acting as an antioxidant.

Vitamin E

Vitamin E is a general name for a group of compounds, of which alpha-tocopherol is the most important free radical scavenger within membrane and lipoproteins. During the past decade, the health effects of vitamin E have been examined in several epidemiological studies, with a clear reduction in risk of CVD being shown in many. These studies include the Health Professional Follow-Up Study (23); Cambridge Heart Antioxidant Study (CHAOS) (26); Antioxidant Vitamins and Coronary Heart Disease in Women (27); Cross-Culture Survey of four European populations (28); Edinburgh Case-Controlled Study (29); and Nurses Health Study in United States (30). Clinical trials have also shown certain benefits from supplemental vitamin E. Furthermore, these studies support the findings on the efficacy of a vitamin E intake above currently recommended amounts (8 to 10 mg alpha-tocopherol equivalents per day). A high intake of vitamin E from foods or supplements may modulate atherogenesis through a variety of mechanisms, including inhibition of LDL oxidation (31), cytokine release, platelet reactivity (32), and smooth muscle cell proliferation (33).

Vitamin C

Although vitamin C has antioxidant properties, the evidence for a cardioprotective effect of vitamin C is weak and inconsistent. Results from cross-cultural studies suggest a strong inverse correlation between plasma levels of vitamin C and cardiovascular motility (34). In another cross-sectional study of diet and carotid wall thickness, men and women above age 55 with lower intake of vitamin C had significantly higher average arterial wall thickness than those with the highest intake (35). Vitamin C may still be important in the prevention of vascular disease among population with near-deficient intake. Recently, vitamin C was considered as a cofactor probably assisting alpha-tocopherol in inhibiting lipid peroxidation by recycling the tocopherol radical (36).

Flavonoids

Flavonoids are a large group of polyphenolic antioxidants that occur naturally in vegetables and fruits and in beverages such as tea and wine. They were first identified as vitamin P, and, along with vitamin C, were found to be important in the maintenance of capillary wall integrity and capillary resistance (37,38). Epidemiological studies have revealed that flavonoid-rich foods correlate with increased longevity and decreased incidence of CVD among the general population (39). Flavonoids are scavengers of superoxide anions, singlet oxygen, and lipid peroxy radicals (40). They can inhibit not only oxidation and cytotoxicity of LDL (41) but also cyclo-oxygenase in vitro, leading to lower platelet aggregation and reduced thrombotic tendencies (42).

Besides all the dietary antioxidants mentioned above, selenium, an essential trace mineral, functions as a cofactor for the antioxidant enzyme glutathione peroxidase. Population studies have shown the risk of CVD to be inversely related to serum levels of selenium (43). In addition, the hormone dehydroepiandrosterone (DHEA) and melatonin (MLT) could also be another source of antioxidants that have been shown to have health benefits (44,45). Recently, an in vivo study of tocopherol-mediated peroxidation and its prevention by coantioxidants indicated that dietary coantioxidants in combination—as opposed to single antioxidants—may be superior in protecting lipoproteins from oxidation (46).

EFFECT OF ANTIOXIDANTS IN HIV INFECTION

The HIV-infected population is known to be oxidatively stressed and deficient in antioxidant micronutrients such as vitamin C, vitamin E, beta-carotene, and selenium. Thus, supplemented antioxidants would be expected to overcome this situation in patients with AIDS. So far, few trials have addressed this issue with regard to humans infected. However, animal studies have demonstrated that supplementation with the antioxidant hormones dehydroepiandrosterone (DHEA) and melatonin (MLT) or with vitamin E could prevent cytokine dysregulation, lipid oxidation, and tissue loss of vitamin E induced by retroviral infection (47,48). In vitro experiments found that the addition of antioxidant vitamins blocked activation of NF-κB and inhibited HIV replication (49). Such knowledge was also supported by a study in human AIDS (19). In an HIV-positive population, daily supplementation of 800 IU vitamin E and 1000 mg vitamin C significantly decreases oxidative stress and produces a trend toward a reduction in HIV viral load.

HYPOTHESIS: ANTIOXIDANTS COULD REDUCE THE RISK OF CVD IN HIV-INFECTED POPULATIONS

Infection with HIV is accompanied by antioxidant deficiency, a decrease in the $CD4^+$ cell count, and the ultimate disruption of immunological function. Elevated levels of interferon gamma lead to the expression of various proinflammatory cytokines and enhanced macrophage capacity to secrete reactive oxygen intermediates. Consequently, excess production of RONS is involved in a series of oxidative reactions in the body. In murine AIDS, increased lipid peroxidation together with decreased phospholipids and elevated cholesterol levels may be responsible for reduced membrane fluidity and elevated membrane viscosity, interfering with signal transduction. Such changes could help explain increased risk for CVD in HIV patients. Thus, it may be that substances that prevent oxidative stress—for example, antioxidants—may slow the process of heart disease and decrease the incidence of CVD among patients with HIV, although few papers have mentioned this to date. Fortunately, some researchers have attempted to confirm the effects of antioxidants on HIV infection. Animal studies seem to clearly demonstrate that supplementation with antioxidants may prevent cytokine dysregulation, lipid oxidation, and tissue vitamin E loss induced by retroviral infection. On the other hand, in uninfected populations, many epidemiological and clinical trails have substantiated the role of dietary antioxidants in the prevention of CVD. From the evidence above, we can propose the hypothesis that dietary antioxidants may also reduce the risk of CVD in AIDS patients. Further studies are required to test this hypothesis. Animal studies alone cannot give us the exact and complete information; we therefore await the confirmation of the benefits of antioxidants to CVD in AIDS populations from epidemiological and clinical trails.

In conclusion, oxidized LDL and oxidative by-products contribute to early atherogenesis, which leads to considerable structural and functional damage to the heart. Antioxidants have been shown to reduce the risk of CVD in most experimental models. Since an excessive production of RONS in the HIV-infected populations and CVD appear to be an important complication of HIV infection, dietary antioxidants combined with traditional therapy would provide an effective way to empower HIV-infected patients to prevent CVD and attain optimal health.

REFERENCES

1. Autran BR, Gorin I, Leibowitch M, et al. AIDS in Haitian women with cardiac Kaposi's sarcoma and Whipple's disease. Lancet 1983; 1:767–768.
2. Patel RC, Frishman WH. Cardiac involvement in HIV infection. Med Clin North Am 1996; 80:1494–1512.
3. Repeto M, Reides C, Carretero MLG, Costa M, Grienmberg G, Llesuy S. Oxidative stress in blood of HIV infected patients. Clin Chim Acta 1996; 225:107–117.
4. Treitinger A, Spada C, Verdi JC, et al. Decreased antioxidant defence in individuals infected by the human immunodeficiency virus. Eur J Clin Invest 2000; 30:454–459.
5. Walmsley SL, Winn LM, Harrison ML, Uetrecht JP, Wells PG. Oxidative stress and thiol depletion in plasma and peripheral blood lymphocytes from HIV-infected patients: toxicological and pathological implications. AIDS 1997; 11:1689–1697.
6. Schwarz KB. Oxidative stress during viral infection: a review. Free Radic Biol Med 1996; 21:641–649.
7. Steinberg D, Pathasarathy S, Carw TE, Khoo JC, Witztum JL. Modifications of low-density lipoprotein that increase its atherogenicity. N Engl J Med 1989; 320:915–924.
8. Steinberg D. Antioxidants and atherosclerosis: a current assessment. Circulation 1991; 84:1420.
9. Meydani M. Vitamin E. Lancet 1995; 345:170–175.
10. Frei B. Natural Antioxidants in Human Health and Disease. San Diego, CA: Academic Press, 1994.
11. Sies H, Stahl W. Vitamins E and C, beta-carotene and other carotenoids as antioxidants. Am J Clin Nutr 1995; 62:1315S.
12. Verlangieri AJ, Bush M. Effects of d-alpha-tocopherol supplementation on experimentaly induced primate atherosclerosis. J Am Coll Nutr 1992; 11:131–138.
13. Sparrow CP, Doebber TW, Olszewski J, Wu MS, Ventre J, Stevens KA, Chao Y. Low-density lipoprotein is protected from oxidation and the progression of atherosclerosis is slowed in cholesterol-fed rabbits by the antioxidant N, N′-diphenyl-phenylenediamine. J Clin Invest 1992; 89:1885–1891.
14. Marche C, Trophilme D, Moyrga R, et al. Cardiac involvement in AIDS: a pathologic study. IV International Conference on AIDS, Stockholm, 1998.
15. Herskowitz A, Vlahov D, Willoughby S, et al. Prevalence and incidence of left ventricular dysfunction in patients with human immunodeficiency virus infection. Am J Cardiol 1993; 71:955–958.
16. Cotton P. AIDS giving rise to cardiac problems JAMA 1990; 263:2149.
17. Grody WW, Cheng L, Lewis W. Infection of the heart by the human immunodeficiency virus. Am J Cardiol 1990; 66:203–206.
18. Das UN, Podma M, Sogar PS, Ramesh G, Koratkar R. Stimulation of free radical

generation in human leukocytes by various agents including tumor necrosis factor is a calmodulin-dependent process. Biochem Biophys Res Commun 1990; 67:1030–1036.

19. Allard JP, Aghdassi E, Chau J, Salit I, Walmsley S. Oxidative stress and plasma antioxidant micronutrients in humans with HIV infection. Am J Clin Nutr 1998; 67:143–147.

20. Patrick L. Nutrients and HIV: Part 1. beta carotene and selenium. Alt Med Rev 1999; 4:403–413.

21. Hoff HF, Hoppe G. Structure of cholesterol-containing particles accumulating in atherosclerotic lesions and the mechanisms of their derivation. Curr Opin Lipidol 1995; 6:317–325.

22. Ziegler EE, Filer LJ. Present Knowledge in Nutrition. Washington, DC: ILSI Press, 1996.

23. Rimm EB, Stampfer MJ, Ascherio A, Giovannucci E, Colditz GA, Willett WC. Vitamin E consumption and the risk of coronary heart disease in men. N Engl J Med 1993; 328:1450–1456.

24. Kardinaal AF, Kok FJ, Ringstad J. Antioxidants in adipose tissue and risk of myocardial infarction. The EURAMIC study. Lancet 1993; 342:1379.

25. Street DA, Comstock GW, Salkeld RM, Schuep W, Klag MJ. Serum antioxidants and myocardial infarction: are low levels of carotenoids and alpha-tocopherol risk factors for myocardial infarction? Circulation 1994; 90:1154.

26. Stephens NG, Parsons A, Schofield PM, Kelly F, Cheeseman K, Mitchinson MJ. Randomised controlled trial of vitamin E in patients with coronary disease: Cambridge Heart Antioxidant Stud (CHAOS). Lancet 1996; 347:781–786.

27. Kushi LH, Folsom AR, Prineas RJ, Mink PJ, Wu Y, Bostick RM. Dietary antioxidant vitamins and death from coronary heart disease in postmenopausal women. N Engl J Med 1996; 334:1156–1162.

28. Riemersma RA, Oliver M, Elton RA, Alfthan G, Vartiainen E, Salo M, Rubba P. Plasma antioxidants and coronary heart disease: vitamin C and E, and selenium. Eur J Clin Nutr 1990; 44:143–150.

29. Riemersma RA, Wood DA, MacIntyre CCH. Risk of angina pectoris and plasma concentrations of vitamin A, C, E and carotene. Lancet 1991; 337:1–5.

30. Stampfer MJ, Hennekens CH, Manson JE, et al. Vitamin E consumption and the risk of coronary disease in women. N Engl J Med 1993; 328:1444–1449.

31. Fuller CJ, Huet BA, Jialal I. Effects of increasing doses of alpha-tocopherol in providing protection of low-density lipoprotein from oxidation. Am J Cardiol 1998; 81:231.

32. Calzada C, Bruckdorfer KR, Rice-Evans CA. The influence of antioxidant nutrients on platelet function in healthy volunteers. Atherosclerosis 1997; 128:97.

33. Boscoboinik D, Szewczyk A, Hensey C, et al. Inhibition of cell proliferation by alpha-tocopherol: role of protein kinase C. J Biol Chem 1991; 266:6188.

34. Huges K, Ong CN. Vitamins, selenium, iron, and coronary heart disease risk in Indians, Malays, and Chinese in Singapore. J Epidemiol Community Health 1998; 52:181.

35. Kritchevsky SB, Shimakawa TS, Tell GS, et al. Dietary antioxidants and carotid artery wall thickness. Circulation 1995; 92:2142–2150.

36. Petsky KL, Frei B. Vitamin C prevents metal ion-dependent initiation and propagation of lipid peroxidation in human low-density lipoprotein. Biochem Biophys Acta 1995; 1257:279.

37. Gabor M. Szent-Gyorgyi and the bioflavonoids: new results and perspectives of pharmacological research into benzo-pyrone derivatives. Commemoration of the 50th anniversary of the award of the Nobel Prize. Progress in Clinical & Biological Research 1988; 280:1–15.

38. Harsteen B. Flavonoids, a class of natural products of high pharmacological potency. Biochemi Pharma 1983; 32:1141–1448.

39. Frankel EN, Kanner J, German JB, Parks E, Kinsella JE. Inhibition of oxidation of human low-density lipoprotein by phenolic substance in red wine. Lancet 1993; 341:454–457.

40. Hertog MGL, Hollman PCH, Katan MB, Kromhout D. Estimation of daily intake of potentially anticarcinogenic flavonoids and their determinants in adults in The Netherlands. Nutr Cancer 1993; 20:21–29.

41. Negre-Salvagyre A, Salvagyre R. Quercetin prevents the cytotoxicity of oxidized low-density by macrophages. Free Radic Biol Med 1992; 12:101–106.

42. Laughton MJ, Evans PJ, Morony MA, Hoult JRS, Halliwell B. Inhibition of mammalian 5-lipoxygenase and cyclo-oxygenase by flavonoids and phenolic dietary additives: relationship to antioxidant activity and to ion-reducing ability. Biochem Pharm 1991; 42:1673–1681.

43. Halbert SC. Diet and nutrition in primary care. Primary Care 1997; 24:825–843.

44. Aragno M, Tamagno E, Boccuzz G, et al. Dehydroepiandrosterone pretreatment protects rats against the pro-oxidant and necrogenic effects of carbon tetrachloride. Biochem Pharmacol 1993; 46:168.

45. Pieri C, Marra M, Moroni P, Recchioni R, Marchesell F. Melatonin: a peroxyl radical scavenger more effective than vitamin E. Life Sci 1994; 55:271.

46. Upston JM, Terentis AC, Stocker R. Tocopherol-mediated peroxidation of lipoproteins: implications for vitamin E as a potential antiatherogenic supplement. FASEB J 1999; 13:977–994.

47. Wang Y, Huang DS, Liang B, Watson RR. Nutritional status and immune responses in mice with murine AIDS are normalized by vitamin E supplementation. J Nutr 1994; 124:2024–2032.

48. Araghi-Niknam M, Zhang Z, Jiang S, Call O, Eskelson CD, Watson RR. Cytokine dysregulation and increased oxidation is prevented by dehydroepiandrosterone in mice infected with murine leukemia retrovirus. Proc Soc Exp Biol Med 1997; 216:386–391.

49. Allard JP, Aghdassi E, Chau J, et al. Effects of vitamin E and C supplementation on oxidative stress and viral load in HIV-infected subjects. AIDS 1998; 12:1653–1659.

18

Antioxidant Vitamins and Antiretroviral Therapy During HIV Infection: Effects on Oxidative Damage

Jin Zhang
Brigham and Women's Hospital and Harvard Medical School, Boston, Massachusetts, U.S.A.

Ronald Ross Watson
University of Arizona, Tucson, Arizona, U.S.A.

INTRODUCTION

Micronutrient deficiencies and early immune responses such as activation of phagocytes and microphages in human immunodeficiency virus (HIV) infection are responsible for an increased oxidative stress and a weakened antioxidant defense in HIV patients. The oxidative stress associated with HIV infection is important for the progression of the disease because the generation of reactive oxygen species (ROS) activates the nuclear transcription factor (NF-κB), which is obligatory for HIV replication. Antioxidants are known to improve immune function and inhibit activation of NF-κB, so they may play important role in HIV prevention. In a murine AIDS (MAIDS) model, vitamin E and multiple antioxidant vitamins were showed to improve immune function and to inhibit activation of NF-κB. EPC-K1, a phosphodiester compound of vitamin E and vitamin C, is considered one of the inhibitory agents of NF-κB.

Azidothymidine (AZT) is a potent inhibitor of the replication of the HIV virus at the point of reverse transcription. The incorporation of AZT monophosphate into viral DNA results in premature termination of DNA synthesis. The major limitation in the use of AZT is the occurrence of severe side effects resulting from mitochondrial myopathy. This might be due to oxidative damage to mitochondria. Mitochondrial myopathy may affect a number of organs, including the heart, liver, muscle, brain, and so forth. In animal studies, dietary supplementation with vitamins C and E at high doses protected against oxidative damage caused by AZT to skeletal muscle and liver mitochondria. The pathogenesis of heart disease in AIDS patients is to a certain extent related to the toxicity of antiretroviral chemotherapy. Studies that related AZT therapy to ultrastructural changes in striated muscle also suggested a potential for cardiotoxicity of AZT, since the structures of cardiac and skeletal muscle are similar in many ways (1). However, preclinical and clinical pharmacological studies have focused on AZT's efficacy in inhibiting retroviruses rather than on its cardiac toxicity. As clinical experience grew, evidence for the toxicity of AZT to striated muscle became more abundant (2). Yet no data were presented on whether antioxidant vitamins can protect the heart against AZT-induced myopathy.

Our hypotheses are the following: (1) AZT-antiviral therapy can work simultaneously with antioxidant vitamins for more efficient treatment for HIV and (2) antioxidant vitamins may have cardioprotective effects on AZT treatment in HIV-infected patients.

DISTURBANCE OF THE ANTIOXIDANT DEFENSE IN HIV

HIV infection continues to increase worldwide, with over 90% of new cases occurring in developing countries, where nutritional problems are commonplace and expensive drugs are generally unavailable (3). Epidemiological and clinical evidence indicates that micronutrient deficiencies are common during HIV infection. Insufficient dietary intake, malabsorption, diarrhea, impaired storage, and altered metabolism of micronutrients can contribute to the development of micronutrient deficiencies (4). Low plasma or serum levels of vitamins A, E, B_6, B_{12}, and C, carotenoids, selenium (Se) and zinc (Zn) are common in many HIV-infected populations (4). Furthermore, early immune responses to HIV infections contribute to ROS production. Activated macrophages and neutrophils generate ROS such as superoxide radicals (O_2^-), hydrogen peroxide (H_2O_2), and hydroxyl radicals (HO). These ROS can induce cellular injury and lysis because free radicals have the potential to cause oxidation of nucleic acids, chromosomal breaks, peroxidation of lipids in cell membranes, and damage to collagen, proteins, and enzymes. ROS can also damage bystander cells and induce pathology. Fortunately, the generation of ROS by immune effector cells or injured tissue is balanced by the antioxidant defense system. As the balance between pro-oxidants and antioxidants is upset and there is overproduction of ROS and resulting pathology, the condition referred to as oxidative stress arises (5), along with HIV infection. Furthermore, the micronutrient deficiencies mentioned above may contribute to the pathogenesis of HIV infection through increased oxidative stress and compromised immunity.

Accumulating evidence suggests HIV-infected patients are under chronic oxidative stress. Perturbations to the antioxidant defense system—including changes in levels of ascorbic acid, tocopherols, carotenoids, selenium, superoxide dismutase, and glutathione—have been observed in the tissues of these patients (6). Elevated serum levels of hydroperoxides and malondialdehyde have also been noted and are indicative of oxidative stress during HIV infection (7). Indications of oxidative stress are observed in asymptomatic HIV-infected patients early in the course of the disease. Cells are protected against oxidative damage by defense systems, including enzymes (superoxide dismutase, glutathione peroxidase, and catalase) and other molecules (e.g., ascorbate, glutathione, alpha-tocopherol and beta-carotene) that interact directly with reactive species to neutralize them. Among the antioxidant enzymes, superoxide dismutase (SOD) acts by dismutating the superoxide anion radical to hydrogen peroxide, which is scavenged by glutathione peroxidase (GPx) and catalase (8). One study has shown that the activity of SOD of blood plasma and mononuclear cells is decreased in the course of HIV infection and that SOD activity is directly correlated with the number of CD4+ lymphocytes in peripheral blood. However, in another study, superoxide dismutase activity of erythrocytes was increased by 24% in asymptomatic HIV infection and 65% in patients with AIDS ($p < 0.05$). In contrast, there was no difference in catalase activity between patients and controls. Glutathione was decreased by 20% in patients with asymptomatic of infection and by 32% in AIDS patients ($p < 0.05$). Total plasma antioxidant capacity was increased by 30 and 57% for the asymptomatic and AIDS patient groups, respectively ($p < 0.05$). These data indicate that the erythrocytes' oxidative stress is associated with the progressive development of HIV disease (9). Further work is necessary to establish the full extent of altered defense system enzymes and to reconcile these apparently conflicting observations.

Oxidative stress may contribute to several aspects of HIV disease pathogenesis, including viral replication, inflammatory response, decreased immune cell proliferation, loss of immune function, apoptosis, chronic weight loss, and increased sensitivity to drug toxicities (7). ROS may potentially be involved in the pathogenesis of HIV infection through direct effects of cells and through interactions with NF-κB and activation of HIV replication. NF-κB is a transcriptional promotor of proteins, which are involved in the inflammatory response and the acute-phase response. NF-κB is bound to factor I κB in the cytoplasm in its inactive form, but various factors, such as tumor necrosis factor alpha (TNF-α) and reactive oxygen intermediates (ROI), can cause the release of NF-κB from factor I κB, and NF-κB translocates to the nucleus and binds to the HIV long terminal repeat (LTR) enhancer element to activate HIV gene expression (10).

ANTIOXIDANT VITAMIN SUPPLEMENTS IN AIDS

There have been few clinical trials of micronutrient supplementation during HIV infection. Most of the studies consist of pilot interventions with single micronutrients. A reduction in oxidative stress and an apparent decrease in viral load were noted in a clinical trial of vitamins E (800 mg/day) and C (1 g/day) in HIV-infected adults in Toronto (11). Diverse antioxidants inhibit HIV-LTR transactivation by blocking NF-κB activation in lymphoblastoid T and monocytic cell lines (12). Ascorbic acid reduced the levels of extracellular reverse transcriptase activity and the expression of p24 antigen in an HIV-infected T-lymphocyte cell line (13). Researchers examined the virological and immunological effects of antioxidant combination treatment for 6 days with high doses of N-acetylcysteine (NAC) and vitamin C in 8 patients with HIV infection (7). The following parameters were assayed before, during, and after antioxidant treatment: HIV RNA plasma levels; numbers of CD4+, CD8+, and CD14+ leukocytes in blood; plasma thiols; intracellular glutathione redox status in CD4+ lymphocytes and CD14+ monocytes; lymphocyte proliferation; lymphocyte apoptosis and plasma levels of tumor necrosis factor alpha (TNF-α); soluble TNF-α receptors and neopterin in plasma. No significant changes in HIV RNA plasma levels or CD4+ lymphocyte counts in blood were noted during antioxidant treatment in the patient group. However, in the 5 patients with the most advanced immunodeficiency (CD4+ lymphocyte counts $< 200 \times 10^6 \, L^{-1}$), a significant rise in CD4+ lymphocyte count, a reduction in HIV

RNA plasma level of 0.8 log, enhanced lymphocyte proliferation, and an increased level of intracellular glutathione in CD4+ lymphocytes were found. No change in lymphocyte apoptosis was noted. These data suggest that short-term, high-dose combination treatment with NAC and vitamin C in patients with HIV infection and advanced immunodeficiency leads to immunological and virological effects that might be of therapeutic value.

LP-BM5 retrovirus induces murine AIDS (MAIDS), characterized by spleno-megaly, lymphadenopathy, T-cell dysfunction, and cytokine dysregulation. These symptoms resemble those of human AIDS. In the MAIDS studies, researchers investigated the inhibitory effect of vitamin E (VE; D-tocopherol acetate) on the development of LP-BM5 retrovirus–induced MAIDS in comparison with AZT (14). Both a high-VE diet and AZT treatment significantly inhibited the increase in spleen weight following the development of MAIDS. The lipid peroxide levels in spleno-cytes of infected mice were lowered by a high-VE diet or AZT treatment. In addition, high-VE diet and AZT treatment enhanced interferon gamma (IFN-γ) and dimin-ished TNF-α production from splenic lymphocytes of infected mice. In splenic lymphocytes of infected mice, the expression of NF-κB was strongly inhibited in both the cytoplasma and the nucleus by a high-VE diet, whereas AZT treatment had almost no effect. These results suggest that vitamin E inhibits the development of MAIDS through the inhibition of NF-κB expression, which mechanism was different from that of AZT.

Previous studies done in our research group showed that supplementation of multiple antioxidants significantly normalized cytokine production by T-helper cells (Th1 and Th2) and restored T- and B-cell proliferation in murine AIDS. It also restored hepatic vitamin E levels, which had been reduced by retroviral infection. Multiple antioxidants were shown to be more effective at restoring or maintaining the immune system than was supplementation with vitamin E alone. These results suggest that multiple antioxidants may have other health benefits beside their antioxidant activities (15). Hirano and coworkers investigated the effect of a phosphodiester compound of vitamins E and C (chemical name, L-ascorbic acid 2-[3,4-dihydro-2,5,7,8-tetramethyl-2-(4,8,12-trimethyltridecyl)-2H-1-benzopyran-6-hydrogen phosphate] potassium salt; code name, EPC-K1), on NF-κB activity in human cultured astrocytoma cells T98G (16). EPC-K1 was shown to inhibit both DNA binding activity and transactivation of NF-κB in a dose-dependent manner. The suppressive effect of EPC-K1 was stronger than that of either vitamin E or vitamin C. Moreover, EPC-K1 had a suppressive effect on the activation of the HIV-1 promoter. It is known that the administration of an optimal combination of vitamins E and C can substantially enhance tissue protection against oxidative stress (17–19). Wefers and Sies demonstrated that vitamin C could act as an antioxidant or as a pro-oxidant in microsomal lipid peroxidation and vitamin E played an out-standing role in switching vitamin C from a potentially damaging agent to a protective agent (19). Vitamin C, therefore, may contribute to anti-NF-κB action of EPC-K1, not by itself but in conjunction with vitamin E.

AZT IN HIV THERAPY AND AZT-INDUCED OXIDATIVE DAMAGE

AZT is a potent inhibitor of the replication of HIV and one of the drugs of choice for the treatment of AIDS (20). Reverse transcriptase (RT) catalyzes the formation of a

DNA copy of the viral RNA genetic information. It is possible to inhibit the action of RT using drugs. AZT is one of the earliest and best known of these drugs; it was approved under the brand name Retrovir by the U.S. Food and Drug Administration (FDA) in 1987. AZT functions as an analogue for thymidine, one of the nucleotide building blocksof DNA. Because AZT has the same shape as thymidine, it can be incorporated into the developing nucleic acid in place of a thymidine molecule. The phosphate group attached to thymidine or AZT forms a bond with the 3'-OH group of the proceeding nucleotide in the developing DNA chain. When thymidine is incorporated into the DNA chain, its 3'-OH becomes the binding site for the next nucleotide's phosphate group. However, AZT lacks the -OH functional group that is necessary to form a bond with the next nucleotide; in its place is an azido $(-N_3)$ group. Therefore, no additional nucleotides can be added once AZT is incorporated into the DNA chain. Hence, the incorporation of AZT into viral DNA results in reverse transcription termination. However, the major limitation in the use of AZT is the occurrence of severe side effects (21). AIDS patients who receive long-term therapy with AZT frequently suffer from toxic mitochondrial (mt) myopathy. This has been attributed to damage in mitochondria and to mtDNA depletion (21). mtDNA depletion in muscles is probably due to the AZT-induced inhibition of DNA polymerase gamma, which is responsible for the replication of mtDNA. Moreover, decreased mtDNA and mt polypeptide synthesis were found in vitro (22). A single animal study in 1991 proposed that AZT causes oxidation of deoxyguanosine to yield 8-oxo-7,8-dihydro-2'-deoxyguanosine (8-oxo-dG) in DNA from the mitochondria (21). The role of mtDNA in cell physiology and medicine was emphasized previously (23). Manifestations of mt diseases are thought to be due, at least in part, to increased free radical formation (23,24). The work done by the researchers shows that AZT causes oxidative damage to the mitochondria of skeletal muscle and that this kind of damage can be prevented by administration of supranutritional doses of antioxidant vitamins. Another study done by the same group of researchers shows that mouse liver mtDNA treated with AZT had 40% more of the oxidized, mutagenic nucleoside 8-oxo-dG than untreated controls (25). This oxidative damage to mtDNA is caused by a significant increase (of over 240%) in peroxide production by liver mitochondria from AZT-treated mice, which was prevented by dietary administration of vitamins C and E. It is proposed that vitamin E, which was added extracellularly, accumulated in the plasma membrane, whereas vitamin E acetate traveled through the cytoplasm where it was deesterified to the active form of vitamin E, which may reach mitochondria, where it scavenges mitochondrial radical intermediates and reduced the production of ROI (26). And vitamin C showed cooperative effects with vitamin E as well a role in preventing oxidative damage to mitochondrial DNA. Other related research shows consistent results in terms of the oxidative damage to mitochondrial DNA. The short-term cardiac side effects of AZT were studied in rats to elucidate the biochemical events contributing to the development of AZT-induced cardiomyopathy (27). The AZT treatment of rats significantly increased ROS and peroxynitrite formation in heart tissues and induced single-strand DNA breaks. Lipid peroxidation and oxidation of cellular proteins were increased as well. Thus, ROS-mediated oxidative damage, in part, plays a role in the development of AZT-induced cardiomyopathy in animal models. These findings suggest that ROS-mediated processes can be important factors in the development of myopathy and cardiomyopathy in AZT-treated AIDS patients. Human trials in this area have been limited. A trial done by Asuncion et al.

indicates that asymptomatic HIV-infected patients treated with AZT have a higher urinary excretion (355 ± 100 pmol/kg/day) of 8-oxo-dG (a marker of oxidative damage to DNA) than untreated controls (asymptomatic HIV-infected patients) (182 ± 29 pmol/kg/day) (21). This was prevented (110 ± 79 pmol/kg/day) by simultaneous oral treatment with AZT plus antioxidant vitamins C and E (ascorbate 1 g/day, α-tocopherol 0.6 g/day). However, so far there are no data to support the value of antioxidant vitamins in the prevention cardiomyopathy induced by AZT.

SUMMARY

Oxidative stress in HIV-positive subjects is fairly common, indicated by the increase in lipid peroxidation, lower plasma concentrations of antioxidant micronutrients, and altered antioxidant enzyme activities. Antioxidant vitamins as a complementary therapy have shown positive effects in HIV treatment, although human trials are still in process. On the one hand, the combination of different antiretroviral therapies may have an impact on increasing resistance to gastrointestinal microsporidiosis and cryptosporidiosis (28). Thus, micronutrient supplementation has largely been adapted to the sphere of complementary therapies in industrialized countries (29). Billions of dollars are spent each year on vitamin and mineral supplements in industrialized countries, and many individuals with HIV infection take such supplements. However, there are no clear data showing that such health expenditures are worthwhile.

On the other hand, AZT treatment is helpful in terminating retroviral transcription. But once AZT ceases being effective and the reverse transcription starts, the replication of HIV virus will be beyond control. Supplementation of antioxidants at this point can inhibit the formation of ROS and block activation of NF-κB, so that HIV gene expression can be inhibited. Additionally, antioxidant vitamins may attenuate AZT toxicity to the mitochondria by eliminating ROS production, which

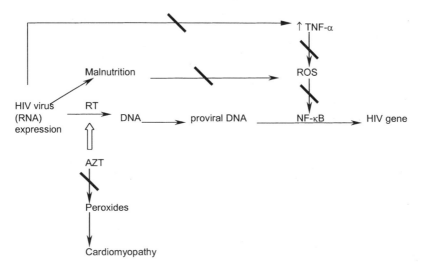

Figure 1 Mechanisms of blockage whereby antioxidant vitamins inhibit HIV replication and AZT-induced cardiomyopathy. Possible blocking sites are shown by the symbol \.

offers a new strategy for the prevention of AZT-induced cardiomyopathy in HIV patients. Animal studies are strongly encouraged to prove this hypothesis, and human trials could then be conducted sequentially (Fig. 1).

REFERENCES

1. Lewis W, Papoian T, Gonzalez B, Louie H, Kelly DP, Payne RM, Grody WW. Mitochondrial ultrastructural and molecular changes induced by zidovudine in rat hearts. Lab Invest 1991; 65:228–236.
2. Gerschenson M, Erhart SW, Paik CY, St Claire MC, Nagashima K, Skopets B, Harbaugh SW, Harbaugh JW, Quan W, Poirier MC. Fetal mitochondrial heart and skeletal muscle damage in *Erythrocebus patas* monkeys exposed in utero to 3'-azido-3'-deoxythymidine. AIDS Res Hum Retrovir 2000; 16:635–644.
3. Quinn TC. Global burden of HIV pandemic. Lancet 1996; 348:99–106.
4. Semba RD, Tang AM. Micronutrients and the pathogenesis of human immunodeficiency virus infection. Br J Nutr 1999; 81:181–189.
5. Baruchel S, Waniberg MA. The role of oxidative stress in disease progression in individuals infected by the human immunodeficiency virus. J Leuk Biol 1992; 52:111–114.
6. Allard JP, Aghdassi E, Chau J, Salit I, Walmsley S. Oxidative stress and plasma antioxidant micronutrients in humans with HIV infection. Am J Clin Nutr 1998; 67:143–147.
7. Muller F, Svardal AM, Nordoy I, Berge RK, Aukrust P, Froland SS. Virological and immunological effects of antioxidant treatment in patients with HIV infection. Eur J Clin Invest 2000; 30:905–914.
8. Sies H. Biochemistry of oxidative stress. Angew Chem Int Ed Engl 1986; 25:1058–1071.
9. Repetto M, Reides C, Gomez Carretero ML, Costa M, Griemberg G, Llesuy S. Oxidative stress in blood of HIV infected patients. Clin Chim Acta 1996; 255:107–117.
10. Schreck R, Rieber P, Baeuerle PA. Reactive oxygen intermediates as apparently widely used messengers in the activation of the NF-κB transcription factor and HIV-1. EMBO J 1991; 10:2247–2258.
11. Allard JP, Aghdassi E, Chau J, Tam C, Kovacs CM, Salit IE, Walmsley SL. Effects of vitamin E and C supplementation on oxidative stress and viral load in HIV-infected subjects. AIDS 1998; 12:1653–1659.
12. Israel N, Gougeror-Pocidalo MA, Aillet F, Virelizier JL. Redox status of cells influences constitutive or reduced NF-κB translocation and HIV long terminal repeat activity in human T and monocytic cell lines. J Immunol 1992; 149:3386–3393.
13. Harakeh S, Jarriwalla RJ, Pauling L. Suppression of human immunodeficiency virus replication by ascorbate in chronically and acute infected cells. Proc Natl Acad Sci USA 1990; 87:1745–1749.
14. Hamada M, Yamamoto S, Kishino Y, Moriguchi S. Vitamin E suppresses the development of murine MAIDS through the inhibition of nuclear factor-kappa B expression. Nutr Res 2000; 20:1163–1171.
15. Lee J, Jiang S, Liang B, Paula I, Zhang Z, David S, Watson RR. Antioxidant supplementation in prevention and treatment of immune dysfunction and oxidation induced by murine AIDS in old mice. Nutr Res 1998; 18:327–339.
16. Hirano F, Tanaka H, Miura T, Hirano Y, Okamoto K, Makino Y, Makino I. Inhibition of NF-κB–dependent transcription of human immunodeficiency virus 1 promoter by a phosphodiester compound of vitamin C and vitamin E, EPC-K1. Immunopharmacology 1998; 39:31–38.

17. McCay PB. Vitamin E; Interactions with free radicals and ascorbate. Annu Rev Nutr 1985; 55:323–340.
18. Chen LH, Thacker RR. Effect of ascorbic acid and vitamin E on biochemical changes associated with vitamin E deficiency in rats. Int J Vitam Nutr Res 1987; 57:385–390.
19. Wefers H, Sies H. The protection by ascorbate and glutatione against lipid peroxidation is dependent on vitamin E. Eur J Biochem 1988; 174:353–357.
20. Rigourd M, Lanchy JM, Le Grice SF, Ehresmann B, Ehresmann C, Marquet R. Inhibition of the initiation of HIV-1 reverse transcription by 3′-azido-3′-deoxythymidine. Comparison with elongation. J Biol Chem 2000; 275:26944–26951.
21. de la Asuncion JG, del Olmo ML, Sastre J, Millan A, Pellin A, Pallardo FV, Vina J. AZT treatment induces molecular and ultrastructural oxidative damage to muscle mitochondria. Prevention by antioxidant vitamins. J Clin Invest 1998; 102:4–9.
22. Lewis W, Gonzalez B, Chomyn A, Paporan T. Zidovudine induces molecular, biochemical, and ultrastructural changes in rat skeletal muscle mitochondria. J Clin Invest 1992; 89:1354–1360.
23. Luft R. The development of mitochodrial medicine. Proc Natl Acad Sci USA 1994; 91:8731–8738.
24. Johns DR. Mitochondrial DNA and disease. N Engl J Med 1995; 333:636–644.
25. de la Asuncion JG, del Olmo ML, Sastre J, Pallardo FV, Vina J. Zidovudine (AZT) causes an oxidation of mitochondrial DNA in mouse liver. J Hepatology 1999; 29:985–987.
26. Packer L, Suzuki YJ. Vitamin E and alpha-lipoate: Role in antioxidant recycling and activation of the NF-κB transcription factor. Mol Aspects Med 1993; 14:229–239.
27. Szabados E, Fischer GM, Toth K, Csete B, Nemeti B, Trombitas K, Habon T, Endrei D, Sumegi B. Role of reactive oxygen species and poly-ADP-ribose polymerase in the development of AZT-induced cardiomyopathy in rat. Free Radic Biol Med 1999; 26:309–317.
28. Carr A, Marriott D, Field A, Vasak E, Cooper DA. Treatment of HIV-1-associated microsporidosis and cryptosporidiosis with combination antiviral therapy. Lancet 1998; 351:256–261.
29. Kotler DP. Antioxidant therapy and HIV infection. Am J Clin Nutr 1998; 67:7–9.

19

Vitamin E Retards Heart Disease in AIDS Patients

Jennifer J. Ravia and Ronald Ross Watson
University of Arizona, Tucson, Arizona, U.S.A.

INTRODUCTION

When the disease now known as acquired immunodeficiency syndrome (AIDS) was first isolated in the early 1980s, little was known about its cause or subsequent effects. The AIDS disease and the virus that causes it, human immunodeficiency virus (HIV), have since been extensively studied. The major debilitating effects of the virus are due to opportunistic infections. While many organ systems sustain damage caused by opportunistic agents, the heart was one of the last to be studied. In many cases, other disorder will give rise to severe symptoms and cause death before the cardiac region has been investigated. In recent years, it has been determined that the number of AIDS and HIV patients suffering from cardiac disorders is larger that previously thought and cardiovascular disease (CVD) is typically referred to as common. Because there is no cure for HIV infection, treatments are based on the alleviation of symptoms and the prolongation of life. If cardiac problems in HIV patients can be successfully treated, their expectancies may increase.

In patients without AIDS/HIV, many treatments exist for preventing or treating heart disease. One of the most popular nutritional therapies is the supplementation of vitamin E. This approach has been shown to be advantageous in patients at high risk for CVD. Therefore, supplementation of vitamin E in AIDS and HIV patients is worth investigating to determine whether it can have a positive effect.

CARDIAC DISEASE IN AIDS/HIV PATIENTS

Although heart disease can and will affect patients at all stages of HIV infection, cardiac problems are more prevalent in patients with advanced AIDS (1). For example, cardiac involvement in male homosexuals was found to be greater during the later stages of the disease and are usually due to an opportunistic infection (3). Heart conditions are more common in AIDS patients who abuse injection drugs, though the side effects typically associated with these drugs are usually within normal limits (1). While all forms of cardiac disorders have somewhat specific symptoms, a differential diagnosis is important because the symptoms of pulmonary infections can mimic those of heart disease (1). Treatment of the appropriate disorder is always of importance, but it becomes a more crucial issue in the AIDS patient. Treatment of the wrong disorder due a misdiagnosis can potentially cause irreversible harm to the immunocompromised patient.

Pericardial Disease

Pericardial disease in AIDS patients can be found in chronic, acute, or asymptomatic stages and can be caused by viral, fungal, and bacterial agents (1). As many as 20 to 40% of AIDS patients have pericardial effusion, but without symptoms (1,2). Current research seeks to determine whether pericardial disease can be caused by AIDS alone or if it is always secondary to an opportunistic infection. A cardiac tamponade is compression of the heart as a result of an effusion, or escape of fluid, in the pericardium. It is not always possible to determine the causes of these effusions and tamponades; however, low pressure tamponades are characteristic in AIDS pericardial disease when the patient is dehydrated or cachectic (1,2). In this phenomenon, the lower blood volume can decrease right ventricular pressure during the filling stage of the cardiac cycle. This disruption of the cardiac cycle allows a small effusion to lead to a significant tamponade (1). The preferred therapy of this condition is immediate catherization to drain the excess fluid.

Myocardial Disease

Myocardial disease in the AIDS patient occurs in four different forms (1):

1. Myocarditis
2. Noninflammatory myocardial necrosis
3. Dilated cardiomyopathy
4. Infiltrative myocardial disease

Myocarditis results from invasive infections or lymphocytic infiltration and is found in up to one-third of all AIDS patients (1,2). Because the HIV virus as well as its proteins have been found within the cardiac tissue in AIDS patients regardless of their cardiac status, it can be concluded that myocarditis can be caused by the HIV virus (2). Noninflammatory myocardial necrosis is due to long-term physiological stress, which leads to the increased secretion of catecholamines. This increase in the levels of catecholamines leads to the degradation of myocardial tissue, but without inflammation (1). This is of interest because the typical response to an increased catecholamine level would be inflammation. In dilated cardiomyopathy, the heart simultaneously becomes dilated in all four chambers, thus disturbing the heart's ability to beat properly. While this condition may be caused by myocarditis, it is thought that the HIV gene can also alter the surfaces of cardiac muscle fibers (1,2). This adjustment leads to the formation of cardiac autoantibodes, which have the ability to cause an autoimmune attack within the body. In vivo, selenium and thiamine deficiencies are thought to be secondarily involved in the dilated cardio-myopathy (1). Furthermore, selenium supplementation has been found to improve cardiac function in pediatric AIDS patients (2). This form of myocarditis generally occurs in the later stages of infection, but ventricular decline has not been found to be related to a decrease in the CD4 cell count (2). Many drugs used to alleviate the manifestations of AIDS can have side effects that may lead to dilated cardiomyopathy as well as atherosclerosis or atherothrombosis (2). Therefore, agents such as vitamin E, that can decrease the risk of myocardial infarction, should be investigated for their possible use in the treatment of cardiomyopathy (2). Infiltrative myocardial disease is most likely the result of a neoplasia or lymphoma taking over portions of the cardiac tissue.

Endocardial Disease

Endocardial disease occurs in three different forms: Marantic or nonbacterial thrombotic, Bacterial, and Fungal (1).

The most common endocardial lesion in AIDS patients is marantic endocarditis, a nonbacterial thrombotic endocardial disease (1). Patients with this disorder usually present with fibrous clumps of red blood cells and platelets that form into a thrombus and adhere to the cardiac valves (2). Marantic endocarditis can become infected and is usually associated with a hypercoagulation disorder (1). This condition is often found in patients over the age of 50 (2). This is of interest because the same age group is typically deficient in serum vitamin E levels, which would normally work to prevent the formation of thrombotic clots. Bacterial endocarditis is more prevalent in immunocompromised patients. Fungal endocarditis is often secondary to systemic fungal disorders (1).

ECHOCARDIOGRAPHY

Echocardiography has proved to be very useful for the early detection of cardiac abnormalities. Echocardiographic abnormalities correlate strongly with those patients who have decreased CD4 counts. Therefore echocardiography should be useful in determining who is at risk for developing cardiac disease (3). Because heart problems generally occur late in the course of AIDS, treatment of the infections and virus early on is better than late treatment of the heart (3). From autopsy studies, lymphocytic myocarditis has been found in all patients with previously abnormal echocardiographs (2). It may therefore be possible, via routine echocardiographs to detect cardiac problems before they develop into deadly illnesses (3).

PROGNOSIS AND CARDIAC DISEASE IN THE AIDS PATIENT

Heart disease in AIDS/HIV patients has also been studied as a prognostic factor. Although many cases of effusion may resolve spontaneously, a long-term left ventricular dysfunction typically indicates a poor prognosis (4). Left ventricular dysfunction could possibly explain the decreased survival rate in AIDS patients with pericardial effusions (4). Pericardial effusions are typically associated with decreased CD4 cell counts. This, and the fact that pericardial effusion is often caused by agents appearing in the later stages of the infection, suggests that the presence of pericardial effusion may act as a marker of the stage of disease (2). While prognosis is not affected by the size of pericardial effusions, it is affected by their presence (2). Although cardiac malfunction has not been implicated as a definitive cause of death in AIDS patients, the survival time for those without cardiac problems may be longer than for those with cardiac abnormalities (5).

VITAMIN E AND HEART DISEASE

Vitamin E has long been thought to have beneficial effects in relation to heart disease. Vitamin E supplementation has been found to prevent the progression of atherosclerosis to myocardial infarction (MI). Thus, those patients who previously presented with plaque accumulation in the arteries can reduce their risk of MI by supplementing with vitamin E (6).

The antioxidant properties of vitamin E allow it to function as a free radical scavenger and thus to reduce plaque formation. When LDLs become oxidized, the fragments are used as constituents of foam cell formation. The foam cells go on to contribute to the fatty streak in the arterial lumen that is the beginning of atherosclerosis. Free radicals, which destroy cell membranes and oxidize various compounds, are allowed to initiate oxidation when available vitamin E begins to decline (7). With enough vitamin E available, the foam cells cannot proliferate. Supplementation of vitamin E has also been shown to reduce the adhesion of immune cells such as monocytes to the endothelial cell wall in the aorta as well as other vessels (8).

Vitamin E helps to maintain the vasodilatory effects of heart vessels by inhibiting PGE_2 synthesis and increasing PGI_2 synthesis (7). The prostaglandin PGI_2 is known for vasodilatory and antiaggregating properties (9). Thus, supplementation of vitamin E promotes vasodilation. Inflammatory cytokines produced by the endothelial aortic cells can be decreased in production with the supplementation of vitamin E. Protein kinase C stimulation in platelet cells encourages aggregation but can be inhibited by vitamin E (8). The collective actions of vitamin E serve to inhibit the formation of blood clots as well as fatty streaks within the vessels. These effects have been shown to be important in the prevention of heart disease and atherosclerosis. Although vitamin E supplementation is beneficial, the results appear to be preventive, not curative.

FACTORS THAT INFLUENCE VITAMIN E STATUS

Several factors can influence the vitamin E status of an individual. Serum vitamin E levels have been recorded to be lower in subjects with cardiovascular disease as compared to healthy subjects (10). Age can also affect vitamin E status, which correlates with the fact that cardiovascular disease develops over time. This is further supported by the fact that the serum vitamin E levels of patients over the age of 51 were lower than those of patients under the age of 40 (10). Activity level appears to have some influence on vitamin E status as well. While average exercise does not affect the levels of serum vitamin E, individuals with cardiovascular endurance training sustained higher levels of vitamin E than at baseline (11). This suggests that there may be an inverse relationship between heart disease and endurance training.

VITAMIN E AND IMMUNE RESPONSE

Vitamin E has been found to be immunoenhancing by increasing lymphocyte count, natural killer (NK) cell activity, and phagocytosis (8). This increases the body's ability to ward off infection. Protein kinase C, when stimulated by agents such as surface proteins on the HIV virus, can transfer the HIV replication state from latent to active as well as stimulate upregulation of HIV. Vitamin E has the ability to inhibit protein kinase C, which may decrease viral replication.

One of the characteristics of the HIV virus is to decrease T-cell activity. This action can be inhibited by vitamin E (12). Arachadonic acid metabolites have also been shown to cause a decrease in T-cell division and the activity of NK cells (12). These metabolites can be rendered inactive with the antioxidant effects of vitamin E.

Prostaglandin synthesis is also influenced by vitamin E. Mice supplemented with vitamin E showed lower levels of PGE_2 than nonsupplemented mice. Prostaglandin E_2 has a positive effect on the immune system; thus vitamin E can stimulate the immune response by inhibiting PGE_2 regulation (12). Studies of murine vitamin E supplementation have shown that such supplementation led to higher interleukin-2 (IL-2) activity than in controls.

IL-2 is a cytokine or protein signal also known as T-cell growth factor. The IL-2 cytokine stimulates production of T cells, thus increasing the collective ability of the immune system to fight infection (9). Cytokines have positive regulatory effects on B and T immune cells as well. This further supports the immunostimulatory effects of vitamin E.

VITAMIN E AND IgE IN THE AIDS/HIV PATIENT

The gastrointestinal tract is often compromised in the AIDS patient, which may lead to a decrease in vitamin E absorption as well as anorexia and cachexia (8). The vitamin E intakes of AIDS patients often falls below 50% of the recommended daily allowance (RDA). When tested for serum vitamin E levels, HIV-positive groups had lower plasma vitamin E than HIV-negative groups. Immunoglobulin E or IgE is an antibody that participates in the immune response to fight the HIV/AIDS virus. Although the mechanism of action is unclear, IgE levels are influenced by vitamin E in the body (13). During the initial stages of HIV infection, high levels of plasma IgE are detectable before CD4 cell count begins to fall (13). As the infection progresses, the IgE levels continue to rise. IgE is unique in that other immunoglobulins do not increase in this manner. Therefore, IgE may be used as a tool to assess HIV progression (13). IgE rose in many different high risk groups such as alcoholics, homosexuals, and intravenous drug users (IDUs) who were HIV+, but IDUs saw the largest increase. IDUs coincidentally had the lowest serum levels of vitamin E (13). These low vitamin E levels can be attributed to an ongoing antigenis response as well as poor intake. Furthermore, HIV+ groups had lower plasma vitamin E levels than the HIV-groups (13). This further explains the relationship between IgE and vitamin E.

CONCLUDING REMARKS

Although heart disease has not been a traditional focus in AIDS and HIV research, clearly the ramifications of the disease if it is left unchecked are consequential. Heart disease in the AIDS patient can be detected long before the symptoms become noticeable by routine echocardiography. Because heart disease has been found to decrease life span in AIDS patients, its early detection may help to prolong lives and improve prognosis. Vitamin E has been widely used to treat heart disease in patients without AIDS or HIV and therefore may be useful in the treatment of cardiac problems in patients with the virus. Vitamin E has numerous effects on vascular integrity as well as immune function. For these reasons, it should be studied for its ability to retard the progression of cardiac abnormalities in HIV/AIDS patients.

REFERENCES

1. Yunis NA, Stone VE. Cardiac manifestations of AIDS. J AIDS 1998; 18:145–154.
2. Rerkpattanapipat P, Wongpraparut N, Joacobs LE, Kotler MN. Cardiac manifestations of AIDS. Arch Intern Med 2000; 160:602–608.
3. Akhras F, Dubrey S, Gazzard B, Noble MM. Emerging patterns of heart disease in HIV infected homosexual subjects with and without opportunistic infections: a prospective color flow Doppler echocardiography study. Eur Heart J 1994; 15:68–75.
4. Blanchard DG. Reversibility of cardiac abnormalities in HIV infected indviduals: a serial echocardiographic study. J Am Coll 1991; 17:1270–1276.
5. Monsuez JJ, Kinney EL, Vittecoq D, Kitzis M, Rosenbaum W, d'Agay MF, Wolff M, Marche C, Janier M, Gorin I, Evans J, Autran B. Comparison among AIDS patients with and without evidence of cardiac disease. Am J Cardiol 1988; 62:1311–1313.
6. Stephens NG, Parsons A, Schofield PM, Kelly F, Cheeseman K, Mitchinson MJ, Brown MJ. Randomised controlled trial of vitamin E in patients with coronary disease: Cambridge Heart Antioxidant Study (CHAOS). Lancet 1996; 347:781–786.
7. Emmert DH, Kirchner JT. The role of vitamin E in the prevention of heart disease. Arch Fam Med 1999; 8:537–542.
8. Liang B, Chung S, Araghinikham M, Lane L, Watson RR. Vitamins and immunomodulation in AIDS. Nutrition 1996; 12:1–7.
9. Sherwood L. Human Physiology: From Cells to Systems. 3d ed. Belmont, CA: Wadsworth, 1997.
10. Torun M, Avci N, Yardim S. Serum levels of vitamin E in relation to cardiovascular diseases. J Clin Pharm and Therapeutics 1995; 20:335–340.
11. Thomas JR, Ziogas G, Yan P, Schmitz P, LaFontaine T. Influence of activity level on vitamin E status in healthy men and women and cardiac patients. J Cardiopulm Rehab 1998; 18:52–59.
12. Meydani SN, et al. Vitamin E supplementation suppresses prostaglandin E2 synthesis and enhances the immune response in aged mice. Mech Ageing Dev 1986; 34:191.
13. Miguez-Burbano MJ, Shor-Posner G, Fletcher MA, Lu Y, Moreno JN, Carcamo C, Page B, Quesada J, Sauberlich H, Baum MK. Immunoglobulin E levels in relatiionship to HIV-1 disease, route of infection, and vitamin E status. Allergy 1995; 50:157–161.

20

HIV- and Cocaine-Induced Subclinical Atherosclerosis

Shenghan Lai and João A. C. Lima
Johns Hopkins Medical Institutions, Baltimore, Maryland, U.S.A.

Qingyi Meng
Chinese PLA General Hospital, Beijing, China

INTRODUCTION

The acquired immunodeficiency syndrome (AIDS) is caused by the human immuno-deficiency virus (HIV-1 or HIV). The primary targets of these infections include the lungs, skin, gastrointestinal tract, and central nervous system. Cardiac involvement was thought to be rare during the early years of the HIV epidemic. In recent years, however, a growing body of evidence has accumulated indicating that cardiac dysfunction can occur in persons infected with HIV. Among the complications associated with HIV disease are pericarditis, myocarditis, ventricular tachycardia, endocarditis, metastatic involvement from Kaposi's sarcoma, and dilated cardiomy-opathy (1). As antiretroviral treatment has improved and prevention of opportunistic infections has become more effective, cardiac disease has emerged as an important component of AIDS. Early data from those treated with highly active antiretroviral therapy (HAART) have raised concerns about a possible increase in both vascular and coronary heart disease (2–4). Some patients receiving protease inhibitors (PIs), key components of HAART, develop various forms of risk factors for coronary artery disease (CAD), such as hyperlipidemia, hyperglycemia, central obesity, and endothe-lial dysfunction (5,6).

Cocaine, like AIDS, is another important public health problem in the United States. As its use has become increasingly widespread, especially among urban populations, the number of cocaine-related cardiovascular events—including angina pectoris, myocardial infarction, cardiomyopathy, and sudden death from cardiac causes—has increased dramatically (7–11). Studies have shown that cocaine use causes structural defects in the endothelial cell barrier, thereby increasing its permeability to low-density lipoprotein and escalating the expression of endothelial adhesion mole-cules and leukocyte migration—effects associated with the progression of atheroscle-rosis (12,13).

Most studies on the effect of cocaine use on cardiovascular complications have focused on clinical diseases, and its effect on subclinical CAD has not yet been thoroughly investigated. Quantification of coronary artery calcification, as determined by electron-beam computed tomography or high-speed spiral computed tomography (CT), measured as a coronary calcification score, is correlated with total plaque size and coronary risk factors and is strongly associated with maximal stenosis in the epicardial arteries. Coronary calcification has been shown to be a marker of atherosclerosis (14,15).

Because both HIV and cocaine can independently produce cardiac complications, it has been hypothesized that the combination of these two toxic agents in a single patient might exacerbate some of the adverse effects of each and increase the incidence of heart and vessel pathology (1). This study was designed to investigate the effects of HIV infection and cocaine use on subclinical atherosclerosis.

METHODS

Study Participants

Between May 2000 and July 2001, a total of 187 study participants from Baltimore, Maryland, were enrolled in a longitudinal study of subclinical atherosclerosis as related to HIV infection and cocaine use. Of these, 137 (73.3%) were recruited from the AIDS Link to Intravenous Experience (ALIVE) study, which is an ongoing prospective study of the natural history of HIV infection among injection drug users in Baltimore (16). The other 26.9% of the study participants were recruited from the eastern part of Baltimore, where most of the ALIVE study participants resided. Inclusion criteria for the longitudinal study were age between 25 and 45 years and black race. Exclusion criteria for the longitudinal study were (1) any evidence of hypertension or ischemic heart disease on the basis of clinical history, previous hospitalization for myocardial infarction, angina pectoris, or electrocardiographic (ECG) and/or echocardiographic evidence of previous myocardial damage by ischemic heart disease; (2) any symptoms believed to be related to cardiovascular disease; and (3) pregnancy. For this investigation, we excluded from analysis those who reported recent opportunistic infection; who were taking anabolic steroids, immunomodulators, and lipid-lowering medications prior to any antiretroviral treatment; who smoked >1 pack of cigarettes daily; or who had any known respiratory, severe hepatic, or renal abnormality or diabetes mellitus. The Committee on Human Research at the Johns Hopkins University approved the study protocol, and all study participants provided informed consent. Information about sociodemographics and drug use behaviors was obtained by interviewer-administered questionnaires. An echocardiographic examination, lipid profile, C-reactive protein and other blood tests, and spiral CT (Siemens Somatom Plus 4 Volume Zoom) were performed to quantify coronary artery calcification, a marker of subclinical coronary atherosclerosis.

Of the total 187 enrolled candidates, 98 (69 males and 29 females) who had had HIV$-$1 infection for >6 months and were receiving stable doses of antiretroviral medications were included in this analysis. Participants in the PI group ($n = 55$) had taken stable doses of commercially available PIs (indinavir, ritonavir, nelfinavir, saquinavir) for >6 months. Participants in the non-PI group ($n = 43$) had undergone stable antiretroviral regimens that did not include a PI, and they had not taken any PIs for >1 month before their current stable non-PI regimens.

Blood Pressure Determinations

Systolic and diastolic blood pressure was measured twice with a standard mercury sphygmomanometer. A nurse at the ALIVE clinic measured each study participant's arm circumference and applied a correctly sized cuff. The participant sat quietly for 5 min; then the nurse obtained the systolic and diastolic blood pressure measurements; a second measurement was made 3 min later. The average of the two readings was used as the screening or baseline reading.

Prospective ECG-Gated Cardiac CT-Scan Protocol

Scanning was performed with a Siemens Somatom Plus 4 Volume Zoom Multislice (Siemens AG, Forchheim, Germany). Subjects were scanned in the nonspiral 240-degree partial sequence scan mode (SEQ): slice thickness was 2.5 mm, tube current was 50 mA, and tube voltage was 140 kV with electrocardiographic (ECG) triggering. Images were acquired by means of a single-breath-hold technique on full inspiration, with an average breath-hold time of 20 to 30 sec. Each scan took 0.36 sec, and the cycle time was 1.3 sec. Four slices 2.5 mm thick were taken by each scan. On average, a total of 12 scans—equal to 48 slices—was obtained on each patient. The scans started just below the carina, and the entire coronary tree was imaged. Scoring was by the Agatston method (17), with a threshold of 130 Hounsfield units (HU). The lesion score was calculated by multiplying the lesion area by a density factor derived from the maximal HU within this area, as originally described by Agatston for EBT scanning (17). A total calcium score was determined by summing individual lesion scores from each of four anatomic sites (left main, left anterior descending, circumflex, and right coronary arteries) in all 48 slices. The spiral CT scans were scored by a radiologist in the Department of Radiology, Johns Hopkins Hospital, with extensive experience in cardiac anatomy and coronary calcium.

Statistical Analysis

Statistical analyses were performed with SAS statistical software (18). Data are reported as mean ± standard deviation (SD) values. The statistical significance of between-subgroup differences was tested by two-way ANOVA followed by hoc t tests with the appropriate corrections. Categorical variables were compared by chi-square or Fisher's exact test. The associations between the continuous data were examined by linear regression analysis. Logistic regression analyses were performed to describe relationships between the categorical parameters. Odds ratios (OR) were presented with 95% confidence intervals (CI). Factors that exhibited statistical significance ($p < 0.050$) in univariate models were jointly entered into a multiple regression model; those that ceased to be significant were deleted in a stagewise manner, thus yielding the final model backwards. A significance level was set at $p < 0.050$, and all p values reported were two-sided.

RESULTS

Of 187 study participants, 91 individuals were HIV-1 seropositive and used cocaine (HIV + /cocaine + group), 7 were HIV-1 positive and did not use cocaine (HIV + /

cocaine– group), 57 were HIV seronegative and used cocaine (HIV–/cocaine+ group), and 32 were HIV-1 negative and did not use cocaine (HIV–/cocaine– group). There were no statistically significant differences in age, sex, systolic blood pressure (SBP), diastolic blood pressure (DBP), and heart rate (HR) among the four groups defined by cocaine use and HIV serostatus except that the body mass index (BMI) in HIV+/cocaine+ group was significantly lower than among those in the HIV–/cocaine– ($p = 0.022$) and HIV+/cocaine– groups ($p = 0.032$) (Table 1). No significant difference in alcohol use was observed among these four groups. The proportion of participants who currently smoked cigarettes was significantly lower in the HIV–/cocaine– group than in the other three groups (all $p < 0.050$) (Table 1). Among the two cocaine-positive groups, no differences were found in the duration of cocaine, heroin, and speedball (a heroin-cocaine mixture) use. The proportions of current cocaine, heroin, and speedball use and frequency of daily drug use were also similar (Table 2).

Of 187 study participants, 161 (86.1%) completed lipid examinations and interviewer-administered questionnaires by the end of July 2001 and were included for analysis. There were no statistically significant differences between those who underwent the lipid examination and those 26 (13.9%) who did not in terms of age, sex, HIV-1 serostatus, BMI, SBP, DBP, HR, and cigarette, alcohol, cocaine, heroin, and speedball use (all $p > 0.05$). No statistically significant differences were found among the four groups in serum total cholesterol (TC), low-density-lipoprotein cholesterol (LDL-C) and very low density lipoprotein cholesterol (VLDL-C), high-density-lipo-protein cholesterol/total cholesterol (HDL-C/TC) and low-density-lipoprotein cho-lesterol/high-density-lipoprotein (LDL-C/HDL-C) ratios. The mean triglyceride (TG) level of the HIV+/cocaine– group was significantly higher than that of the HIV–/cocaine– ($p = 0.021$) and HIV–/cocaine+ groups ($p = 0.033$). The mean TG level in the HIV+/cocaine+ group was also higher than that in HIV–/cocaine– group ($p = 0.019$). Participants in the two HIV-positive groups had significantly lower HDL-C levels than those in the two HIV-negative groups (HIV+/cocaine+ versus HIV–/cocaine–, $p = 0.016$; versus HIV–/cocaine+, $p = 0.021$; and HIV+/

Table 1 General Characteristics of 187 Study Participants in Baltimore, Maryland

	HIV–/cocaine– ($N=32$)	HIV–/cocaine+ ($N=57$)	HIV+/cocaine– ($N=7$)	HIV+/cocaine+ ($N=91$)
Age (years)	33.8 ± 6.2	39.5 ± 4.1	39.0 ± 4.1	38.9 ± 4.9
Sex, male/female (n)	16/16	38/19	5/2	65/26
Cigarette use (n)	14(43.8%)	51(89.5%)[a]	5(71.4%)[b]	81(89.0%)[a]
Alcohol use (n)	17(53.1%)	42(73.7%)	5(71.4%)	63(69.2%)
BMI (kg/m^2)	27.7 ± 5.7	24.9 ± 4.7	33.5 ± 11.4	24.1 ± 4.0[c,d]
SBP (kPa)	15.3 ± 1.8	15.5 ± 1.6	16.0 ± 1.5	14.7 ± 1.8
DBP (kPa)	10.6 ± 1.2	10.2 ± 1.1	11.5 ± 2.4	10.5 ± 1.2
HR (beart/minute)	64.0 ± 9.8	63.0 ± 7.7	66.0 ± 9.4	62.9 ± 8.4

[a] $p < 0.01$ vs. change in HIV–/cocaine– group.
[b] $p < 0.05$ vs. HIV–/cocaine+ group.
[c] $p < 0.05$.
[d] $p < 0.05$ vs. HIV+/cocaine– group.

Table 2 Drug Use Behaviors Among Those Who Used Cocaine

	HIV−/cocaine+ N=57 (%)	HIV+/cocaine+ N=91 (%)	p value
Current drug use (n)			
Cocaine	57(100.0)	91(100.0)	1.000
Heroin	51(89.5)	74(81.3)	0.183
Speedball	49(86.0)	75(82.4)	0.569
Duration of drug use (years)			
Cocaine	11.6 ± 7.7	12.3 ± 11.3	0.676
Heroin	14.0 ± 8.3	13.2 ± 12.0	0.693
Speedball	9.1 ± 8.2	11.0 ± 12.0	0.312
Daily use of cocaine			
Cocaine	13(22.8)	16(17.6)	0.436
Heroin	5(8.8)	3(3.3)	0.152
Speedball	9(15.8)	14(15.4)	0.947

cocaine− versus HIV−/cocaine−, $p = 0.020$; versus HIV−/cocaine+, $p = 0.029$, respectively) (Table 3).

Although differences in the proportions of abnormal TC (>5.2 mmol/L) and LDL-C (>3.12 mmol/L) were found among those four groups, differences were not statistically significant. The proportions of abnormal TG (>1.65 mmol/L) in the HIV+/cocaine+ (15.8%) and the HIV+/cocaine− groups (42.9%) were significantly higher than that in the HIV−/cocaine− group (0%) (HIV−/cocaine− versus HIV+/cocaine+, $p = 0.044$; versus HIV+/cocaine−, $p = 0.011$). The proportion of abnormal TG in the HIV+/cocaine+ group (15.8%) appeared somewhat higher than that in the HIV−/cocaine+ group (8.8%; $p = 0.230$). The proportions of abnormal HDL-C level (<1.04 mmol/L) in the two HIV-positive groups were also

Table 3 Lipids and Lipoproteins in 187 Study Participants

HIV+	HIV−/cocaine− (N=21)	HIV−/cocaine+ (N=57)	HIV−/cocaine− (N=7)	HIV+/cocaine+ (N=76)
TG (mmol/L)	0.7 ± 0.3	1.0 ± 0.5	2.0 ± 1.7[a,b]	1.2 ± 0.6[a]
TC (mmol/L)	4.5 ± 0.8	4.7 ± 0.9	4.3 ± 0.6	4.4 ± 1.0
HDL-C (mmol/L)	1.6 ± 0.4	1.5 ± 0.6	0.9 ± 0.3[a,b]	1.3 ± 0.5[a,b]
LDL-C (mmol/L)	2.6 ± 0.7	2.7 ± 0.9	3.2 ± 0.8	2.6 ± 0.9
VLDL-C (mmol/L)	0.3 ± 0.1	0.5 ± 0.2	0.5 ± 0.4	0.5 ± 0.2
HDL-C/TC (%)	35.5 ± 8.0	33.2 ± 11.4	20.0 ± 7.8	29.0 ± 9.2
LDL-C/HDL-C	1.7 ± 0.6	2.1 ± 1.2	2.4 ± 2.6	3.0 ± 6.2
TG > 1.65 mmol/L (n, %)	0(0)	5(8.8)	3(42.9)[a]	12(15.8)[a]
TC > 5.2 mmol/L (n, %)	4(19.1)	13(22.8)	1(14.3)	14(18.4)
HDL-C < 1.04 mmol/L (n, %)	1(4.8)	11(19.3)	4(57.1)[b,c]	24(31.6)[a]
LDL-C > 3.12 mmol/L (n, %)	3(14.3)	14(24.6)	2(28.6)	17(22.4)

[a] $p < 0.05$.
[b] $p < 0.05$ vs. change in HIV+/cocaine+ group.
[c] $p < 0.01$ vs. HIV−/cocaine− group.

significantly higher than those in the two HIV-negative groups, respectively (HIV+/cocaine+ versus HIV−/cocaine−, $p = 0.012$; versus HIV−/cocaine+ $p = 0.156$; and HIV+/cocaine− versus HIV−/cocaine−, $p = 0.008$; versus HIV−/cocaine+, $p = 0.044$). The proportion of abnormal HDL-C level in the HIV−/cocaine+ group tended to be higher than that in the HIV−/cocaine− group (19.3% versus 4.8%; $p = 0.090$) (Table 3).

In the red blood cell analyses, no difference was found among the four groups in hemoglobin (Hb), hematocrit (HCT), mean cell volume (MCV), mean corpuscular hemoglobin concentration (MCHC), red blood cell counts (RBC), standard deviation of red blood cell distribution width (RDW-SD), and platelet counts (Table 4). In the white blood cell count analyses, neutrophile, lymphocyte, monocyte and total white blood cell counts were similar among the four groups. In the differential count analyses, neutrophils, lymphocytes, and monocytes were also similar among those four groups with one exception. The monocyte percentage in the HIV+/cocaine+ group was significantly higher than that in the HIV−/cocaine− group ($p = 0.032$) (Table 4).

Of the 187 study participants, 139 (74.3%) completed spiral CT examinations and interviewer-administered questionnaires by the end of July 2001 and were included for analyses. There were no statistically significant differences between those who underwent the CT examinations and those who did not (48, or 26%) in terms of age, sex, HIV-1 serostatus, BMI, SBP, DBP, HR, and cigarette, alcohol, cocaine, heroin, and speedball use (all $p > 0.05$).

Although differences in mean calcium scores were found among the four groups, they were not statistically significant. The mild coronary artery calcification (scores >2.5, upper limit of the HIV−/cocaine− group) in the HIV+/cocaine− group (28.6%) seemed somewhat higher than that in the HIV−/cocaine+ (10.3%; $p =$

Table 4 Results of Blood Cell Analyses in 187 Study Participants

HIV+	HIV−/cocaine− (N=32)	HIV−/cocaine+ (N=57)	HIV−/cocaine− (N=7)	HIV+/cocaine+ (N=91)
Hb (g/dL)	12.7 ± 1.3	13.4 ± 1.5	12.3 ± 0.5	12.7 ± 1.9
RBC (10^{12}/L)	4.5 ± 0.6	4.5 ± 0.5	4.3 ± 0.5	4.2 ± 0.6
HCT (vol%)	38.1 ± 3.3	40.1 ± 4.1	36.3 ± 1.4	37.9 ± 4.7
MCV (μm^3)	84.9 ± 9.8	89.5 ± 7.3	86.0 ± 10.9	89.8 ± 8.0
MCH (pg)	28.5 ± 3.8	30.0 ± 2.7	29.0 ± 4.1	30.1 ± 3.1
MCHC (g/dL)	33.5 ± 0.8	33.5 ± 0.7	33.8 ± 0.4	33.5 ± 0.7
RDW-SD (%)	14.0 ± 1.2	14.1 ± 1.4	14.8 ± 2.3	14.4 ± 1.8
WBC (10^9/L)	4.9 ± 1.4	5.8 ± 1.7	5.6 ± 2.5	4.7 ± 3.5
Neutrophil (%)	48.9 ± 9.5	54.5 ± 9.5	56.0 ± 22.6	52.3 ± 14.2
Lymphocyte (%)	38.5 ± 7.8	34.1 ± 8.0	30.5 ± 17.7	33.1 ± 12.5
Monocyte (%)	8.5 ± 2.6	8.9 ± 2.2	11.3 ± 3.7	10.4 ± 3.9[a]
Neutrophil count (10^9/L)	2.4 ± 1.0	3.2 ± 1.2	3.5 ± 2.7	2.6 ± 2.2
Lymphocyte count (10^9/L)	1.9 ± 0.6	2.0 ± 0.7	1.4 ± 0.5	1.5 ± 1.4
Monocyte count (10^9/L)	0.4 ± 0.2	0.4 ± 0.2	0.5 ± 0.1	0.4 ± 0.2
Platelet (10^{10}/L)	26.8 ± 4.6	24.4 ± 6.6	23.6 ± 9.9	23.1 ± 7.7

[a] $p < 0.05$ vs. HIV−/cocaine+ group.

0.327) and the HIV−/cocaine− groups (0%; p = 0.056). The proportion of mild coronary artery calcification in the HIV+/cocaine+ group (23.6%) was also higher than that in the HIV−/cocaine+ (10.3%; p = 0.086) and the HIV−/cocaine− groups (0%; p = 0.010). The mild coronary artery calcification in the HIV−/cocaine+ group tended to be higher than that in the HIV−/cocaine− group (10.3% versus 0%; p = 0.169) (Table 5).

Logistic regression analyses suggested cocaine use might be associated with calcium score (OR = 2.86; 95% CI = 0.63–13.03; p = 0.173). HIV-1 infection was significantly associated with coronary artery calcification (OR = 4.13; 95% CI = 1.32–12.95; p = 0.015). Multivariate regression analyses indicated that only age >35 years (OR = 16.18; 95% CI = 1.62–161.26; p = 0.018), BMI (OR = 4.76; 95% CI = 1.07–1.29; p = 0.001), and HIV-1 infection (OR = 4.76; 95% CI = 1.29–17.48; p = 0.019) were significantly associated with calcium scores. The final model suggests that after adjustment for age and BMI, HIV-1 infection remains independently associated with coronary calcification.

Of the 187 study participants, 156 (83.4%) completed serum CRP measurements and interviewer-administered questionnaires by the end of July 2001 and were included for analysis. There were no statistically significant differences between those who underwent the CRP measurements and those who did not (31, or 17.6%) in terms of age, sex, HIV-1 serostatus, BMI, SBP, DBP, HR, and cigarette, alcohol, cocaine, heroin, and speedball use (all p > 0.05).

The mean levels of C-reactive protein (CRP) were different among these four groups. The proportion of abnormal CRP (>1.9 mg/L) in the HIV+/cocaine+ group was 58.7%, which was higher than that in the HIV−/cocaine+ (37.0%; p = 0.015)

Table 5 Coronary Artery Calcium Scores and C-reactive Protein in 187 Study Participants

HIV+	HIV−/cocaine−	HIV−/cocaine+	HIV−/cocaine−	HIV+/cocaine+
Coronary artery calcium scores				
(N)	(21)	(39)	(7)	(72)
Mean ± SD	0.3 ± 0.7	16.1 ± 72.1	2.9 ± 5.2	7.1 ± 22.8
Ranges	0–2.5	0–422.3	0–13.6	0–131.2
Score positive (%)	4(19.0)	11(28.2)	4(57.1)[a]	25(34.7)
Scores > 2.5(%)	0(0)	4(10.3)[b]	2(28.6)[c]	17(23.6)[d,e]
Scores > 5(%)	0(0)	4(10.3)[b]	2(28.6)[c]	15(20.8)[d]
Scores > 10(%)	0(0)	4(10.3)[b]	1(14.3)	9(12.5)
C-reactive protein				
(N)	(21)	(54)	(6)	(75)
Mean ± SD (mg/L)	2.9 ± 4.3	8.5 ± 29.1	2.4 ± 1.8	5.0 ± 11.1
Ranges (mg/L)	0.2–19.2	0.1–208.0	0–4.4	0.2–87.2
>1.9 mg/L (%)	8(38.1)	20(37.0)	4(66.7)	44(58.7)[d,f]

[a] p = 0.053.
[b] p = 0.169 vs. change in HIV−/cocaine− group.
[c] p = 0.056.
[d] p < 0.05.
[e] p = 0.06 vs. HIV−/cocaine+ group.
[f] p = 0.094.

and the HIV−/cocaine− group (38.1%; $p = 0.094$) (Table 5). The total proportion of abnormal CRP in the two HIV-positive groups (59.3%, or 48 of 81) was also significantly higher than that in the two HIV-negative groups (37.3%, or 28 of 75; $p = 0.006$). No significant difference in abnormal CRP was found between the cocaine-positive (50.4%, or 64 of 129) and the other negative groups (12 of 27, or 55.6%; $p = 0.625$).

Logistic regression analyses showed that cocaine use was not associated with abnormal CRP when users were compared with nonusers: OR = 1.21 (95% CI = 0.53 to 2.79; $p = 0.651$). However, HIV-1 infection was significantly associated with elevated CRP (OR = 2.37; 95% CI = 1.25 to 4.50; $p = 0.008$). Multiple logistic regression analyses indicated that BMI (OR = 1.09; 95% CI = 1.00 to 1.14; $p = 0.051$) and HIV-1 infection (OR = 2.45; 95% CI = 1.27 to 4.77; $p = 0.008$) were associated with abnormal CRP levels. The final model suggests that after adjustment for BMI, HIV-1 infection remains independently associated with CRP abnormalities.

DISCUSSION

To our knowledge, this is the first report to investigate the effects of simultaneous cocaine use and HIV-1 infection on subclinical coronary atherosclerosis. In agreement with prior studies, our study revealed that cocaine abusers had atherogenic lipid changes characterized by elevated levels of serum TG and a reduction of HDL-C; accompanying HIV-1 infection exacerbated those lipid changes in a black population (19–25). Calcium scores, which are markers for coronary heart disease, were elevated in cocaine abusers, and those users with HIV-1 infection had significantly higher calcium scores than cocaine-positive individuals alone and both HIV- and cocaine-negative individuals. Those scores suggest that conjoint cocaine use and HIV-1 infection can exacerbate coronary artery atherosclerosis. Although HIV-1 infection was associated with serum CRP, a marker of inflammation, no association was noted between cocaine use and serum CRP. This finding implies that coincident cocaine abuse and HIV-1 infection exacerbated the atherosclerotic progress, although not by the mechanism of inflammation.

It has been demonstrated that HIV-1 infection induces a decrease in total cholesterol and a late increase of triglycerides with a reduction of HDL, and drug addicts are frequently characterized by hypercholesterolemia and hypertriglyceridemia (19–21). Similar results were found in this study with regard to individuals either using cocaine or having HIV-1 infection. We also found that the coincident conditions of cocaine use and HIV-1 infection could induce a marked increase in triglycerides with a pronounced reduction of HDL-C levels and no significant change of total cholesterol. This finding suggests a synergetic effect on atherosclerosis and also implies the positive effects on serum TG and HDL-C and the antagonistic effects on serum total cholesterol levels with these two entangled epidemics.

In view of the relatively high rates of HIV-1 infection among inner-city drug users and increased longevity among those receiving antiviral therapy, CAD has become an important cause of cardiac morbidity and mortality in the HIV-1-infected population. There have been recent reports of coronary atherosclerosis and myocardial infarctions in young HIV-1-infected patients, thereby renewing interest in examining the associations between HIV infection, cocaine use, and subclinical CAD (1). There are many case reports of young HIV-infected patients or cocaine abusers who present with myocardial infarction and CAD (26–29). These case reports have raised the question of whether subclinical atherosclerosis may be related to cocaine use and HIV-1 infection. In addition to retrospective analyses of coronary events from existing databases, investigations have studied surrogate markers of subclinical atherosclerosis in HIV-infected subjects (2,30). Recent studies have shown that coronary artery calcium is a good marker of underlying atherosclerotic disease that has accumulated in vascular walls (31). Calcium screening is best employed in asymptomatic subjects at intermediate risk of CAD to address the presence of atherosclerotic disease and to assess the risk of individual patients (32). In this study, we found calcium scores were elevated in cocaine abusers; those users who also had HIV-1 infection had even higher calcium scores. That provided strong evidence that conjoint cocaine use and HIV-1 infection can exacerbate coronary artery subclinical atherosclerosis.

In recent studies, the serum levels of CRP, a marker of the reactant serum protein component of the inflammatory response, were associated with the risk of future ischemic heart disease (33–35). Our present study showed that serum CRP levels, which had no marked relation with the cocaine use, were significantly associated with HIV-1 infection. These findings provide evidence of a link between atherosclerosis and HIV-1 infection and imply that coincident cocaine use and HIV-1 infection aggravated by coronary atherosclerosis may not be associated with inflammation.

No conjoint effects were found in this study in terms of the red blood cell and white blood cell analyses except that cocaine users with HIV-1 infection had higher monocyte differential counts than those of either cocaine- or HIV-negative individuals. That is in agreement with prior reports suggesting that monocytes are major targets of HIV-1 infection in patients with AIDS (36–37).

One limitation of our study was the small sample size of the HIV-positive/cocaine-negative group (only 7 cases) because of the nature of the study enrollment criteria and the distribution of risk in the populations. Second, unmeasured differences in socioeconomic status between participants in each group may have affected outcome parameters as a result of the cross-sectional design. In our study, all groups were similar in major risk factors for CAD except for cigarette use, which was confirmed to be related with recent drug use (38). No significant differences, however, were found among the three cocaine– or HIV-positive groups; it is unlikely that differences in cigarette use accounted for the large differences in lipids, serum CRP levels, and calcium scores. Finally, it must be emphasized that these observational findings are preliminary. Some confounding factors, which are related to the epidemics of cocaine use and HIV-1 infection, may associated with the coronary artery events and should be considered in further studies.

CONCLUSION

This study indicates that coincident cocaine use and HIV-1 infection produce atherogenic lipid and CRP changes and exacerbate coronary artery calcificattion, thus suggesting that cocaine users who are infected with HIV-1 may be at elevated risk for coronary artery subclinical atherosclerosis. It shows that both HIV infection and cocaine abuse may have serious cardiovascular complications. It also suggests that cocaine use by an HIV-infected person places that individual at an increased risk of cardiac complications. Because this study is an ongoing one, we will be able, in the near future, to test the hypothesis that there are synergistic effects on subclinical athero-sclerosis between these two agents.

ACKNOWLEDGMENT

This work was supported by grants from the National Institute on Drug Abuse (DA 12777, DA04334, and DA12568).

REFERENCES

1. Soodini G, Morgan JP. Can cocaine abuse exacerbate the cardiac toxicity of human immunodeficiency virus? Clin Cardiol 2001; 24:177–181.
2. Barbaro G. Cardiovascular manifestations of HIV infection. J R Soc Med 2001; 94:384–390.
3. Passalaris JD, Sepkowitz KA, Glesby M. Coronary artery disease and human immunodeficiency virus infection. Clin Infect Dis 2000; 31:787–797.
4. Carr A, Cooper DA. Adverse effects of antiretroviral therapy. Lancet 2000; 356:1423–1430.
5. Carr A, Samaras K, Thorisdottir A, Kaufmann GR, Chisholm DJ, Cooper DA. Diagnosis, prediction, and natural course of HIV protease-inhibitor-associated lipodystrophy, hyperlipidaemia, and diabetes mellitus. Lancet 1999; 353:2893–2899.
6. Stein JH, Klein MA, Bellehumeur JL, McBride PE, Wiebe DA, Otvos JD, Sosman JM. Use of human immunodeficiency virus-1 protease inhibitors is associated with atherogenic lipoprotein changes and endothelial dysfunction. Circulation 2001; 104(3):257–262.
7. Lange RA, Hillis LD. Cardiovascular complications of cocaine use. N Engl J Med 2001; 345:351–358.
8. Kolodgie FD, Virmani R, Cornhill JF, Herderick EE, Smialek J. Increase in atherosclerosis and adventitial mast cells in cocaine abusers: an alternative mechanism of cocaine associated coronary vasospasm and thrombosis. J Am Coll Cardiol 1991; 17:1553–1560.
9. Simpson R, Edwards W. Pathogenesis of cocaine induced ischemic heart disease. Arch Pathol Lab Med 1986; 110:479–484.
10. Roh L, Hamele-Bena D. Cocaine-induced ischemic myocardial disease. Am J Forens Med Pathol 1990; 11:130–135.
11. Majid PA, Patel B, Kim HJ, Zimmerman JL, Dellinger RP. An angiographic and histologic study of cocaine-induced chest pain. Am J Cardiol 1990; 65:812–814.
12. Kolodgie FD, Wilson PS, Mergner WJ, Virmani R. Cocaine-induced increase in the permeability function of human vascular endothelial cell monolayers. Exp Mol Pathol 1999; 66(2):109–122.
13. Gan X, Zhang L, Berger O, Stins MF, Way D, Taub DD, Chang SL, Kim KS, House SD, Weinand M, Witte M, Graves MC, Fiala M. Cocaine enhances brain endothelial adhesion molecules and leukocyte migration. Clin Immunol 1999; 91(1):68–76.
14. Sangiorgi G, Rumberger JA, Severson A, Edwards WD, Gregoire J, Fitzpatrick LA, Schwards RS. Arterial calcification and not lumen stenosis is highly correlated with atherosclerotic plague burden in humans: a histologic study of 723 coronary artery segments using nondecalcifying methodology. J Am Coll Cardiol 1998; 31:126–133.
15. Wexler L, Brundage B, Crouse J, Detrano R, Fuster V, Maddahi J, Rumberger J, Stanford

W, White R, Taubert K, and AHA staff. Coronary artery calcification: pathophysiology, epidemiology, imaging methods, and clinical implications. Circulation 1996; 94:1175–1192.

16. Anthony JC, Vlahov D, Celentano DD, Menon AS, Margolick JB, Cohn S, Nelson KE, Polk BF. Self-reported interview data for a study of HIV-1 infection among intravenous drug users: description of methods and preliminary evidence on validity. J Drug Issues 1991; 21(4):739–757.

17. Agatston AS, Janowitz WR, Hildner FJ, Zusmer NR, Viamonte M Jr, Detrano R. Quantification of coronary artery calcium using ultrafast computed tomography. J Am Coll Cardiol 1990; 15(4):827–832.

18. SAS Institute, Inc. SAS/STAT User Guide. Version 8. Cary, NC: SAS Institute, Inc, 1999.

19. Muga R, Tor J, Rey-Joly C, Pardo A, Llobet P, Foz M. Dyslipemia and HIV-1 infection in intravenous drug addicts. Med Clin 1993; 100(5):161–163.

20. Ducobu J, Payen MC. Lipids and AIDS. Rev Med Brux 2000; 21(1):11–17.

21. Rogowska-Szadkowska D, Borzuchowska AK, Obserwacyjno ZB. The level of triglicerides, total cholesterol and HDL cholesterol in various stages of human immunodeficiency virus (HIV) infection. Pol Arch Med Wewn 1999; 101(2):145–150.

22. Mercie P, Tchamgoue S, Thiebaut R, Vialard JF, Faure I, Dancourt V, Marimoutou C, Dabis F, Rispal P, Darmon Y, Leng B, Pellegrin JL. Atherogen lipid profile in HIV-1-infected patients with lipodystrophy syndrome. Eur J Int Med 2000; 11(5):257–263.

23. Braun BL, Murray DM, Sidney S. Lifetime cocaine use and cardiovascular characteristics among young adults: the Cardia study. Am J Public Health 1997; 87(4):629–634.

24. Chen K, Scheier LM, Kandel DB. Effects of chronic cocaine use on physical health: a prospective study in a general population sample. Drug Alcohol Depend 1996; 43(1–2):23–37.

25. Fernandez-Miranda C, Pulido F, Carillo JL, Larumbe S, Gomez Izquierdo T, Ortuno B, Rubio R, del Palacio A. Lipoprotein alterations in patients with HIV infection: relation with cellular and humoral immune markers. Clin Chim Acta 1998; 274(1):63–70.

26. Minor RL, Scott BD, Brown DD, Winniford MD. Cocaine-induced myocardial infarction in patients with normal coronary arteries. Ann Intern Med 1991; 115:797–806.

27. Passalaris JD, Sepkowitz KA, Glesby MJ. Coronary artery disease and human immunodeficiency virus infection. Clin Infect Dis 2000; 31:787–797.

28. Tabib A, Leroux C, Mornex JF, Loire R. Accelerated coronary atherosclerosis and arteriosclerosis in young human-immunodeficiency-virus–positive patients. Coron Artery Dis 2000; 11(1):41–46.

29. Flynn TE, Bricker LA. Myocardial infarction in HIV infected men receiving protease inhibitors. Ann Intern Med 1999; 131:548.

30. Margolin A, Avants SK, Setaro JF, Rinder HM, Grupp L. Cocaine, HIV, and their cardiovascular effects: is there a role for ACE-inhibitor therapy? Drug Alcohol Depend 2000; 61:35–45.

31. Raggi P. Coronary calcium on electron beam tomography imaging as a surrogate maker of coronary artery disease. Am J Cardiol 2001; 87(suppl A):27A–34A.

32. Haberl R, Becker A, Knez A, Becker C, Lang C, Bruning R, Reiser M, Steinbeck G. Correlation of coronary calcification and angiographically documented stenoses in patients with suspected coronary artery disease: results of 1,764 patients. J Am Coll Cardiol 2001; 37(2):451–457.

33. Lower GDO, Yarnell, Rumley A, Bainton D, Sweetnam PM. C-reactive protein, fibrin D-dimer, and incident ischemic heart disease in the speedwell study. Arterioscler Thromb Vasc Biol 2001; 21:603–610.

34. Kiechl S, Egger G, Mayr M, Wiedermann CJ, Bonora E, Oberhollenzer F, Muggeo M, Xu Q, Wick G, Poewe W, Willeit J. Chronic infections and the risk of carotid atherosclerosis. Circulation 2001; 103:1064–1071.

35. Ridker PM. High-sensitivity C-reactive protein. Potential adjunct for global risk assess-

ment in the primary prevention of cardiovascular disease. Circulation 2001; 103:1813–1821.

36. Lafrenie RM, Wahl LM, Epstein JS, Hewlett IK, Yamada KM, Dhawan S. HIV-1-Tat modulates the function of monocytes and alters their interactions with microvessel endothelial cells. A mechanism of HIV pathogenesis. J Immunol 1996; 156(4):1638–1645.

37. Lafrenie RM, Wahl LM, Epstein JS, Yamada KM, Dhawan S. Activation of monocytes by HIV-Tat treatment is mediated by cytokine expression. J Immunol 1997; 159(8):4077–4083.

38. Lai S, Lai H, Page JB, McCoy CB. The association between cigarette smoking and drug abuse in the United States. J Addict Dis 2000; 19(4):11–24.

21

Cocaine, HIV, and Heart Disease: Research at NIDA and Recommendations for Future Research

Jag H. Khalsa
National Institute on Drug Abuse, National Institutes of Health, Bethesda, Maryland, U.S.A.

Sander G. Genser
Uniformed Services University of the Health Sciences, Bethesda, Maryland, U.S.A.

This short chapter briefly describes (1) the effects of cocaine and the human immunodeficiency virus (HIV) on the cardiovascular system; (2) the ongoing research at the National Institute on Drug Abuse, a part of the National Institutes of Health; and (3) directions for future research on the subject. Additionally, the reader is referred to more extensive reviews by Das and Laddu (1), Kloner et al. (2), and Wilkins (3).

EPIDEMIOLOGY OF COCAINE USE

In the United States cocaine has been in use for the past several decades. Initially it was used as an anesthetic, included in some over-the-counter preparations, and used as a recreational agent. But over the subsequent years its use has increased to an extent that, according to the National Household Survey (4), there were an estimated 1.2 million Americans who were current users of cocaine in 2000. This represents 0.5 % of the population aged 12 and older. There were 265,000 current crack cocaine users. The 2000 Drug Abuse Warning Network (DAWN) (5) data on the emergency department (ED) drug-related episodes show that there were 71 cocaine-related mentions per 100,000 population. (A drug "mention" is an instance of a particular drug being recorded—"mentioned"—in an ED visit reported to DAWN. As many as five drugs can be recorded for a single visit.) The reference population comprises persons aged 6 to 97 who were treated in a hospital ED for a drug abuse–related condition.

PHARMACOLOGY OF COCAINE

Cocaine is a powerful anesthetic agent with strong vasoconstrictive properties. It can be absorbed from all mucous membrane sites and has the potential to cause severe cardiovascular complications ranging from chest pain to myocardial infarction, arrhythmias, cardiomyopathy, and myocarditis. Many of these cardiac effects may be related to cocaine's physiological/pharmacological action. Acute doses of cocaine suppress myocardial contractility, reduce coronary caliber and coronary blood flow, increase vascular resistance, induce electrical abnormalities in the heart, and, in conscious animals (dogs), increase heart rate and blood pressure. These effects decrease myocardial oxygen supply and may increase demand, due to tachycardia and hypertension. Thus, myocardial ischemia and/or infarction may occur, leading to necrosis. Myocardial infarction has been reported after cocaine is smoked as well as after intranasal use. Ischemia and/or infarction may also result from increased aggregation of platelets. Moreover, acute depression of left ventricular (LV) function by cocaine may lead to the a transient cardiomyopathy. Chronic cocaine use can lead to the cardiovascular complications mentioned above as well as acceleration of atherosclerosis and, in high-risk chronic cocaine abusers, left ventricular hypertrophy. Acute or chronic cocaine use can also cause arrhythmias. On the other hand, direct cardiotoxic effects may include myocardial toxicity, myocyte necrosis, myocarditis, and foci of myocyte fibrosis, all of which can lead to cardiomyopathy. Other cardiovascular effects may include ruptured aorta and endocarditis. Cocaine cardiotoxicity may be due to its ability to block sodium channels, leading to a local anesthetic or membrane-stabilizing effect, and/or its ability to block reuptake of catecholamines in the presynaptic neurons of the central and peripheral nervous system, resulting increased levels of catecholamines and hence increased sympathetic output. Other potential mechanisms of cocaine cardiotoxicity include (1) a possible direct calcium effect, leading to contraction of vessels and contraction bands in myocytes, and (2) hypersensitivity and increased platelet aggregation, which may be related to increased catecholamines (2). Additionally, cocaine alters circulating levels of the catecholamines (norepinephrine, epinephrine), adrenocorticotropic hormone (ACTH), and cortisol. Research suggests that the effects of increases in steroid-potentiated actions of catecholamines on vascular tissues contribute to the etiology of cocaine-related medical complications such as coronary ischemia and ischemia-based renal failure (3).

Cocaine abuse is also associated with electrocardiographic (T-wave) abnormalities in people 50 years of age or older, suggesting the need for frequent screening for cardiovascular disease among aging cocaine abusers (6). The effect of other licit or illicit drugs on cocaine cardiotoxicity is not clear. However, there is increasing evidence that the combined use of alcohol and cocaine produces enhanced behavioral and cardiotoxic effects, possibly resulting from the direct actions of each and also from cocaethylene, a cocaine metabolite formed in the presence of alcohol (7,8). In terms of treatment, the correct therapy for cocaine cardiotoxicity remains unknown. However, calcium channel blockers, alpha blockers, nitrates, and thrombolytic therapy show some promise for the treatment of acute toxicity. The use of the angiotensin-converting enzyme (ACE) inhibitor fosinopril has been reported to be somewhat effective in the treatment of cardiotoxicity of cocaine and HIV (9). Beta blockade is controversial and may worsen coronary blood flow. In patients who develop cardiomyopathy, the usual therapy for this entity is appropriate (2).

HUMAN IMMUNODEFICIENCY VIRUS (HIV) AND CARDIOVASCULAR COMPLICATIONS

The HIV infects CD4 lymphocytes and macrophages, causing profound immunosuppression that eventually develops into acquired immunodeficiency syndrome (AIDS). An estimated 34.3 million people worldwide were living with HIV/AIDS at the end of 1999 (10,11). On the other hand, the most recent United Nations AIDS Programme (UNAIDS) update shows that at the end of 2001, an estimated 40 million people globally were living with HIV (12). In developed countries in Europe and North America, an estimated 1.5 million were living with HIV. Since 1981, when AIDS was first identified, approximately 1 million Americans have become infected with HIV, resulting in serious morbidity and mortality. However, with the increase in survival time and more effective antiviral therapy, new complications and manifestations of late-stage HIV infection are being reported, including cardiovascular disease. Since the first reported case of fatal dilated cardiomyopathy in an AIDS patient in 1986 (13), numerous echocardiographic studies have reported a high incidence of symptomatic cardiovascular complications in HIV-infected individuals. These complications include pericardial effusion, myocarditis, dilated cardiomyopathy, endocarditis, malignant neoplasms, coronary artery disease, and drug-related cardiotoxicity. In 1991, the prevalence of cardiac manifestations in AIDS patients ranged between 28 and 73% (14). In 1996, HIV cardiomyopathy was reported to be the fourth leading cause of dilated cardiomyopathy in adults in the United States. Half of these patients died of this disease within 6 to 12 months.

HIV AND COCAINE

The combined effects of cocaine and HIV coinfection remain unclear, although one may find exacerbated events of cardiac dysfunction (15). The effects include cardiomyopathies, left ventricular dysfunction, increased myocardial infarction, blood pressure dysregulation, and other vascular changes. An increase in ventricular wall thickness, considered a possibility in chronic cocaine abusers (16), has been reported in association with antiretroviral therapy in HIV-infected patients (17). Coronary atherosclerosis and increased calcium levels in the coronary arteries have been reported among African-American cocaine abusers coinfected with HIV (18).

COCAINE AND CARDIOVASCULAR RESEARCH AT NIDA

The National Institute on Drug Abuse (NIDA), a part of the National Institutes of Health (NIH), supports 85% of world's research on drug addiction, comorbidity, and associated medical and health consequences. Currently NIDA supports basic and clinical research on cardiovascular complications of substance abuse including abuse of cocaine, and infections in substance-abusing populations, such as HIV, hepatitis C, and sexually transmitted diseases. Following are examples that illustrate the breadth of drug abuse–related cardiovascular research at NIDA, which supports studies in the following areas: causes of varying sensitivity to cocaine-induced cardiovascular complications; differences in cocaine-related patterns of autonomic activity; endomorphins and cardiopulmonary control; roles of cocaine in central mechanisms of cardiomyopathy and cardiac function; sympathetic nerve activity of cocaine; efficacy of ACE-inhibitor therapy in the treatment of cardiovascular complications of HIV infection in cocaine abusers; subclinical atherosclerosis in HIV-infected cocaine abusers; cardiovascular complications in cocaine-exposed infants; maternal exposure to cocaine and fetal cardiotoxicity; efficacy of selenium therapy for cardiovascular disease in HIV-infected cocaine abusers; effects of cocaine on the sympathetic regulation of endotoxemia, which predisposes individuals to cardiovascular dysfunction; and mechanisms of cocaine-induced exacerbation of viral myocarditis.

FUTURE RESEARCH ON COCAINE AND HIV-RELATED HEART DISEASE

Based on recommendations from recent meetings cosponsored by NIDA and the National Heart, Lung, and Blood Institute (NHLBI), (see Chap. 24), where leading clinician/scientists discussed the most current research on HIV, substance abuse, and heart disease, NIDA encourages research to (1) Determine the incidence, prevalence, and pathophysiology of HIV related cardiovascular disease in vulnerable populations such as women, infants, and youth exposed to HIV and substance abuse; (2) study the role of other pathogens in HIV-related cardiovascular complications; (3) study autoimmune mechanisms in HIV-related cardiac conditions, particularly in combination with other pathogens; (4) determine the genetic predisposition for transition to dilated cardiomyopathy; (5) study the influence on cardiovascular disease of other conditions such as diabetes, atherosclerosis, and lifestyle in conjuction with behaviors such as smoking and recreational drug abuse, which are increasingly common among HIV-positive patients.

Recommendations include study of the following contributing to the mechanisms of cellular injury in HIV related cardiovascular complications: (1) interactions of viral replication, immune system activation, and inflammatory pathways in HIV/AIDS-related cardiovascular disease (CVD); (2) metabolic/energetic mechanisms such as the role of mitochondrial ATP production, cardiac myocyte energetics, increased reactive oxygen species, altered oxygen utilization, and changes in gene expression in HIV-related CVD; (3) the role of both acute and chronic highly active antiretroviral therapies (HAART) in HIV/AIDS-related CVD; and pharmacokinetic drug interactions between HAART and pharmaceuticals use in the treatment of cardiac disease; (4) the role of HIV components (gp120, tat, etc.) in cardiac myocyte function; (5) interactions between immune cells (infected and/or uninfected), parenchymal cells, and cardiac myocytes; (6) study of the role of cytokines in the modulation of cardiac myocyte function; (7) mechanisms such as recruitment, gene expression, and signaling events among cells; and (8) the role of the hypothalamic-pituitary-adrenal (HPA) axis in HIV-related cardiovascular disease.

On the subject of therapies for HIV/AIDS cardiovascular complications, recommendations include the following: (1) undertake preclinical investigations; (2) develop animal models to study the effects of antiretroviral therapies for HIV cardiovascular complications that would provide a basis for large clinical trials; and (3) in clinical therapeutics and prevention trials, determine (1) optimal therapies for treating HIV-related cardiomyopathy; (2) if these therapies should be different for other forms of cardiomyopathy; (3) if early intervention is possible and advantageous; and (4) if the early changes in left ventricular performance can be prevented or reversed. Finally, studies of alternative therapies (e.g., antioxidants, immunomodulators, nutritional therapies) in HIV CVD were recommended for increased support.

REFERENCES

1. Das G, Laddu A. Cocaine: friend or foe? Part 1. Int J Clin Pharmacol Ther Toxicol 1993; 31(9):449–455.
2. Kloner RA, Hale S, Alker K, Rezkalla S. The effects of acute and chronic cocaine use on the heart. Circulation 1992; 85(2):407–419.
3. Wilkins JN. Brain, lung, and cardiovascular interactions with cocaine and cocaine-induced catecholamine effects. J Addict Dis 1992; 11(4):9–19.
4. Substance Abuse and Mental Health Services Administration (SAMHSA). Household Survey of Drug Abuse. Rockville, MD: SAMSA, 2001.
5. Substance Abuse and Mental Health Services Administration, Drug Abuse Warning Network. Rockville, MD: SAMSA, 2001.
6. Hollister LE. Electrocardiographic screening in psychiatric patients. J Clin Psychiatry 1995; 56(1):26–29.
7. Fowler JS, Volkow ND, Logan J, MacGregor RR, Wang GJ, Wolf AP. Alcohol intoxication does not change [11C]cocaine pharmacokinetics in human brain and heart. Synapse 1992; 12(3):228–235.
8. Henning RJ, Wilson LD, Glauser JM. Cocaine plus ethanol is more cardiotoxic than cocaine or ethanol alone. Crit Care Med 1994; 22(12):1896–1906.
9. Morgolin A, Avants SK, Setaro JF, Rinder HM, Grupp L. Cocaine, HIV, and their cardiovascular effects: is there a role of ACE-inhibitor therapy? Drug Alcohol Depend 2000; 61(1):35–45.
10. Gayle HD, Hill GL. Global impact of human immunodeficiency virus and AIDS. Clin Microbiol Rev 2001; 14:327–335.
11. Gayle HD. An overview of the global HIV/AIDS epidemic, with a focus on the United States. AIDS 2000; 14:S8–S17.
12. United Nations AIDS (UNAIDS). AIDS Epidemic Update, December 2001. UNAIDS/ 01.74E-WHO/CS/CSR/NCS 2001.2, English Original, Dec 2001, ISBN 92-9173–132-3, Joint United Nations Programme on HIV/AIDS/WHO.
13. Cohen IS, Anderson DW, Vermani R, Reen BM, Macher AM, Sennesh J, DiLorenzo P, Redfield RR. Congestive cardiomyopathy in association with the acquired immunodeficiency syndrome. N Engl J Med 1986; 315(10):628–630.
14. Rerkpattanapipat P, Wongpraparut N, Jacobs LE, Kotler MN. Cardiac manifestations of acquired immunodeficiency syndrome. Arch Intern Med 2000; 160:602–608.
15. Soodini G, Morgan JP. Can cocaine abuse exacerbate the cardiac toxicity of human immunodeficiency virus? Clin Cardiol 2001; 24(3):177–181.
16. Eisenberg MJ, Jue J, Mendelson J, Jones RT, Schiller NB. Left ventricular morphologic features and function in nonhospitalized cocaine users: a quantitative two-dimensional echocardiographic study. Am Heart J 1995; 129(5):941–946.
17. Meng Q, Lima JAC, Lai H, Vlahov D, Celentano D, Strathdee S, Nelson K, Tong W, Lai S. Use of HIV protease inhibitors is associated with left ventricular morphologic changes and diastolic dysfunction. J AIDS 2002; 30:306–310.
18. Lai S, Lai H, Meng Q, Tong W, Vlahov D, Celentano D, Strathdee S, Nelson K, Fishman EK, Lima JAC. Effect of cocaine use on coronary calcium among black adults in Baltimore, Maryland. Am J Cardiol 2002; 90:326–328.

22

Cocaine-Induced Exacerbation of Viral Myocarditis

Jufeng Wang and James P. Morgan
Beth Israel Deaconess Medical Center, Harvard Medical School, Boston, Massachusetts, U.S.A.

BACKGROUND

HIV and Myocarditis

Infectious myocarditis is an inflammatory process of the heart that is due to an infectious agent, usually a virus. The inflammation may not be confined to the myocardium and sometimes involves the pericardium as well, in which case it is referred to as myopericarditis. Although myocarditis is commonly associated with infections, an inflammatory reaction may follow a variety of insults, including exposure to drugs, chemicals, physical agents, bites and stings, and endogenous or exogenous catecholamines. Myocarditis occurs in acute, subacute, and chronic forms. It may be reversible, stable, or relentlessly progressive. In acute viral myocarditis the heart is dilated, the papillary muscles and trabeculae carneae are flattened, and the myocardium is pale and often yellow-gray, with yellow-brown streaks of minute hemorrhages. Microscopically, there may be serous effusion with only a few inflammatory cells, or there may be destruction and loss of muscle fibers, with polymorphonuclear leukocytes early and mononuclear cells later, including histiocytes and sometimes eosinophils. Necrosis of myofibers occurs and may be either patchy or diffuse and may be found at any site, including the conduction system. Chronic and healed lesions show interstitial fibrosis and have evidence of loss of myofibers (92,93,95–97). After 7 to 10 days from the onset of symptoms, viruses can sometimes be cultured from the myocardium. For many years, reports on myocarditis were plagued by lack of uniform histological criteria. In order to provide a common approach, the Dallas criteria were developed in 1984 in hopes that a uniform histopathological classification would improve our understanding of myocarditis and its therapy (1–6).

Evidence from animal experiments, primarily in mice, indicates two possible mechanisms of injury to the heart. In viral myocarditis, direct invasion by the virus and replication are found early after the onset of infection and result in myocardial necrosis. The infectious phase is usually 7 to 14 days, during which virus is recoverable from the heart; this is usually followed by a complete recovery. In this acute phase, a direct cytotoxic effect of the virus on the myocardium is postulated. Serum neutralizing antibody (IgM) develops within a week, and it is thought that this, together with mononuclear cell invasion, limits viral replication.

Severe myocarditis may result from more virulent viral strains; alternatively a "conditioned response" to viruses that are ordinarily benign may result in an acute infectious phase with severe congestive heart failure, ventricular arrhythmias, cardiac tamponade, and death. A substantial body of evidence suggests that in some individuals, acute viral myocarditis may evolve into chronic dilated cardiomyopathy. The mechanism may be an immune-mediated injury. This hypothesis is attractive in view of the potential benefit of immunosuppressive therapy, but further evidence will be needed to establish an unequivocal cause-and-effect relationship (74–90). Experimental evidence in animals and circumstantial evidence in humans support the concept that myocardial injury from infection is not always a simple process. Instead, it has multiple causes deriving from the convergence of several conditioning factors, one of which may be infection. Possible conditioning factors include familial predisposition, peripartum state, hypoxia, exercise, malnutrition, bacterial infection, ethanol intake, ionizing radiation, and exposure to heat or cold, among others (1–6). Much of the recent work in our laboratory has been related to the hypothesis that catecholamines may play an important conditioning role in patients abusing cocaine (7,8).

A variety of viruses have been reported as causative agents of myocarditis in humans, including coxsackie, echo and influenza viruses, cytomegalovirus, poliomyelitis virus, infectious mononucleosis virus, herpes simplex virus, adenovirus, and several others (1–6). In recent years, a growing body of evidence has accumulated indicating that cardiac dysfunction can occur in patients infected with HIV (9–14). Among the complications associated with HIV disease are pericarditis, myocarditis, ventricular tachycardia, endocarditis, cardiac malignancy (Kaposi's sarcoma, lymphoma), and dilated cardiomyopathy. In an autopsy series, lymphocytic myocarditis was seen in 35 to 52% of cases, and lymphocytic myocarditis has been associated with left ventricular dysfunction and ventricular tachycardia (1,9). The cause of lymphocytic myocarditis is not known but could be related to opportunistic infection with viral, protozoan, bacterial, fungal, or microbacterial pathogens. It is not known whether HIV can itself infect or damage cardiac muscle.

Cocaine, HIV, and Myocarditis

An increasing amount of evidence suggests that cocaine abusers have an increased incidence of HIV infection and HIV-related myocarditis (15–20). These data suggest but do not prove a cause-and-effect relationship. Possible mechanisms of this effect include enhanced infectivity of the virus through a diminished immune response or through cocaine-induced damage to the endothelial/endocardial cells or myocytes themselves, thereby reducing structural barriers to cellular penetration of the virus and increasing the vascular permeability and diffusability of viral particles. Evidence supporting this possibility includes reports in the literature suggesting that cocaine can damage the endothelial lining of cells after even a single exposure, thereby accelerating atherosclerosis in animal models (21–24). In addition, cocaine has been reported to cause myocardial cell damage through direct and catecholamine- mediated effects as well as by producing myocardial ischemia and infarction (25–32). Both lymphocytic and eosinophilic myocarditis has been reported in cocaine abusers (33–35). Alternatively, cocaine may exacerbate viral myocarditis by enhancing the toxicity of the viral agent once it has penetrated the cell membrane. Such an effect may occur through a direct or catecholamine-mediated alteration in the cellular milieu that in turn could alter viral transcription and replication. Such effects could include a change in cellular pH, shift in osmolarity, or depletion of high-energy stores necessary for protective proteolytic enzyme activity. Of course, it is likely that the effects of cocaine on the animal or patient with myocarditis are complex and involve several mechanisms or conditioning factors, as described above (98–115). However, the observation that exacerbation of myocarditis seems to occur with cocaine but not other commonly abused drugs without prominent cardiac effects, including heroin and phencyclidine, suggest that cocaine may have a unique combination of properties that make its use in patients exposed to or infected with viral pathogens susceptible to developing myocarditis. We have proposed that the unique ability of cocaine to increase local release and circulating levels of catecholamines is the primary effect responsible for exacerbation of myocarditis (7,8). There are four major mechanisms that are likely to account for cocaine-mediated exacerbation of viral myocarditis, via its direct or indirect actions (116–138):

1. General impairment of cellular integrity, making the myocardium more susceptible to any additional insult. For example, generalized necrosis/ stunning of myocardial cells secondary to an ischemic insult might conceivably impair cardiac reserve sufficiently to produce clinical expression of superimposed myocarditis that would be masked by the considerable functional reserve of normal hearts.

2. The myocardial pathogenicity of the virus may be enhanced leading to an increased initial viral load per cell or a greater number of infected cells.

3. The myocardial cell pathogenicity of the virus may be enhanced, consequently resulting in an enhanced replication of the virus within the cell.

4. The myocardial cell pathogenicity of the virus may be enhanced, consequently resulting in decreased cellular defenses against viral induced cytotoxins.

Catecholamines, Cocaine, and Myocarditis

The hypothesis that catecholamines may exacerbate viral myocarditis in both animals and humans is based on evidence from several different sources. The most direct evidence arises from carefully controlled studies of murine myocarditis indicating that hypercatecholaminergic states, such as pheochromocytoma, and sympathomimetic drugs can cause or significantly exacerbate myocarditis (33–49). Moreover, sympatholytic agents and states may ameliorate the manifestations of myocarditis and decrease mortality, although this effect is controversial (49–54). It is provocative that many of the interventions shown to ameliorate viral myocarditic pathogenicity including calcium channel blockers act predominately to modulate the cellular effects of catecholamines, perhaps by enhancing NO levels, which has been shown to markedly enhance sympathomimetic effects on the heart (55–58). Additional evidence includes the observation that, among commonly abused substances in the HIV and general populations [alcohol, nicotine, caffeine, marijuana, and cocaine most notably (25,27)], cocaine alone has been associated with an increased incidence of reportable cases of myocarditis, suggesting that its unique sympathomimetic properties, not shared with these other agents, may be the causative factor (139–145). Moreover, in the clinical arena, it has been accepted clinical practice for many years to restrict the activities of patients with myocarditis based on circumstantial evidence that exercise exacerbates the disease (1–6). In addition to directly increasing the work of the heart, normal exercise is associated with a marked increase in circulating catecholamine levels (59–73). The availability of reproducible animal models of myocarditis has allowed us to directly test the catecholamine hypothesis with regard to cocaine (8).

HYPOTHESIS TESTED: COCAINE IN MYOCARDITIS

Methodology

We used mice to test our hypothesis that cocaine can increase the incidence and exacerbate viral myocarditis. BALB/c mice were divided into eight groups: saline control, encephalomyocarditis virus (EMCV), cocaine 10 mg/kg (coc-10), cocaine 30 mg/kg (coc-30), cocaine 50 mg/kg (coc-50), EMCV + coc-10, EMCV + coc-30, EMCV + coc-50. After inoculation with EMCV, the mice were treated daily with cocaine or saline for 90 days. Mice were sacrificed on day 3, 7, 14, 21, 35, 60, or 90 after EMCV inoculation. Mortality was recorded and myocarditis was evaluated by hematoxylin/eosin staining. The mortality of the myocarditis mice treated with cocaine increased significantly, from 22% (EMCV) to 25.7% (coc-10 + EMCV), 41.4% (coc-30 + EMCV), and 51.4% (coc-50 + EMCV) ($p < 0.05$), respectively. The incidence and severity of inflammatory cell infiltration and myocardial lesions was higher in infected mice exposed to cocaine. Cocaine administered only before infection did not exacerbate myocarditis. Norepinephrine (NE) assay showed that cocaine exposure significantly increased myocardial NE concentration, but this increase was partially inhibited in infected animals. Adrenalectomy abolished the effect of cocaine on mortality. Furthermore, propranolol, a beta blocker, significantly decreased the enhancing effects of cocaine on myocarditic mice. We find that cocaine increased the severity and mortality of viral myocarditis in mice. Increased catecholamines may be a major factor responsible for this effect.

Results

Experiment One

Morbidity and Mortality. Three days after the virus inoculation, the mice appeared ill; some developed coat ruffling, weakness, and irritability. After day 7, myocardial necrosis and inflammatory cell infiltration were more extensive. RT-PCR results showed the presence of EMCV RNA in the mouse hearts 7 days after inoculation of virus. Some mice developed paralysis of the hind legs. The mortality of the virus control group was 22%. Infection with EMCV produced pathological changes similar to those reported previously (76,94). Cocaine alone did not produce death in any of the three doses studied.

After exposure to cocaine, mortality of the myocarditic mice significantly increased ($p < 0.05$ compared with the untreated group). The total survival rate (Fig. 1) in each group was 78% for the virus group (11 of 50), 74.3% for EMCV + coc-

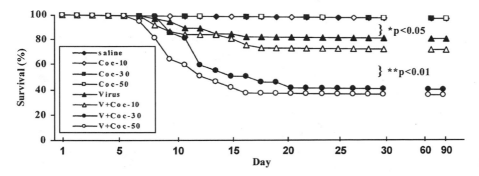

Figure 1 Survival in murine myocarditis model induced by EMCV. Animals were treated with cocaine daily. The percent survival in the cocaine-treated groups was significantly lower than in the EMCV alone group from days 5 through 12, $p < 0.05$. Coc-10, cocaine 10mg/kg; coc-30, cocaine 30 mg/kg; coc-50, cocaine 50 mg/kg. Each treated group consisted of 50 to 70 mice, and each cocaine alone group consisted of 20 mice. (From Ref. 8.)

10 (18 of 70), 58.6% for EMCV + coc-30 (36 of 70), and 48.6% for EMCV + coc-50 (41 of 70). As the dose of cocaine was increased, the mortality from myocarditis significantly increased; there was a significant dose-response relationship among the cocaine-treated groups ($p < 0.05$). Moreover, in the EMCV + coc-50 group, death occurred earlier than in the other groups. There were no significant pathological findings in the myocardia of mice treated with cocaine alone. As indicated in Figure 1, the deaths of mice occurred within 4 to 16 days of virus inoculation.

Histological Examination. On day 3, few scattered foci of myocyte necrosis associated with inflammatory cells were noted in viral infected mice. By days 7, 14, and 35, myocyte necrosis and accompanying inflammation had become extensive, confluent in some areas and multifocal in others. Inflammatory cells were predominantly mononuclear. On day 60, there was obvious cavity dilatation and a decrease in wall thickness. In cocaine-treated groups, the pathological changes were exacerbated in both acute and subacute phases of myocarditis. During the chronic phase of myocarditis, some areas showed fibroblastic and vascular proliferation in the regions of necrotic, focally calcified myocytes. Also, a mild degree of fibrosis was recognized in the areas of fibroblastic proliferation. On day 35 and later, the major histological findings were multifocal fibroblastic and vascular proliferation and fibrosis in the myocardium associated with necrotic calcified myocytes. Cavity dilatation was observed in the EMCV-plus-cocaine group. However, inflammatory cell infiltration was not prominent (Fig. 2). On day 60, in addition to clear cavity dilatation, hearts showed a decrease in ventricular wall thickness. On day 90, the pathological changes were similar to day 60. These results showed that cocaine exposure exacerbated the course and severity of myocarditis. At the subacute phase, the histopathological scores for necrosis and inflammatory cell infiltration were significantly higher in comparison with those of the virus control. In the chronic phase, the score for inflammatory cell infiltration and necrosis decreased in both groups; however, the percent of mice with cavity dilatation increased (Figure 3A to C) ($p < 0.05$).

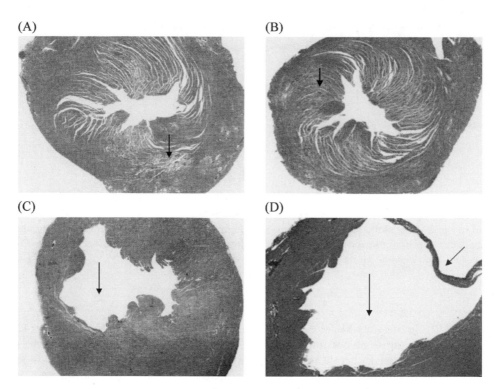

Figure 2 Myocardial sections from cocaine-treated myocarditic mice. Panels A and B: days 7 and 14 after cocaine treatment in infected mice. The arrows point to inflammatory cell infiltration and necrosis. Panel C: enlarged ventricular chamber at day 35. Panel D: dilatation of left ventricular chamber and decreased wall thickness at day 60. (Hematoxylin/eosin stain; original magnification ×2.) (From Ref. 8.)

Experiment Two

Acute (5-day), subacute (15-day), and chronic (30-day) preexposure to cocaine did not increase the mortality or exacerbate the severity of myocarditis. There were no marked differences in pathological changes between the preexposure and saline control mice.

Experiment Three

Cocaine exposure markedly increased norepinephrine (NE) concentrations in mouse hearts (Fig. 4). An 80% increase in the content of NE was seen after 3 days' administration compared to saline controls ($p < 0.05$). NE reached the peak concentration during the early period of cocaine administration. As administration of cocaine continued, the NE content decreased but was still significantly higher than in the saline controls. In the EMCV group, NE concentration was significantly lower than saline control ($p < 0.05$). Cocaine exposure, however, significantly elevated the content of NE in EMCV mouse hearts ($p < 0.05$ compared to EMCV control).

Experiment Four

After adrenalectomy, cocaine's effects to increase mortality or exacerbate the severity of myocarditis were abolished (Fig. 5). These data indicate that removal of the adrenal

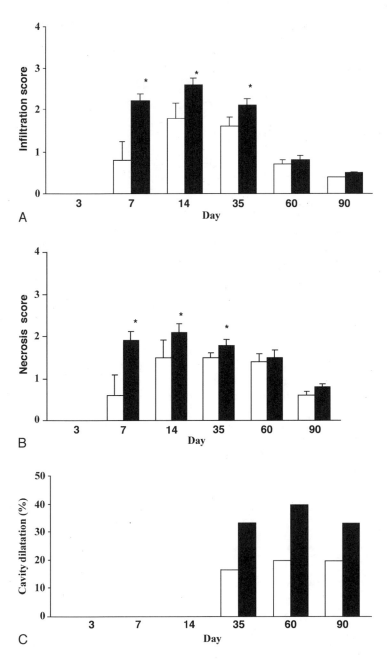

Figure 3 Histological grading according to experimental group and time. Histological scoring of hearts ranged from 0 to 4 in each of the categories of inflammation, necrosis, and chamber enlargement. The enhancing effect of cocaine upon myocarditis through day 35 is evident. Dilatation of the left ventricle became evident only on day 35. Data are displayed as group mean $\pm$ SEM. *$p < 0.05$ compared to virus group. Open bar: EMCV group; Solid bar: EMCV plus cocaine 30 mg/kg. Panel A: infiltration, □ Saline; ■ Cocaine. Panel B: necrosis, Panel C: cavity dilatation. □ Saline; ■ Cocaine. (From Ref. 8.)

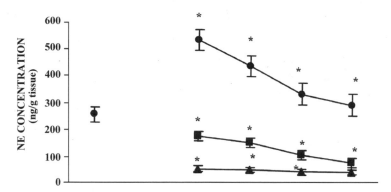

Figure 4 Myocardial concentration of norepinephrine (NE). Mice were infected with EMCV and treated with cocaine (30 mg/kg) $n = 6$, $p > 0.05$ compared with saline control. Circle: cocaine group; square: cocaine plus EMCV; triangle: EMCV. The results show that cocaine exposure significantly increased the concentration of NE. (From Ref. 8.)

gland, a major source of catecholamine in mice, ameliorated cocaine's toxicity in the EMCV group.

Experiment Five

Figure 6 shows that propranolol significantly decreased the mortality of myocarditic mice ($p < 0.05$ compared to EMCV control) and also attenuated the enhancing effect of cocaine on viral myocarditis ($p < 0.05$ compared to EMCV + coc-30 group). The necrosis and inflammatory cell infiltration were less than that in the EMCV group. These data indicate that beta-adrenergic blockade ameliorated the toxic effect of cocaine on myocarditic mice.

In conclusion, cocaine increased the severity and mortality of viral myocarditis in the mouse model, supporting the hypothesis that catecholamines may be a major factor responsible for this effect.

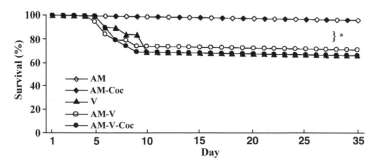

Figure 5 Survival in myocarditic mice with bilateral adrenalectomy. Mice were infected with EMCV after a 2-week recovery from the surgery and treated with cocaine 30 mg/kg. *$p < 0.05$ compared to EMCV-infected mice. AM, adrenalectomy; AM-Coc, adrenalectomy plus cocaine (30 mg/kg); V, EMCV; AM-V, adrenalectomy plus EMCV; AM-V-Coc, adrenalectomy plus EMCV and cocaine (30 mg/kg). Each group consisted of 30 mice. All of the mice in the AM and AM-Coc groups survived; the survival curves overlapped. (From Ref. 8.)

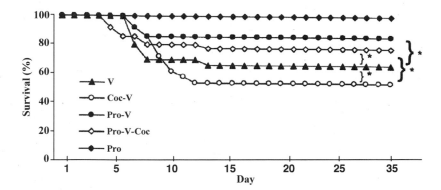

Figure 6 Survival in myocarditic mice treated with either propranolol (Pro) or cocaine daily. The percent survival in Pro was significantly higher than that in the V (EMCV) alone group. Also, Pro significantly decreased the mortality of myocarditic mice treated with cocaine. *$p < 0.05$. Pro, propranolol 3 mg/kg; Pro-V, EMCV plus pro; Pro-V-Coc, EMCV plus cocaine 30 mg/kg and Pro. Each treated group consisted of 40 to 60 mice. (From Ref. 8.)

ACKNOWLEDGMENT

This work supported in part by DA 63030-03 NIH/NHLBI.

REFERENCES

1. Rodeheffer RJ, Gersh BJ. Cardiomyopathy and biopsy. A. Dilated cardiomyopathy and the myocarditides. In: Giuliani ER, Gersh BJ, McGoon MD, Hayes DL, Schaff HU, eds. Mayo Clinic Practice of Cardiology. St. Louis: Mosby, 1996:636–671.
2. Ensley RD, Renlund DG, Mason JW. Myocarditis. In: Willerson JT, Cohn JN, eds. Cardiovascular Medicine. New York: Churchhill Livingstone, 1995:894–923.
3. Brown CA, O'Connell JB. Myocarditis and idiopathic dilated cardiomyopathy. Am J Med 1995; 99(3):309–314.
4. Pisani B, Taylor DO, Mason JW. Inflammatory myocardial diseases and cardiomyopathies. Am J Med 1997; 102(5):459–469.
5. Abelmann WH. Myocarditis. N Engl J Med 1966; 275(17):944–945.
6. Liu P, Martino T, Opavsky MA, Penninger J. Viral myocarditis: balance between viral infection and immune response. Can J Cardiol 1996; 12(10):935–943.
7. Soodini G, Morgan JP. Can cocaine abuse exacerbate the cardiac toxicity human immunodeficiency virus? Clin Cardiol 2001; 24:177–181.
8. Wang J-F, Zhang J, Min J-Y, Sullivan MF, Crumpacker CS, Abelmann WH, Morgan JP. Cocaine enhances myocarditis induced by encephalomyocarditis virus in murine model. Am J Physiol Heart Circ Physiol 2002; 282:H956–H963.
9. Patel RC, Frishman WH. Cardiac involvement in HIV infection. Med Clin North Am 1996; 80(6):1493–1512.
10. Levy WS, Varghese J, Anderson D, et al. Myocarditis diagnosed by endomyocardial biopsy in human immunodeficiency virus infection with cardiac dysfunction. Am J Cardiol 1998; 62:658–659.
11. Hale GS, Kainer M, Wright E, Mijch A. HIV associated myocarditis: clinical course and response to corticosteroid therapy. Annu Conf Australas Soc HIV Med 1995; 7:68.

12. Barbaro G, DiLorenzo G, Grisorio B, Barbarini G. Clinical meaning of ventricular ectopic beats in the diagnosis of HIV-related myocarditis: a retrospective analysis of Holter electrocardiographic recordings, echocardiographic parameters, histopathological and virologic findings. Cardiologia 1996; 41(12):1199–1207.

13. Beschorner WE, Baughman K, Turnicky RP, Hutchins GM, Rowe SA, Kavanaugh-McHugh AL, Suresch DL, Herskowtiz A. HIV-associated myocarditis. Pathology and immunopathology. Am J Pathol 1990; 137(6):1365–1371.

14. Herskowtiz A, Willoughby SB, Vlahov D, Baughman KL, Ansari AA. Dilated heart muscle disease associated with HIV infection. Eur Heart J 1995; 16:50–55.

15. Larrat EP, Zierler S. Entangled epidemics: cocaine use and HIV disease. J Psychoact Drugs 1993; 25(3):207–221.

16. Goodkin K, Shapshak P, Metsch LR, McCoy CB, Crandall KA, Kumar M, Fujimura RK, McCoy V, Zhang BT, Reyblat S, Xin KQ, Kuman AM. Cocaine abuse and HIV-1 infection: epidemiology and neuropathogenesis. J Neuroimmunol 1998; 83(1-2):88–101.

17. Wilson T, DeHovitz JA. STDs, HIV, and crack cocaine: a review. Aids Patient Care STDS 1997; 11(2):62–66.

18. Peterson PK, Gekker G, Schut R, Hu S, Balfour HH, Chao CC. Enhancement of HIV-1 replication by opiates and cocaine: the cytokine connection. Adv Exp Med Biol 1993; 335:181–188.

19. Shapshak P, Crandall KA, Xin KQ, Goodkin K, Fujimura RK, Bradley W, McCoy CB, Nagano I, Yoshioka M, Petito C, Sun NC, Srivastava AK, Weatherby N, Steward R, Delgado S, Matthews A, Douyon R, Okuda K, Yang J, Zhangl BT, Cao XR, Shatkovsky S, Fernandez JB, Shah SM, Perper J. HIV-1 neuropathogenesis and abused drugs: current reviews, problems, and solutions. Adv Exp Biol 1996; 402:171–186.

20. Donahoe RM, Falek A. Neuroimmunomodulation by opiates and other drugs of abuse: relationship to HIV infection and AIDS. Adv Biochem Psychopharmacol 1988; 44:145–158.

21. Kolodgie FD, Virmani R, Cornhill JF, Herderick EE, Smialek J. Increase in atherosclerosis and adventitial mast cells in cocaine abusers: an alternative mechanism of cocaine-associated coronary vasospasm and thrombosis. J Am Coll Cardiol 1991; 17(7):1553–1560.

22. Egashira K, Pipers FS, Morgan JP. Effects of cocaine on epicardial coronary artery reactivity in minature swine after endothelial injury and high cholesterol feeding. In vivo and in vitro analysis. J Clin Invest 1991; 88(4):1307–1314.

23. Bacharach JM, Colville DS, Lie JT. Accelerated atherosclerosis, aneurysmal disease, and aortitis: possible pathogenetic association with cocaine abuse. Int Angiol 1992; 11(1):83–86.

24. Kolodgie FD, Wilson PS, Cornhill JF, Herderick EE, Mergner WJ, Virmani R. Increased prevalence of aortic fatty streaks in cholesterol-fed rabbits administered intravenous cocaine: the role of vascular endothelium. Toxicol Pathol 1993; 21(5):425–435.

25. Kloner RA, Hale S, Alker K, Rezkalla S. The effects of acute and chronic cocaine use on the heart. Circulation 1992; 85(2):407–419.

26. Karch SB, Billingham ME. The pathology and etilogy of cocaine-induced heart disease. Arch Pathol Lab Med 1988; 112(3):225–230.

27. Isner JM, Shokshi SK. Cardiac complications of cocaine abuse. Annu Rev Med 1991; 42:133–138.

28. Peng SK, French WJ, Pilikan PC. Direct cocaine cardiotoxicity demonstrated by endomyocardial biopsy. Arch Pathol Lab Med 1989; 113(8):842–845.

29. Lange RA, Hillis LD. Cardiovascular complications of cocaine use. N Engl J Med 2001; 345:351–358.

30. Rezkalla SH, Hale S, Kloner RA. Cocaine-induced heart diseases. Am Heart J 1990; 120:1403–1408.

31. Om A. Cardiovascular complication of cocaine. Am J Med Sci 1992; 303(5):333–339.

32. Knuepfer MM, Branch CA, Gan Q, Fischer VW. Cocaine-induced myocardial ultrastructural alterations and cardiac output responses in rat. Exp Mol Pathol 1993; 59(2):155–168.

33. Jentzen JM. Cocaine-induced myocarditis. Am Heart J 1989; 117(6):1398–1399.

34. Virmani R, Robinowitz M, Smialek JE, Smyth DF. Cardiovascular effects of cocaine: an autopsy study of 40 patients. Am Heart J 1988; 115(5):1068–1076.

35. Talebzadeh VC, Chevrolet JC, Chatelain P, Helfer C, Cox JN. Eosinophilic myocarditis and pulmonary hypertension in a drug-addict. Anatomo-clinical study and brief review of the literature. Ann Pathol 1990; 10(1):40–46.

36. Nash CB, Carter JR. Hemorrhagic myocarditis and cardiovascular collapse induced by catecholamine infusion. Arch Int Pharmacodyn Ther 1967; 166(1):172–180.

37. Cho T, Tanimura A, Saito Y. Catecholamine-induced cardiopathy accompanied with pheochromocytoma. Acta Pathol Jpn 1987; 37(1):123–132.

38. Van Vliet PD, Burchell HB, Titus JL. Focal myocarditis associated with pheochromocytoma. N Engl J Med 1966; 274(20):1102–1108.

39. Bindoli A, Rigobello MP, Deeble DJ. Biochemical and toxicological properties of the oxidation products of catecholamines. Free Radic Biol Med 1992; 13(4):391–405.

40. Kammermeier M, Grobecker HF. Cardiotoxicity of catecholamines after application of L-DOPA in Wistar-Kyoto (WKY) and spontaneously hypertensive rats (SHR). Hypertens Res 1995; 18(suppl 1):S165–S168.

41. Davila DF, Gottenberg CF, Torres A, Holzhaker G, Barrios R, Ramoni P, Donis JH. Cardiac sympathetic-parasympathetic balance in rats with experimentally-induced acute chagasic myocarditis. Rev Inst Med Trop Sao Paulo 1995; 37(2):155–159.

42. Prichard BN, Owens CW, Smith CC, Walden RJ. Heart and catecholamines. Acta Cardiol 1991; 46(3):309–322.

43. Van Vliet PD, Burchell HB, Titus JL. Focal myocarditis associated with pheochromocytoma. N Engl J Med 1966; 274(20):1102–1108.

44. Brown CA, O'Connell JB. Myocarditis and idiopathic dilated cardiomyopathy. Am J Med 1995; 99(3):309–314.

45. Siltanen P, Penttila O, Merikallio E, Kyosola K, Klinge E, Pispa J. Myocardial catecholamines and their biosynthetic enzymes in various human heart diseases. Acta Med Scand Suppl 1982; 660:24–33.

46. Haft JI. Cardiovascular injury induced by sympathetic catecholamines. Prog Cardiovasc Dis 1974; 17(1):73–86.

47. Noda M, Kawano O, Uchida O, Sawabe T, Saito G. Myocarditis induced by sympathomimetic amines. I. Jpn Circ J 1970; 34(1):7–12.

48. Morin Y, Cote G. Toxic agents and cardiomyopathies. Cardiovasc Clin 1972; 4:245–267.

49. Seta Y, Kanda T, Yokoyama T, Kobayashi I, Suzuki T, Nagai R. Effect of amrinone on murine viral myocarditis. Res Commun Mol Pathol Pharmacol 1997; 95(1):57–66.

50. Rezkalla S, Kloner RA, Khatib G, Smith FE, Khatib R. Effect of metoprolol in acute coxsackievirus B3 murine myocarditis. J Am Coll Cardiol 1988; 12(2):412–414.

51. Anandasabapathy S, Frishman WH. Innovative drug treatments for viral and auto-immune myocarditis. J Clin Pharmacol 1998; 38(4):295–308.

52. Mehes G, Rajkovits K, Papp G. Effect of various types of sympathicolytics on isoproterenol- induced myocardial lesions. Acta Physiol Acad Sci Hung 1966; 29(1):75–85.

53. Dunn AJ, Vickers SL. Neurochemical and neuroendocrine responses to Newcastle disease virus administration in mice. Brain Res 1994; 645(1-2):103–112.

54. Dong R, Liu P, Wee L, Butany J, Sole MJ. Verapamil ameliorates the clinical and pathological course of murine myocarditis. J Clin Invest 1992; 90(5):2022–2030.

55. Hiraoka Y, Kishimoto C, Takada H, Nakamura M, Kurokawa M, Ochiai H, Shiraki K.

Nitric oxide and murine coxsackievirus B3 myocarditis: aggravation of myocarditis by inhibition of nitric oxide snythase. J Am Coll Cardiol 1996; 28(6):1610–1615.

56. Lowenstein CJ, Hill SL, Lafond-Walker A, Wu J, Allen G, Landavere M, Rose NR. Herskowitz A Nitric oxide inhibits viral replication in murine myocarditis. J Clin Invest 1996; 97(8):1837–1843.

57. Wang WZ, Matsumori A, Yamada T, Shioi T, Okada I, Matsui S, Sato Y, Suzuki H, Shiota K, Kasayama S. Beneficial effects of amlodipine in a murine model of congestive heart failure induced by viral myocarditis. A possible mechanism through inhibition of nitric oxide production. Circulation 1997; 95(1):245–251.

58. Keaney JF, Hare JM, Ballingand JL, Loscalzo J, Smith TW, Colucci WS. Inhibition of nitric oxide synthase augments myocardial contractile responses to beta-adrenergic stimulation. Am J Physiol 1996; 271(6 Pt 2):H2646–H2652.

59. Conlee RK, Barnett DW, Kelly KP, Han DH. Effects of cocaine on plasma catecholamine and muscle glycogen concentrations during exercise in the rat. J Appl Physiol 1991; 70(3):1323–1327.

60. Bracken ME, Bracken DR, Nelson AG, Conlee RK. Effect of cocaine on exercise endurance and glycogen use in rats. J Appl Physiol 1988; 64(2):884–887.

61. Cigarroa CG, Boehrer JD, Brickner ME, Eichhorn EJ, Grayburn PA. Exaggerated pressor response to treadmill exercise in chronic cocaine abusers with left ventricular hypertrophy. Circulation 1992; 86(1):226–231.

62. Cabinian AE, Kiel RJ, Smith F, Ho KL, Khatib R, Reyes MP. Modification of exercise-aggravated coxsackie virus B3 murine myocarditis by T lymphocyte suppression in an inbred model. J Lab Clin Med 1990; 115(4):454–462.

63. Gatmaitan BG, Chason JL, Lerner AM. Augmentation of the virulence of murine coxsackie-virus B-3 myocardiopathy by exercise. J Exp Med 1970; 131(6):1121–1136.

64. Friman G, Larsson E, Rolf C. Interaction between infection and exercise with special reference to myocarditis and the increased frequency of sudden deaths among young Swedish orienteers 1979-92. Scan J Infect Dis Suppl 1997; 104:41–49.

65. Christensen NJ, Galbo H. Sympathetic nervous activity during exercise. Annu Rev Physiol 1983; 45:139–153.

66. Hosenpud JD, Campbell SM, Niles NR, Lee J, Mendelson D, Hart MV. Exercise induced augmentation of cellular and humoral autoimmunity associated with increased cardiac dilatation in experimental autoimmune myocarditis. Cardiovasc Res 1987; 21(3):217–222.

67. Pagliari R, Peyrin L. Physical conditioning in rats influences the central and peripheral catecholamine responses to sustained exercise. Eur J Appl Physiol 1995; 71(1):41–52.

68. Kiel RJ, Smith FE, Chason J, Khatib R, Reyes MP. Coxsackievirus B3 myocarditis in C3H/HeJ mice: description of an inbred model and the effect of exercise on virulence. Eur J Epidemiol 1989; 5(3):348–350.

69. Ilback NG, Friman G, Squibb RL, Johnson AJ, Balentine DA, Beisel WR. The effect of exercise and fasting on the myocardial protein and lipid metabolism in experimental bacterial myocarditis. Acta Pathol Microbiol Immunol Scand 1984; 92(4):195–204.

70. Friman G, Wesslen L, Karjalainen J, Rolf C. Infectious and lymphocytic myocarditis: epidemiology and factors relevant to sports medicine. Scan J Med Sci Sports 1995; 5(5):269–278.

71. Gwathmey JK, Slawsky MT, Perreault CL, Briggs GM, Morgan JP, Wei JY. Effect of exercise conditioning on excitation-contraction coupling in aged rats. J Appl Physiol 1990; 69(4):1366–1371.

72. Han DH, Kelly KP, Fellingham GW, Conlee RK. Cocaine and exercise: temporal changes in plasma levels of catecholamines, lactate, glucose, and cocaine. Am J Physiol 1996; 270(3 Pt 1):E438–E444.

73. Conlee RK, Barnett DW, Kelly KP, Han DH. Effects of cocaine, exercise, and resting conditions on plasma corticosterone and catecholamine concentrations in the rat. Metabolism 1991; 40(10):1043–1047.

74. Abelmann WH. Viral myocarditis and its sequelae. Ann Rev Med 1973; 24:145–152.

75. Kishimoto C, Abelmann WH. In vivo significance of T cells in the development of coxsackievirus B3 myocarditis in mice. Immature but antigen-specific T cells aggravate cardiac injury. Circ Res 1990; 67(3):589–598.

76. Kishimoto C, Kuribayashi K, Fukuma K, Masuda T, Tomioka N, Abelmann WH, Kawai C. Immunologic identification of lymphocyte subsets in experimental murine myocarditis with encephalomyocarditis virus. Different kinetics of lymphocyte subsets between the heart and the peripheral blood, and significance of Thy 1.2+ (pan T) and Lyt 1+, 23+ (immature T) subsets in the development of myocarditis. Circ Res 1987; 61(5):715–725.

77. Kishimoto C, Thorp KA, Abelmann WH. Immunosuppression with high doses of cyclophosphamide reduces the severity of myocarditis but increases the mortality in murine Coxsackievirus B3 myocarditis. Circulation 1990; 82(3):982–989.

78. Kishimoto C, Abelmann WH. Monoclonal antibody therapy for prevention of acute coxsackievirus B3 myocarditis in mice. Circulation 1989; 79(6):1300–1308.

79. Abelmann WH. Virus and the heart. Circulation 1971; 44(5):950–956.

80. Gwathmey JK, Nakao S, Come PC, Goad ME, Serur JR, Als AV, Abelmann WH. An experimental model of acute and subacute viral myocarditis in the pig. J Am Coll Cardiol 1992; 19(4):864–869.

81. Kishimoto C, Hung GL, Ishibashi M, Khaw BA, Kolodny GM, Abelmann WH, Yasuda T. Natural evolution of cardiac function, cardiac pathology and antimyosin scan in a murine myocarditis model. J Am Coll Cardiol 1991; 17(3):821–827.

82. Adesanya CO, Goldberg AH, Phear WP, Thorp KA, Young NA, Abelmann WH. Heart muscle performance after experimental viral myocarditis. J Clin Invest 1976; 57(3):569–575.

83. Kishimoto C, Abelmann WH. Absence of effects of cyclosporine on myocardial lymphocyte subsets in coxsackievirus B3 myocarditis in the aviremic stage. Circ Res 1989; 65(4):934–945.

84. Abelmann WH, Adesanya CO, Goldberg AH, Phear WP, Young NA. Depressed myocardial function in subacute experimental viral myocarditis. Recent Adv Stud Cardiac Struct Metab 1975; 6:535–542.

85. Abelmann WH. Myocarditis and dilated cardiomyopathy. West J Med 1989; 150(4):458–459.

86. Yamada T, Matsumori A, Sasayama S. Therapeutic effect of anti-tumor necrosis factor-α antibody on the murine model of viral myocarditis induced by encephalomyocarditis virus. Circulation 1994; 89:846–851.

87. Matsumori A, Kawai C. An animal model of congestive (dilated) cardiomyopathy: dilation and hypertrophy of the heart in the chronic stage in DBA/2 mice with myocarditis caused by encephalomyocarditis virus. Circulation 1982; 66(2):355–360.

88. Matsumori A, Sasyama S. Immunomodulating agents for the management of heart failure with myocarditis and cardiomyopathy—lessions from animal experiments. Eur Heart J 1995; 16(suppl 0):140–143.

89. Yamamoto N, Shiramori M, Ogura M, Seko Y, Kikuchi M. Effects of intranasal administration of recombinant murine interferon-gamma on murine acute myocarditis caused by encephalomyocarditis virus. Circulation 1998; 97:1017–1023.

90. Matsumori A, Ohkusa T, Matoba Y, Okada I, Yamada T, Kawai C, Tamaki N, Watanabe Y, Yonekura Y, Endo K, et al. Myocardial uptake of antimyosin monoclonal antibody in a murine model of viral myocarditis. Circulation 1989; 79(2):400–405.

91. Araki M, Kanda T, Imai S, Suzuki T, Murata K, Kobayashi I. Comparative effects of losartan, captopril, and enalapril on murine acute myocarditis due to encephalomyocarditis virus. J Cardiovasc Pharmacol 1995; 26(1):61–6589.

92. Burch GE, Harb JM, Colcolough HL, Tsui CY. Encephalomyocarditis infection of the newborn mouse myocardium. An electron microscopic study. Arth Intern Med 1971; 127(1):148–156.

93. Harb JM, Burch GE. Ultrastructural cytopathology of mouse myocardium associated with EMC viral infection. J Mol Cell Cardiol 1973; 5(1):55–62.

94. Hirasawa K, Han JS, Takeda M, Itagaki S, Doi K. Encephalomyocarditis (EMC) virus-induced myocarditis by different virus variants and mouse strains. J Vet Med Sci 1992; 54(6):1125–1129.

95. Manning WJ, Wei JY, Katz SE, Douglas PS, Gwathmey JK. Echocardiography detected myocardial infarction in the mouse. Lab Anim Sci 1993; 43:583–585.

96. Cittadini A, Mantzoros CS, Hampton TG, Katz SE, Travers KE, Flier JS, Morgan JP, Douglas PS. Cardiovascular phenotype of transgenic mice with reduced brown fat. Circulation 1997; 96:1–465.

97. Tanaka N, Dalton N, Mao L, Rockman HA, Peterson KL, Gottshall KR, Hunter JJ, Chien KR, Ross J. Transthoracic echocardiography in models of cardiac disease in the mouse. Circ 1996; 94:1109–1117.

98. Hampton TG, Kranias EG, Morgan JP. Simultaneous measurement of intracellular calcium and ventricular function in the phospholamban-deficient mouse heart. Biochem Biophys Res Commun 1996; 226(3):836–841.

99. Hampton TG, Amende I, Travers KE, Morgan JP. Intracellular calcium dynamics in mouse model of myocardial stunning. Am J Physiol 1998; 274:H1821–H1827.

100. Perreault CL, Morgan KG, Morgan JP. Effects of cocaine on intracellular handling in cardiac and vascular smooth muscle. NIDA Res Monogr 1991; 108:139–153.

101. Stambler BS, Morgan JP, Mietus J, Moody GB, Goldberger AL. Cocaine alters heart rate dynamics in conscious ferrets. Yale J Biol Med 1991; 64(2):143–153.

102. Miao L, Qiu Z, Morgan JP. Cholinergic stimulation modulates negative inotropic effect of cocaine on ferret ventricular myocardium. Am J Physiol 1996; 270:H678–H684.

103. Huang L, Woolf JH, Ishiguro Y, Morgan JP. Effect of cocaine and methylecgonidine on intracellular Ca2+ and myocardial contraction in cardiac myocytes. Am J Physiol 1997; 273:H893–H901.

104. Egashira K, Pipers FS, Morgan JP. Effects of cocaine on epicardial coronary artery reactivity in miniature swine after endothelial injury and high cholesterol feeding. In vivo and in vitro analysis. J Clin Invest 1991; 88(4):1307–1314.

105. Egashira K, Morgan KG, Morgan JP. Effects of cocaine on excitation-contraction coupling of aortic smooth muscle from the ferret. J Clin Invest 1991; 87(4):1322–1328.

106. Xiao YF, Morgan JP. Cocaine blockade of the acetylcholine-activated muscarinic K+ channel in ferret cardiac myocytes. J Pharmacol Exp Ther 1998; 284(1):10–18.

107. Nunez BD, Mial L, Ross JN, Nunez MM, Baim DS, Carrozza JP, Morgan JP. Effects of cocaine on carotid vascular reactivity in swine after balloon vascular injury. Stroke 1994; 25(3):631–638.

108. Perreault CL, Hague NL, Ransil BJ, Morgan JP. The effects of cocaine on intracelluar Ca2+ handling and myofilament Ca2+ responsiveness of ferret ventricular myocardium. Br J Pharmacol 1990; 101(3):679–685.

109. Miao L, Nunez BD, Susulic V, Wheeler S, Carrozza JP, Ross JN, Morgan JP. Cocaine-induced microvascular vasoconstriction but differential systemic haemodynamic responses in Yucatan versus Yorkshire varieties of swine. Br J Pharmacol 1996; 117(3):559–565.

110. Qiu Z, Morgan JP. Differential effects of cocaine and cocaethylene on intracellular Ca2+ and myocardial contraction in cardiac myocytes. Br J Pharmacol 1993; 109(2):293–298.

111. Nunez BD, Miao L, Kuntz RE, Ross JN, Gladstone S, Baim DS, Gordon PC, Morgan JP, Carrozza JP. Cardiogenic shock induced by cocaine in swine with normal coronary arteries. Cardiovasc Res 1994; 28(1):105–111.

112. Perreault CL, Hague NL, Morgan KG, Allen PD, Morgan JP. Negative inotropic and relaxant effects of cocaine on myopathic human ventricular myocardium and epicardialcoronary arteries in vitro. Cardiovasc Res 1993; 27(2):262–268.

113. Wang SY, Nunez BD, Morgan JP, Dai HB, Ross JN, Sellke FW. Cocaine and the porcine coronary microcirculation: effects of chronic cocaine exposure and hypercholesterolemia. J Cardiothorac Vasc Anesth 1995; 9(3):290–296.

114. Nunez BD, Miao L, Klein MA, Nunez MM, Travers KE, Ross JN, Carrozza JP, Morgan JP. Acute and chronic cocaine exposure can produce myocardial ischemia and infarction in Yucatan swine. J Cardiovasc Pharmacol 1997; 29(2):145–155.

115. Woolf JH, Huang L, Ishiguro Y, Morgan JP. Negative inotropic effect of methylecgonidine, a major product of cocaine base pyrolysis, on ferret and human myocardium. J Cardiovasc Pharmacol 1997; 30(3):352–359.

116. Fliss H, Gattinger D. Apoptosis in ischemic and reperfused rat myocardium. Cir Res 1996; 79:949–956.

117. Bialik S, Geene DL, Saaaon IE, Cheng R, Horner JW, Evans SM, Lord EM, Koch CJ, Kitsis RN. Myocyte apoptosis during acute myocardial infarction in the mouse localizes to hypoxic regions but occurs independent of p53. J Clin Invest 1997; 100:1363–1372.

118. Berger MM, See DM, Redl B, Aymard M, Lina B. Comparison of procedures for the detection of enteroviruses in murine heart samples by in situ polymerase chain reaction. Res Virol 1997; 148(6):409–416.

119. Matsuzawa H, Shimizu K, Okada K, Ando K, Hashimoto K, Koga Y. Analysis of target organs for the latency of murine cytomegalovirus DNA using specific pathogen free and germ free mice. Arch Virol 1995; 140(5):853–864.

120. Adachi K, Muraishi A, Seki Y, Yamaki K, Toshizuka M. Coxsackievirus B3 genomes detected by polymerase chain reaction: evidence of latent persistency in the myocardium in experimental murine myocarditis. Histol Histopathol 1996; 11(3):587–596.

121. Wee L, Liu P, Penn L, Butany JW, McLaughlin PR, Sole MJ, Liew CC. Persistence of viral genome into late stages of murine myocarditis detected by polymerase chain reaction. Circulation 1992; 86(5):1605–1614.

122. Kyu B, Matsumori A, Sato Y, Okada I, Champman NM, Tracy S. Cardiac persistence of cardioviral RNA detected by polymerase chain reaction in a murine model of dilated cardiomyopathy. Circulation 1992; 86(2):522–530.

123. Matsumori A, Okada I, Yamada T, Maruyama S, Kawai C. Pathogenesis of myocardial injury in myocarditis and cardiomyopathy. Jpn Circ J 1991; 55(11):1132–1137.

124. Wolff D, Skourtopoulos M, Hornschemeyer D, Wolff C, Korner M, Korfer R, Kleesiek K. Longitudinal monitoring of latent and active human cytomegalovirus infections in peripheral blood of heart transplant receipients by single-tube nested RT-PCR. Microbiol Res 1996; 151(4):343–349.

125. Manning WJ, Wei JY, Katz SE, Litwin SE, Douglas PS. In vivo assessment of LV mass in mice using high-frequency cardiac ultrasound: necropsy validation. Am J Physiol 1994; 266:H1672–1675.

126. Bachmaier K, Mair J, Offner F, Pummerer C, Neu N. Serum cardiac troponin T and creatine kinase-MB elevations in murine autoimmune myocarditis. Circulation 1995; 92(7):1927–1932.

127. Robson RD. The action of adrenergic neurone blocking agents and other drugs on the pressor responses of various agents in the anaesthetized rat. Br J Pharmacol 1967; 29(2):194–203.

128. Spencer PS. Amitriptyline and the "cheese" reaction to MAOIs. Lancet 1982; 2(8294):385.

129. Lee WC, Yoo CS. The role of monoamine oxidase in the cardiac accumulation of norepinephrine. Arch Int Pharmacodyn Ther 1967; 169(1):221–236.

130. Hutchins DA. The effect of pargyline and desmethylimipramine on monoamine concentrations and amphetamine-induced glycogenolysis in the mouse brain. Br J Pharmacol 1979; 65(3):489–494.

131. Gainer JH. Viral myocarditis in animals. Adv Cardiol 1974; 13:94–105.

132. Kolattukudy PE, Quach T, Bergese S, Breckenridge S, Hensley J, Altshuld R, Gordillo G, Klenotic S, Orosz C, Parker-Thornburg J. Myocarditis induced by targeted expression of the MCP-1 gene in murine cardiac muscle. Am J Pathol 1998; 152(1):101–111.

133. Liu P, Penninger J, Aitken K, Sole M, Mak T. The role of transgenic knockout models in defining the pathogenesis of viral heart disease. Eur Heart J 1995; 16(Suppl 0):25–27.

134. Rockman HA, Koch WJ, Lefkowitz RJ. Cardiac function in genetically engineered mice with altered adrenergic receptor signaling. Am J Physiol 1997; 272:H1553–H1559.

135. Stevenson M. Molecular mechanisms for the regulation of HIV replication, persistence and latency. AIDS 1997; 11:AS25–AS33.

136. Heard I, Costagliola D, Kazatchkine M, Orth G. High rate of persistence of HPV infection in HIV-seropositive women [abstr 332]. Fourth Conference on Retroviral and Opportunistic Infection, 1997:125.

137. Wong JK, Hezareh M, Gunthard HF, Havlir DV, Ignacio CC, Furtado M, Wolinsky SM, Spina CA, Richman DD. Persistence of replication competent HIV in patients with undetectable plasma virus [abstr 519]. Fifth Conference on Retroviral and Opportunistic Infection, 1998:233.

138. Soudeyns H, Pantaleo G. New mechanims of viral persistence in primary human immunodeficiency virus (HIV) infection. J Biol Regul Homeost Agents 1997; 11:37–39.

23

Role of the Catecholamine–Nitric Oxide System in Cocaine- and HIV-Induced Vascular Inflammation and Its Pharmacological Implications

David S. Chi and William L. Stone
James H. Quillen College of Medicine, East Tennessee State University, Johnson City, Tennessee, U.S.A.

Hiren B. Patel
Holston Valley Medical Center, Kingsport, Tennessee, U.S.A.

Guha Krishnaswamy
James H. Quillen College of Medicine, East Tennessee State University, and James H. Quillen VA Medical Center, Johnson City, Tennessee, U.S.A.

INTRODUCTION

Increasing evidence suggests that atherosclerosis is an inflammatory disease. Since HIV-infected individuals often develop opportunistic infections and immune activation, the resulting inflammatory response could be an important factor contributing to an accelerated form of atherosclerosis. The mechanism whereby inflammation in HIV infection contributes to atherosclerosis is not fully understood. HIV-infected individuals show evidence of increased nitric oxide (NO) production, suggesting that NO-dependent mechanisms may regulate vascular inflammatory responses. For example, peroxynitrite, a highly reactive chemical species formed from the generation of NO and superoxide radicals, is known to convert low-density lipoprotein (LDL) to an atherogenic oxLDL form, which can then induce endothelial activation. In the case of cocaine, a common drug of abuse, the elaboration of catecholamines may further contribute to endothelial injury and atherosclerosis. We believe the response to cocaine may be mediated partially by effects of catecholamines on the generation of NO. There is evidence suggesting that human atherosclerotic plaques contain the inducible form of nitric oxide synthase (iNOS), which produces NO. Preliminary studies from our laboratory have shown that catecholamines can increase the production of NO in lipopolysaccharide (LPS)-stimulated macrophages by promoting the expression of iNOS. Although speculative, these data provide a potential link between cocaine abuse in HIV-infected individuals and accelerated atherosclerosis.

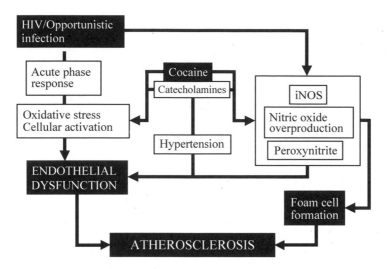

Figure 1 Mechanisms of cocaine- and HIV-induced vascular dysfunction and atherosclerosis. Cocaine use can increase levels of catecholamines, which in turn can promote nitric oxide (NO) production via inducible NO synthase (iNOS). In excess, NO can directly cause vascular dysfunction and can facilitate the conversion of LDL to more atherogenic forms, thereby enhancing foam cell formation. HIV and/or opportunistic infection enhances NO production and induces the acute-phase response, which leads to oxidative stresses and cellular activation, resulting in endothelial dysfunction and atherosclerosis.

Cocaine use could result in increased levels of catecholamines, which in turn could promote NO production. In excess, NO can directly cause vascular dysfunction and can facilitate the conversion of LDL to more atherogenic forms, thereby enhancing foam cell formation. These interactions are summarized in Figure 1. This chapter discusses the possible links between the catecholamine–nitric oxide system and cocaine- and HIV-induced vascular dysfunction and offers some implications for therapy.

INFLAMMATION, HIV INFECTION, AND CARDIOVASCULAR DISEASE

Atherosclerosis is the underlying cause of most cardiovascular disease and is caused by gradual buildup of "plaque" in the arterial wall. LDL is the major source of the lipids occurring in these plaques. There is now considerable evidence that LDL lipids (primarily cholesteryl esters) make their way into plaques by entering macrophages resident in the arterial wall. These macrophage cells take up so much LDL that they become "foamy" in appearance and are, therefore, called foam cells. This is the very first step in atherosclerosis, termed fatty streak formation, and this process begins in childhood. It is surprising, however, that macrophages incubated with LDL are not transformed into foam cells. Only after LDL is oxidized (oxLDL) will it cause macrophages to become foam cells. These observations have led to the "LDL oxidative modification hypothesis." Although most in vitro experiments uphold this hypothesis, not all evidence is supportive (1). Oxidative stress caused by any inflammatory process in the arterial wall should be expected to accelerate atherogenesis.

An ever-increasing body of information supports the view that atherosclerosis is associated with infection and inflammatory processes (2–12). For example, Mayr et al. (13) found a significant correlation between atherosclerosis in the carotid and femoral arteries and IgA antibodies to *Chlamydia pneumoniae*, and this correlation was not significantly changed after adjustment for established risk factors. For those individuals who were seropositive to *C. pneumoniae*, the prevalence of carotid atherosclerosis dramatically increased with both increasing levels of C-reactive protein (CRP) and clinical evidence of chronic respiratory infection. In general, elevated markers of systemic inflammation—such as soluble adhesion molecules, circulating bacterial endotoxin, soluble heat-shock protein 60, and antibodies to mycobacterial heat-shock protein 65—are predictive of increased atherosclerotic risk (4). The molecular mechanisms whereby increased infections could accelerate atherosclerosis are not yet known with certainty. It is likely that increased local inflammation and the resulting oxidative stress could contribute to atherogenesis by oxidative modification to LDL.

A hallmark of AIDS is a dramatically increased rate of opportunistic infections, many of which are only rarely seen in individuals with a normal immune system. It is reasonable, therefore, to suggest that these opportunistic infections could contribute to accelerated atherosclerosis in HIV-positive individuals. Accelerated coronary atherosclerosis has indeed been observed even among young HIV-positive patients (14). *C. pneumoniae* infections, which are implicated in atherogenesis, are a possible cause of severe respiratory infection in HIV-infected patients (15,16).

In addition to increased opportunistic bacterial infections, HIV-infected individuals have increased susceptibility to viral infections such as cytomegalovirus, hepatitis, and herpes simplex. Although not universal (13,17), there is considerable evidence suggesting that cytomegalovirus plays a role in atherosclerosis (18,19). Similarly, hepatitis A virus may play a causal role in atherogenesis (20). Despite the fact that herpes simplex virus induces an inflammatory response in endothelial cells (21), antibody levels against this virus have not been associated with an increased risk of coronary heart disease (CHD) (22). It is likely that infection and inflammation, by inducing NO production, in addition to causing oxidative stress, could alter the arterial endothelium from an anticoagulant surface to a procoagulant surface, thereby promoting the adhesion of neutrophils, macrophages, and platelets, which are known to play a proatherogenic role (23).

COCAINE-INDUCED VASCULAR DYSFUNCTION

Both cocaine and HIV-1 infection could potentiate the development of coronary artery disease (CAD) by divergent mechanisms but with certain essentially common pathways. In both cases, mast cell, macrophage, and endothelial activation can occur, either directly or through intermediary pharmacological or pathological processes involving circulating neurohumoral or cytokine mediators.

Cocaine (benzoyl-methylecgonine) is an alkaloid derived from the leaves of *Erythoroxylon coca*. As summarized by Zafar and coworkers, cocaine for smoking is cheap and has the ability to deliver the drug in high concentrations to the central nervous system. However, the short half-life of cocaine's euphoric effect leads to repeated use, resulting in a rapid development of cumulative toxicity (24). A unique sequence of cardiovascular events, referred to as the "Casey Jones reaction," can occur with acute cocaine overdose, resulting in early stimulation (hypertension, tachycardia), advanced stimulation (cardiorespiratory failure, arrhythmia), and late depression (circulatory collapse and cardiac arrest). It is likely that, by functioning as an agonist for the catecholamine reuptake transporter, cocaine increases the concentration of neurotransmitters at the postsynaptic receptor. This leads to increased activation of the sympathetic nervous system, resulting in a hyperadrenergic state (24).

It is well documented that increasing use of cocaine is frequently associated with acute cardiovascular events, including stroke, myocardial infarction (MI), coronary thrombosis, arrhythmia, and sudden death. One study, done by He et al. (25), showed the direct cytotoxic effect of cocaine on human coronary artery endothelial cells (HCAECs) by documenting that cocaine induced a time- and dose-dependent increase in apoptosis in cultured HCAECs, which is calcium-dependent and is likely to be mediated by the release of cytochrome *c* and subsequent activation of caspase 9 and caspase 3. Increased apoptosis of endothelial cells results in endothelial dysfunction, which has a key role in cocaine-induced coronary artery vasoconstriction, leading to myocardial ischemia and infarction. Cocaine also increases intracellular calcium (26–28) and impairs mitochondrial function by dissipating the mitochondrial membrane potential (26,29,30). In addition, cocaine enhances leukocyte-endothelial interactions by inducing adhesion molecules on endothelium and enhancing monocyte cytokine release and transendothelial migration (31).

The widespread use of cocaine has been linked with an increased prevalence of infectious disease (32–34), particularly HIV. Mao et al. (35) demonstrated that cocaine downregulates endothelial interleukin 8 (IL-8) production by increasing transforming growth factor beta (TGF-β). IL-8 is one of the key neutrophil activators and chemoattractants (36) produced by a variety of cell types, including endothelial cells (37). Alteration of IL-8 production by cocaine may lead to derangement of the immune response to pathogens, thus increasing susceptibility to infectious disease and cancer. Peterson et al. (38) demonstrated that cocaine potentiated HIV-1 replication in human peripheral blood mononuclear cell cultures through the involvement of TGF-β. Thus, reduction of IL-8 by cocaine may be important in the natural history of HIV infection, and TGF-β may play an important role in enhancing the effect of cocaine on HIV infection.

ROLE OF CATECHOLAMINE IN COCAINE- AND HIV-INDUCED VASCULAR DYSFUNCTION

Cocaine increases levels of norepinephrine and epinephrine. Sustained increases in circulating catecholamines by infusion of epinephrine or norepinephrine have been shown to cause moderate cardiovascular and metabolic effects (39). These catecholamines are thought to play a direct role in atherogenesis and cardiovascular disease (40,41). Epinephrine has been found to accelerate the development of atherosclerosis in monkeys fed an atherogenic diet (40). Both norepinephrine and epinephrine stimulate the growth of aortic smooth muscle cells and aortic endothelial cells (41).

Catecholamines also increase blood pressure, the release of free fatty acids by adipose tissue, and plasma levels of triglyceride and very low density lipoprotein (VLDL). The report of Kolodgie et al. (42) showed that cocaine causes a rapid concentration-dependent increase in endothelial cell permeability to peroxidase and LDL but has no effect on resting levels of intracellular cyclic adenosine monophosphate (cAMP). Cell morphology in cocaine-treated endothelial monolayers showed a marked recognition of F-actin and the formation of intercellular gaps, which were essentially neutralized by pretreatment with forskolin. Moreover, elevated levels of catecholamines increase blood clotting, thereby increasing the risk of arterial obstruction and MI.

Catecholamines are elaborated in stress responses to mediate vasoconstriction, thus elevating systemic vascular resistance and blood pressure. Activation of the sympathetic nervous system together with microbial infection exerts a synergistic interaction that could result in the enhancement of the inflammatory processes (43). In addition, it has been suggested that catecholamines stimulate macrophage secretion of NO via inducible nitric oxide synthase (44,45). Excess production of NO unbalances the concentration of NO in the endothelial environment and causes endothelial dysfunction.

Chi et al. (45) have recently found that epinephrine and norepinephrine but not dopamine enhance nitric oxide production in stimulated murine macrophages via increased levels of iNOS protein. Under pathophysiological conditions of inflammation and infection, NO can produce peroxynitrite (Fig. 2). Endothelial cells are probably critically situated to suffer from much of the peroxynitrite-mediated oxidative damage in inflammatory conditions. It is also interesting that macrophages isolated from stressed mice demonstrate an increased secretion of NO after stimula-

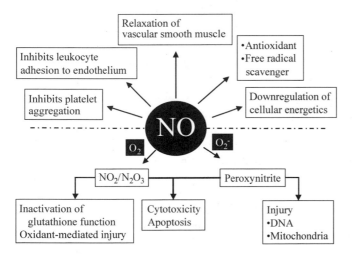

Figure 2 Possible effects of nitric oxide (NO) on vascular responses. NO is an antioxidant and free-radical scavenger. Physiological effects of NO mainly include relaxation of vascular smooth muscle and inhibition of leukocyte adhesion to endothelium and platelet aggregation. NO also downregulates cellular energetics. In addition, NO reacts with oxygen and superoxide to generate NO_2/N_2O_3 and peroxynitrite, respectively, which, in turn, inactivate glutathione function, cause oxidant-mediated injury and cytotoxicity, impair mitochondria, and damage DNA.

tion with lipopolysaccharide (LPS) (46). These results suggest that macrophage function can be altered by catecholamines.

In a key paper, Kohut et al. (47) reported that adrenal catecholamines modulate the antiviral function of alveolar macrophages. These investigators divided mice into exercise and control groups treated with saline or propranolol, a beta-receptor antagonist. They found a suppression of macrophage antiviral function in the saline-treated exercise group but not in the saline-treated controls or the exercise group treated with propranolol. In contrast, isoproterenol, a beta-receptor agonist, suppressed antiviral function in cultured alveolar macrophages. The authors suggest that the decreased antiviral function may be due to catecholamines. Further evidence for a role of catecholamines in regulating macrophage function comes from the work of Petty et al. (48). These investigators found that the phagocytic function of RAW264 macrophages was suppressed by epinephrine and that this inhibition could be blocked by propranolol.

Although the biological mechanisms have not yet been defined, the presence of adrenergic receptors on macrophages would present a reasonable molecular link. Abrass et al. (49) have, in fact, presented compelling evidence for a beta-adrenergic receptor on rat peritoneal macrophages, indicating that catecholamines could modulate macrophage function through a beta-adrenoceptor. Several reports have also shown that the effect of catecholamines on immune function is due to beta adrenoceptors (45,50–54).

The picture that emerges as a working model is one in which catecholamines, released as a result of cocaine use, stimulate macrophage secretion of NO (and thereby the ability to promote oxidized and atherogenic forms of LDL), and diminish both macrophage antiviral and phagocytic functions. A diminished antiviral and phagocytic function would not bode well for the ability of macrophages to deal with opportunistic infections in HIV-infected individuals.

ROLE OF NO IN COCAINE- AND HIV-INDUCED VASCULAR PATHOLOGY

It is established that cocaine causes inhibition of catecholamine reuptake, which is the main basis for cocaine-induced cardiovascular toxic effects (55–57). The report by Mo et al. (44) showed that vasoconstriction caused by cocaine is blocked by pretreatment with N^G-monomethyl-L-arginine (L-NMMA), an arginine analogue, and the authors hypothesized a cocaine-induced inhibiting activity on local vasodilator endothelium-derived NO (EDNO). Togna et al. (58) have shown that cocaine significantly reduced endothelium-dependent relaxations induced by acetylcholine, or substance P, but significantly increased endothelium-dependent relaxation response to 2,5-di-tert-butylhydroquinone, a sarcoplasmic Ca^{2+}-ATPase pump inhibitor, in the aortic rings. They suggested that cocaine reduces NO release from vascular endothelium apparently through the inhibiting action of the Ca^{2+}-ATPase pump. Recent studies indicate that NO modulates vascular permeability under both physiological and pathological conditions (59). Since NOS inhibitors influence cocaine induced toxicity (60–62), it is clear that cocaine-induced increases in permeability may be affected by NO. Because cocaine acts by preventing catecholamine reuptake, it is not clear why the effect of cocaine was totally prevented by L-NMMA, which would suggest that NO is also involved in the release or maintenance of catecholamine levels at the peripheral nerve terminals.

It is very possible that an excessive generation of NO and superoxide radicals in the arteries of HIV-infected individuals could contribute to an accelerated form of atherosclerosis by promoting the formation of oxidized and atherogenic forms of LDL. Indeed, LDL isolated from human (HIV-negative) aortic atherosclerotic intima has extremely high levels of 3-nitrotyrosine (63), which likely forms by the reaction of peroxynitrite with tyrosine residues. Furthermore, Buttery et al. (64) found that human atherosclerotic lesions (but not normal arteries) contain iNOS protein, which was localized to macrophages, foam cells, and vascular smooth muscle cells. Significantly, the distribution of nitrotyrosine in the atherosclerotic lesions was identical to that observed for iNOS (64). Wilcox et al. (65) have also found increased levels of iNOS (as well as neuronal NOS) in macrophages, endothelial cells, and mesenchymal-appearing intimal cells from human atherosclerotic lesions.

Collins and coworkers (66) showed that NOS inhibitors are capable of increasing the potency of acutely administered cocaine and other stimulants without themselves having cocaine-like discriminative stimulant effects. NOS inhibitors also modify the psychomotor stimulant and reinforcing effects of cocaine. Together, these actions support the view that NO may play a role in the cocaine addiction process (67).

NO Generation

Vascular endothelium, a semipermeable barrier between blood and tissue for the exchange of the substrates and products of metabolism, constitutes a multifunctional organ with a broad spectrum of properties and activities. In addition to controlling vascular tone by releasing EDNO, it also regulates vascular homeostasis through the release of a large number of other factors that influence vasomotor tone, fibrinolysis, thrombosis, vascular growth, and vascular inflammation. EDNO production by endothelial cells is stimulated by mechanical forces (68) and following exposure to acetylcholine, adenosine diphosphate (ADP), bradykinin, thrombin, and serotonin (5-HT) (69). EDNO causes a vasodilatory effect by two mechanisms: one is by increasing intracellular cyclic guanosine monophosphate (cGMP) in vascular smooth muscle cells and the other is by activation of calcium-dependent potassium channels in vascular smooth muscle cells (70). Endothelium also produces other vasodilator substances, including prostacyclin (71), adenosine (72), and endothelium-derived hyperpolarizing factor (EDHF) (73). In addition, endothelium also produces vaso-constrictor substances including endothelin (74), angiotensin II (75), thromboxane A_2 (76) and other prostanoid vasoconstrictors (77).

NO is produced in a variety of tissues by nitric oxide synthase (NOS). Based on the location and the mechanism of regulation, three isoforms of NOS have been identified. They are neuronal NOS (nNOS, also termed NOS I), inducible NOS (iNOS, also termed NOS II), and endothelial NOS (eNOS, also termed NOS III). nNOS is a 155-kDa protein found in the cytoplasm of various cell types, including neurons, skeletal muscle fibers, and lung epithelium (78). eNOS is a 140-kDa protein and exists in endothelial cells, some neurons, and cardiac myocytes (79). Both nNOS and eNOS constitutively produce low levels of NO in neurons and endothelium, providing for neurosignaling and helping to maintain vascular homeostasis and tissue perfusion. Since nNOS and eNOS are constitutively expressed, they are also

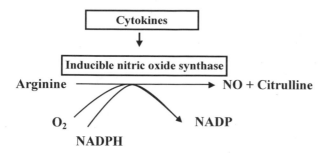

Figure 3 NO synthesis. Cytokines, acting through the nuclear factor kappa B transcription factor, induce the synthesis of inducible nitric oxide synthase, which utilizes oxygen, nicotinamide-adenine dinucleotide phosphate (NADPH), and the amino acid arginine to synthesize nitric oxide (NO).

collectively called constitutive NOS (cNOS). iNOS is a 130-kDa protein and is expressed in macrophages in both cytosolic and membrane-associated forms (80,81). NO is generated in macrophages by iNOS following exposure to cytokines such as interferon gamma (INF-γ), TNF-α and IL-1 and /or microbial products, such as LPS (Fig. 3).

Effects of NO on Vascular Responses

NO, a short-lived, gaseous radical, is a potent multifunctional reactive metabolite that can act as a neurotransmitter and vasodilator and is a major effector molecule of immune cells against tumor cells and pathogens. Physiological responses of NO mainly include relaxation of vascular and nonvascular smooth muscle and inhibition of platelet aggregation and leukocyte adhesion to the endothelium. These physiological responses are mediated by the activation of soluble guanylyl cyclase, leading to the formation of cGMP, which, in turn, proceeds through several downstream elements, including cGMP-dependent protein kinases, cGMP-regulated phosphodiesterases, and cGMP-gated ion channels (82). Directly, NO exerts biological effects from protective to deleterious activity, depending on the amount produced and the specific chemical environment (83) (Fig. 2). NO, as an antioxidant and scavenger of free radicals, may be protective against oxidative stress. On the other hand, NO down-regulates the activity of cytochrome oxidase (84) and mitochondrial aconitase (85), resulting in a profoundly negative influence on cellular energetics. Indirect effects of NO include reactions with oxygen and superoxide. When NO reacts with O_2, it decays to nitrite (NO_2^-) and generates NO_2 and N_2O_3. In the situation of high NO production, formation of N_2O_3, a potent nitrosating species, increases by a factor of 15,000 (86). This nitrosative stress enhances the cellular susceptibility to oxidant-mediated damage. Reports have shown that excessive NO production during infections often causes damage to tissues, especially of the vascular system (87,88). In septic shock, NO has been found to be involved in vascular collapse, which is a major contributor to mortality (83). In addition, generation of N_2O_3 can lead to the formation of N-nitrosamines, which are carcinogenic compounds (89), and S-nitrosothiols. Furthermore, because EDNO blunts platelet aggregation and the constrictor responses to serotonin, thrombin, and other products of aggregating platelets (90,91), loss of

EDNO may contribute to the severity of thrombosis and vasoconstriction under these circumstances. Feihl et al. (83) have done an excellent review of the biology of NO.

Role of NO in Oxidant Stress

NO reacts with the superoxide radical (O_2^-) to yield peroxynitrite, a highly reactive oxidant species, which mediates oxidative damage. Peroxynitrite formation in biological systems has been found to be mostly restricted to conditions of abnormally high and approximately equal fluxes of NO and O_2^- (92,93) (Fig. 2). The reaction of peroxynitrite with glutathione inactivates this key element of antioxidant defenses (94). Peroxynitrite also damages mitochondria by irreversibly inhibiting several steps in the mitochondrial electron transport chain via binding to Fe-S clusters (84,95). Furthermore, peroxynitrite impairs cellular energetics by incriminating DNA damage and activation of the nuclear enzyme poly-(ADP-ribose) polymerase (PARP), a pathway increasingly recognized as a major mechanism of NO/peroxynitrite mediated cytotoxicity (96,97).

Several reports have shown that NO directly induces apoptosis (98–100) in a variety of cell lines, such as macrophages (101), vascular endothelial cells (102), and ventricular myocytes (103). Recent data indicate that peroxynitrite rather than NO may be the species responsible for NO-dependent apoptosis (83). Peroxynitrite-dependent apoptosis is dependent on the energy state and redox status of the cell, with significant protection provided by high levels of glutathione or ascorbic acid (104,105). NO, however, has also been reported to protect cells against apoptosis by upregulating antiapoptotic proteins, such as Bcl-2 and heme oxygenase-1 and inhibiting mitochondrial release of cytochrome *c* and activation of caspase 3 (98–100).

PHARMACOLOGICAL IMPLICATIONS

An improved understanding the molecular mechanisms of cocaine- and HIV-induced vascular dysfunction could provide the basis for the development of drugs and rational therapeutic strategies and improve care for a broader range of patients. Since over-production of NO is caused by enhancing the effect of iNOS synthesis by catecholamines via beta adrenoceptors (45,50–54), beta-adrenoceptor antagonists may be potential candidate drugs for prevention of atherogenesis in cocaine abuse and HIV infection.

Beta-carotene and antioxidants may be helpful in the prevention of atherogenesis. In patients infected with HIV, therapy with beta-carotene and antioxidant selenium for 1 year was found to be associated with lower levels of the endothelial activation markers, soluble thrombomoduline (sTM) and von Willebrand factor (vWF) (106). Ascorbic acid treatment has been shown to improve EDNO action in patients with CAD (107), hypercholesterolemia (108), and hypertension (109). In addition, there is some intriguing evidence suggesting that CRP is not just a marker for cardiovascular disease but is actually a causative factor. CRP may play a direct role in promoting the inflammatory component of atherosclerosis and presents a potential target for the treatment of atherosclerosis due to inflammation.

Since NO is implicated in the cardiovascular abnormalities of endotoxic shock, studies have been carried out to treat endotoxic shock by inhibiting NO production via the administration of agents able to block NOS activity. To that effect, the most widely used compounds have been analogues of L-arginine, such as N^G-nitro-L-arginine (L-NA), L-NMMA, and N^G-monomethyl-L-arginine methyl ester (L-NAME) (83). However, while the results were encouraging, a range of deleterious effects occurred in the experimental animals. It appears that while targeting iNOS-mediated overproduction of NO might be useful, concomitant inhibition of eNOS is likely counterproductive by impairing essential functions of the endothelium, such as agonist-stimulated vasodilatation and downregulation of activated blood cell adherence (83). Thus, a more suitable approach in managing septic shock in particular and infection/inflammation-induced atherogenesis in general would be the use of agents able to selectively inhibit the activity of iNOS.

Several compounds with relative selectivity towards iNOS have been developed. They are either amino acid–based (e.g., L-canavanine and L-N-iminoethly-lysine) or non–amino acid–based (e.g., amidines, guanidines, and S-alkyl-isothioureas) inhibitors. The selectivity for iNOS of all these agents is only relative and they may block all NOS isoforms when used at sufficiently high doses (83). Selective inhibitors improved arterial blood pressure and the vascular reactivity to vasoconstrictors, as demonstrated by an increase in the pressor responses to norepinephrine administration in vivo (83). Data from two studies also support the notion that in endotoxemia, iNOS-derived NO may inhibit eNOS, leading to an endothelial dysfunction that may be reversed by selective iNOS inhibitors (83,110,111). However, several studies failed to show any beneficial effect of selective iNOS inhibitors on LPS-induced organ damage (112–114).

Overproduction of NO may be modulated by other means. Low substitution doses of corticosteroids have been found to be beneficial in septic patients (115). The inhibition of iNOS expression by pretreatment with specific blockers of nuclear factor kappa B (NF-κB)–dependent transcription, such as pyrrolidine dithiocarbamate, has been reported with favorable results (116–118). In addition, for overproduced NO, scavenging by agents such as carboxy-PTIO, hydroxocobalamin, trivalent iron chelates, or solutions of modified hemoglobin has been reported to be effective (119–122). The consequences of NO overproduction on vascular tone may be counteracted with inhibitors of guanylate cyclase, such as methylene blue (123–126).

CONCLUSION

Endothelial activation has been shown to be associated with atherogenesis and leads to the development of CAD. Cocaine, by its inhibitory effects on catecholamine reuptake, by increasing vascular permeability, by formation of intercellular gaps, and at least in part by its inhibitory effect on endothelial NO, causes endothelial dysfunction. Cocaine also shows a direct cytotoxic effect on endothelial cells by apoptosis. Cocaine induces a catecholamine surge, which in turn induces NO overproduction in macrophages via iNOS synthesis. NO serves as a neurotransmitter and vasodilator under physiological conditions but causes oxidant-mediated damage and cytotoxicity to endothelium and facilitates formation of atherogenic LDL under pathological conditions. In addition, cocaine downregulates endothelial IL-8 production by increasing TGF-β, leading to derangement of the immune response to pathogens. Furthermore, by increasing permeability of vascular endothelium, cocaine promotes HIV-induced endothelial activation. In HIV infection, endothelium is activated by viral invasion, action of the HIV-associated proteins tat and gp12, and the effect of secreted cytokines. HIV and opportunistic infection cause chronic inflammation, which can lead to atherosclerosis by (1) overproduction of NO, inflammatory cytokines, and other mediators; (2) the acute-phase response; (3) procoagulant change; and (4) foam-cell formation. Thus, cocaine and HIV, by way of catecholamine and NO, exert a synergistic effect on endothelial dysfunction and promote each other's action in the development of premature CAD among cocaine abusers who are infected with HIV.

ACKNOWLEDGMENTS

Funded by NIH grants, AI-43310 and HL-63070, the Ruth R. Harris Endowment, the Cardiovascular Research Institute, and the Research Development Committee of East Tennessee State University.

REFERENCES

1. Asmis R, Jelk J. Vitamin E supplementation of human macrophages prevents neither foam cell formation nor increased susceptibility of foam cells to lysis by oxidized LDL. Arterioscler Thromb Vasc Biol 2000; 20:2078–2086.
2. Mehta JL, Saldeen TG, Rand K. Interactive role of infection, inflammation and traditional risk factors in atherosclerosis and coronary artery disease. J Am Coll Cardiol 1998; 31:1217–1225.
3. Elghannam H, Tavackoli S, Ferlic L, Gotto AM Jr, Ballantyne CM, Marian AJ. A prospective study of genetic markers of susceptibility to infection and inflammation, and the severity, progression, and regression of coronary atherosclerosis and its response to therapy. J Mol Med 2000; 78:562–568.
4. Kiechl S, Egger G, Mayr M, Wiedermann CJ, Bonora E, Oberhollenzer F, Muggeo M, Xu Q, Wick G, Poewe W, Willeit J. Chronic infections and the risk of carotid atherosclerosis: prospective results from a large population study. Circulation 2001; 103:1064–1070.
5. Noll G. Pathogenesis of atherosclerosis: a possible relation to infection. Atherosclerosis 1998; 140(suppl 1):S3–S9.
6. Sinisalo J, Paronen J, Mattila KJ, Syrjala M, Alfthan G, Palosuo T, Nieminen MS, Vaarala O. Relation of inflammation to vascular function in patients with coronary heart disease. Atherosclerosis 2000; 149:403–411.
7. Jousilahti P, Salomaa V, Rasi V, Vahtera E, Palosuo T. The association of C-reactive protein, serum amyloid a and fibrinogen with prevalent coronary heart disease—baseline findings of the PAIS project. Atherosclerosis 2001; 156:451–456.
8. Mehta JL, Romeo F. Inflammation, infection and atherosclerosis: do antibacterials have a role in the therapy of coronary artery disease? Drugs 2000; 59:159–170.
9. Van Lente F. Markers of inflammation as predictors in cardiovascular disease. Clin Chim Acta 2000; 293:31–52.
10. de Boer OJ, van der Wal AC, Becker AE. Atherosclerosis, inflammation, and infection. J Pathol 2000; 190:237–243.
11. Libby P. What have we learned about the biology of atherosclerosis? The role of inflammation. Am J Cardiol 2001; 88:3J–6J.

12. Albert NM. Inflammation and infection in acute coronary syndrome. J Cardiovasc Nurs 2000; 15:13–26.

13. Mayr M, Kiechl S, Willeit J, Wick G, Xu Q. Infections, immunity, and atherosclerosis: associations of antibodies to *Chlamydia pneumoniae, Helicobacter pylori*, and cytomeg-alovirus with immune reactions to heat-shock protein 60 and carotid or femoral atherosclerosis. Circulation 2000; 102:833–839.

14. Tabib A, Leroux C, Mornex JF, Loire R. Accelerated coronary atherosclerosis and arteriosclerosis in young human-immunodeficiency-virus-positive patients. Coron Artery Dis 2000; 11:41–46.

15. Comandini UV, Maggi P, Santopadre P, Monno R, Angarano G, Vullo V. *Chlamydia pneumoniae* respiratory infections among patients infected with the human immunode-ficiency virus. Eur J Clin Microbiol Infect Dis 1997; 16:720–726.

16. Blasi F, Boschini A, Cosentini R, Legnani D, Smacchia C, Ghira C, Allegra L. Outbreak of *Chlamydia pneumoniae* infection in former injection-drug users. Chest 1994; 105:812–815.

17. Saetta A, Fanourakis G, Agapitos E, Davaris PS. Atherosclerosis of the carotid artery: absence of evidence for CMV involvement in atheroma formation. Cardiovasc Pathol 2000; 9:181–183.

18. Memon RA, Staprans I, Noor M, Holleran WM, Uchida Y, Moser AH, Feingold KR, Grunfeld C. Infection and inflammation induce LDL oxidation in vivo. Arterioscler Thromb Vasc Biol 2000; 20:1536–1542.

19. Musiani M, Zerbini ML, Muscari A, Puddu GM, Gentilomi G, Gibellini D, Gallinella G, Puddu P, La Placa M. Antibody patterns against cytomegalovirus and Epstein-Barr virus in human atherosclerosis. Microbiologica 1990; 13:35–41.

20. Zhu J, Quyyumi AA, Norman JE, Costello R, Csako G, Epstein SE. The possible role of hepatitis A virus in the pathogenesis of atherosclerosis. J Infect Dis 2000; 182:1583–1587.

21. Visser MR, Vercellotti GM. Herpes simplex virus and atherosclerosis. Eur Heart J 1993; 14(suppl K):39–42.

22. Sorlie PD, Nieto FJ, Adam E, Folsom AR, Shahar E, Massing M. A prospective study of cytomegalovirus, herpes simplex virus 1, and coronary heart disease: the atherosclerosis risk in communities (ARIC) study. Arch Intern Med 2000; 160:2027–2032.

23. Vercellotti GM. Effects of viral activation of the vessel wall on inflammation and thrombosis. Blood Coagul Fibrinolysis 1998; 9(suppl 2):S3–S6.

24. Zafar H, Vaz A, Carlson RW. Acute complications of cocaine intoxication. Hosp Pract (Off Ed) 1997; 32:167–181.

25. He J, Xiao Y, Zhang L. Cocaine induces apoptosis in human coronary artery endothelial cells. J Cardiovasc Pharmacol 2000; 35:572–580.

26. Grant RL, Acosta D Jr. A digitized fluorescence imaging study on the effects of local anesthetics on cytosolic calcium and mitochondrial membrane potential in cultured rabbit corneal epithelial cells. Toxicol Appl Pharmacol 1994; 129:23–35.

27. He GQ, Zhang A, Altura BT, Altura BM. Cocaine-induced cerebrovasospasm and its possible mechanism of action. J Pharmacol Exp Ther 1994; 268:1532–1539.

28. Zhang A, Cheng TP, Altura BT, Altura BM. Acute cocaine results in rapid rises in intracellular free calcium concentration in canine cerebral vascular smooth muscle cells: possible relation to etiology of stroke. Neurosci Lett 1996; 215:57–59.

29. Masini A, Gallesi D, Giovannini F, Trenti T, Ceccarelli D. Membrane potential of hepatic mitochondria after acute cocaine administration in rats—the role of mitochondrial reduced glutathione. Hepatology 1997; 25:385–390.

30. Yuan C, Acosta D Jr. Cocaine-induced mitochondrial dysfunction in primary cultures of rat cardiomyocytes. Toxicology 1996; 112:1–10.

31. Fiala M, Gan XH, Zhang L, House SD, Newton T, Graves MC, Shapshak P, Stins M, Kim KS, Witte M, Chang SL. Cocaine enhances monocyte migration across the blood-brain barrier. Cocaine's connection to AIDS dementia and vasculitis? Adv Exp Med Biol 1998; 437:199–205.

32. Brudney K, Dobkin J. Resurgent tuberculosis in New York City. Human immunodeficiency virus, homelessness, and the decline of tuberculosis control programs. Am Rev Respir Dis 1991; 144:745–749.

33. Rubin RB, Neugarten J. Medical complications of cocaine: changes in pattern of use and spectrum of complications. J Toxicol Clin Toxicol 1992; 30:1–12.

34. Weiss SH. Links between cocaine and retroviral infection. JAMA 1989; 261:607–609.

35. Mao JT, Zhu LX, Sharma S, Chen K, Huang M, Santiago SJ, Gulsurd J, Tashkin DP, Dubinett SM. Cocaine inhibits human endothelial cell IL-8 production: the role of transforming growth factor-beta. Cell Immunol 1997; 181:38–43.

36. Hebert CA, Baker JB. Interleukin-8: a review. Cancer Invest 1993; 11:743–750.

37. Strieter RM, Kunkel SL, Showell HJ, Marks RM. Monokine-induced gene expression of a human endothelial cell-derived neutrophil chemotactic factor. Biochem Biophys Res Commun 1988; 156:1340–1345.

38. Peterson PK, Gekker G, Chao CC, Schut R, Molitor TW, Balfour HH Jr. Cocaine potentiates HIV-1 replication in human peripheral blood mononuclear cell cocultures. Involvement of transforming growth factor-beta . J Immunol 1991; 146:81–84.

39. Tulen JH, Moleman P, Blankestijn PJ, Man i V, van Steenis HG, Boomsma F. Psychological, cardiovascular, and endocrine changes during 6 hours of continuous infusion of epinephrine or norepinephrine in healthy volunteers. Psychosom Med 1993; 55:61–69.

40. Kukreja RS, Datta BN, Chakravarti RN. Catecholamine-induced aggravation of aortic and coronary atherosclerosis in monkeys. Atherosclerosis 1981; 40:291–298.

41. Bauch HJ, Grunwald J, Vischer P, Gerlach U, Hauss WH. A possible role of catecholamines in atherogenesis and subsequent complications of atherosclerosis. Exp Pathol 1987; 31:193–204.

42. Kolodgie FD, Wilson PS, Mergner WJ, Virmani R. Cocaine-induced increase in the permeability function of human vascular endothelial cell monolayers. Exp Mol Pathol 1999; 66:109–122.

43. Chen L, Boomershine C, Wang T, Lafuse WP, Zwilling BS. Synergistic interaction of catecholamine hormones and *Mycobacterium avium* results in the induction of interleukin-10 mRNA expression by murine peritoneal macrophages. J Neuoimmunol 1999; 93:149–155.

44. Mo W, Singh AK, Arruda JA, Dunea G. Role of nitric oxide in cocaine-induced acute hypertension. Am J Hypertens 1998; 11:708–714.

45. Chi DS, Qui M, Krishnaswamy G, Li C, Stone W. Regulation of nitric oxide production from macrophages by lipopolysaccharide and catecholamines. Nitric Oxide 2003; 8: 127–132.

46. Shapira L, Frolov I, Halabi A, Ben-Nathan D. Experimental stress suppresses recruitment of macrophages but enhanced their *P. gingivalis* LPS-stimulated secretion of nitric oxide. J Periodontol 2000; 71, 476–481.

47. Kohut ML, Davis JM, Jackson DA, Colbert LH, Strasner A, Essig DA, Pate RR, Ghaffar A, Mayer EP. The role of stress hormones in exercise-induced suppression of alveolar macrophage antiviral function. J Neuroimmunol 1998; 81:193–200.

48. Petty HR, Berg KA. Combinative ligand-receptor interactions: epinephrine depresses RAW264 macrophage antibody-dependent phagocytosis in the absence and presence of met-enkephalin. J Cell Physiol 1988; 134:281–286.

49. Abrass CK, O'Connor SW, Scarpace PJ, Abrass IB. Characterization of the beta-adrenergic receptor of the rat peritoneal macrophage. J Immunol 1985; 135:1338–1341.

50. Sigola LB, Zinyama RB. Adrenaline inhibits macrophage nitric oxide production through beta1 and beta2 adrenergic receptors. Immunology 2000; 100:359–363.

51. Christensen JD, Hansen EW, Frederiksen C, Molris M, Moesby L. Adrenaline influences the release of interleukin-6 from murine pituicytes: role of beta2-adrenoceptors. Eur J Pharmacol 1999; 378:143–148.

52. Ben-Eliyahu S, Shakhar G, Page GG, Stefanski V, Shakhar K. Suppression of NK cell activity and of resistance to metastasis by stress: a role for adrenal catecholamines and beta-adrenoceptors. Neuroimmunomodulation 2000; 8:154–164.

53. Boomershine CS, Lafuse WP, Zwilling BS. Beta2-adrenergic receptor stimulation inhibits nitric oxide generation by *Mycobacterium avium* infected macrophages. J Neuoimmunol 1999; 101:68–75.

54. Hasko G, Shanley TP, Egnaczyk G, Nemeth ZH, Salzman AL, Vizi ES, Szabo C. Exogenous and endogenous catecholamines inhibit the production of macrophage inflammatory protein (MIP) 1 alpha via a beta adrenoceptor mediated mechanism. Br J Pharmacol 1998; 125:1297–1303.

55. Billman GE. Mechanisms responsible for the cardiotoxic effects of cocaine. FASEB J 1990; 4:2469–2475.

56. Isner JM, Chokshi SK. Cardiovascular complications of cocaine. Curr Probl Cardiol 1991; 16:89–123.

57. Om A. Cardiovascular complications of cocaine. Am J Med Sci 1992; 303:333–339.

58. Togna GI, Graziani M, Russo P, Caprino L. Cocaine toxic effect on endothelium-dependent vasorelaxation: an in vitro study on rabbit aorta. Toxicol Lett 2001; 123:43–50.

59. Draijer R, Atsma DE, van der LA, van Hinsbergh VW. cGMP and nitric oxide modulate thrombin-induced endothelial permeability. Regulation via different pathways in human aortic and umbilical vein endothelial cells. Circ Res 1995; 76:199–208.

60. Itzhak Y. Modulation of cocaine- and methamphetamine-induced behavioral sensitization by inhibition of brain nitric oxide synthase. J Pharmacol Exp Ther 1997; 282:521–527.

61. Pudiak CM, Bozarth MA. L-NAME and MK-801 attenuate sensitization to the locomotor-stimulating effect of cocaine. Life Sci 1993; 53:1517–1524.

62. Brogan WC III, Lange RA, Kim AS, Moliterno DJ, Hillis LD. Alleviation of cocaine-induced coronary vasoconstriction by nitroglycerin. J Am Coll Cardiol 1991; 18:581–586.

63. Leeuwenburgh C, Hardy MM, Hazen SL, Wagner P, Oh-ishi S, Steinbrecher UP, Heinecke JW. Reactive nitrogen intermediates promote low density lipoprotein oxidation in human atherosclerotic intima. J Biol Chem 1997; 272:1433–1436.

64. Buttery LD, Springall DR, Chester AH. Inducible nitric oxide synthase is present within human atherosclerotic lesions and promotes the formation and activity of peroxynitrite. Lab Invest 1996; 75:77–85.

65. Wilcox JN, Subramanian RR, Sundell CL, Tracey WR, Pollock JS, Harrison DG, Marsden PA. Expression of multiple isoforms of nitric oxide synthase in normal and atherosclerotic vessels. Arterioscler Thromb Vasc Biol 1997; 17:2479–2488.

66. Collins SL, Edwards MA, Kantak KM. Effects of nitric oxide synthase inhibitors on the discriminative stimulus effects of cocaine in rats. Psychopharmacology (Berl) 2001; 154:261–273.

67. Wolf ME. The role of excitatory amino acids in behavioral sensitization to psychomotor stimulants. Prog Neurobiol 1998; 54:679–720.

68. Olesen SP, Clapham DE, Davies PF. Haemodynamic shear stress activates a K+ current in vascular endothelial cells. Nature 1988; 331:168–170.

69. Moncada S, Higgs A. The L-arginine-nitric oxide pathway. N Engl J Med 1993; 329:2002–2012.

70. Bolotina VM, Najibi S, Palacino JJ, Pagano PJ, Cohen RA. Nitric oxide directly activates calcium-dependent potassium channels in vascular smooth muscle. Nature 1994; 368:850–853.

71. Oates JA, FitzGerald GA, Branch RA, Jackson EK, Knapp HR, Roberts LJ. Clinical implications of prostaglandin and thromboxane A2 formation (1). N Engl J Med 1988; 319:689–698.

72. Pearson JD, Gordon JL. Vascular endothelial and smooth muscle cells in culture selectively release adenine nucleotides. Nature 1979; 281:384–386.

73. Chen G, Suzuki H, Weston AH. Acetylcholine releases endothelium-derived hyperpolarizing factor and EDRF from rat blood vessels. Br J Pharmacol 1988; 95:1165–1174.

74. Yanagisawa M, Kurihara H, Kimura S, Tomobe Y, Kobayashi M, Mitsui Y, Yazaki Y, Goto K, Masaki T. A novel potent vasoconstrictor peptide produced by vascular endothelial cells. Nature 1988; 332:411–415.

75. Dzau VJ. Circulating versus local renin-angiotensin system in cardiovascular homeostasis. Circulation 1988; 77:I4–I13.

76. Tesfamariam B, Brown ML, Deykin D, Cohen RA. Elevated glucose promotes generation of endothelium-derived vasoconstrictor prostanoids in rabbit aorta. J Clin Invest 1990; 85:929–932.

77. Luscher TF, Vanhoutte PM. Endothelium-dependent contractions to acetylcholine in the aorta of the spontaneously hypertensive rat. Hypertension 1986; 8:344–348.

78. Bredt DS, Snyder SH. Isolation of nitric oxide synthetase, a calmodulin-requiring enzyme. Proc Natl Acad Sci USA 1990; 87:682–685.

79. Pollockm JS, Forstermann U, Mitchell JA, Warner TD, Schmidt HHHW, Nakane M, Murad F. Purification and characterization of particulate endothelium-derived relaxing factor synthase from cultured and native bovine aortic endothelial cells. Proc Natl Acad Sci USA 1991; 88:10480–10484.

80. Stuehr DJ, Cho HJ, Kwon NS, Weise M, Nathan CF. Purification and characterization of the cytokine-induced macrophage nitric oxide synthase: An FAD-and FMN-containing flavoprotein. Proc Natl Acad Sci USA 1991; 88:7773–7777.

81. Yui Y, Hattori R, Kosuga K, Eizawa H, Hiki K, Kawai C. Purification of nitric oxide synthase from rat macrophages. J Bio Chem 1991; 226:12544–12547.

82. Denninger JW, Marletta MA. Guanylate cyclase and the .NO/cGMP signaling pathway. Biochim Biophys Acta 1999; 1411:334–350.

83. Feihl F, Waeber B, Liaudet L. Is nitric oxide overproduction the target of choice for the management of septic shock? Pharmacol Ther 2001; 91:179–213.

84. Brown GC. Nitric oxide and mitochondrial respiration. Biochim Biophys Acta 1999; 1411:351–369.

85. Gardner PR, Costantino G, Szabo C, Salzman AL. Nitric oxide sensitivity of the aconitases. J Biol Chem 1997; 272:25071–25076.

86. Miller MJ, Sandoval M. Nitric oxide. III. A molecular prelude to intestinal inflammation. Am J Physiol 1999; 276:G795–G799.

87. Cobb JP, Danner RL. Nitric oxide and septic shock. JAMA 1996; 275:1192–1196.

88. MacMicking JD, Nathan C, Hom G, Chartrain N, Fletcher DS, Trumbauer M, Stevens K, Xie QW, Sokol K, Hutchinson N. Altered responses to bacterial infection and endotoxic shock in mice lacking inducible nitric oxide synthase. Cell 1997; 8:641–650.

89. Hecht SS. Approaches to cancer prevention based on an understanding of N-nitrosamine carcinogenesis. Proc Soc Exp Biol Med 1997; 216:181–191.

90. Golino P, Piscione F, Willerson JT, Cappelli-Bigazzi M, Focaccio A, Villari B, Indolfi C, Russolillo E, Condorelli M, Chiariello M. Divergent effects of serotonin on coronary-artery dimensions and blood flow in patients with coronary atherosclerosis and control patients. N Engl J Med 1991; 324:641–648.

91. Shimokawa H, Vanhoutte PM. Impaired endothelium-dependent relaxation to aggregating platelets and related vasoactive substances in porcine coronary arteries in hypercholesterolemia and atherosclerosis. Circ Res 1989; 64:900–914.

92. Miles AM, Bohle DS, Glassbrenner PA, Hansert B, Wink DA, Grisham MB. Modulation of superoxide-dependent oxidation and hydroxylation reactions by nitric oxide. J Biol Chem 1996; 271:40–47.

93. Rubbo H, Radi R, Trujillo M, Telleri R, Kalyanaraman B, Barnes S, Kirk M, Freeman BA. Nitric oxide regulation of superoxide and peroxynitrite-dependent lipid peroxidation. Formation of novel nitrogen-containing oxidized lipid derivatives. J Biol Chem 1994; 269:26066–26075.

94. Arteel GE, Briviba K, Sies H. Protection against peroxynitrite. FEBS Lett 1999; 445:226–230.

95. Hausladen A, Fridovich I. Superoxide and peroxynitrite inactivate aconitases, but nitric oxide does not. J Biol Chem 1994; 269:29405–29408. .

96. Szabo C, Dawson VL. Role of poly(ADP-ribose) synthetase in inflammation and ischaemia-reperfusion. Trends Pharmacol Sci 1998; 19:287–298.

97. Szabo C, Zingarelli B, O'Connor M, Salzman AL. DNA strand breakage, activation of poly (ADP-ribose) synthetase, and cellular energy depletion are involved in the cytotoxicity of macrophages and smooth muscle cells exposed to peroxynitrite. Proc Natl Acad Sci USA 1996; 93:1753–1758.

98. Kim YM, Bombeck CA, Billiar TR. Nitric oxide as a bifunctional regulator of apoptosis. Circ Res 1999; 84:253–256.

99. Liaudet L, Soriano FG, Szabo C. Biology of nitric oxide signaling. Crit Care Med 2000; 28:N37–N52.

100. Shen YH, Wang XL, Wilcken DE. Nitric oxide induces and inhibits apoptosis through different pathways. FEBS Lett 1998; 433:125–131.

101. Albina JE, Cui S, Mateo RB, Reichner JS. Nitric oxide-mediated apoptosis in murine peritoneal macrophages. J Immunol 1993; 150:5080–5085.

102. Lopez-Collazo E, Mateo J, Miras-Portugal MT, Bosca L. Requirement of nitric oxide and calcium mobilization for the induction of apoptosis in adrenal vascular endothelial cells. FEBS Lett 1997; 413:124–128.

103. Pinsky DJ, Aji W, Szabolcs M, Athan ES, Liu Y, Yang YM, Kline RP, Olson KE, Cannon PJ. Nitric oxide triggers programmed cell death (apoptosis) of adult rat ventricular myocytes in culture. Am J Physiol 1999; 277:H1189–H1199.

104. Bolanos JP, Almeida A, Stewart V, Peuchen S, Land JM, Clark JB, Heales SJ. Nitric oxide-mediated mitochondrial damage in the brain: mechanisms and implications for neurodegenerative diseases. J Neurochem 1997; 68:2227–2240.

105. Sandoval M, Zhang XJ, Liu X, Mannick EE, Clark DA, Miller MJ. Peroxynitrite-induced apoptosis in T84 and RAW 264.7 cells: attenuation by L-ascorbic acid. Free Radic Biol Med 1997; 22:489–495.

106. Constans J, Seigneur M, Blann AD, Renard M, Resplandy F, Amiral J, Guerin V, Boisseau MR, Conri C. Effect of the antioxidants selenium and beta-carotene on HIV-related endothelium dysfunction. Thromb Haemost 1998; 80:1015–1017.

107. Levine GN, Frei B, Koulouris SN, Gerhard MD, Keaney JF Jr, Vita JA. Ascorbic acid reverses endothelial vasomotor dysfunction in patients with coronary artery disease. Circulation 1996; 93:1107–1113.

108. Ting HH, Timimi FK, Haley EA, Roddy MA, Ganz P, Creager MA. Vitamin C improves endothelium-dependent vasodilation in forearm resistance vessels of humans with hypercholesterolemia. Circulation 1997; 95:2617–2622.

109. Taddei S, Virdis A, Ghiadoni L, Magagna A, Salvetti A. Vitamin C improves endothelium-dependent vasodilation by restoring nitric oxide activity in essential hypertension. Circulation 1998; 97:2222–2229.

110. Schwartz D, Mendonca M, Schwartz I, Xia Y, Satriano J, Wilson CB, Blantz RC. Inhibition of constitutive nitric oxide synthase (NOS) by nitric oxide generated by inducible NOS after lipopolysaccharide administration provokes renal dysfunction in rats. J Clin Invest 1997; 100:439–448.

111. Fischer LG, Horstman DJ, Hahnenkamp K, Kechner NE, Rich GF. Selective iNOS inhibition attenuates acetylcholine. Anesthesiology 1999; 91:1724–1732.

112. Gundersen Y, Corso CO, Leiderer R, Dorger M, Lilleaasen P, Aasen AO, Messmer K. Use of selective and nonselective nitric oxide synthase inhibitors in rat endotoxemia: effects on hepatic morphology and function. Shock 1997; 8:368–372.

113. Ou J, Carlos TM, Watkins SC, Saavedra JE, Keefer LK, Kim YM, Harbrecht BG, Billiar TR. Differential effects of nonselective nitric oxide synthase (NOS) and selective inducible NOS inhibition on hepatic necrosis, apoptosis, ICAM-1 expression, and neutrophil accumulation during endotoxemia. Nitric Oxide 1997; 1:404–416.

114. Vos TA, Gouw AS, Klok PA, Havinga R, van Goor H, Huitema S, Roelofsen H, Kuipers F, Jansen PL, Moshage H. Differential effects of nitric oxide synthase inhibitors on endotoxin-induced liver damage in rats. Gastroenterology 1997; 113:1323–1333.

115. Bollaert PE, Charpentier C, Levy B, Debouverie M, Audibert G, Larcan A. Reversal of late septic shock with supraphysiologic doses of hydrocortisone. Crit Care Med 1998; 26:645–650.

116. Hong HJ, Wu CC, Yen MH. Pyrrolidine dithiocarbamate improves the septic shock syndromes in spontaneously hypertensive rats. Clin Exp Pharmacol Physiol 1998; 25:600–606.

117. Kishnani NS, Tabrizi-Fard MA, Fung HL. Diethyldithiocarbamate prolongs survival of mice in a lipopolysaccharide-induced endotoxic shock model: evidence for multiple mechanisms. Shock 1999; 11:264–268.

118. Nathan C. Inducible nitric oxide synthase: what difference does it make? J Clin Invest 1997; 100:2417–2423.

119. Bone HG, Waurick R, Van Aken H, Booke M, Prien T, Meyer J. Comparison of the haemodynamic effects of nitric oxide synthase inhibition and nitric oxide scavenging in endotoxaemic sheep. Intens Care Med 1998; 24:48–54.

120. Greenberg SS, Xie J, Zatarain JM, Kapusta DR, Miller MJ. Hydroxocobalamin (vitamin B12a) prevents and reverses endotoxin-induced hypotension and mortality in rodents: role of nitric oxide. J Pharmacol Exp Ther 1995; 273:257–265.

121. Kazmierski WM, Wolberg G, Wilson JG, Smith SR, Williams DS, Thorp HH, Molina L. Iron chelates bind nitric oxide and decrease mortality in an experimental model of septic shock. Proc Natl Acad Sci USA 1996; 93:9138–9141.

122. Yoshida M, Akaike T, Wada Y, Sato K, Ikeda K, Ueda S, Maeda H. Therapeutic effects of imidazolineoxyl N-oxide against endotoxin shock through its direct nitric oxide–scavenging activity. Biochem Biophys Res Commun 1994; 202:923–930.

123. Cheng X, Pang CC. Pressor and vasoconstrictor effects of methylene blue in endotoxaemic rats. Naunyn Schmiedebergs Arch Pharmacol 1998; 357:648–653.

124. Paya D, Gray GA, Stoclet JC. Effects of methylene blue on blood pressure and reactivity to norepinephrine in endotoxemic rats. J Cardiovasc Pharmacol 1993; 21:926–930.

125. Keaney JF Jr, Puyana JC, Francis S, Loscalzo JF, Stamler JS, Loscalzo J. Methylene blue reverses endotoxin-induced hypotension. Circ Res 1994; 74:1121–1125.

126. Zhang H, Rogiers P, Preiser JC, Spapen H, Manikis P, Metz G, Vincent JL. Effects of methylene blue on oxygen availability and regional blood flow during endotoxic shock. Crit Care Med 1995; 23:1711–1721.

24

Cardiovascular Complications of HIV/AIDS and Substance Abuse

Jag H. Khalsa
National Institute on Drug Abuse, National Institutes of Health, Bethesda, Maryland, U.S.A.

INTRODUCTION

The human immunodeficiency virus (HIV) infects CD4 lymphocytes and macrophages, causing profound immunosuppression that eventually develops into acquired immunodeficiency symdrome (AIDS). An estimated 34.3 million people worldwide were living with HIV/AIDS at the end of 1999 (1,2). Since 1981, when AIDS was first identified, approximately 1 million Americans have become infected with HIV, with serious outcomes of morbidity and mortality (3). However, with the increased survival due to more effective antiviral therapy, new complications and manifestations of late-stage HIV infection are being reported, including cardiovascular disease. Since the first reported case of fatal dilated cardiomyopathy in AIDS patients in 1986, numerous echocardiographic studies have reported a high incidence of symptomatic cardiovascular complications in HIV-infected individuals (4). These complications include pericardial effusion, myocarditis, dilated cardiomyopathy, endocarditis, malignant neoplasms, coronary artery disease, and drug-related cardiotoxicity. In 1991, the prevalence of cardiac manifestations in AIDS patients ranged from 28 to 73%. In 1996, HIV cardiomyopathy was reported to be the fourth leading cause of dilated cardiomyopathy in adults in the United States. Half of these patients died of this disease within 6 to 12 months. Similar cardiovascular complications have also been reported with substance abuse, in particular with cocaine abuse (see Chap. 21).

To encourage further research on cardiovascular disease in HIV infection, the National Heart, Lung, and Blood Institute (NHLBI) released Requests for Applications (RFAs) on the following topics: "Etiology of Cardiovascular Complications in HIV Infection," "Endothelial Dysfunction in HIV Infection," and "Genesis of Cardiomyopathy with HIV Infection and Alcohol Abuse" in 1996, 1997, and 1998, respectively. In 1998, to encourage research on cardiovascular disease in HIV infection and substance abuse, in particular cocaine, the National Institute on Drug Abuse (NIDA) joined with the NHLBI and cosponsored an RFA on the topic "Cardiovascular Complications from Cocaine Abuse in HIV Infection"; it also supported additional innovative studies. The funding of this cardiovascular research was followed by two excellent NHLBI and NIDA cosponsored meetings in September 2000 and May 2002, where several leading clinician-scientists (see a complete list at end of chapter) discussed (1) the most current data on etiology and underlying pathophysiology of cardiovascular complications of HIV/AIDS and substance abuse (cocaine, alcohol); (2) in vitro tests and in vivo models for the study of cardiovascular complications (e.g., cardiomyopathy) of HIV and substance abuse; (3) endothelial function in HIV infection; and (4) the problems of design and conducting such studies in clinical populations. They also made recommendations for supporting innovative research on the subject.

ETIOLOGY OF CARDIOVASCULAR COMPLICATIONS IN HIV INFECTION

Jolicoeur (Clinical Research Institute of Montreal, Quebec, Canada) reported on cardiac disease in transgenic mice, expressing only Env, Rev, and Nef (neurite extension factor) accessory proteins of HIV-1, which developed disease similar to human AIDS. He pointed out that other transgenic lines expressing only Nef also developed cardiac disease and that coronary vascular function was compromised in the transgenic mice. Jolicoeur argued that there was a strong resemblance between the cardiac lesions in transgenic mice and those found in humans with AIDS, and the fact that these lesions arise not as a consequence of Nef expression in cardiomyocytes but rather in CD4+ T cells and in cells of the macrophagic/dendritic lineage make this mouse model quite suitable for studying the pathogenesis of these lesions.

AIDS-related cardiomyopathy (AIDS-CM) is an important clinical problem, but its pathogenesis is poorly understood. To define the role of a specific HIV-1 regulatory protein in the development of AIDS-CM, Lewis (Emory U) studied HIV-1 Tat in cardiac ventricular myocytes in the mouse model. He showed that the cardiac mitochondria of these transgenic mice were significantly enlarged and elongated, with fragmented cristae at 10 months of age, and suggested that this model may serve effectively for studying AIDS-CM and may also offer insights into mechanisms of normal and defective cardiac mitochondrial biogenesis.

By using the murine AIDS model (LPBM5 retrovirus–infected mice), Watson (U. Arizona) demonstrated significantly dilated cardiomyopathy with diminished contractile function at 12 weeks following the retroviral treatment of mice. He concluded that there was a virally induced dilated cardiomyopathy in the murine AIDS model without chronic involvement of the inflammatory mediators inducible nitric oxide synthase (iNOS) and tumor necrosis factor-alpha (TNF-α).

On the basis of earlier work showing that the murine AIDS model mimics the time-dependent cardiac dysfunction and pathological changes seen in HIV-infected patients, Bauer (Ohio State U.) showed that the combination of retroviral infection with nonseptic lipopolysaccharide (LPS) caused a further reduction of cardiac output and fractional shortening detected in retrovirus-infected mice. The exposure to subseptic levels of gram-negative bacteria enhanced cardiovascular pathogenesis in the murine model, suggesting that bacterial coinfection might augment HIV-related cardiac complications in humans.

Lymphocytic myocarditis is a common pathological lesion in AIDS cardiomyopathy, yet the role of direct retroviral infection of cardiomyocytes and the mechanisms of myocyte injury remain controversial. Shannon (Harvard Medical School) found that simian immunodeficiency virus (SIV) viral remnants were commonly present in the myocardia from SIV-infected rhesus macaques but were always found in association with CD4+/CD68+ macrophages in the presence of myocarditis or cardiac dendritic cells in the absence of inflammation. The mechanism of myocardial injury appeared to be apoptosis mediated through the Fas death receptor.

ENDOTHELIAL DYSFUNCTION AND HIV TAT

Transmigration of the HIV-infected cells from the bloodstream into tissues is not well defined. However, Groopman (Harvard Medical School) showed that HIV-1 Tat, a protein secreted by infected cells, might act as a protocytokine by causing release of monocyte chemoattractant protein-1 (MCP-1) from the endothelial monolayer and thereby might facilitate monocyte transmigration into tissue via a protein kinase c signaling pathway. He also demonstrated that HIV-1 Tat was able to activate apoptosis in microvascular endothelium by a mechanism distinct from the secretion of TNF or the Fas pathway.

Flores (U. Colorado) reported on the mechanism of myocardial inflammation in AIDS. She found that purified Tat upregulated E-selectin in human umbilical vein endothelial cells. This effect was mediated through changes in redox status and NF-κB. She also found that another NF-κB family member, ReIB, was upregulated in response to either Tat or TNF-α. According to Flores, ReIB might be more important in regulating a chronic than an acute inflammatory response.

Terada (U. Texas) hypothesized that the secreted HIV transcription factor Tat acts, in concert with TNF-α, to modify endothelial cell phenotype through an oxidant-dependent activation of MAP kinase signaling cassettes. He reported that expression of p47phox, a signal-receiving NADPH oxidase subunit, is higher in endothelial cells than in several epithelial cell lines and in whole tissues. Overexpression of a mutant p47phox-defective gene in the first SH3 binding domain diminished TNF-induced JNK activation, further suggesting a role for a vascular homolog of the phagocyte oxidase in JNK activation.

HIV-1 Tat acts in synergy with suboptimal levels of bFGF or combined inflammatory cytokines to induce angiogenesis. Whether the transcriptional activation function of intracellular Tat has proangiogenic effects has not been determined. Since CDK9, a cellular protein kinase, interacts with the activation domain of Tat and mediates transactivation in other cell types, Morris (Louisiana State U.) proposed the existence of a functional endothelial cell-derived CDK9 cell. She showed that human umbilical vein endothelial cell induced by bFGF demonstrated a modest increase in CDK9 cell expression and activity. These data suggest that CDK9 activity might be regulated in endothelial cells induced to proliferate and differentiate. Experiments are in progress to determine whether CDK9 activity participates in Tat-mediated angiogenesis.

ENDOTHELIAL DYSFUNCTION IN HIV INFECTION

Clements (Johns Hopkins U.) showed that cell-free SIV virus could cross the intact human endothelial cell monolayers, but not epithelial cell monolayers in an in vitro transwell culture system, suggesting specificity of virus–endothelial cell interaction. She also indicated that virions that transversed the endothelial cell monolayers were capable of infecting susceptible cells.

The molecular mechanisms of AIDS-cardiovascular disease are unknown. Chen (Emory U.) incubated SIV virus–like particles (VLPs), which contain gag and gp120, with iliac arteries of rhesus macaque monkeys and showed that SIV VLPs reduced vessel relaxation in response to acetylcholine and that SIV VLP-treated vessels decreased eNOS expression and increased superoxide anion production. These data suggest that SIV VLP-gp120 impaired endothelium-mediated vasorelaxation.

Vpr is an accessory regulatory protein of HIV-1 produced in the late phase of the HIV-1 life cycle and packaged into the HIV-1 virion. Zhao (St. Louis U.) argued that despite the suggestive evidence that Vpr affected the cytoskeletal structure, the mechanism involved and the role of cytoskeletal molecules in Vpr-induced cellular changes remain unknown. He identified a Vpr-interacting kinase (RIK) that specifically phosphorylates the myosin regulatory light chain at Ser19, a residue critical for the regulation of actomyosin contraction. Zhao also showed that Vpr mutants incapable of interaction with RIK failed to inhibit RIK.

The recent discovery of Toll-like receptor (TLR), a new class of receptors that play a central role in the recognition of microbial macromolecules, such as LPS from gram-negative bacteria and cell-wall constituents from gram-positive bacteria, and triggering of innate cell activation, raises the question of whether viruses such as HIV might interact with TLRs. Ho (Aaron Diamond Center, NY) described his ongoing functional studies that will delineate whether HIV triggers cellular activation through TLRs and whether lipophosphoglycan could block this interaction.

CARDIOVASCULAR COMPLICATIONS WITH COCAINE ABUSE

Agrawal (Tulane U.) reported on the effects of cocaine on HERG-(human-ether-a-go-go-gene)-encoded K channel. He showed that cocaine and two of its metabolites, cocaethylene and methylecgonine, blocked HERG-encoded K channels in HERG transfected cells, but cocaine's other major metabolites, ecgoninemethylester and benzoylecgonine, did not. These results suggest that both cocaine and cocaethylene could contribute to cardiac repolarization in patients who abused cocaine.

Bauer (Ohio State U.) discussed the role of oxidative stress in cocaine-induced cardiac and vascular toxicity. He showed that acute cocaine dosing causes lasting cardiac and vascular dysfunction via oxidative mechanisms in vivo and in vitro. These changes were associated with cardiac NOS II induction, protein nitration, and selective impairment of vascular endothelium. Bauer suggested that intracellular oxidant production (in the absence of ischemia) might be an important mechanism in cocaine cardiovascular toxicity.

CARDIOVASCULAR COMPLICATIONS FROM COCAINE ABUSE IN HIV INFECTION

By using cocultures of peripheral blood mononuclear cells and human cardiac micro-vascular endothelial cells, Ansari (Emory U.) studied the effects of cocaine, catechol-amines, and HIV infection on leukocyte-endothelial cell interactions. He showed that leukocytes adhered to endothelial cells in both HIV- and norepinephrine-treated cocultures, with an increase in the levels of E-selectin and matrix metalloproteinases (MMPs). These data suggest a model in which cocaine-induced catecholamines primed HIV-infected lymphocytes for adhesion and localization in cardiac micro-vessels, where they could induce MMP-mediated vascular injury.

Fiala (UCLA) reported on the effects of cocaine on coronary artery endothelial permeability and HIV-1 invasion. He found that HIV-1 penetration across a coronary artery endothelial cell barrier model was 17 times higher at 24 hr postinfection than at 2 hr postinfection. This level of penetration was associated with vacuolization of endothelial cell, increased ICAM-1 protein level (ICAM is intercellular adhesion molecule), and penetration of virions into the vacuoles. Cocaine treatment enhanced apoptosis of endothelial cell, produced vacuolization of endothelial cell, and disrupted tight junctions. Data suggest that cocaine might cause the rapid progression of HIV-1 heart and brain infection by decreasing the barrier function of endothelia to the virus and monocyte/macrophages.

Krishnaswamy (East Tennessee State U.) demonstrated that endothelial cell and mast cell activation by cocaine, catecholamines, and HIV glycoproteins could activate inflammatory function in these cells. However, in macrophages, epinephrine synergized with LPS to induce nitrite synthesis. Since nitrite is a vasodilator, it might mitigate some of the harmful effects of vasoactive cytokines and catecholamines in this system. Mono-kines, cocaine, catecholamines, and HIV-associated secreted proteins were capable of endothelial cell and mast cell activation, which might result in some of the observed abnormalities in the vasculopathy, such as atherogenesis, of AIDS and cocaine use.

Lewis (Emory U.) discussed whether cocaine abuse in AIDS increased the risk of sudden cardiac death, the pathological changes of cocaine cardiotoxicity, and changes of cardiac remodeling. He showed that survival period was shorter in the gag/pol AIDS transgenic mice treated with cocaine than in the wild-type mice treated with cocaine. Histological examination showed the presence of focal cardiac myocyte contraction band changes and periarterial fibrosis in the left ventricles of the cocaine-treated mice. These changes appeared worse in the cocaine-treated transgenic mice. Lewis concluded that cocaine administration and viral infection were associated with cardiac remodeling and accelerated mortality in transgenic mice.

Morgan (Harvard Medical School) used encephalomyocarditis virus (EMCV)-infected mice to test his hypothesis that cocaine could increase the incidence and exacerbate the cardiac effects of viral myocarditis. He showed that in mice inoculated with EMCV, incidence of viral myocarditis, inflammatory cell infiltration, myocardial lesion, and mortality increased with cocaine administration. Furthermore, interferon-induced GTPase was significantly decreased in cocaine-treated mice with myocarditis after EMCV inoculation. Thus, Morgan concluded that interferon-induced GTPase-related signal pathways might be involved in the enhanced susceptibility to viral myocarditis seen in cocaine-treated mice.

GENESIS OF CARDIOMYOPATHY WITH HIV INFECTION AND ALCOHOL ABUSE

Coxsackievirus B3 (CVB3), an enterovirus in the Picornaviridae, is an etiological agent of virus-induced myocarditis. Watson (U. Arizona) observed that a murine AIDS model with CBV3-infection showed significant heart lesions. This was because retroviral infection suppressed the response of type 1 T-helper (Th1) cells, which caused cytokine dysregulation and immunosuppression and facilitated coxsackievirus-induced myocarditis. He also showed that murine AIDS facilitated severe cardiotoxicity during coxsackievirus infection, while nonretrovirus-infected mice were resistant. These effects were exaggerated by ethanol, possibly from a shift in the cytokine balance in favor of a Th2 response by enhancing Th2 and/or by suppressing Th1 function.

Wallace (Emory U.) discussed whether there was a relationship between ethanol consumption, mitochondrial malfunction, and AIDS cardiomyopathy. He hypothesized that ethanol and HIV acted synergistically to produce heart disease, because both agents inhibited cardiac mitochondrial function through inhibiting mitochondrial oxidative phosphorylation and increasing the production of mitochondrial oxygen radicals. Wallace treated mice harboring various genetic defects in mitochondrial energy production and antioxidant defenses with toxic levels of ethanol, the murine AIDS virus, and the two in combination. He argued that if the mitochondria were important in the combined ethanol and AIDS toxicity, then these mitochondrial mutant strains should show an increased sensitivity to both agents, and the effects should be synergistic. Further studies are in progress.

CLINICAL RESEARCH

Since chronic cardiac disease is a major health problem in children with HIV infection, particularly those living past 5 years of age, it is important to understand the pathophysiology of heart failure in children. Bowles (Baylor College of Medicine) and his group (Towbin et al.) described their ongoing study of analyzing retrospective and prospective myocardial tissue samples for HIV viral genome and other viral genomes, inflammatory mediators, and other potential causes of cardiac dysfunction (such as apoptosis) in HIV-infected children. Preliminary data show the presence of common viral (especially adenoviral) DNA sequences in heart muscle of HIV-infected children.

Lima (Johns Hopkins U.) and his colleagues (Lai et al., Johns Hopkins U.) described their ongoing study of atherosclerosis among cocaine abusers infected with HIV. The overall goals of the study were to (1) describe prospectively the etiology and natural history of atherosclerosis and the ability of noninvasive tools to measure atherosclerotic burden in cocaine-abusing, HIV-infected black men and women and (2) investigate whether HIV infection, cocaine abuse, and protease inhibitor treatment accelerate atherosclerosis. The study subjects are being reexamined 2 years later and followed up for at least 2 years. The study may provide critical information about the impact of HIV, cocaine abuse, and antiviral protease inhibitors on the development of atherosclerosis.

Rinder (Yale U.) and his colleagues (Margolin et al.) briefly described their ongoing study to determine whether fosinopril [an angiotensin-converting enzyme (ACE) inhibitor] would reduce cocaine use and reduce or prevent the cardiotoxicity of cocaine and HIV infection via its effects on the heart and cardiovascular system in HIV-positive, cocaine-dependent, methadone-maintained patients. Urine toxicology screens, two-dimensional and Doppler echocardiograms, and platelet reactivity of physiological agonists are being studied. In addition, the investigators plan to examine biological and psychosocial risk factors for cardiovascular disorders among cocaine abusers infected with HIV.

Overall, the participants made excellent presentations and offered recommendations for future research (see Chap. 21). They also recommended that NHLBI/ NIDA/NIH should maintain and enhance the momentum already established by this group of clinicians and scientists by issuing additional solicitations or encouraging this type of research by providing additional funding for resource sharing or access to core facilities.

PARTICIPANTS IN NHLBI AND NIDA MEETINGS IN SEPTEMBER 2000 AND MAY 2002

Krishna C. Agrawal, Ph.D., Tulane University School of Medicine; Aftab A. Ansari, Ph.D., Emory University School of Medicine; Sheila A. Barber, Ph.D., Johns Hopkins University School of Medicine; John A. Bauer, Ph.D., Ohio State University; Neil E. Bowles, Ph.D., Baylor College of Medicine; Changyi J. Chen, M.D., Ph.D., Emory University School of Medicine; Zheng W. Chen, M.D., Ph.D., Harvard Medical School; Janice E. Clements, Ph.D., Johns Hopkins University; Adela Cota-Gomez, Ph.D., University of Colorado Health Sciences Center; Milan Fiala, M.D., UCLA School of Medicine; Sonia Flores, Ph.D., University of Colorado; Jerome E. Groopman, M.D., Harvard Medical School; Chandrasekhar Gujuluva, Ph.D., UCLA School of Medicine; Sandra Colombini Hatch, M.D., NHLBI/NIH; Winnie W. Henderson, M.S., Oregon Health Sciences University; John L. Ho, M.D., Cornell University/ Aaron Diamond AIDS Research Center; Paul Jolicoeur, M.D., Ph.D., Clinical Research Institute of Montreal, Montreal, Quebec, Canada; Jag H. Khalsa, Ph.D., NIDA/NIH; Guha Krishnaswamy, M.D., East Tennessee State University/Veterans Affairs Medical Center, Johnson City, TN; Douglas F. Larson, Ph.D., University of Arizona Health Sciences Center; William Lewis, M.D., Emory University School of Medicine; Joao Lima, M.D., Johns Hopkins University School of Medicine; Nancy Q. Liu, M.D., UCLA School of Medicine; Clifford R. Lyons, M.D., University of New Mexico; James P. Morgan, M.D., Ph.D., Harvard Medical School/Beth Israel Deaconess Medical Center; Eugene Morkin, M.D., University of Arizona Health Sciences Center; Cindy A. Morris, Ph.D., Louisiana State University Medical Center; Ashlee V. Moses, Ph.D., Oregon Health Sciences University; Hannah H. Peavy, M.D., NHLBI/ NIH; Henry M. Rinder, M.D., Yale University School of Medicine; Richard P. Shannon, M.D., Harvard Medical School; Deborah E. Sullivan, Ph.D., Louisiana State University Medical Center; J. Bruce Sundstrom, Ph.D., Emory University School of Medicine; Roy Sutliff Ph.D., Emory University School of Medicine; Lance S. Terada, M.D., University of Texas Southwestern/Dallas VA Medical Center; Douglas C. Wallace, Ph.D., Emory University School of Medicine; Lan-Hsiang Wang, Ph.D., NHLBI/NIH; Ronald R. Watson, Ph.D., University of Arizona School of Medicine; Mark D. Wewers, M.D., Ohio State University; Ling-Jun Zhao, Ph.D., Saint Louis University Medical Center.

REFERENCES

1. Gayle HD, Hill GL. Global impact of human immunodeficiency virus and AIDS. Clin Microbiol Rev 2001; 14:327–335.

2. Gayle HD. An overview of the global HIV/AIDS epidemic, with a focus on the United States. AIDS 2000; 14:S8–S17.
3. United Nations AIDS (UNAIDS). AIDS Epidemic Update, December 2001. UNAIDS/ 01.74E-WHO/CS/CSR/NCS 2001.2, English Original, December 2001, ISBN 92-9173-132-3, Joint United Nations Programme on HIV/AIDS/WHO.
4. Cohen IS, Anderson DW, Vermani R, Reen BM, Macher AM, Sennesh J, DiLorenzo P, Redfield RR. Congestive cardiomyopathy in association with the acquired immunodeficiency syndrome. N Engl J Med 1986; 315(10):628–630.

25

Lipids, Lipodystrophy, and AIDS

Jean Ducobu
CHU Tivoli, La Louvière, Belgium

M. C. Payen
Saint-Pierre Hospital, Université Libre de Bruxelles, Brussels, Belgium

INTRODUCTION

The widespread use of combined antiretroviral therapies has greatly reduced morbidity and mortality in HIV-infected patients. Although the success of combination therapy has created hope for long-term treatment, the extensive use of these highly active antiretroviral therapies (HAART) has also uncovered previously uncharacterized adverse drug reactions.

One of the most common adverse effects of HAART is lipodystrophy, including peripheral fat wasting and central fat accumulation. While evidence of the role of protease inhibitors (PI) treatment in lipodystrophy is significant, other results point to independent contributions from nucleoside reverse transcriptase inhibitors (NRTI) or even to the natural history of HIV infection itself. Moreover, investigations into the etiology of this disorder have revealed complicated metabolic changes in many patients, contributing to hyperglycemia, insulin resistance, mitochondrial toxicity, and hyperlipidemia, with associated risks of diabetes and cardiovascular disease. Since these represent significant health risks, the mechanisms of these changes must be elucidated to prevent and treat HIV-related lipodystrophy while maintaining effective antiretroviral therapy.

The impact on lipid parameters of HIV and AIDS without treatment is first briefly reviewed in this chapter, followed by the metabolic consequences of highly active antiretroviral therapies. The management of these deleterious drawbacks is also described.

LIPIDS AND AIDS

The acquired immunodeficiency syndrome (AIDS) is frequently accompanied by changes in lipid concentrations. The observed increase in plasma triglyceride (TG) levels is due to increased very low density lipoproteins (VLDL) and also to TG-enriched low-density lipoproteins (LDL) and high-density lipoproteins (HDL) (1,2).

In many cohorts, subjects who were HIV positive but who yet have AIDS did not have significantly elevated levels of TG (3) (Table 1).

Hypertriglyceridemia due to increased VLDL has been reported in many bacterial, parasitic, and viral infections. These infections can decrease the clearance of circulating lipoproteins, resulting from reduced lipoprotein lipase (LPL) activity, or they can stimulate hepatic lipid synthesis through in either hepatic fatty acid synthesis or in the reesterification of fatty acids derived from lipolysis. These alterations in TG metabolism are thought to be induced by an increase in the cytokines that mediate the immune response, including tumor necrosis factor (TNF), interleukin-1 (IL-1), and the interferons (IFNs).

In AIDS, there is a significant correlation between levels of plasma TG and INF-α (4–6). In contrast, no significant relationship was found between levels of TNF-α and plasma TG. It is therefore possible that increases in TNF-α levels were missed, as TNF-α is secreted in a pulsatile manner and is rapidly cleared from the circulation (Table 2).

Of importance, TG clearance is markedly reduced in HIV-positive and AIDS patients. A highly significant correlation was observed between IFN-α levels and the rate of TG clearance. Total postheparin lipase, hepatic lipase, and LPL activities were all decreased in patients with AIDS (3) (Table 3).

In addition, a close correlation was found between TG clearance and serum TG in both HIV-positive and AIDS patients. Slower TG clearance could contribute to approximately one-third of the variance in plasma TG levels in HIV-positive and AIDS subjects. It is possible that other aspects of TG metabolism are disturbed in AIDS and HIV infection. De novo lipogenesis was found to be increased in such patients, with a significant correlation to circulating IFN-α levels (4). In summary, increased circulating levels of IFN-α in AIDS likely influence TG metabolism and plasma TG levels.

Additionally, in AIDS, the levels of apolipoprotein E (apo-E) are significantly elevated in proportion to levels of plasma triglycerides (7). Furthermore, an increase in the sialylation of apoE in VLDL was seen with qualitative alteration in function. Increases in the more sialylated forms of apoE have also been found in diabetes and renal failure.

Decreased concentrations of LDL and HDL are found in patients with AIDS as well as in asymptomatic HIV-infected individuals (Tables 1 and 2).

Table 1 Plasma Lipid and Apolipoprotein Levels Expressed by Mean +/− SEM

	Control $n = 16$	HIV + $n = 14$	AIDS $n = 15$
TG (mmol/L)	1.15 ± 0.12	1.24 ± 0.17	2.29 ± 0.28
Cholesterol (mmol/L)	4.73 ± 0.17	3.88 ± 0.20	3.90 ± 0.29
HDL cholesterol (mmol/L)	1.27 ± 0.07	0.80 ± 0.04	0.80 ± 0.05
Apo-A-1 (mg/dL)	124.00 ± 8.24	90.40 ± 4.50	86.80 ± 5.40
LDL cholesterol (mmol/L)	3.13 ± 0.17	2.64 ± 0.19	2.18 ± 0.27
Apo-B-100 (mg/dL)	74.5 ± 4.28	58.00 ± 3.38	59.50 ± 6.40

Source: Ref. 3.

Table 2 Mean Value (Standard Deviation) of Lipidic Parameters in the Four Groups (Stratified According to CD_4 Cell Values) of HIV-Positive Patients and in Controls

Group	1	2	3	4	Control
CD4 cells/mm	<50	50–200	200–400	>400	
Patients (n)	32	25	22	15	20
TG (mmol/L)	1,97 (1.27)	1.32 (0,71)	1.56 (0,84)	1.42 (1)	1 (0,35)
CH (mmol/L)	4 (0.93)	4,6 (0.9)	4.9 (1)	5.2 (1.3)	5.2 (0.66)
HDL-C (mmol/L)	0,75 (0.24)	1.12 (0.37)	1.01 (0.3)	1.09 (0.46)	1.38 (0.31)
LDL-C (mmol/L)	2.79 (1.01)	2.89 (0.76)	3.15 (0.91)	3.52 (1.10)	3.73 (0.66)
TNF-α(pg/mL)	45 (33)	36 (22)	26 (25)	12 (16)	5 (5)
INF-α(mƱ/mL)	4,6 (9.09)	0,6 (1.5)	0.25 (0.65)	0 (0)	0 (0)

Source: Ref. 6.

Total cholesterol, HDL cholesterol (including HDL2 and HDL3), Apo A-1, and Apo-B-100 were all decreased to a similar extent in both AIDS and HIV (8). LDL cholesterol was significantly decreased in AIDS, while LDL cholesterol in HIV-positive patients fell in between values in AIDS and those in control subjects. The striking decreases in cholesterol, apolipoproteins, and, especially HDL cholesterol in HIV-positive subjects who had not yet developed hypertriglyceridemia imply that disturbances in cholesterol metabolism precede alteration of TG metabolism during HIV infection.

Patients without HIV receiving injections of IFN-α, IFN-γ, IL-2, or TNF-α showed decreased plasma LDL and/or HDL cholesterol levels. Decreased plasma cholesterol levels were also reported after administration of granulocyte-macrophage colony-stimulating factor. In contrast to its correlation with TG levels, circulating levels of IFN-α do not correlate with HDL or LDL cholesterol in AIDS patients. Consistent with previous reports, decreased levels of LDL and HDL cholesterol were found in all stages of HIV infection but more frequently and to a greater extent in those with a lower CD4+ T-cell count. This held particularly true for HDL cholesterol (Table 2).

The postulated mechanisms explaining the low LDL levels include a increase in LDL receptor activity and/or an increase in scavenger receptors in macrophages. However, experimental data on these issues are contradictory (6). Low HDL levels can be in part explained by the decreased apo-A1 concentrations often observed in AIDS.

Table 3 Triglyceride Clearance and Plasma Postheparin Lipase Activity[a]

	Control	HIV +	AIDS
TG clearance time ($t_{1/2}$ in minutes)	15.2 ± 1.37	25.0 ± 2.50	41.5 ± 5.16
Total lipase	15.1 ± 0.93	12.4 ± 1.40	11.0 ± 1.01
Hepatic lipase	11.2 ± 0.95	9.20 ± 1.30	8.16 ± 0.90
Lipoprotein lipase (LPL)	3.86 ± 0.28	3.23 ± 0.28	2.83 ± 0.19

[a] Activity for lipases is expressed as nanomoles free fatty acids per milliliter produced per hour (FFA/mL) of plasma-h.
Source: Ref. 3.

Table 4 Lipid Hydroperoxide and Total Antioxidant Capacity in Serum Samples of Patients Infected with HIV

	HIV-Infected patients ($n = 14$)	Control subjects ($n = 14$)
Lipid hydroperoxide (mmol/L)	1.44	0.25
Total antioxidant capacity (mmol/L)	1.04	1.66

Source: Ref. 10.

AIDS is associated with two- to threefold increases in the concentration of small dense LDL, resulting in a B phenotypic pattern. The prevalence of large LDL (subclass A phenotype) is decreased in the subjects with AIDS (9). Subjects with AIDS who have the LDL-B phenotype, generally have a marked increase in plasma TG levels compared to AIDS subjects with the LDL A phenotype. On the basis of multiple regression analysis, plasma TG levels appear to be the strongest independent predictor of the LDL-B phenotype in AIDS subjects. In individuals with the LDL B phenotype, HDL concentrations are reduced. In parallel, apolipoprotein-B levels are increased and apolipoprotein-A1 levels decreased. Given such atherogenic alterations in the lipid profile, it is not surprising that LDL phenotype B is associated with an approximately threefold increased risk of myocardial infarction. Moreover lipoprotein (a) [Lp(a)] is higher in AIDS than in controls.

Patients infected with HIV show lower concentrations of antioxidant compounds (10). Because lipid hydroperoxide products were also elevated in the asymptomatic stage of AIDS, the determination of lipid hydroperoxide and total antioxidant status in serum may be clinically helpful (Table 4).

Depleted concentrations of tocopherol, ascorbic acid, and beta-carotene in patients with HIV may lead to higher oxidative stress. Moreover, recent research indicates that overproduction of free radicals may favor replication of HIV-1.

Table 5 summarises the major changes in plasma lipids, lipoproteins, and apolipoproteins observed in patients with HIV and AIDS.

Table 5 Dyslipidemia in HIV + and AIDS
Patients

↗ TG (late)
↗ VLDL (late)
↘ Cholesterol (early)
↘ LDL (early)
↘ HDL (early)
↗ Lp (a)
Presence of small, dense LDL (phenotype B)
↘ Apo B and ↘ Apo A
↗ Apo E (sialylated)
↘ Antioxidant capacity
↗ Lipid peroxidation

Plasma lipids may influence cellular function through changes in lipid membrane composition. Low HDL cholesterol and high TG levels may impair immunocompetence of both humoral and cellular systems. Apo-A-1 (the major apolipoprotein of HDL) and its amphipathic helix peptide analogues inhibit HIV-induced syncytium formation. Rather than being deleterious, the changes in circulating lipoproteins may represent, like the rest of the acute-phase response, part of host defense. Indeed, TG-rich lipoproteins have been shown to prevent endotoxin-induced toxicity in vivo and to neutralize a variety of viruses (5). But if some of the changes may be beneficial, other lipid modifications (small dense LDL, lipid peroxydation, and so on) are likely to be detrimental in chronic process.

LIPODYSTROPHY AND AIDS

Features and Prevalence

Definition

After the publication of several case reports, abnormal fat distribution in HIV-1-infected patients receiving HAART was formally described as a clinical entity in 1998, under the name of lipodystrophy syndrome or fat redistribution syndrome (FRS) (11–13). Although this was initially described as a single entity, at least two different syndromes seem to coexist: lipoatrophy or loss of subcutaneous fat and lipodystrophy. The common physical manifestations of the lipodystrophy syndrome are subcutaneous fat loss in the face and limbs, visceral fat accumulation causing increased abdominal girth, enlargement of the dorsocervical fat pad ("buffalo hump"), and enlargement of the breasts (14) (Table 6).

Lipodystrophy was initially considered to be due only to HIV-1 protease inhibitors (PIs). However, lipodystrophy does not (invariably) develop in all patients treated with PIs and was also reported in patients who had never received them (15–17). Moreover, reversion of lipodystrophy does not occur after withdrawal of PIs. More recently, several studies have also linked the development of lipodystrophy with specific nucleoside reverse transcriptase inhibitors (NRTI). The assessment of the lipodystrophy syndrome ranges from clinical examination and measurements of waist-to-hip ratio to bioelectrical impedance analysis, sonography, and computed tomography (CT) scans.

Table 6 Features of Lipodystrophy Syndrome

Clinical (lipodystrophy)
Peripheral lipoatrophy: face, arms, legs, buttocks
Central fat accumulation: intra-abdominal, dorsocervical spine, breasts, other lipomata
Metabolic
Hypertriglyceridemia
Hypercholesterolemia
Insulin resistance (increases in insulin and C-peptide concentrations)
Type 2 diabetes mellitus/impaired glucose tolerance
Lactic acidemia

Prevalence

Many authors from different countries have reviewed the prevalence of HIV-associated FRS.

In his study, Basdevant (Table 7) shows different prevalences of HIV-FRS with a very extensive range, from 6.4 to 58.6% in HIV-associated FRS (18). Prospective cohorts were specifically designed to identify risk factors for lipodystrophy, including NRTI and PIs.

In a prospective study, Martinez et al. observed that after a median follow-up of 18 months, 85 (17%) of 494 followed patients developed both types of lipodystrophy (19). The incidences of any lipodystrophy, with subcutaneous lipoatrophy and lipodystrophy with central obesity, were respectively 11.7, 9.2, and 7 per patient-year. An increased risk for any lipodystrophy was found among women as compared with men with intravenous versus oral drug use, with increasing age and with the duration of exposure to antiretroviral therapy, but not with any individual antiretroviral agent (19).

Manfredi et al. observed that lipodystrophy and hypertriglyceridemia [present in 75 of 200 patients (37.5%)] was significantly more frequent with ritonavir as compared with indinavir ($p < 0.001$), while isolated saquinavir use was associated with higher TG levels than NRTI treatment alone or no antiretroviral therapy ($p < 0.03$) (20). Hypercholesterolemia was found in 27 subjects (13.5%), more after treatment with indinavir as compared with ritonavir or saquinavir ($p < 0.05$).

Thiebaut et al. prospectively followed 925 patients and found that 27% on a PI regimen and 48% on HAART developed hypertriglyceridemia (HTG) (4.2 cases per 100 person-years). Male sex, baseline TG levels, low CD4 counts, and overweight are the main risk factors for HTG (21). The prevalence of hyperlipidemia in HIV-infected patients taking PIs was reported to be up to 74%, compared with 28% in those not taking the drugs.

Hence, the lipodystrophy syndrome is unlikely to be a direct consequence of HIV-1, given that the syndrome is seen mainly in patients receiving HAART, that lipodystrophy and its severity are independent of plasma HIV-1 load, and that lipodystrophy can occur in recently infected patients who receive HAART. Studies to date have suggested that risk factors may include low body weight before therapy, overweight after therapy, baseline TG concentrations, total duration of HAART, use of the dual PI combination ritonavir-saquinavir (rather than the individual

Table 7 Prevalence of HIV-Associated Fat Redistribution Syndrome (FRS) in France

Author	Therapy	*n*	Atrophic	Hypertrophic	Combined	Total	%
APROCO	PI	116	17	23	20	68	58.6
Rozenbaum	PI	624	14	15	55	84	13.5
GECSA	PI and other anti-HIV drugs	581	15	22	0	37	6.4
Saint-Marc	PI and other anti-HIV drugs	154	22	6	25	53	34.4
Viard	PI	196	7	3	15	25	12.3

Source: Ref. 18.

PI such as saquinavir, indinavir, or nelfinavir), and use of a nucleoside analogue (mainly stavudine). Whether there is a definite hierarchy of causative drugs is not yet known.

Insulin Resistance

The use of PIs in the treatment of HIV is also associated with insulin resistance. Peripheral insulin resistance has been suggested to contribute to the described changes in the lipid and glucose metabolism of HIV patients. In the studies of Wally et al., 67 patients treated with PIs, 13 therapy-naive patients, and 18 HIV-negative controls were tested for insulin sensitivity by performing an intravenous insulin tolerance test, a well established alternative to the euglycemic clamp technique. (22,23). Patients on PIs had a significantly decreased insulin sensitivity when compared with therapy-naive patients, and PI treatment led to a significant increase in total TG and cholesterol levels by 113 and 37 mg/dL, respectively (Fig. 1, Table 8).

The most striking finding in that study was the significantly lower insulin sensitivity in the patients treated with PIs compared with therapy-naive patients. Impairment of insulin sensitivity associated with the use of PIs largely differs in severity. Minor decreases in insulin sensitivity can be compensated, resulting in normal oral glucose tolerance. The prevalence of diabetes mellitus is about 8 to 10%, with most cases being identified after oral glucose loading.

HIV protease inhibitors are also capable of selectively inhibiting the transport function of glucose transporters (Glut 4). This effect may be partly responsible for the insulin resistance frequently observed in HIV-treated patients (24).

Many HIV-treated patients develop the so-called polymetabolic syndrome (syndrome X) with visceral obesity, insulin resistance, impaired glucose tolerance, increased TG; decreased HDL; increased small, dense LDL; increased diastolic BP; and increased plasminogen activator inhibitor-1 (PAI-1). This polymetabolic syndrome is well known to confer an increased risk of CAD.

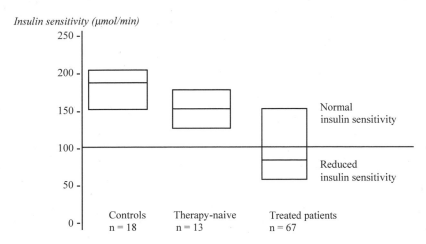

Figure 1 Insulin sensitivity (*) in patients on protease inhibitors, therapy-naive patients, and HIV-negative controls. (*) The insulin sensitivity was analyzed by the intravenous insulin tolerance test. (From Ref. 23.)

Table 8 Comparison of Patients on Protease Inhibitors, Therapy-Naive Patients, and HIV-Negative Controls

	HIV-negative controls ($n = 18$)	Therapy-naive patients ($n = 13$)	Patients treated with protease inhibitors ($n = 67$)
Age (years)	30(20–56)	35(28–81)	44(25–97)
Body mass index (kg/m^2)	22.3(18.8–27.7)	22.3(17.6–29.4)	24.0(17.5–32.6)
CD4 cell count (x10^6/L)	ND[a]	428(9–782)	321(75–1075)
Insulin sensitivity (μmol/L/min)	177(107–261)	156(114–209)	75(0–206)
Number normal/ pathological	18/0	13/0	26/41
Basal glucose (mg/dL)	72(62–82)	76(69–89)	80(59–221)
Total triglycerides (mg/dL)	ND	138(47–317)	294(46–1176)
Total cholesterol (mg/dL)	ND	177(139–221)	203(62–359)

[a] ND = not done.
Source: Ref. 23.

Mechanisms of Metabolic Changes Induced by HAART

Many pathogenic mechanisms have been explored to explain the metabolic changes observed in AIDS patients during their treatment (Table 9).

Glucocorticoïd Excess

The association of buffalo hump and truncal obesity suggests a Cushing-like syndrome. However, elevations in serum cortisol were never observed during PI or HAART treatment (14). Neither lipodystrophy nor PI therapy has been associated with significant differences in concentrations of testosterone, sex-hormone-binding globulin, or prolactin. Leptin concentrations are low, consistent with a reduced fat mass (25).

Protease Inhibitors Homology

Despite the evidence that drugs other than PIs may contribute to HAART-associated lipid abnormalities, the incidence and severity of lipid elevations are most dramatic with PI treatment.

Table 9 Potential Mechanisms of HIV-HAART Lipodystrophy Phenotype

Glucocorticoïd excess
Protease inhibitors (PI) homology theory
NRTI mitochondrial toxicity
Combination of mechanisms

NRTI, Nucleoside reverse transcriptase inhibitors.

The clearance of lipoprotein particles from the vascular compartment is mediated by receptors such as the LDL receptor and the LDL receptor-related protein (LRP), which mainly acts on hepatic uptake of TG-rich particles. Hence, reduced LRP activity may result in decreased lipoprotein-remnant clearance and two- to threefold elevations in plasma triglycerides. This is very similar to the changes observed with HAART in humans.

Indeed, Carr et al. suggested an association between low LRP and PI-related hyperlipidemia (15). The catalytic region of HIV-1 protease, to which PIs bind, has a molecular homology to regions within two proteins that regulate lipid metabolism: 58% with cytoplasmic retinoic-acid binding protein type 1 (CRABP-1) and 63% with low-density-lipoprotein receptor–related protein (LRP). Protease inhibitors could inhibit CRABP-1 and cytochrome P450 3A-mediated synthesis of cis-9-retinoic acid, a key activator of the retinoid X receptor and a peroxisome proliferator activated receptor type gamma (PPARγ) heterodimer, an adipocyte receptor that regulates peripheral adipocyte differentiation and apoptosis. PI binding to LRP would impair chylomicron and VLDL uptake by the liver. The resulting hyperlipidemia could contribute to central fat deposition (and in the breasts in the presence of estrogen), insulin resistance, and, in susceptible individuals, type 2 diabetes.

But the molecular homology between the protease inhibitor and LRP is relatively modest and restricted to a domain of the molecule not directly implicated in lipid metabolism. Moreover, the role of LRP in vivo is essentially relevant to remnant metabolism in the context of diminished LDL-receptor activity.

In addition, PIs may inhibit the synthesis of cis-9-retinoic acid, which is catalyzed by cytochrome P450-3A. Within adipocyte nuclei, cis-9-retinoic acid functions as a heterodimer with peroxisome proliferator activated receptor type gamma (PPARγ). The fact that the PPARγ is mainly expressed in peripheral rather than in central fat might explain the preferential wasting of peripheral fat. Excessive release of fatty acids from peripheral sites can lead to hyperlipidaemia. However, Gagnon et al. observed opposite results in cell cultures (i.e., decreased released of free fatty acids) (26). Therefore other pathogenic theories must be proposed and tested.

Mitochondrial Toxicity

Mitochondrial toxicity of the nucleoside-analogue reverse-transcriptase inhibitors can also play an essential role in the development of the lipodystrophy syndrome, similar to that of mitochondrial defects in the development of multiple symmetrical lipomatosis (27). Recently, a similarity was noted between HAART-related lipodystrophy and benign or multiple symmetrical lipomatosis (MSL), also called Madelung's disease or Launois-Bensaude adenolipomatosis. Clinically, this syndrome has been distinguished into two types. In MSL type 1, patients generally have a low body-mass index and show symmetrical accumulation of fatty masses, especially in the subcutaneous regions of the neck and shoulders and inside the mediastinum. In addition, there is pronounced atrophy of subcutaneous fat in the extremities, somehow similar to HAART-related lipodystrophy. In contrast, patients with MSL type 2 are usually overweight and show a more diffuse lipomatosis. Since both MSL types 1 and 2 may associated with hypertriglyceridemia and insulin resistance, MSL has been considered as a TG storage disease.

Several reports on MSL have shown point mutations at the nucleotide position 8344 in the mitochondrial DNA (mtDNA) or multiple or single mtDNA deletions, leading to impaired function of the oxidative phosphorylation complex IV.

Apart from the inherited mtDNA defects, depletion of mtDNA may also be acquired. The only enzyme that is responsible for mtDNA replication, DNA polymerase γ, is inhibited to a varying extent by NRTIs used in HAART (28). A decrease in muscle and in subcutaneous adipose tissue mitochondrial DNA content was found in HAART-treated HIV-infected patients (29) but also in the blood cells of HIV-infected but never treated individuals as well as in patients treated with antiretroviral drugs (30). Studies of NRTIs in enzyme assays and cell cultures demonstrate the following hierarchy in mitochondrial DNA polymerase gamma inhibition: stavudine > lamivudine > zidovudine > abacavir. In vitro investigations have documented impairment of the mitochondrial enzymes adenylate kinase and the adenosine diphosphate/adenosine triphosphate translocator (31). Recently, PI therapy was reported to lead to mitochondrial respiratory chain dysfunction and to mitochondrial DNA deletions. Some proteases are essential for mitochondrial function (32). Inhibition of DNA-polymerase gamma and other mitochondrial enzymes can gradually lead to mitochondrial dysfunction and cellular toxicity and could be responsible for nearly all the side effects—such as polyneuropathy, myopathy, cardiomyopathy, pancreatitis, bone marrow suppression, and lactic acidosis—that have been attributed to the use of NRTIs.

Combination of Mechanisms

Another possible mechanism of hypertriglyceridemia induced by HAART involves hepatic lipid synthesis. In vitro cell culture models have been extensively used to characterize triglyceride rich lipoprotein production. Nascent VLDL is formed in the endoplasmic reticulum by the microsomal triglyceride transfer protein (MTP) mediated assembly of newly synthesized TGs, cholesteryl ester, and other lipids with apoprotein B100 (apoB100). The rate of VLDL secretion is regulated by proteasomal degradation of apoB in response to lipid availability and MTP activity (17).

Liang et al. tested whether ritonavir (RTV) or saquinavir (SQV) could inhibit proteasome-mediated degradation of apoB100 and demonstrated an accumulation of full-length apo-B100 in cells treated with both PIs (33). Surprisingly, despite such apo B accumulation a significant blockade in apoB secretion was observed in these cells and was attributed to inhibition of MTP activity and neutral lipid synthesis. Addition of fatty acids (oleic acid) resulted in a net increase in secretion of apo B lipoproteins. Given that the PIs are often taken before of with meals, a potential mechanisms for RTV mediated lipid and lipoprotein increases could be the accumulation and net increased secretion of apo B lipoproteins due to fat loading during meals (34).

In their excellent review of HIV lipodystrophy, Mooser and Carr discussed recent experimental data (17). PI-associated hyperlipidemia may also be due to accelerated hepatic production of VLDL particles (35). PIs can stimulate in vitro the production of triglycerides-rich lipoproteins in HepG2 cells. Moreover an approximately 30% increase in plasma triglycerides and cholesterol levels was associated with a strong activation in the liver of lipogenic genes under the control of sterol regulatory element-binding protein (SREBP)-1c. The abundance of SREBP-1c protein in the nucleus of liver cells was increased in ritonavir-treated animals. This effect was associated with increased abundance of SREBP-1c transcripts, which suggests a retarded degradation of the active form of SREBP-1c, possibly through a ritonavir-mediated inhibition of proteasome activity (36,37).

Additional mechanisms may account for the observed accumulation of SREBP-1c in liver cells during therapy. First, improved nutritional status may contribute to the activation of SREBP-1c in the liver. Next, insulin has been shown to markedly transactivate the SREBP expression in animals, and hyperinsulinemia is frequently encountered in HAART-associated lipodystrophy (38). Finally, intense cross talk has recently been demonstrated between the SREBP system and nuclear receptors. Retinoid X receptor (RXR) plays a pivotal role in this process by forming heterodimers with a variety of partners, including retinoid acid receptor, peroxisome proliferator-activated receptors (PPARs), and liver X receptor (LXR) (39). It is conceivable that PIs displace the equilibrium from RXR-PPARα heterodimers toward RXR-LXR heterodimers in the liver. A reduced heterodimerization of RXR with PPARα would have an effect opposite to that of fibrates, which, by liganding PPARα, induce a reduction in plasma concentration of triglyceride-rich lipoproteins.

Increased transient abundance of the active cleaved form of SREBP-1c has recently been documented in 3T3 preadipocytes exposed to ritonavir (40). Moreover, HAART-associated lipodystrophy shares a series of features with one particular mouse model of congenital lipodystrophy, that is generated by overexpressing of the nuclear portion of SREBP-1c under the control of the adipocyte-specific aP2 promoter. These mice are lipodystrophic, hyperlipidemic, diabetic, and hypoleptinemic (41). Interestingly, hyperlipidemia and diabetes in these animals can be entirely corrected by administration of leptin, indicating a direct role for leptin in insulin sensitivy in these animals. Whether this scenario is applicable to HAART-

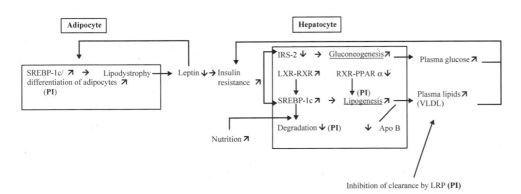

Figure 2 Model for lipodystrophy-insulin resistance-hyperlipidemia syndrome. On the right (hepatocyte), augmented activity of SREBP-1c results from protease inhibitor (PI)–mediated inhibition of degradation SREBP-1c, from hyperinsulinemia and from improved nutrition. PI displace the RXR-PPAR α equilibrium to RXR-liver X receptor (LXR), which stimulates SREBP. Accelerated lipogenesis and reduced clearance of TG-rich lipoproteins due to PI inhibition of LRP increase lipid levels. On the left (adipocyte), PI increase the differentiation of preadipocytes to adipocytes, which leads to lipodystrophy; resulting reduced leptin levels contribute to insulin resistance. Elevated insulin levels downregulate insulin receptor substrate (IRS-2) with an increase in gluconeogenesis and overexpression of SREBP-1c in the liver and in the adipocyte, thus generating two vicious circles. (Adapted from Ref. 17.)

treated humans and the role of PPARγ in this syndrome remains to be established (42,43).

In humans, both clinical patterns—increase in truncal fat and loss of peripheral fat—could be due respectively to increased adipocyte differentiation (40) and to decreased adipocyte differentiation (44).

In summary, HAART-related lipodystrophy could result from a multifactorial, cascadic process in which both NRTIs and PIs play a pathogenic role (Fig. 2).

Clinical Consequences of Lipodystrophy Syndrome

Many efforts have been undertaken to alleviate the clinical and psychological consequences of these physical abnormalities. A critical component of this syndrome is the changes in body habitus, which could modify the compliance of patients with dramatic consequences on HIV development and therapeutic failure.

Several case reports have described premature coronary artery disease (CAD) in patients with few or no risk factors receiving PI therapy (Fig. 3) (10,46). However, a causal link has not been shown, and there are no data estimating the prevalence of cardiovascular disease in patients receiving HAART. Some cases have developed in patients who received very brief PI therapy, which may indicate a prothrombotic rather than an atherosclerotic effect of therapy. The increase in risk has been estimated from available metabolic data (by use of the Framingham equations) (47). It

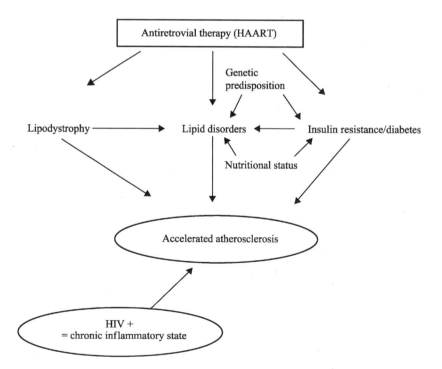

Figure 3 Interplay of metabolic causes in relation to atherosclerosis in patients receiving antiretroviral therapy.

Table 10 Absolute 5-Year Coronary Risk (%)

			No FRS[a]	FRS (+)
Men	Nonsmoker	30 years	<1	2
		50 years	4	9
	Smoker	30 years	1	4
		50 years	6	14
Women	Nonsmoker	30 years	<1	<1
		50 years	2	9
	Smoker	30 years	<1	1
		50 years	4	14

[a] FRS = fat redistribution syndrome.
Source: Ref. 43.

has been shown that the absolute 5-year coronary risk is particularly increased in males, those above 50 years of age, and smokers, according to the presence of the FRS (Table 10).

In another study, Rickerts et al. have shown, that after the introduction of HAART, the incidence of myocardial infarction among HIV patients increased in their cohort from 0.86 in 1983–1986 to 3.41 per 1000 patients-years in 1995–1998 (48) (Table 11).

A worldwide cohort study (the DAD project) will prospectively address this issue.

One further risk of severe hypertriglyceridemia with PI therapy is acute pancreatitis, but this association remains rare. Patients with diabetes mellitus or impaired glucose tolerance are also at increased risk of microvascular diabetic disease such a retinopathy, neuropathy, and nephropathy over the medium to long term.

Management

There is no proven therapy for any component of lipodystrophy syndrome. Factors that affect a decision to treat would include presence of symptoms, the patient's

Table 11 MI Incidence in the Frankfurt HIV Cohort (1983–1998)

4993 subjects	
MI[a] per 1000 patients-years	
1983–1986	0.86
1987–1990	1.14
1991–1994	0.59
1995–1998	3.41

[a] MI = myocardial infarction.
Source: Ref. 48.

status, the likelihood that a particular HAART regimen would extend over the long term, the severity of the disease, and the presence of one or more cardiovascular risk factors (Table 12).

Cessation of smoking as well as dietary measures and physical activity should be recommended for all patients and may be sufficient when lipid values are only modestly elevated.

A diet low in fat (<30% of total calories) and low saturated fat (<10%) is recommended for patients with Fredrickson types IIa and IIb abnormalities, with the addition of a low-carbohydrate diet for those with types IV to V and IIb disorders who have elevated triglycerides. Weight control and an exercise program are appropriate in all patients with lipid disorders and are essential in those who have elevated triglycerides. Short-term exercise contributes to improve body composition in HIV-lipodystrophy patients (49).

Lipid-lowering drugs are necessary if diet and exercise fail to control LDL or triglyceride values adequately. The choice should be based not only on traditional considerations but also on aspects that are specific to the HIV-infected population.

Therapy of the lipid disorders is based on levels of LDL-C and/or TG and the number of CAD risk factors. The target value for LDL-C is less than 160 mg/dL for those with one or no risk factors and below 130 mg/dL for those with two or more risk factors. If CAD is present, target LDL is below 100 mg/dL. Normal triglycerides should be less than 150 mg/dL (50).

Hydroxymethylglutaryl-coenzyme A (HMG-CoA) reductase inhibitors are recommended for treatment of Fredrickson types IIa and IIb abnormalities. Care is recommended when one of these drugs is being considered in patients receiving PIs, since most inhibit the CYP enzyme, particularly CYP 3A4. Pravastatin is not metabolized by CYP 3A4, unlike lovastatin, simvastatin, and atorvastatin.

All PIs are metabolized by CYP3A4 and are also inhibitors of CYP3A4, with ritonavir being the most potent inhibitor. Although drug-drug interactions have not been reported between HMG-CoA reductase inhibitors and PIs, the potential does exist for inhibition of metabolism of the former by the latter, with a resulting risk of toxic effects on muscles.

No toxic effects were observed in a study with atorvastatin and gemfibrozil (51). Of the 20 patients initially treated with diet or exercise, 12 were judged treatment failures and were started on lipid-lowering agents (4 on gemfibrozil only and 8 on atorvastatin). Nineteen patients were judged to have a suboptimal response to

Table 12 Prevention and Therapy of HIV-FRS

Diet and exercise	
Drugs:	Protease inhibitors (PI) switch
	Alternating sequences
	Fibrates or/and statins
	Metformin
	Peroxisome proliferator activated receptors (PPAR-γ) activators (thiazolidinediones)
	Others

PI, protease inhibitors; PPAR-γ, peroxisome proliferator activated receptors.

gemfibrozil alone and had atorvastatin added. Among patients receiving both gemfibrozil and atorvastatin, in the group with the highest lipids, the mean cholesterol concentration fell 30% and the triglycerides concentration 60% over 6 months ($p = 0.0004$ and $p = 0.01$). Although these concentrations are still high, they likely reflect a significant decrease in potential cardiac risk. The guidelines of the National Cholesterol Education Program (NCEP) advise caution in the use of gemfibrozil and statins together due to a concern about an increased risk of myopathy.

Fibric acids are the first-line drugs for HIV-infected patients with primary hypertriglyceridemia undergoing PI therapy. Fenofibrate, like gemfibrozil, inhibits triglyceride synthesis and increases lipoprotein lipase activity (52). Bezafibrate was administered once daily for 6 to 18 months in 49 patients with hyperlipidemia due to ritonavir or indinavir (19). This drug reduced TG and cholesterol levels by 37 an 25% respectively. Thirty-three patients (67.3%) reached normal triglyceridemia after 6 to 9 months and normal cholesterol was obtained in all subjects. Bezafibrate was safe in all the patients.

One theoretical treatment option is withdrawal or substitution of HAART. Usually PI withdrawal improves metabolic perturbations but not the FRS. Uncontrolled data suggest that protease-inhibitor substitution with nevirapine and stavudine withdrawal may improve fat accumulation and lipoatrophy, respectively. Several ongoing randomized studies are currently assessing this strategy (53,54).

Some potential agents can cause problems. Anabolic steroids are anabolic for muscle, not for fat, although increased muscle mass may partly disguise fat loss. Subcutaneous or intralesional growth hormone can reduce intra-abdominal adiposity and the size of buffalo humps, respectively, but can worsen lipoatrophy or precipitate diabetes when given parentally.

Two new medical options are now being investigated. Two insulin sensitizers usually used in type 2 diabetes (metformin and glitazone) have been tested (43,55).

Hadigan et al. have shown in a placebo-controlled trial that 500 mg of metformin twice a day reduces insulin resistance and related cardiovascular parameters in HIV-infected patients with lipodystrophy. Moreover, metformin decreases PAI-1 and tissue plasminogen activator (t-PA), markers of impaired fibrinolysis and cardiovascular risk. These parameters are increased in lipodystrophy and polymetabolic syndrome (56,57).

PPAR γ activator, 400 mg/day (troglitazone) was given over 3 months to 6 patients (43). A clear improvement in insulin sensitivity, with an increase in lean body mass and a decrease in visceral adipose tissue was observed in 4 patients. Total TG decreased and HDL increased. No adverse effect, such as hepatotoxicity, was noted.

A large prospective study is ongoing to test on a large HIV patients cohort the impact of this promising drug class. Surgery (excision or liposuction) has been done in some patients with severe fat accumulation, although the fat can reaccumulate within a matter of months. Implant surgery for fat wasting (an approach used for some forms of congenital lipodystrophy) has also been reported (45).

CONCLUSION

A better understanding of HAART-associated lipid disorders, lipodystrophy, and insulin resistance is crucial because of the impact on quality of life, the potential cardiovascular risks, and the social and psychological consequences in AIDS (58). Identification of an active HIV drug without metabolic side effects are highly desirable.

Not only more data on lipid lowering drugs in the context of HAART but also results from intervention studies on clinical events are urgently needed. The long-term management of HIV infection depends of the successful meeting of these challenges.

REFERENCES

1. Grunfeld C, et al. Hypertriglyceridemia in the acquired immmunodeficiency syndrome. Am J Med 1989; 86:27–31.
2. Kereveur A, Cambillau M, Kazatchkine M, Moatti N. Lipoprotein anomalies in HIV infections. Ann Med Interne 1996; 147:333–343.
3. Grunfeld C, Pang M, Doerrler W, Shigenaga JK, Jensen P, Feingold KR. Lipids, lipoproteins, triglyceride clearance and cytokines in human immunodeficiency virus infection and the acquired immunodeficiency syndrome. J Clin Endocrinol Metab 1992; 74:1045–1052.
4. Grunfeld C, et al. Circulating interferonalpha levels and hypertriglyceridemia in the acquired immunodeficiency syndrome. Am J Med 1991; 90:154–162.
5. Weinroth SE, Parenti DM, Simon GL. Wasting syndrome in AIDS: Pathophysiologic mechanisms and therapeutic approaches. Infect Agents Dis 1995; 4:76–94.
6. Constans J, Pellegrin JL, Peuchant E, et al. Plasma lipids in HIV infected patients: a prospective study in 95 patients. Eur J Clin Invest 1994; 24:416–420.
7. Grunfeld C, Doerrler W, Pang M, Jennsen P, Weisgraber KH, Feingold KR. Abnormalities of apolipoprotein E in the acquired immunodeficiency syndrome. J Clin Endocrinol Metab 1997; 82:3734–3740.
8. Zangerle R, Sarcletti M, Gallati H, Reibnegger G, Wachter H, Fuchs D. Decreased plasma concentrations of HDL-cholesterol in HIV-infected individuals are associated with immune activation. J AIDS 1994; 7:1149–1156.
9. Feingold KR, Krauss RM, Pang M, Doerrler W, Jensen P, Grunfeld C. The hypertriglyceridemia of acquired immunodeficiency syndrome is associated with an increased prevalence of low density lipoprotein subclass pattern B. J Clin Endocrinol Metab 1993; 76:1423–1427.
10. MacLemore J, Beeley P, Thorton K, Morrisroe K, Blackwell W, Dasgupta A. Rapid automated determination of lipid hydroperoxide concentrations and total antioxydant status of serum samples from patients infected with HIV. Am J Clin Pathol 1998; 109:268–273.
11. Miller KD, Jones E, Yanovski JA, Shan Kar R, Feverstein I, Falloon J. Visceral abdominal fat accumulation associated with use of indinavir. Lancet 1998; 351:871–875.
12. Churchill DR, Pym AS, Babiker AG, Back DJ, Weber JN. Hyperlipidaemia following treatment with protease inhibitors in patients with HIV-1 infection. Br J Clin Pharmacol 1998; 46:518–519.
13. Lo JC, Mulligan K, Tail VW, Algren H, Schambelan M. "Buffalo hump" in men with HIV-1 infection. Lancet 1998; 351:867–870.
14. Stocker DN, Meier PJ, Stoller R, Fattinger KE. "Buffalo hump" in HIV-1 infection. Lancet 1998; 352:320–321.
15. Carr A, Samaras K, Chisholm DJ, Cooper DA. Pathogenesis of HIV-1 protease inhibitor–associated peripheral lipodystrophy, hyperlipidaemia, and insulin resistance. Lancet 1998; 351:1881–1883.

16. Ducobu J, Payen MC. Lipids and AIDS. Rev Med Brux 2000; 1:11–17.
17. Mooser V, Carr A. Antiretroviral associated hyperlipidemia in HIV disease. Curr Opin Lipidol 2001; 12:313–319.
18. Basdevant A. Metabolic anomalies after antiretroviral treatment. J Ann Diabeto Hotel Dieu 2000; 167–177.
19. Martinez E, Mocroft A, Garcia-Viejo MA, Perez-Cuevas JB, Blanco JL. Risk of lipodystrophy in HIV-1 infected patients treated with protease inhibitors: a prospective cohort study. Lancet 2001; 357:592–595.
20. Manfredi R, Chiodo F. Disorders of lipid metabolism in patients with HIV disease treat with antiretroviral agents: frequency, relationship with administered drugs, and role of hypolipidaemic therapy with bezafibrate. J Infect 2001; 42(3):181.
21. Thiebaut R, Dequae-Merchadou L, Ekouevi DK, Mercie P, Malvy D, No D, Dabis F. The Groupe d'Epidemiologie Clinique du SIDA en Aquitaine (GECSA). HIV Med 2001; 2(2):84–88.
22. Walli R, Goebel FD, Demant T. Impaired glucose tolerance and protease inhibitors. Ann Intern Med 1998; 129:837–838.
23. Walli R, Herfort O, Michl GM, et al. Treatment with protease inhibitors associated with peripheral insulin resistance and impaired oral glucose tolerance in HIV-1 infected patients. AIDS 1998; 11:F167–F173.
24. Murata H, Hruz PW, Mueckler M. The mechanism of insulin resistance caused by HIV protease inhibitor therapy. J Biol Chem 2000; 7; 275(27):20251–20254.
25. Estrada V, Serrano-Rios M, Larrad MT, Villar NG, Lopez AG, Tellez M, Fernandez C. Leptin and adipose tissue maldistribution in HIV-infected male patients with predominant fat loss treated with antiretroviral therapy. J AIDS 2002; 29(1):32–40.
26. Gagnon AM, Angel J, Sorisky A. Protease inhibitors and adipocyte differentiation in cell culture. Lancet 1998; 352:1032.
27. Brinkman K, Smeitink JA, Romeijn JA, Reiss A. Mitochondrial toxicity induced by nucleosideanalogue reversetranscriptase inhibition is a key factor in the pathogenesis of antiretroviral therapy related lipodystrophy. Lancet 1999; 354:1112–1118.
28. Cossarizza A, Mussini C, Vigano A. Mitochondria in the pathogenesis of lipodystrophy induced by anti-HIV antiretroviral drugs: actors or bystanders? Bioessays 2001; 23 (11):1070–1080.
29. Shikuma CM, HU N, Milne C, Yost F, Waslien C, Shimizu S, Shiramizu B. Mitochondrial DNA decrease in subcutaneous adipose tissue of HIV-infected individuals with peripheral lipoatrophy. AIDS 2001; 15:1801–1809.
30. Côté HC, Brumme ZL, Kevin JP, Alexander C, Wynhoven B, et al. Changes in mito-chondrial DNA as a marker of nucleoside toxicity in HIVinfected patients. N Engl J Med 2002; 811–820.
31. Kakuda TN. Pharmacology of nucleoside and nucleotide reverse transcriptase inhibitor-induced mitochondrial toxicity. Clin Ther 2000; 22(6):685–708.
32. Zaera MG, Miro O, Pedrol E, Soler A, Picon M, Cardellach F, Casademont J, Nunes V. Mitochondrial involvement in antiretroviral therapyrelated lipodystrophy. AIDS 2001; 15:1643–1651.
33. Liang JS, Distler O, Cooper DA, Jamil H, Deckelbaum RJ, Ginsberg HM, Sturley SL. HIV protease inhibitors protect apolipoprotein B from degradation by the proteasome: a potential mechanism for protease inhibitorinduced hyperlipidemia. Nat Med 2001; 7(12):1327–1331.
34. Distler O, Cooper DA, Delckelbaum RJ, Sturley SL. Hyperlipidemia and inhibitors of HIV protease. Curr Opin Clin Nutr Metab Care 2001; 4(2):99–103.
35. Lenhard JM, Croom DK, Weiel JE, Winegar DA. HIV protease inhibitors stimulate hepatic triglyceride synthesis. Arterioscler Thromb Vasc Biol 2000; 20:2625–2629.
36. Kuhel DG, Woollett LA, Fichtenbaum CJ, Hui DY. HIV protease inhibitorinduced

hyperlipidemia and lipodystrophy is mediated through regulation of sterol responsive element binding protein (SREBP) responsive genes [abstr]. Circulation 2000; 102(suppl II):11–36.

37. André P, Groettrup M, Klenerman P, et al. An inhibitor of HIV-1 protease modulates proteasome activity, antigen presentation, and T cell responses. Proc Natl Acad Sci USA 1998; 95:13120–13124.

38. Shimomura I, Bashmakof Y, Ikemoto S, et al. Insulin selectively increases SREBP-1c mRNA in the livers of rats with streptozotocin-induced diabetes. Proc Natl Acad Sci USA 1999; 96:13656–13661.

39. Repa JJ, Liang G, Ou J, et al. Regulation of mouse sterol regulatory element-binding protein-1c gene (SREBP-1c) by oxysterol receptors, LXRalpha and LXRbeta. Genes Dev 2000; 14:2819–2830.

40. Nguyen AT, Gagnon AM, Angel JB, Sorisky A. Ritonavir increases the level of active ADD-1/SREBP-1 protein during adipogenesis. ADIS 2000; 14:2467–2473.

41. Shimomura I, Hammer RE, Ikemoto S, et al. Leptin reverses insulin resistance and diabetes mellitus in mice with congenital lipodystrophy. Nature 1999; 401:73–76.

42. Shimomura L, Matsuda M, Hammer RE, et al. Decreased IRS2 and increased SREBP-1c lead to mixed insulin resistance and sensitiviy in livers of lipodystrophic and ob/ob mice. Mol Cell 2000; 6:77–86.

43. Walli R, Michl GM, Muhlbayer D, et al. Effects of troglitazone on insulin sensitivity in HIV-infected patients with protease inhibitor-associated diabetes mellitus. Res Exp Med 2000; 199:253–262.

44. Wentworth JM, Burris TP, Chatterjee VKK. HIV protease inhibitors block human preadipocyte differentiation, but not via the PPARγ/RXR heterodimers. J Endocrinol 2000; 164:R7–510.

45. Carr A, Cooper DA. Adverse effects of antiretroviral therapy. Lancet 2000; 356:1423–1430.

46. Flynn TE, Bricker LA. Myocardial infarction in HIV-infected men. Ann Intern Med 1999; 131:258–262.

47. Egger M, et al. HAART and coronary disease: the need for perspective. AIDS 2001; 15(suppl 5):5193–5201.

48. Rickerts V, Brodt H, Staszewski S, Stille W. Incidence of myocardial infarctions in HIV-infected patients between 1983 and 1993: the Frankfurt HIV-cohort study. Eur J Med Res 2000; 5(8):329–333.

49. Jones SP, Doran DA, Leatt PB, Maher B, Pirmohamed M. Short-term exercise training improves body composition and hyperlipidaemia in HIV-positive individuals with lipodystrophy. AIDS 2001; 15(15):2049–2051.

50. The Expert Panel on Detection, Evaluation and Treatment of High Blood-Cholesterol in Adults. Executive summary of the third report of the National Cholesterol Education Program (Adult Treatment Panel III). JAMA 2001; 285:2486–2497.

51. Henry K, Melroe H, Huebesch J, Hermundson J, Simpson J. Atorvastatin and gemfibrozil for protease inhibitor-related lipid abnormalities. Lancet 1998; 352:1031–1032.

52. James C, Maria F, Victor E, Joli D, Kelly B, Laura S, Nanette C. Use of fenofibrate in the management of protease inhibitor-associated lipid abnormalities. Pharmacotherapy 2000; 20(6):727–734.

53. Moyle G. Clinical manifestations and management of antiretroviral nucleoside analog-related mitochondrial toxicity. Clin Ther 2000; 22(8):911–936.

54. Carr A, Hudson J, Chuah J, Mallal S, Law M, Hoy J, Doong N, French Smith D, Cooper DA, and the PIILR Study Group. HIV protease inhibitor substitution in patients with lipodystrophy: a randomized, controlled, open-label, multicentre study. AIDS 2001; 15(14):1811–1822.

55. Saint-Marc T, Touraine JL. Effects of metformin on insulin resistance and central

adiposity patients receiving effective protease inhibitor therapy. AIDS 1999; 13(18):1000–1002.

56. Hadigan C, Corcoran C, Basgoz N, Davis B, Sax P, Grinspoon S. Metformin in the treatment of HIV lipodystrophy syndrome: a randomized controlled trial. JAMA 2000; 284(4):472–477.

57. Hadigan C, Meigs JB, Rabe J, D'Agostino RB, Wilson PW, Lipinska I, Tofler GH, Grinspoon SS. Framingham Heart Study: increased PAI-1 and tPA antigen levels are reduced with metformin therapy in HIV-infected patients with fat redistribution and insulin resistance. J Clin Endocrinol Metab 2001; 86(2):939–943.

58. Hoffmann C, Jaeger H. Cardiology and AIDS-HAART and the consequences. Ann N Y Acad Sci 2001; 946:130–144.

26

Pathogenesis of HIV-Associated Cardiovascular Complications in the HAART Era

Giuseppe Barbaro
University La Sapienza, Rome, Italy

INTRODUCTION

Studies published before the introduction of highly active antiretroviral therapy (HAART) have tracked the incidence and course of HIV infection in relation to both pediatric and adult cardiac illnesses (1). These studies show that subclinical echocardiographic abnormalities independently predict adverse outcomes and identify high-risk groups to target for early intervention and therapy.

The introduction of HAART has significantly modified the course of HIV disease, with longer survival and improved quality of life. Though inconclusive at this time, early data raised concerns about an increase in both peripheral and coronary arterial disease with HAART. A variety of potential etiologies have been postulated for HIV-related heart disease, including myocardial infection with HIV itself, opportunistic infections, viral infections, autoimmune response to viral infection, drug related cardiotoxicity, nutritional deficiencies, and prolonged immunosuppression (Table 1).

DILATED CARDIOMYOPATHY

The estimated annual incidence of dilated cardiomyopathy with HIV infection before introduction of HAART was 15.9 per 1000 (1). Symptoms of heart failure may be masked in HIV-infected patients by concomitant illnesses such as diarrhea or malnutrition, or it may be disguised by bronchopulmonary infections. The gross and microscopic findings with HIV-associated dilated cardiomyopathy are similar to those for idiopathic dilated cardiomyopathy in immunocompetent persons, with four-chamber dilation and patchy myocardial fibrosis. Additional echocardiographic findings include diffuse left ventricular hypokinesis and decreased fractional shortening.

Compared to patients with idiopathic dilated cardiomyopathy, those with HIV infection and dilated cardiomyopathy have markedly reduced survival (hazard ratio for death from congestive heart failuire: 5.86) (2). The median survival to AIDS-related death is 101 days in patients with left ventricular dysfunction and 472 days in

Table 1   Principal HIV-Associated Cardiovascular Abnormalities

Type	Possible etiologies and associations	Incidence

Dilated cardiomyopathy	Infectious
	  HIV, *Toxoplasma gondii*,
	  coxsackievirus group B,
	  Epstein-Barr virus,
	  Cytomegalovirus, *Adenovirus*
	  Autoimmune response to
	  infection
	Drug-related
	  Cocaine, possibly nucleoside
	  analogues
	  IL-2, doxorubicin, interferon
	Metabolic/Endocrine
	  Nutritional deficiency/wasting
	  selenium, B_{12}, carnitine
	  Thyroid hormone, growth
	  hormone
	  Adrenal insufficiency,
	  hyperinsulinemia
	Cytokines
	  TNF-α, nitric oxide, TGF-β,
	  endothelin-1
	  Hypothermia
	  Hyperthermia
	  Autonomic insufficiency
	  Encephalopathy
	  Acquired immunodeficiency
	  HIV viral load, length of
	  immunosuppression
		15.9 patients/1000 asymptomatic HIV-infected persons before the introduction of HAART (1)

Coronary heart disease	Protease inhibitors–induced metabolic and coagulative disorders, arteritis	Contrasting data reported after the introduction of protease inhibitors containing HAART
Systemic arterial hypertension	HIV-induced endothelial dysfunction; vasculitis in small, medium, and large vessels in the form of leukocytoclastic vasculitis; atherosclerosis secondary to HAART; aneurysms of the large vessels such as the carotid, femoral, and abdominal aorta with impairment of flow to the renal arteries; PI-induced insulin resistance with increased sympathetic activity and sodium retention	20–25% of HIV-infected persons before the introduction of HAART (60); up to 74% in HIV-infected persons with HAART-related metabolic syndrome (61)

Table 1 Continued

Type	Possible etiologies and associations	Incidence
Pericardial effusion	Bacteria: Staphylococcus, Streptococcus, Proteus, Nocardia, Pseudomonas, Klebsiella, Enterococcus, Listeria *Mycobacteria (Mycobacterium tuberculosis, Mycobacterium avium intracellulare, Mycobacterium kansasii)* Viral pathogens HIV, herpes simplex virus, herpes simplex virus type 2, cytomegalovirus Other pathogens *Cryptococcus, Toxoplasma, Histoplasma* Malignancy Kaposi's sarcoma Malignant lymphoma Capillary leak/wasting/ malnutrition Hyopthyroidism Prolonged acquired immunodeficiency	11%/year in asymptomatic AIDS patients before the introduction of HAART (74)
HIV-associated pulmonary hypertension	Recurrent bronchopulmonary infections; pulmonary arteritis; microvascular pulmonary emboli due to thrombus or drug injection; plexogenic pulmonary arteriopathy; mediator release from endothelium	1/200 of HIV-infected persons before the introduction of HAART (75)
AIDS-related tumors	Kaposi's sarcoma	12–28% of AIDS patients before the introduction of HAART (75,76)
	Non-Hodgkin's lymphomas	Mostly limited to case reports before the introduction of HAART

patients with a normal heart at a similar stage of HIV infection (1). There is no evidence from prospective studies to suggest that HAART has a beneficial effect on HIV-associated cardiomyopathy. However, some retrospective studies suggest that by preventing opportunistic infections and improving the immunological parameters, HAART might reduce the incidence of HIV-associated heart disease and improve its course (3,4).

Myocarditis and Viral Myocardial Infection as Causes of Cardiomyopathy

Myocarditis and myocardial infection with HIV are the best-studied causes of dilated cardiomyopathy in HIV disease (5). HIV-1 virions appear to infect myocardial cells in a patchy distribution with no direct association between the presence of the virus and myocyte dysfunction (5). The myocardial fiber necrosis is usually minimal, with accompanying mild to moderate lymphocytic infiltrates. It is unclear how HIV-1 enters myocytes, which do not have CD4 receptors, although dendritic reservoir cells may play a role by activating multifunctional cytokines that contribute to progressive and late tissue damage, such as tumor necrosis factor alpha (TNF-α), interleukin-1 (IL-1), interleukin-6 (IL-6), and interleukin-10 (IL-10) (2). Coinfection with other viruses (usually coxsackievirus B3 and cytomegalovirus) may also play an important pathogenetic role) (2,5).

AUTOIMMUNITY AS A CONTRIBUTOR TO CARDIOMYOPATHY

Cardiac-specific autoantibodies (anti–alpha myosin autoantibodies) are more common in HIV-infected patients with dilated cardiomyopathy than in those with healthy hearts. Currie et al. have reported that HIV-infected patients were more likely to have specific cardiac autoantibodies than were HIV-negative controls (6). Those with echocardiographic evidence of left ventricular dysfunction were particularly likely to have cardiac autoantibodies, supporting the theory that cardiac autoimmunity plays a role in the pathogenesis of HIV-related heart disease and suggesting that cardiac autoantibodies could be used as markers of left ventricular dysfunction in HIV-positive patients with previously normal echocardiographic findings (6).

In addition, monthly intravenous immunoglobulin in HIV-infected pediatric patients minimizes left ventricular dysfunction, increases left ventricular wall thickness, and reduces peak left ventricular wall stress, suggesting that both impaired myocardial growth and left ventricular dysfunction may be immunologically mediated (7). These effects may be the result of immunoglobulins inhibiting cardiac autoantibodies by competing for Fc receptors, or they could be the result of immunoglobulins dampening the secretion or effects of cytokines and cellular growth factors (7). These findings suggest that immunomodulatory therapy might be helpful in adults and children with declining left ventricular function, although further study of this possible therapy is needed.

Myocardial Cytokine Expression as a Factor in Cardiomyopathy

Cytokines play a role in the development of HIV-related cardiomyopathy (2). Myocarditis and dilated cardiomyopathy are associated with markedly elevated cytokine production, but the elevations may be highly localized within the myocardium, making peripheral cytokine levels uninformative (2).

When myocardial biopsies from patients with HIV-associated cardiomyopathy are compared to samples from patients with idiopathic dilated cardiomyopathy, the former stain more intensely for both TNF-α and inducible nitric oxide synthase (iNOS). Staining is particularly intense in samples from patients with a myocardial viral infection, independent of antiretroviral treatment (2). Staining is also more intense in samples from patients with HIV-associated cardiomyopathy coinfected with coxsackievirus B3, cytomegalovirus, or other viruses (2). Moreover, staining for iNOS is more intense in samples from patients coinfected with HIV-1 and coxsackievirus B3 or cytomegalovirus than in samples from patients with idiopathic dilated cardiomyopathy and myocardial infection with coxackievirus B3 or who had adenovirus infection alone (2).

In patients with HIV-associated dilated cardiomyopathy and more intense iNOS staining the survival rate was significantly lower: those whose samples stained more than 1 optical density unit had a hazard ratio of mortality of 2.57 (95% confidence interval: 1.11 to 5.43). Survival in HIV-infected patients with less intense staining was not significantly different from survival in patients with idiopathic dilated cardiomyopathy (2).

The inflammatory response may be enhanced by HIV-1 myocardial infection, by the interaction between HIV-1 and cardiotropic viruses, and by immunodeficiency. These factors may increase both the expression and the cytotoxic activity of specific cytokines such as TNF-α and iNOS and blunt the expected increase of antiinflammatory cytokines such as IL-10 (8).

Relationship Between HIV-Associated Cardiomyopathy and Encephalopathy

HIV-infected patients with encephalopathy are more likely to die of congestive heart failure than are those without encephalopathy (hazard ratio: 3.4) (9–11). Cardiomyopathy and encephalopathy may both be traceable to the effects of HIV reservoir cells in the myocardium and the cerebral cortex. These cells may hold HIV-1 on their surfaces for extended time periods even after antiretroviral treatment, and they may chronically release cytotoxic cytokines (TNF-α, IL-6, and endothelin-1), which contribute to progressive and late tissue damage in both systems (11). Because the reservoir cells are not affected by treatment, the effect is independent of whether the patient receives HAART.

Nutritional Deficiencies as a Factor in Left Ventricular Dysfunction

Nutritional deficiencies are common in HIV infection and may contribute to ventricular dysfunction independently of HAART. Malabsorption and diarrhea can both lead to trace element deficiencies, which have been directly or indirectly associated with cardiomyopathy (12–14). Selenium replacement may reverse cardiomyopathy and restore left ventricular function in selenium-deficient patients (12–14). HIV infection may also be associated with altered levels of vitamin B_{12}, carnitine, growth hormone, and thyroid hormone, all of which have been associated with left ventricular dysfunction (14).

Left Ventricular Dysfunction Caused by Drug Cardiotoxicity

Studies of transgenic mice suggest that zidovudine is associated with diffuse destruction of cardiac mitochondrial ultrastructure and inhibition of mitochondrial DNA replication (15,16). This mitochondrial dysfunction may result in lactic acidosis, which could also contribute to myocardial cell dysfunction. However, in a study of infants born to HIV-positive mothers followed from birth to age 5, perinatal exposure to zidovudine was not found to be associated with acute or chronic abnormalities in left ventricular structure or function (17). Other nucleoside reverse transcriptase inhibitors, such as didanosine and zalcitabine, do not seem to either promote or prevent dilated cardiomyopathy (1).

Treating HIV-Associated Cardiomyopathy

Standard treatment regimens for heart failure are generally recommended for HIV-infected patients with dilated cardiomyopathy and congestive heart failure even though these regimens have not been tested in this specific population. Patients with systolic dysfunction and symptoms of fluid retention should receive a loop diuretic and an aldosterone antagonist as well as an angiotension-converting enzyme (ACE) inhibitor. ACE inhibitors are recommended based on general heart failure studies, but they may be poorly tolerated due to low systemic vascular resistance from diarrheal disease, infection, or dehydration. Digoxin may be added to therapy for patients with persistent symptoms or rapid atrial fibrillation (18). In euvolumic patients, a beta blocker may be started for its beneficial effects on circulating levels of inflammatory and anti-inflammatory cytokines (19).

HIV INFECTION, OPPORTUNISTIC INFECTIONS, AND VASCULAR DISEASE

A wide range of inflammatory vascular disease—including polyarteritis nodosa, Henoch-Schönlein purpura, and drug-induced hypersensitivity vasculitis—may develop in HIV-infected individuals. A Kawasaki-like syndrome (20) and Takayasu's arteritis (21) have also been described. The course of vascular disease may be accelerated in HIV-infected patients because of atherogenesis stimulated by HIV-infected monocyte-macrophages, possibly via altered leukocyte adhesion or arteritis (22).

Some patients with AIDS have a clinical presentation resembling systemic lupus erythematosus (SLE)—including vasculitis, arthralgias, myalgias, and auto-immune phenomena with a low titer positive antinuclear antibody; coagulopathy with lupus anticoagulant; hemolytic anemia; and thrombocytopenic purpura. Hyper-gammaglobulinemia from polyclonal B-cell activation may be present but often diminishes in the late stages of AIDS. Specific autoantibodies to double-stranded DNA, Sm antigen, RNP antigen, SSA, SSB, and other histones may be found in a majority of HIV-infected persons, but their significance is unclear (22).

Endothelial Dysfunction

Endothelial dysfunction and injury have been described in HIV infection (23). Circulating markers of endothelial activation, such as soluble adhesion molecules and procoagulant proteins, are elaborated in HIV infection. HIV may enter endothelium via CD4 or galactosyl-ceramide receptors (23). Other possible mechanisms of entry include chemokine receptors (24). Endothelium isolated from the brain of HIV-infected subjects strongly expresses both CCR3 and CXCR4 HIV-1 coreceptors, whereas coronary endothelium strongly expresses CXCR4 and CCCR2A coreceptors (24). CCR5 is expressed at a lower level in both types of endothelium. The fact that CCR3 is more common in brain endothelium than in coronary endothelium could be significant in light of the different susceptibilities of heart and brain to HIV-1 invasion (24). These chemokine receptors could play a role in endothelial migration and repair (24).

Endothelial activation in HIV infection may also be caused by cytokines secreted in response to mononuclear or adventitial cell activation by the virus or may be a direct effect of the secreted HIV-associated proteins gp 120 (envelope glycoprotein) and Tat (transactivator of viral replication) on endothelium (23). Opportunistic agents, such as cytomegalovirus, frequently coinfect HIV-infected patients and may contribute to the development of endothelial damage. Moreover, a retrospective analysis of postmortem reports revealed a strong correlation between Kaposi's sarcoma (KS), the most frequent AIDS-related neoplasm, and the presence of atheroma (25). On the basis of this observation and of previous experimental data, the authors hypothesize that human herpesvirus-8 (HHV-8, a virus that is found in all forms of KS) may trigger or accelerate the development of atheroma in the presence of hyperlipidemia (25). In spite of all these observations, the clinical effects of HIV-1 and opportunistic agents on endothelial function have not been elucidated.

HIV Infection and Coronary Arteries

The association between viral infection (cytomegalovirus or HIV-1 itself) and coronary artery lesions is not clear. HIV-1 sequences have recently been detected by in situ hybridization in the coronary vessels of an HIV-infected patient who died from acute myocardial infarction (26). Potential mechanisms through which HIV-1 may damage coronary arteries include activation of cytokines and cell-adhesion molecules and alteration of major-histocompatibility-complex (MHC) class I molecules on the surface of smooth muscle cells (26).

Opportunistic Infections

Toxoplasma gondii can produce a gross pattern of patchy, irregular, white infiltrates in myocardium similar to those of non-Hodgkin's lymphoma (1). Microscopically, the myocardium shows scattered mixed inflammatory cell infiltrates with polymorphonuclear leukocytes, macrophages, and lymphocytes. True *T. gondii* cysts or pseudocysts containing bradyzoites are often hard to find, even if inflammation is extensive. Immunohistochemical staining may reveal free tachyzoites, otherwise difficult to distinguish, within the areas of inflammation. *T. gondii* myocarditis can produce focal myocardial fiber necrosis and heart failure can ensue (1).

Other opportunistic infections of the heart are infrequent. They are often incidental findings at autopsy, and cardiac involvement is probably the result of widespread dissemination, as exemplified by *Candida* and by the dimorphic fungi *Cryptoccocus neoformans*, *Coccidioides immitis*, and *Histoplasma capsulatum*. Patients living in endemic areas for *Trypanosoma cruzi* may rarely develop a pronounced myocarditis (1).

ANTIRETROVIRAL THERAPY AND METABOLIC DISORDERS

The introduction in recent years of HAART has significantly modified the course of HIV disease, prolonging survival and improving the quality of life. However, early data have raised concern that HAART regimens, especially those including protease inhibitors (PIs), are associated with an increased incidence of metabolic and somatic changes that in the general population are associated with an increased risk for both peripheral and coronary artery disease, producing an intriguing clinical scenario. Many studies have shown that a high proportion of patients treated with PIs have a significant increase of circulating triglycerides, total and low-density-lipoprotein (LDL) cholesterol, insulin, and fasting glucose (27–30). Of note is that also an increase of lipoprotein (a) was reported (31). In non-HIV patients the increase of lipoprotein (a) has been associated with premature atherosclerosis independent of the levels of cholesterol (32).

Pathogenesis of PI-Related Metabolic Disorders

PIs are designed to target the catalytic region of HIV-1 protease. This region is homologous with regions of two human proteins that regulate lipid metabolism: cytoplasmic retinoic acid–binding protein 1 (CRABP-1) and low-density lipoprotein receptor–related protein (LRP) (33,34). It has been hypothesized, although without strong experimental support, that this homology may allow PIs to interfere with these proteins, which may be the cause of the metabolic and somatic alterations that develop in PI-treated patients (i.e., dyslipidemia, insulin resistance, increased C-peptide levels, and lipodystrophy) (33,34). The hypothesis is that PIs inhibit CRABP-1-modified and cytochrome P450-3A-mediated synthesis of cis-9-retinoic acid and peroxisome proliferator–activated receptor type gamma (PPAR-α) hetero-dimer. This inhibition increases the rate of apoptosis of adipocytes and reduces the rate at which preadipocytes differentiate into adipocytes, with the final effect of reducing triglyceride storage and increasing lipid release. PI-binding to LRP would impair hepatic chylomicron uptake and endothelial triglyceride clearance, resulting in hyperlipidemia and insulin resistance (33,34).

Recent data indicate that dyslipidemia may, at least in part, be caused either by PI-mediated inhibition of proteasome activity and accumulation of the active portion of sterol regulatory element–binding protein 1c in liver cells and adipocytes (35) or to apo C-III polymorphisms in HIV-infected patients (36). Fauvel et al. described a two- to threefold increase in apo-E and apo C-III, essentially recovered as associated to apo B–containing lipoparticles (37). In this study multivariate analysis revealed that, among the investigated parameters, apo C-III was the only one found strongly associated with the occurrence of lipodystrophy (odds ratio, 5.5) (37). Some nucleoside analogues, such as stavudine, may enhance the effects of PIs when given in combination. Experimental studies have shown that stavudine depletes white adipose tissue and mitochondrial DNA in obese but not lean mice (38).

There is also evidence that PIs directly inhibit the uptake of glucose in insulin-sensitive tissues, such as fat and skeletal muscle, by selectively inhibiting the glucose transporter Glut4 (39). The relationship between the degree of insulin resistance and levels of soluble type 2 TNF-α receptor suggests that an inflammatory stimulus may contribute to the development of HIV-associated lipodystrophy (40). Endothelial dysfunction has recently been described in PI recipients, further supporting the increased risk of cardiovascular disease in these patients (41).

Mitochondrial Damage and Metabolic Disorders

Similarities between HAART-associated fat redistribution and metabolic abnormalities with both inherited lipodystrophies and benign symmetrical lipomatosis could suggest the pathophysiological involvement of nuclear factors like lamin A/C and nucleoside-induced mitochondrial dysfunction (42), although no mutations or polymorphisms in the gene encoding lamin A/C associated with aberant adipocyte tissue distribution or metabolic abnormalities have been detected in HIV-infected patients with lipodystrophy. However, this could explain many of the side effects seen in people taking nucleosides, including peripheral neuropathy, pancreatitis, leukopenia, and possibly lipodystrophy (29,43). It has been suggested that lipodystrophy might also be related to an imbalance in the immune system that remains after triple-drug therapy is started; even though triple-drug therapy prevents HIV from attacking immune system cells, it may not halt the negative effects of HIV on other cells in the body (29,43). However, the temporal and causal relationship between the three major components of the HAART-related metabolic syndrome—i.e., dyslipidemia, visceral adiposity and insulin -resistance—remains to be elucidated (30).

ANTIRETROVIRAL THERAPY AND CARDIOVASCULAR RISK

Risk Stratification and Pharmacological Therapy

For HIV-infected patients on HAART, it may be important to evaluate the traditional vascular risk factors according to the Framingham score and to try to intervene on those that can be modified (44). These factors may be in addition to nonreversible risk factors, such as male gender, age greater than 40 years, and family history of premature coronary heart disease. Patients may also be smokers and may have a sedentary lifestyle, both of which predispose to coronary heart disease and stroke. Existing guidelines for the management of dyslipidemias in the general population, such as those of the National Cholesterol Education Program, currently represent the basis for therapeutic recommendations also in HIV-infected individuals (44). Dietary modification and exercise are general health measures likely to be beneficial in HIV infected patients with a HAART-related metabolic syndrome (44).

Fibric acid derivatives and statins can lower HIV-associated cholesterol and triglyceride levels, although further data are needed on interactions between statins and PIs. Since most statins are metabolized through the CYP3A4 pathway, the inhibition of CYP3A4 by PIs could potentially increase by severalfold the concentrations of statins, thus increasing the risk of skeletal muscle toxicity or hepatic toxicity. The statin that is least influenced by the CYP3A4 metabolic pathway is pravastatin. Moyle et al. (45) recently reported that dietary advice plus pravastatin significantly reduced total cholesterol in HIV-infected patients taking PIs without significant adverse effects through week 24. Fibrates are unlikely to have significant interactions with PIs, since their principal metabolic pathway is CYP4A. In patients with dyslipidemia who do not respond to diet and exercise and eventually to drug treatment with statins or with fibrates, a combined therapy can be tried. However, the concomitant use of statins and fibrates increases the risk of skeletal muscle toxicity and should be carefully monitored. Hypoglycemic agents may have some role in managing glucose abnormalities, but troglitazone cannot be recommended for fat abnormalities alone, and metformin may cause lactic acidosis (46).

Switching from PIs

An approach to the treatment of dyslipidemia in patients treated with PIs is to switch to PI-free combination regimens. Although large randomized trials are lacking, some favorable effects have been shown (47–49). Of interest are data indicating that patients never treated with HAART, who started a PI-sparing regimen including nevirapine showed a significant increase of high-density-lipoprotein (HDL) cholesterol (50). If further confirmed, these findings both may influence the initial choice of therapy for HIV-1 infection and might lead to novel approaches targeted at raising HDL cholesterol for coronary heart disease prevention in patients on HAART.

HAART and Coronary Heart Disease

The patients with preexisting additional risk factors (e.g., hypertension, diabetes, smoking, and increased plasma-homocysteine levels) may have a higher risk of developing coronary heart disease because of accelerated atherosclerosis (51). Contrasting opinions exists about the incidence of acute coronary syndromes (unstable angina, myocardial infarction) among HIV-infected patients receiving PIs, including HAART. In fact, studies on the risk of coronary heart disease among HIV-infected individuals receiving PI therapy have not shown a consistent association.

In the retrospective analysis of the Frankfurt HIV-Cohort Study, Rickerts et al. (52) reported a fourfold increase in the annual incidence of myocardial infarction among HIV-infected patients after the introduction of HAART regimens, including PIs, compared to the pre-HAART period. In this study, previous HAART therapy, including PIs, was significantly associated with the incidence of myocardial infarction both in univariate analysis and in a multiple regression model.

A large multinational joint venture with the partecipation of 11 national HIV cohorts has been in progress since the beginning of 2000 (53). Approximately 22,000 subjects are followed at 180 sites across Europe, Australia, and the United States. The data presently available indicate that HAART-treated subjects with preserved immunity, better viral suppression, lipodystrophy, and greater age are at risk for cardiovascular disease based on lipid profile (53). In this study lipodystrophy was found among both PI users and nonnucleoside reverse transcriptase inhibitors (NNRTIs), although it was was most severe among users of four drugs, including both PIs and NNRTIs (53).

The analysis of the HIV Outpatient Study (HOPS) investigators of 5676 oupatients documented a significant increase in the incidence of myocardial infarction after the introduction of PIs (p value for linear trend = 0.01) with hazard ratio of 5.77 (95% confidence interval: 1.3 to 25.6; $p = 0.009$) (54). In this study the use of

PIs was an independent risk factor in the multivariate analysis (hazard ratio:4.92; 95% confidence interval:1.3 to 32.3; $p = 0.04$) (54).

Other studies that evaluated the relationship between HAART and coronary heart disease found no increase in the risk of coronary heart disease associated with HAART. The largest of these, the U.S. Veterans Administration Study, was reported as a late breaker at the 2002 Conference on Retroviruses and Opportunistic Infections (55). This study, of 36,000 HIV-positive individuals insured by the Veterans Administration, found a decrease in cardiovascular morbidity and mortality among HIV-positive individuals after the introduction of HAART as compared to the period before HAART was available, in spite of the fact that 30 to 40% of HIV-infected individuals were using PIs (55).

A meta-analysis of phase III studies of PIs on 8700 HIV-positive subjects who were randomized to HAART (with or without PIs) was conducted by the first four companies to develop PIs (56). No increase in the risk of myocardial infarction among PI users was reported after an average of 1 year on the drug (56). Similarly, an analysis of phase III of the protease inhibitor indinavir found no increase in risk of coronary heart disease among patients randomized to indinavir-containing therapy as compared to patients randomized to two nucleoside analogues (57).

HAART and Peripheral Vascular Disease

Also, the issue of surrogate markers of subclinical atherosclerosis has been addressed. A study was performed on a cohort of 168 HIV-infected patients to measure the intima-media thickness and assess indirectly the cardiovascular risk. In this population, a high prevalence of atherosclerotic plaques within the femoral or carotid arteries was observed, but their presence was not associated with the use of PIs (58). Different results were reported in another study, in which a higher-than-expected prevalence of premature carotid lesions in PI-treated patients was observed when compared to PI-naive patients (59).

HAART, Hypertension, and Coagulative Disorders

The prevalence of hypertension in HIV disease has been estimated to be about 20 to 25% before the introduction of HAART (60). Recent reports indicate that elevated blood pressure may be related to PI-induced lipodystrophy and metabolic disorders, especially to fasting triglyceride with a prevalence of hypertension in up to 74% of patients with HAART-related metabolic syndrome (61). The prevalence of hypertension associated with erythropoietin therapy is 47%; the effect may be related to the increase in hematocrit and blood viscosity (62). A syndrome of acquired glucocorticoid resistance has been described in HIV-infected patients with hypercortisolism and a lower affinity of the glucocorticoid receptors (60). The syndrome is characterized clinically by weakness, hypertension or hypotension, and changes in skin pigmentation.

Moreover, HIV-infected patients, especially those with fat redistribution, may develop coagulation abnormalities, such as increased levels of fibrinogen, D-dimer, plasminogen activator inhibitor 1, and tissue-type plasminogen activator antigen or deficiency of protein S (63,64). These abnormalities have been associated with

Table 2 Cardiovascular Actions/Interactions of Common HIV Therapies

Class	Drugs	Cardiac drug interactions	Cardiac side effects
Antiretroviral			
Nucleoside reverse transcriptase inhibitors (RTIs)	Abacavir (Ziagen), Zidovudine (AZT, Retrovir)	Dipyridamole	Lactic acidosis (rare), hypotension, skeletal muscle myopathy, (mitochondrial dysfunction hypothesized, but not seen clinically)
Nonnucleoside RTIs	Delavirdine (Rescriptor), efavirenz (Sustiva), nevirapine (Viramune)	Warfarin (class interaction), calcium channel blockers, beta blockers, quinidine, steroids, theophylline	Delavirdine can cause serious toxic effects if given with antiarrythmic drugs and myocardial ischemia if given with vasoconstrictors
Protease inhibitors	Amprenavir (Agenerase), indinavir (Crixivan), nelfinavir (Viracept), ritonavir (Norvir)	All are metabolized by cytochrome p-450 and interact with: sildenafil, amiodarone, lidocaine, quinadine, warfarin, statins	Implicated in premature atherosclerosis, dyslipidemia, insulin resistance, and lipodystrophy/lipoatrophy
	Saquinavir (Invirase, Fortovase)	Calcium channel blockers, beta blockers (1.5-3x increase), prednisone, quinine, theophylline (decrease concentrations)	
Anti-infective			
Antibiotics	Erythromycin, clarithromycin	Cytochrome p-450 metabolism and drug interactions	Orthostatic hypotension, ventricular tachycardia, bradycardia, QT prolongation
	Rifampicin	Reduces therapeutic effect of digoxin by induction of intestinal P-glycoprotein	

Antifungal	Trimethoprim/sulfamethoxazole (Bactrim)	Increases warfarin effects	Orthostatic hypotension, QT prolongation
	Amphotericin B	Digoxin toxicity	Hypertension, renal failure, hypokalemia thrombophlebitis, angioedema–dilated cardiomyopathy, arrhythmias
	Ketoconazole, intraconazole	Cytochrome p-450 metabolism and drug interactions; increase levels of sildenafil, warfarin, "statins," nifedipine, digoxin	
Antiviral	Foscarnet, ganciclovir	Zidovudine	Reversible cardiac failure (dose-related effect), electrolyte abnormalities, ventricular tachycardia (QT prolongation), hypotension
Antiparasitic	Pentamidine (intravenous)		Hypotension, arrhythmias (torsades de pointes, ventricular tachycardia), hyperglycemia, hypoglycemia, sudden death Note: Contraindicated if baseline QTc > 0.48
Chemotherapeutic	Vincristine, doxorubicin (Adriamycin)	Decrease digoxin level	Arrhythmias, myocardial infarction, dilated cardiomyopathy (dose-related effect), autonomic neuropathy
	Recombinant INF-α		Hypertension, hypotension, dilated cardiomyopathy, ventricular and supraventricular arrhythmias, atrioventricular block
	IL-2		Hypotension, arrhythmias, myocardial infarction, cardiac failure, capillary leak, thyroid alterations

Source: Ref. 1.

documented thromboses involving both veins and arteries and seem to be related to PI-containing HAART (63,65). In a large multicenter epidemiological survey, Sullivan et al. reported an incidence of clinically recognized thrombosis of 2.6 per 1000 person-years in a sample of 42,935 HIV-infected adults. Thrombosis was more common in patients who were aged 45 or older, those with opportunistic infections, those who were hospitalized, and those who were prescribed megestrol or indinavir (66). The routine evaluation of coagulation parameters is probably not advisable until the benefit of widespread screening is assessed in prospective studies. However, clinicians should be aware of the increased risk of coagulative disorders in HIV-infected patients receiving HAART.

COMMOM HIV THERAPIES AND THE HEART

In AIDS patients with KS, reversible cardiac dysfunction was associated with prolonged, high-dose therapy with IFN-α (1). Doxorubicin used to treat AIDS-related KS and non-Hodgkin's lymphoma has a dose-related effect on dilated cardiomyopathy, as does foscarnet sodium used to treat cytomegalovirus esophagitis (1). Cardiac arrhythmias have been described with the administration of amphotericin B (67), ganciclovir (68), trimethoprim/sulfamethoxazole (69), and pentamidine (70). The principal cardiovascular actions/interactions of common HIV therapies are reported in Table 2 (1).

CARDIAC INVOLVEMENT WITH AIDS-RELATED NEOPLASMS

The prevalence of cardiac Kaposi's sarcoma (KS) in AIDS patients ranges from 12 to 28% in retrospective autopsy studies in the pre-HAART period (5). Cardiac involvement with KS usually occurs when widespread visceral organ involvement is present. The lesions are typically less than 1 cm in size and may be pericardial or, less frequently, myocardial, and they are only rarely associated with obstruction, dysfunction, morbidity, or mortality (5). Microscopically, there are atypical spindle cells lining slit-like vascular spaces.

Non-Hodgkin's lymphoma (NHL) involving the heart is infrequent in AIDS (5). Most are high-grade B-cell (small and noncleaved) Burkitt-like lymphomas, with the rest classified as diffuse large B-cell lymphomas (in the REAL classification). Lymphomatous lesions may appear grossly as either discrete localized or more diffuse nodular to polypoid masses (71,72). Most involve the pericardium, with variable myocardial infiltration (71,72). There is little or no accompanying inflammation and necrosis. The prognosis of patients with HIV-associated cardiac lymphoma is generally poor because of widespread organ involvement, although some patients treated with combination chemotherapy have experienced clinical remission (73).

The introduction of HAART has reduced the incidence of cardiac involvement by KS and NHL, perhaps attributable to the patients' improved immunological state and to suppression of opportunistic infections with HHV-8 and Epstein-Barr virus, which are known to play an etiological role in these neoplasms (73).

CONCLUSIONS

Cardiac and pulmonary complications of HIV disease are generally late manifestations and may be related to prolonged effects of immunosuppression and a complex interplay of mediator effects from opportunistic infections, viral infections, autoimmune response to viral infection, drug-related cardiotoxicity, nutritional deficiencies, and prolonged immunosuppression (1). It is hoped that HAART, by improving the clinical course of HIV disease, will reduce the incidence of pericardial effusions and myocardial involvement of HIV-associated malignancies and coinfections. However, a careful cardiac screening is warranted for patients who are being evaluated for HAART or are receiving HAART regimens, especially those with other known underlying cardiovascular risk factors as the atherogenic effects of PI—including HAART—may synergistically promote the acceleration of coronary and cerebrovascular disease and increase the risk of death from myocardial infarction and stroke. A close collaboration between cardiologists and infectious disease specialists may be useful for decisions regarding use of antiretrovirals and other therapies for a careful stratification of cardiovascular risk and cardiovascular monitoring.

REFERENCES

1. Barbaro G, Klatt EC. HIV infection and the cardiovascular system. AIDS Rev 2002; 4:93–103.
2. Barbaro G, Di Lorenzo G, Soldini M, et al. Intensity of myocardial expression of inducible nitric oxide synthase influences the clinical course of human immunodeficiency virus–associated cardiomyopathy. Circulation 1999; 100:933–939.
3. Pugliese A, Isnardi D, Saini A, Scarabelli T, Raddino R, Torre D. Impact of higly active antiretroviral therapy in HIV-positive patients with cardiac involvement. J Infect 2000; 40:282–284.
4. Bijl M, Dieleman JP, Simoons M, Van Der Ende ME. Low prevalence of cardiac abnormalities in an HIV-seropositive population on antiretroviral combination therapy. J AIDS 2001; 27:318–320.
5. Barbaro G, Di Lorenzo G, Grisorio B, Barbarini G, and the Gruppo Italiano per lo Studio Cardiologico dei pazienti affetti da AIDS Investigators. Cardiac involvement in the acquired immunodeficiency syndrome: a multicenter clinical-pathological study. AIDS Res Hum Retrovir 1998; 14:1071–1077.
6. Currie PF, Goldman JH, Caforio AL, et al. Cardiac autoimmunity in HIV related heart muscle disease. Heart 1998; 79:599–604.
7. Lipshultz SE, Easley KA, Orav EJ, et al. Cardiac dysfunction and mortality in HIV-infected children. The Prospective P2C2 HIV Multicenter Study. Circulation 2000; 102:1542–1548.
8. Freeman GL, Colston JT, Zabalgoitia M, Chandrasekar B. Contractile depression and expression of proinflammatory cytokines and iNOS in viral myocarditis. Am J Physiol 1998; 274:249–258.

9. Lipshultz SE, Easley KA, Orav EJ, et al. Left ventricular structure and function in children infected with human immunodeficiency virus. The prospective P^2C^2 HIV multicenter study. Circulation 1998; 97:1246–1256.

10. Cooper ER, Hanson C, Diaz C, et al. Encephalopathy and progression of human immunodeficiency virus disease in a cohort of children with perinatally acquired human immunodeficiency virus infection. J Pediatr 1998; 132:808–812.

11. Barbaro G, Di Lorenzo G, Soldini M, et al. Clinical course of cardiomyopathy in HIV-infected patients with or without encephalopathy related to the myocardial expression of TNF-α and iNOS. AIDS 2000; 14:827–838.

12. Miller TL, Orav EJ, Colan SD, Lipshultz SE. Nutritional status and cardiac mass and function in children infected with the human immunodeficiency virus. Am J Clin Nutr 1997; 66:660–664.

13. Miller TL. Cardiac complications of nutritional disorders. In: Lipshultz SE, ed. Cardiology in AIDS. New York: Chapman & Hall, 1998:307–316.

14. Hoffman M, Lipshultz SE, Miller TL. Malnutrition and cardiac abnormalities in the HIV-infected patients. In: Miller TL, Gorbach S, eds. Nutritional Aspects of HIV infection. London: Arnold, 1999:33–39.

15. Lewis W, Simpson JF, Meyer RR. Cardiac mitochondrial DNA polymerase gamma is inhibited competitively and noncompetitively by phosphorylated zidovudine. Circ Res 1994; 74:344–348.

16. Lewis W, Grupp IL, Grupp G, et al. Cardiac dysfunction in the HIV-1 transgenic mouse treated with zidovudine. Lab Invest 2000; 80:187–197.

17. Lipshultz SE, Easley KA, Orav EJ, et al. Absence of cardiac toxicity of zidovudine in infants. N Engl J Med 2000; 343:759–766.

18. Barbaro G, Fisher SD, Giancaspro G, Lipshultz SE. HIV-associated cardiovascular complications: a new challenge for emergency physicians. Am J Emerg Med 2001; 19:566–574.

19. Ohtsuka T, Hamada M, Hiasa G, et al. Effect of beta-blockers on circulating levels of inflammatory and anti-inflammatory cytokines in patients with di8lated cardiomyopathy. J Am Coll Cardiol 2000; 37:412–417.

20. Johnson RM, Little JR, Storch GA. Kawasaki-like syndromes associated with human immonodeficiency virus infection. Clin Infect Dis 2001; 32:1628–1634.

21. Shingadia D, Das L, Klein-Gitelman M, Chadwick E. Takayasu's arteritis in a human immunodeficiency virus-infected adolescent. Clin Infect Dis 1999; 29(2):458–459.

22. Gisselbrecht M. Vasculitis during human acquired immunodeficiency virus infection. Pathol Biol (Paris) 1999; 47(3):245–247.

23. Chi D, Henry J, Kelley J, Thorpe R, Smith JK, Krishnaswamy G. The effects of HIV infection on endothelial function. Endothelium 2000; 7(4):223–242.

24. Berger O, Gan X, Gujuluva C, et al. CXC and CC chemokine receptors on coronary and brain endothelia. Mol Med 1999; 5(12):795–805.

25. Grahame-Clarke C, Alber DG, Lucas SB, Miller R, Vallance P. Association between iruses and Kaposi's sarcoma and atherosclerosis: implications for gammaherpesviruses and vascular disease. AIDS 2001; 15:1902–1905.

26. Barbaro G, Barbarini G, Pellicelli AM. HIV-associated coronary arteritis in a patient with fatal myocardial infarction. N Engl J Med 2001; 344:1799–1800.

27. Behrens GM, Stoll M, Schmidt RE. Lipodystrophy and metabolic disorders in anti-HIV therapy. MMW Fortschr Med 2000; 142(suppl 1):68–71.

28. Vigouroux C, Gharakhanian S, Salhi Y, et al. Diabetes, insulin resistance and dyslipidaemia in lipodystrophic HIV-infected patients on highly active antiretroviral therapy (HAART). Diabetes Metab 1999; 25(3):225–232.

29. John M, Nolan D, Mallal S. Antiretroviral therapy and the lipodystrophy syndrome. Antivir Ther 2001; 6:9–20.

30. Nolan D, Mallal S. Getting to the HAART of insulin resistance. AIDS 2001; 15:2037–2041.

31. Periard D, Telenti A, Sudre P, et al. Atherogenic dyslipidemia in HIV-infected individuals treated with protease inhibitors. The Swiss HIV Cohort Study. Circulation 1999; 100:700–705.

32. Assmann G, Schulte H, Von Eckardstein K. Hypertriglyceridemia and elevated lipoprotein (a) are risk factors for major coronary events in middle-aged men. Am J Cardiol 1996; 77:1178–1179.

33. Carr A, Samaras K, Chisholm DJ, Cooper DA. Pathogenesis of HIV-1-protease inhibitor-associated peripheral lipodystrophy, hyperlipidaemia, and insulin resistance. Lancet 1998; 351(9119):1881–1883.

34. Carr A, Samaras K, Burton S, et al. A syndrome of peripheral lipodystrophy, hyperlipidaemia and insulin resistance in patients receiving HIV protease inhibitors. AIDS 1998; 12(7):F51–F58.

35. Mooser V, Carr A. Antiretroviral therapy-associated hyperlipidemia in HIV disease. Curr Opin Lipidol 2001; 12:313–319.

36. Fauvel J, Bonnet E, Ruidavets JB, et al. An interaction between apo C-III variants and protease inhibitors contributes to high tiglyceride/low HDL levels in treated HIV patients. AIDS 2001; 15:2397–2406.

37. Bonnet E, Ruidavets JB, Tuech J, et al. Apoprotein c-III and E-containing lipoparticles are markedly increased in HIV-infected patients treated with protease inhibitors: association with the development of lipodystrophy. J Clin Endocrinol Metab 2001; 86(1):296–302.

38. Gaou I, Malliti M, Guimont MC, et al. Effect of stavudine on mitochondrial genome and fatty acid oxidation in lean and obese mice. J Pharmacol Exp Ther 2001; 297:516–523.

39. Murata H, Hruz PW, Mueckler M. The mechanism of insulin resistance caused by HIV protease inhibitor therapy. J Biol Chem 2000; 275(27):20251–20254.

40. Mynarcik DC, McNurlan MA, Steigbigel RT, Fuhrer J, Gelato MC. Association of severe insulin resistance with both loss of limb fat and elevated serum tumor necrosis factor receptor levels in HIV lipodystrophy. J AIDS 2000; 25(4):312–321.

41. Stein JH, Klein MA, Bellehumeur JL, et al. Use of human immunodeficiency virus-1 protease inhbitors is associated with atherogenic lipoprotein changes and endothelial dysfunction. Circulation 2001; 104:257–262.

42. Behrens GM, Stoll M, Schmidt RE. Lipodystrophy syndrome in HIV infection: what is it, what causes it and how can it be managed? Drug Saf 2000; 23(1):57–76.

43. Smith D. Clinical significance of treatment-induced lipid abnormalities and lypodystrophy. J HIV Ther 2001; 6:25–27.

44. Dube MP, Sprecher D, Henry WK, et al. Preliminary guidelines for the evaluation and management of dyslipidemia in adults infected with human immunodeficiency virus and receiving antiretroviral therapy: recommendations of the Adult AIDS Clinical Trial Group Cardiovascular Disease Focus Group. Clin Infect Dis 2000; 31(5):1216–1224.

45. Moyle G, Lloyd M, Reynolds B, Baldwin C, Mandalia S, Gazzard BG. Dietary advice with or without pravastatin for the management of hypercholesterolaemia associated with protease inhibitor therapy. AIDS 2001; 15:1503–1508.

46. Currier JS. How to manage metabolic complications of HIV therapy: what to do while we wait for answers. AIDS Read 2000; 10(3):162–169.

47. Carr A, Hudson J, Chuan J, et al. HIV protease inhibitor substitution in patients with lipodystrophy: a randomized, controlled, open-label, multicentre study. AIDS 2001; 15:1811–1822.

48. Clumeck N, Goebel F, Rozenbaum W, Gerstoft J, et al. Simplification with abacavir-based triple nucleoside therapy versus continued protease inhibitor-based highly active anti-

retroviral therapy in HIV-1-infected patients with undetectable plasma HIV-1 RNA. AIDS 2001; 15:1517–1526.

49. Ruiz L, Negredo E, Domingo P, et al. Antiretroviral treatment simplification with nevirapine in protease inhibitor-experienced patients with hiv-associated lipodystrophy: 1-year prospective follow-up of a multicenter, randomized, controlled study. J AIDS 2001; 27:229–236.

50. van der Valk M, Kastelein JJP, Murphy RL, et al. Nevirapine-containing antiretroviral therapy in HIV-1 infected patients results in an anti-atherogenic lipid profile. AIDS 2001; 15:2407–2414.

51. Behrens G, Schmidt H, Meyer D, Stoll M, Schmidt RE. Vascular complications associated with use of HIV protease inhibitors. Lancet 1998; 351:1958.

52. Rickerts V, Brodt H, Staszewski S, Stille W. Incidence of myocardial infarctions in HIV-infected patients between 1983 and 1998: the Frankfurt HIV-cohort study. Eur J Med Res 2000; 5(8):329–333.

53. Friis-Moller N, Reiss P, Kirk O, et al. Cardiovascular risk factors in HIV patients. Association with antiretroviral therapy (abstr 018). The D A D Study. 8th European Conference on Clinical Aspects and Treatment of HIV infection. Athens, 2001.

54. Holmberg S, Moorman A, Tong T, et al. Protease inhibitor use and adverse cardiovascular outcome in ambulatory HIV patients (abstr T698). 9th Conference on Retroviruses and Opportunistic Infections. Seattle, WA, 2002.

55. Bozzette SA, Ake C, Carpenter A, et al. Cardiovascular and cerebrovascular outcomes with changing process of anti-HIV therapy in 36,766 US Veteran (abstr LB9). 9th Conference on Retroviruses and Opportunistic Infections. Seattle, WA, 2002.

56. Coplan P, Cormier K, Japour A, et al. Myocardial infarction incidence in clinical trials of 4 protease inhibitors (abstr 34). 7th Conference on Retroviruses and Opportunistic Infections. San Francisco CA (January 30–February 2), 2000.

57. Coplan P, Nikas A, Leavit RY, et al. Indinavir did not increase the short-term risk of adverse cardiovascular events relative to nucleoside reverse transcriptase inhibitor therapy in four phase III clinical trials. AIDS 2001; 15:1584–1586.

58. Depairon M, Chessex S, Sudre P, et al. Premature atherosclerosis in HIV-infected individuals: focus on protease inhibitor therapy. AIDS 2001; 15:329–334.

59. Maggi P, Serio G, Epifani G, et al. Premature lesions of the carotid vessels in HIV-1-infected patients treated with protease inhibitors. AIDS 2000; 14:F123–F128.

60. Aoun S, Ramos E. Hypertension in the HIV-infected patient. Curr Hypertens Rep 2000; 2(5):478–481.

61. Sattler FR, Qian D, Louie S, et al. Elevated blood pressure in subjects with lipodystrophy. AIDS 2001; 15:2001–2010.

62. Raine AE. Hypertension, blood viscosity and cardiovascular morbidity in renal failure: implication of erythropoietin therapy. Lancet 1988; 1:97–100.

63. Witz M, Lehmann J, Korzets Z. Acute brachial artery thrombosis as the initial manifestation of human immunodeficiency virus infection. Am J Hematol 2000; 64(2):137–139.

64. Hadigan C, Meigs JB, Rabe J, et al. Increased PAI-1 and tPA Antigen levels are reduced with metformin therapy in HIV-infected patients with fat redistribution and insulin resistance. J Clin Endocrinol Metab 2001; 86(2):939–943.

65. Nair R, Robbs JV, Chetty R, Naidoo NG, Woolgar J. Occlusive arterial disease in HIV-infected patients: a preliminary report. Eur J Vasc Endovasc Surg 2000; 20(4):353–357.

66. Sullivan PS, Dworkin MS, Jones JL, Hooper WC. Epidemiology of thrombosis in HIV-infected individuals. The Adult/Adolescent Spectrum of HIV Disease Project. AIDS 2000; 14:321–324.

67. Arsura EL, Ismail Y, Freeman S, Karunakav AR. Amphotericin B-induced dilated cardiomyopathy. Am J Med 1994; 97:560–562.

68. Cohen AJ, Weiser B, Afzal Q, Fuhrer J. Ventricular tachycardia in two patients with AIDS receiving ganciclovir (DHPG). AIDS 1990; 4:807–809.
69. Lopez JA, Harold JG, Rosenthal MC, Oseran DS, Schapira JN, Peter T. QT prolungation and torsades de pointes after administration of thrimethoprim-sulfamethoxazole. Am J Cardiol 1987; 59:376–377.
70. Stein KM, Haronian H, Mensah GA, Acosta A, Jacobs J, Klingfield P. Ventricular tachycardia and torsades de pointes complicating pentamidine therapy of *Pneumocystis carinii* pneumonia in the acquired immunodeficiency syndrome. Am J Cardiol 1990; 66:888–889.
71. Duong M, Dubois C, Buisson M, et al. Non-Hodgkin's lymphoma of the heart in patients infected with human immunodeficiency virus. Clin Cardiol 1997; 20(5):497–502.
72. Sanna P, Bertoni F, Zucca E, et al. Cardiac involvement in HIV-related non-Hodgkin's lymphoma: a case report and short review of the literature. Ann Hematol 1998; 77(1–2):75–78.
73. Dal Maso L, Serraino D, Franceschi S. Epidemiology of HIV-associated malignancies. Cancer Treat Res 2001; 104:1–18.
74. Heidenreich PA, Eisenberg MJ, Kee LL, et al. Pericardial effusion in AIDS. Incidence and survival. Circulation 1995; 92:3229–3234.
75. Barbaro G, Fisher SD, Lipshultz SE. Pathogenesis of HIV-associated cardiovascular complications. Lancet Infect Dis 2001; 1:115–124.
76. Barbaro G, DiLorenzo G, Grisorio B, Barbarini G, and the Gruppo Italiano per lo Studio Cardiologico dei pazienti affetti da AIDS investigators. Cardiac involvement in the acquired immunodeficiency syndrome. A multicenter clinical-pathological study. AIDS Res Hum Retrovir 1998; 14:1071–1077.

27

Lipodystrophy Syndrome and HIV Disease

Aurea Westrick-Thompson
Baptist Medical Center/Wolfson Children's Hospital, Jacksonville, Florida, U.S.A.

Simin Bourchi-Vaghefi
University of North Florida, Jacksonville, Florida, U.S.A.

With the advent of more effective therapies for human immunodeficiency virus (HIV) infection, HIV-positive patients are living symptom-free longer and leading more normal lives. However, new complications such as cardiovascular disease are becoming more prevalent in this population. Patients with HIV infection currently represent one of the most rapidly developing groups with cardiovascular disease globally. Moreover, the protease inhibitors (PIs) used to treat HIV infection induce a syndrome of lipodystrophy and dyslipidemia that may be associated with accelerated atherosclerosis as well as insulin resistance (1).

Altered fat disposition syndrome, also known as lipodystrophy, has become a prominent feature in individuals infected with HIV who are long-term survivors of AIDS and are undergoing highly active retroviral therapy (HAART) (2,3). *Lipodystrophy* is not a new term. Lluis Barraquer-Roviralta, a Spanish neurologist, described the syndrome of progressive lipodystrophy in 1907. This syndrome was subsequently known as Barraquer's syndrome (4). Although the main feature of Barraquer's syndrome is the progressive atrophy of the subcutaneous fat of the face, it is interesting to note how once again lipodystrophy is of interest, but in a completely different complex.

Congenital lipodystrophy is an uncommon autosomal recessive disorder that occurs mainly in females and is characterized by the loss of subcutaneous fat, insulin-dependent diabetes mellitus, and masculinization secondary to defective metabolism of fat. Acquired lipodystrophy and dyslipidemia are now most commonly encountered in patients infected with HIV disease who take PIs.

PROTEASE INHIBITORS

PIs have played a critical role in improving the prognosis of people infected with HIV. Recent findings indicate, however, that PIs may cause significant alterations in lipid metabolism. In one study it was determined that, following initiation of the PI, a significant increase in cholesterol levels resulted in 80% of the patients taking norvir/

saquinovir, 51% of patients taking indinavir, and 47% of patients taking nelfinavir (5). In another study, peripheral lipoatrophy (an estimated 0.35 kg fat loss per month overall from the face, limbs, and upper trunk) was observed after a median of 10 months of PI therapy in association with all licensed PIs. It is thought that the lipodystrophy syndrome may be a result of the inhibition of two proteins involved in lipid metabolism that have significant homology to the catalytic site of HIV protease— specifically, cytoplasmic retinoic acid binding protein type 1 and low-density-lipo-protein (LDL) receptor-related protein (6).

One of the PIs that is specifically becoming associated with lipodystrophy syndrome is Crixivan, or indinavir. Many individuals on Crixivan are noticing to be accumulating fat primarily in the abdominal area, popularly termed the "crix belly" (7) within the HIV community. The weight gain often accompanies muscle wasting in the face, arms, and legs. Resistance weight training, along with a healthy diet consisting of adequate amounts of protein, can help to preserve and improve lean body mass in extremities. Nutritional therapy and exercise for this population are discussed in later sections of this chapter.

LIPODYSTROPHY AND BODY ALTERATION

The prevalence of lipodystrophy syndrome among HIV-infected individuals and the accompanying metabolic disorders have been described since the onset of HAART in HIV-infected patients (8). The introduction of HAART has resulted in a decrease in opportunistic infections but also led to the development of new clinical manifestations such as lipodystrophy and immune reconstitution illnesses. Study of lipid profiles and use of dual energy x-ray absorptiometry (DEXA) to assess lipodystrophy have been necessitated by these changes in the epidemic (9). Sonography has also been studied as a method of regional subcutaneous fat measurement in HIV-infected patients and therefore provided a potential way to better assess and diagnose lipodystrophy in this population (10).

Although AIDS and HIV-related morbidity and mortality rates in patients with advanced HIV infection who are treated with combination of antiretroviral medi-cations have declined, metabolic adverse effects associated with these regimens have been increasingly recognized (11). Alterations in fat distribution are among the most frequent side effects of combined retroviral therapy. They may occur in patients receiving only PIs and in those treated only with combinations of nucleoside reverse transcriptase inhibitors (12). Fat distribution patterns usually appear as central visceral obesity, breast enlargement in women, the development of a "buffalo hump," and loss of peripheral fat (13). The broad variety of alterations in body fat associated with metabolic abnormalities pose the question as to whether they represent different components of the same syndrome or are actually manifestations of different pathogenic mechanisms. Recent clinical evidence in this area is consistent with a higher risk of alterations in body fat in females versus males (12).

Risk factors for the HIV-associated lipodystrophy syndrome were studied in a cross-sectional study with 278 HIV-infected patients in an outpatient German tertiary care center. Changes in body shape were quantified using linear analogue scales. The cumulative treatment duration for each antiretroviral drug, CD4 count, viral load, and age were investigated as potential risk factors for a clinical diagnosis of lipodystrophy

(LD) syndrome. LD syndrome was determined in 88 of the patients as well as significantly higher risk of developing LD with long-term PI treatment. Older age and a history of low CD4 counts were also contributing factors, although nucleoside analogues did not contribute significantly (14).

In a study by Lo and colleagues, antiretroviral therapy was studied as a risk factor for 8 HIV-1–infected men who experienced enlargement of the dorsocervical fat pad, or buffalo hump. Between June 1995 and October 1997, results of total and regional body-composition analysis by DEXA, glucose, cholesterol, triglyceride, and cortisol levels of the morphologically afflicted HIV patients were compared with those obtained in a control population of 15 HIV-1–infected men whose age, body mass index and CD4 lymphocyte counts were within the range of values in the 8 study patients. It was discovered that the 8 patients with buffalo hump were clinically stable on various antiretroviral regimens, 4 or which included a PI. No other signs of Cushing's syndrome were observed, and plasma cortisol values did not differ significantly from those of controls. Compared with controls, men with buffalo hump also had a higher proportion of fat in the trunk region, suggesting central accumulation of fat. Triglyceride but not cholesterol values were higher in the patients than in controls, but this difference was not significant. Fasting glucose levels did not differ significantly. The researchers concluded that the development of a buffalo hump could not be attributed to hypercortisolism in the 8 men and that its occurrence was not unique to patients on PI therapy (15).

In another study, by Thiebaut et al., the prevalence of clinical lipodystrophy and metabolic disorders and risk factors for these in 581 HIV-infected individuals were examined. A cross-sectional survey of the Aquitaine Cohort was performed in January of 1999. In this study, the clinical diagnosis of LD was further categorized as fat wasting (FW), peripheral fat accumulation (FA), or mixed syndromes (MS). Of the total number of patients studied, 61% were treated with protease inhibitors. The overall prevalence of LD was 38%. Of this total, 16% presented with FW, 12% with FA, and 10% with MS. The prevalence of metabolic abnormalities was 49%; of lipid disorders, 20%; and of glucose disorders, 20%. The researchers found that FW was associated more with males and with antiretroviral treatment. Body mass index was more closely associated with both FW and FA, while waist-to-hip ratio was more closely associated with FA and MS (16).

Two cross-sectional studies in 1996 ($n = 247$ participants) and 1997 ($n = 266$ participants) were conducted with HIV-infected outpatients to determine the effects of antiretroviral therapy, including PIs, on body composition and the prevalence of malnutrition. Among the patients who participated in both studies, 111 patients started new antiretroviral treatment, including PIs, between 1996 and 1997 and were studied longitudinally. Total body water, intracellular water, extracellular water, and fat mass were estimated via bioelectrical impedance analysis (BIA). It was determined that the prevalence of malnutrition was reduced by 30 to 50% from 1996 to 1997, depending on the definition used. In the longitudinal study, total body water and the ratio between intracellular water and extracellular water increased, while fat mass decreased. BIA showed a greater increase in intracellular water in 23 (21%) of the patients with clinically apparent fat redistribution than among patients without this syndrome, although estimates of changes in fat mass were not significantly different. It was concluded from this study that antiretroviral treatment may actually protect HIV-positive patients against the development of malnutrition, as whole-body BIA data

suggest an increase in appendicular body cell mass associated with improved antiretroviral therapies. However, the method is unreliable in detecting fat redistribution
and may warrant recalibration of prediction equations for those undergoing antiretroviral treatment (17).

Some researchers have theorized that HAART is responsible for a dysregulation
in the homeostasis of tumor necrosis factor alpha (TNF-α), a cytokine involved in lipid
metabolism. Ledru et al. measured cytokine production in HIV-positive patients
under HAART for a period of 18 months. A dramatic polarization to TNF-α synthesis
of both CD4 and CD8 cells was observed in all patients. Lipodystrophy was found to
be associated with a more dramatic TNF-α dysregulation; a positive correlation was
found between the absolute number of TNF-α CD8 T-cell precursors and lipid parameters usually altered in lipodystrophy syndrome, such as cholesterol and triglyceride
levels. The researchers concluded that HAART dysregulates homeostasis of TNF-α
synthesis and suggest that this inflammatory response, induced by efficient antiretroviral therapy, is a risk factor of lipodystrophy in HIV-infected patients (18).

METABOLIC ABNORMALITIES OF GLUCOSE AND LIPID

The viral burden and stress present in HIV-infected individuals elicit a complex
hormonal and immunological response that may alter various biochemical pathways,
including glucose metabolism. Although not as common before the era of potent
antiretroviral therapies, insulin resistance has now been described as an important
component of the lipodystrophy syndrome. Although the etiology of abnormalities in
glucose metabolism remains unknown, the complex and multifactorial nature of
glucose metabolism makes the management of hyperglycemia or diabetes mellitus a
challenge for HIV-positive individuals and their health care professionals. Because of
similarities to the pathogenesis of diabetes, management of antiretroviral-induced
hyperglycemia could follow the recommendations of the American Diabetes Association (19).

A 5-year historical cohort study followed and trended the serum glucose and
lipid levels in HIV disease after initiation of PI therapy. This study sought to determine
whether changes were independent of virological response and improvement in disease
severity. It also determined risk factors associated with the development of hyperglycemia, hyperlipidemia, and lipodystrophy. This cohort study was performed in a
population of 221 HIV-infected individuals from October 1, 1993 through July 31,
1998. Adjusted incidence rate ratios were estimated by means of Poisson regression. It
was found that the cumulative incidence of new-onset hyperglycemia, hypercholesterolemia, hypertriglyceridemia, and lipodystrophy was 5, 24, 19% and 13% respectively.
It is interesting to note that most of these metabolic events occurred after initiation
of PI therapy. Anabolic steroids and psychotropic drugs were also found to be associated with lipodystrophy syndrome. The inclusion of potential intermediate variables
such as virologic suppression and increased body weight did not reduce the magnitude
of the association with PIs. The association between the incidence of elevated
triglycerides and ritonavir was stronger than for other PIs. However, the incidence
of hyperglycemia, hypercholesterolemia, and lipodystrophy did not vary significantly
across the spectrum of PI therapies. The researchers were able to conclude that there
seemed to be an independent association between PI use and hyperglycemia, hyper-

lipidemia, and lipodystrophy that could not be explained by the antiviral and therapeutic effect of PIs (11). A study by Mercie et al. aimed at estimating the prevalence of lipodystrophy (LD) among 233 HIV-positive patients and defining the associated lipid profiles of these patients. Lipid profiles (cholesterol, atherogenicity ratios, and triglycerides), blood glucose, CD4 count, and plasma viral load were determined, and patients were classified into two groups on the basis of whether they presented with clinical signs of LD. Overall it was found that of the 233 HIV individuals, 61 cases (26.1%) of LD were noted. LD patients were found to be older men with a lower CD4 count and more often at the AIDS stage of the disease (8). Analysis of lipid subfractions and atherogenicity ratios indicated a proatherogenic lipid profile for the LD patients. The researchers concluded that the underlying physiopathological mechanism of LD is still unknown. However, the lipid profile of HIV-infected patients with LD syndrome appears to place them at a higher risk for the progression of atherosclerosis.

In a retrospective review of 232 patient charts, individuals aged 19 through 68 years with HIV disease newly treated with a PI for at least 1 month were studied. Patients were grouped according to their protease inhibitor therapy: indinavir, nelfinavir, ritonavir, ritonavir plus saquinavir, and saquinavir alone. Baseline triglyceride and cholesterol levels were obtained before initiation of PI therapy and were compared at intervals during the study. Ritonavir-containing regimens were found to have the most profound effect on lipid levels, followed by nelfinavir. Fifty-seven percent of patients on single PI ritonavir regimens doubled their triglyceride values within the first 2 months of therapy, and lipid levels reached a plateau after 1 to 2 months, although increases were sustained. Increases in lipid levels did not correlate with gender, age, ethnicity, CD4 count, or viral load (20).

To better understand the metabolic complications of hypertriglyceridemia under PI use, the apoprotein and lipoprotein profiles in male HIV-infected patients undergoing retroviral therapy were studied. In this study, 49 patients received a PI and 14 were given two reverse transcriptase inhibitors. An additional 63 male participants acted as controls. All patients under PI therapy displayed low levels of plasma glucose and increased insulin. PI administration was also associated with moderate hypertrygliceridemia and low levels of high-density lipoprotein (HDL) cholesterol and apolipoprotein (apo) A-1 levels. The most significant change, however, was found in a two- to threefold increase in the apo E and apo C-III levels essentially recovered as associated to apo B–containing lipoparticles. Levels of these lipoparticles were two to eight times control values. Approximately 50% of PI-treated patients had developed a patent lipodystrophy (21). As a final conclusion to the study, 13 of the PI-receiving patients with patent hypertriglyceridemia were given fenofibrate and reevaluated 2 months later. Triglycerides, apo E, apo C-III, and the corresponding lipoparticles had returned to nearly normal levels, which indicated the accumulation of potentially atherogenic lipoparticles under PI therapy.

In contrast, we looked at a longitudinal study that investigated the effect of PIs on insulin sensitivity, glycemia, and serum lipids in 91 consecutive HIV-infected patients treated with PIs for at least 12 months. Fasting glucose levels, lipid-profile insulinemia, CD4 T lymphocytes, and plasma HIV-1 RNA were performed at baseline and on PI therapy. Triglycerides and cholesterol levels were significantly elevated on PI therapy, although it was found that fasting glycemia, insulin sensitivity, and insulin secretion were not modified after PI therapy. PI therapy significantly increased body mass index, and lipodystrophy was observed in 40.6% of patients treated with PIs. Serum lipid changes correlated with changes in the CD4 T-cell count. This longitudinal study found that PIs had no significant effect on fasting glucose levels, insulin sensitivity, or insulin secretion that is not consistent with other cross-sectional studies which did not include baseline measurements before PI initiation. However, there was a similar increase in serum lipids to other studies. The results suggest that PIs could be responsible for the development of hypertriglyceridemia through a mechanism independent of insulin resistance (22).

Some have theorized that the cortisol/dehydroepiendrosterone (DHEA) ratio in HIV-disease is related to the metabolic alterations of lipodystrophy. Christeff et al. studied serum cortisol and DHEA concentrations and the overall ratio of cortisol/ DHEA in HIV-infected men either untreated or undergoing various antiretroviral treatments including HAART. Cortisol levels were found to be elevated in all patients regardless of the stage of the illness and independently of the therapy. In contrast, serum DHEA levels were elevated in the asymptomatic stage and below normal in the "full-blown" AIDS patients, either untreated or treated with monoantiretroviral therapy. The DHEA level was found to be low in HAART-treated patients with lipodystrophy, yet it was highly elevated in HAART-treated patients without symptoms of lipodystrophy. The cortisol/DHEA ratio was similar to controls in patients who were asymptomatic, untreated, or treated with monoantiretroviral therapy, but it was increased in AIDS patients. Likewise, this ratio was increased in those showing positive symptoms of lipodystrophy, yet it was normalized in those showing no indications of lipodystrophy syndrome. Changes in the cortisol/DHEA ratio were negatively correlated with the in vivo CD4 T-cell counts, malnutrition markers (body-cell mass and fat mass) or with increased circulating lipids (cholesterol, triglycerides, and apolipoprotein B) associated with lipodystrophy syndrome. The researchers were able to conclude that the cortisol/DHEA ratio is altered in HIV-infected men, particularly in those with malnutrition or lipodystrophy, and that this ratio remains altered during antiretroviral treatment including HAART. These findings could have important clinical implications since manipulation of this ratio may help to prevent metabolic (protein and lipid) alterations (23).

MORPHOLOGICAL AND METABOLIC ABNORMALITIES

To provide population-based estimates of the prevalence of LD syndrome and constituent symptoms and to identify correlates of prevalent symptomology, participants in a provincewide HIV/AIDS program in Canada reported morphological and metabolic abnormalities. Probable LD was defined as self-report of at least one morphological abnormality or both high cholesterol and triglyceride levels. The variables investigated included age, sex, ethnicity, transmission risk group, CD4 T-cell count, plasma viral load, AIDS diagnosis, duration of infection, alternative therapy use, use of antiretroviral therapy (ART) use (past, current, and duration) by class and specific drug, total duration of ART, and current adherence. Of 1035 participants, 50% appeared to have probable LD, with 36% reporting peripheral wasting, 33% abdominal weight gain, 6% with buffalo hump, 10% with reported increased triglycerides, and 12% with increased cholesterol levels. In this study, LD was associated with older age, use of ingested alternative therapies, use of PIs, and duration of stavudine treatment. In analysis limited to participants exposed to PI, after similar adjustment, the duration of lamivudine rather than stavudine treatment was associated with lipodystrophy (24).

In another study to compare body composition, body fat distribution, and insulin secretion in HIV-infected patients undergoing therapy with nucleoside reverse transcriptase inhibitors (NRTIs), a cross-sectional design method was used. Forty-three HIV-infected patients participated in long-term NRTI therapy including stavudine or zidovudine and another 15 therapy-naive HIV-infected patients served as the control. All patients were assessed for fat wasting by BIA, and regional fat distribution was estimated using caliper measurements of skinfold thickness and evaluated by computed tomography at abdominal and midthigh level. Fasting glucose, insulin, C peptide, triglyceride, cholesterol, free fatty acid, testosterone, follicle-stimulating hormone, luteinizing hormone, cortisol levels, CD4 T-cell count and HIV viral load were determined. Daily caloric and nutrient intakes were evaluated as well. It was found that the zidovudine group and the control group had similar body composition and regional fat distribution. Stavudine therapy was associated with a significantly lower percentage of body fat, markedly decreased subcutaneous to visceral fat ratio, along with a higher mean intake of fat and cholesterol. Fasting plasma glucose, insulin and C-peptide levels were similar among the three groups. Triglyceride levels were significantly higher in the stavudine group than in the controls, but did not differ between the stavudine and the zidovudine group or between the zidovudine and the controls. Free fatty acids were not significantly elevated in any group. Lipodystrophy was observed clinically in 17 (63%) of patients taking stavudine, and in 3 (18.75%) taking zidovudine for a median period of 14 months. The relative risk of developing fat wasting was higher in the group receiving stavudine versus zidovudine. Five out of 12 patients had a major or mild improvement in their lipodystrophy after stavudine treatment was stopped. The researchers concluded that lipodystrophy may be related to long-term NRTI therapy, especially that including stavudine (7).

A prospective study of 26 Caucasian men (median age 43.5 years) with HIV-1 viral loads of <500 copies per milliliter for 12 months while on HAART who interrupted treatment for a median of 7.0 weeks were observed for changes. Seventeen (65.4%) patients reported at least one fat redistribution symptom at baseline. Serum lipids, glucose and insulin levels, cortisol and anthropometric parameters were measured before and after HAART interruption. It was found that a relatively brief interruption of HAART resulted in significant improvements in total cholesterol, LDL cholesterol, and triglyceride levels, suggesting that hyperlipidemia and alterations in cortiosteroid metabolism in the setting of HAART are a direct drug effect that reverses with drug withdrawal. No changes were observed in insulin resistance profiles or anthropometric measurements, possibly because of the brief duration of HAART interruption (25).

MEDICAL NUTRITION THERAPY

Findings have indicated that PIs may significantly increase lipids to levels posing a health risk greater than that of the illness itself. We have reviewed some of the research about lipodystrophy syndrome, and now address some of the nutritional issues surrounding this syndrome as well as the prevention of heart disease and excessive weight gain in the HIV-positive individual.

In the early years of HIV/AIDS, the primary goal of medical nutritional therapy was to prevent wasting—a rapid loss of lean body tissue in the HIV-infected patient. This still remains a challenge for many with HIV disease, along with nutrient imbalances, malabsorption, metabolic disorders, and unwanted side effects from medications. But a new problem is presenting itself as well. Some HIV-positive individuals on HAART are experiencing weight gain beyond what they would like. With the weight gain come escalating triglyceride and cholesterol levels and glucose abnormalities. These prominent features of lipodystrophy are risk factors for cardiovascular disease and the development of insulin resistance. Other side effects of these elevated lipid levels can often lead to acute pancreatitis and another hospital stay. Add the regular risk factors for heart disease such as smoking, sedentary lifestyle, and family history to the HAART regimens and the risk of coronary artery disease increases greatly in these HIV-infected individuals. Acknowledgment of the role that diet plays in heart disease and diabetes may help to lessen the effects of lipodystrophy.

HIV-infected patients displaying elevated serum lipid levels and undesired fat accumulation are therefore being encouraged to:

Consume nutrient-dense foods such as meat, beans/legumes, and other high-protein foods, vegetables, fruits, and low-fat or skim dairy products as well as whole-grain breads and cereals; also to choose lean cuts of meat, water-packed tuna, and cooked eggs for high-quality protein versus high-fat luncheon meats, hot dogs, and bacon.

"Empty-calorie" foods or "simple sugars" are discouraged (such as the sugar contained in soft drinks, candy, frosting, honey, molasses, jams, and sweet desserts) because they are low in vitamins, minerals, and protein.

Refrain from high-calorie drinks such as sodas, sports drinks, flavored water, and sweet tea, which may be needed for sick days.

Exercise regularly for increased caloric expenditure and to help decrease cholesterol and triglyceride levels; exercise also helps build muscle mass, which helps the body to fight illness and infection and provides reserves during illness, especially since the body uses protein reserves as its first line of defense in dealing with infection (26).

It must be noted, however, that even with excess fat accumulation, people with HIV disease are *not* advised to go on weight-reducing "diets." In fact, diets very low in fat may worsen the risk for heart disease, especially in people with elevated triglycerides or low HDL cholesterol levels and type II diabetes. Studies suggest that a high-carbohydrate diet (60% carbohydrate, 25% fat, 15% protein) can elevate both fasting and postprandial triglyceride concentrations (27). The goal of medical nutritional therapy is to simply maintain or build lean body mass while cutting back on saturated fats and simple sugars so as help to lower cholesterol and triglyceride levels and improve with glucose control.

One study investigated the impact of nutritional interventions for the treatment of PI-related hyperlipidemia. Melroe and colleagues wanted to determine if initiation of interventions based on the National Cholesterol Education Program (NCEP) guidelines would be effective in lowering PI hyperlipidemia without disrupting the effectiveness of the HIV therapy. A total of 45 HIV-positive individuals who were taking a PI and had abnormally high lipid levels were studied. Mean serum cholesterol levels prior to starting PI therapy were 170 mg/dL, as compared to the mean cholesterol at time of enrollment of 289 mg/dL and triglycerides of 870 mg/dL. Interventions included diet and exercise regimens as well as the prescription of gemfibrozil alone or in combination with atorvatstatin. Overall, intervention was shown to decrease serum cholesterol levels to 201 mg/dL in a study period of 10 months. With such a small sample size, in combination with both medication and diet interventions simultaneously, one is unable to determine if diet and exercise alone would have had the same lipid-lowering effects (29).

To better understand the possible influence of dietary fat on the metabolic effects of PI therapy, a group of researchers fed high-versus low-fat diets to a study group of mice that were then treated with a PI of either indinavir (IDV), nelfinavir (NFV), saquinavir (SQV), or amprenavir (APV) by subcutaneous delivery for 2 weeks. Serum concentrations of glucose, insulin, triglycerides, free fatty acids, glycerol, pancreatic lipase, bilirubin, alkaline phosphatase, blood urea nitrogen (BUN), and interscapular fat mass and epididymal fat weights were determined. The researchers found that some metabolic effects of PI therapy were dependent on diet. The IDV- and NFV-treated mice had greater serum glucose concentrations and resulting body weight; IDV-treated mice had lower serum insulin; NFV-treated mice had greater interscapular fat mass; and SQV-treated mice had lower serum triglyceride concentrations than control mice fed the low- but not the high-fat diet. In comparison, the NFV- and IDV-treated mice had greater triglyceride concentrations and levels of blood urea nitrogen, and SQV-treated mice had greater serum cholesterol levels than control mice fed the high- but not the low-fat diet. The serum concentration of SQV was lower in mice fed the high-fat compared with the low-fat diet. IDV- and NFV-treated mice had greater fatty acid levels, and IDV-treated mice had greater pancreatic lipase, bilirubin, and alkaline phosphatase than control mice fed either diet. AVP treatment showed little effect on the serum measurements in this study. They were able to conclude that dietary fat did influence some but not all of the effects of PI therapy on metabolism. It also appeared that different therapies produced different effects in vivo, indicating that various PIs affect distinct metabolic pathways (28,29).

EXERCISE AND EFFECTS ON LIPODYSTROPHY

As we have reviewed, increased abdominal fat associated with lipodystrophy may predispose patients with HIV disease to diabetes as well as hypertension and coronary artery disease. One study looked at whether exercise training could reduce truncal fat in men with fat redistribution. Ten men with increasing abdominal girth participated in a 16-week trial of progressive resistance training with an aerobic component three times a week. Total lean body mass, fat mass, and trunk fat mass were assessed using dual-DXA. After 16 weeks of exercise, strength increased in three of the four exercises tested, and there was a significant decline in total body fat by 1.5 kg (in which most of the decline occurred in truncal fat). Weight and lean body mass did not change. No adverse effects were seen from the training. It was recommended that control trials of this approach are warranted (29).

Frequency, intensity, and duration as well as aerobic versus resistance training need to be individualized for people with HIV disease. It is of benefit for the person living with HIV/AIDS to have a good understanding of the different characteristics of both aerobic and anaerobic types of exercise. Aerobic exercise can help with improving the cardiovascular system and insulin sensitivity, while weight-resistance training can help increase lean body mass/total body cell mass and can aid in reshaping the body.

CONCLUSION

The epidemiological, etiopathogenic, laboratory, and clinical features of serum lipid abnormalities occurring in the course of HIV disease are still poorly understood, while limited data are available regarding the management of HIV-related lipodystrophy as well as the efficacy of dietary-exercise programs and that of specific hypolipidemic agents. The HIV-infected patient on antiretroviral therapy PIs should have his or her lipid profile monitored in order to suggest a diet and hyperlipidemic treatment when applicable and to help prevent clinical outcomes related to long-term dyslipidemia. The selection of an appropriate hypolipidemic agent is difficult, and possible increased risks of pharmacologic interactions, toxicity, and impaired patient's adherence should be taken into consideration. Last, the HIV-infected individual with LD syndrome should never be encouraged to go on a weight loss diet, with the risk of losing lean body mass, which the individual may have to rely on at a later time for recovery from opportunistic infections.

REFERENCES

1. Krishnaswamy G, Chi DS, Kelley JL, Sarubbi F, et al. The cardiovascular and metabolic complications of HIV infection. Cardiol Rev 2000; 8(5):260–268.
2. Tinnerello D, Rostler S. Heart healthy food choices in the era of HAART. HIV Res Rev 2000; 4(4):1–22.
3. Tinnerello D, Meyer SA. Heart healthy food choices in the era of HAART: Part Two. HIV Res Rev 2000; 4(5):1, 4, 6–8, 14–17, 22–23.
4. Greene AK, Barraquer-Roviralta Lluis. (1855–1928): Spanish neurologist described progressive lipodystrophy. Plast Reconstr Surg 2001; 107(1):158–162.
5. Melroe NH, Kopaczewski J, Henry K, Huebsch J. Lipid abnormalities associated with protease inhibitors. J Assoc Nurses AIDS Care 1999; 10(2):22–30.
6. Carr A HIV protease inhibitor-related lipodystrophy syndrome. Clin Infect Dis 2000; (suppl 2):S135–S142.
7. www.tufts.edu.
8. Mercie P, Tchamgoue S, Thiebaut R, Viallard J, et al. Atherogen lipid profile in HIV-1-infected patients with lipodystrophy syndrome. Eur J Intern Med 2000; 11(5):257–263.
9. Kingston MA, Bowman CA. The investigation of patients with HIV infection: 10 years of progress. Int J STD AIDS 2001; 12(1):1–7.
10. Martinez E, Bianchi L, Garcia-Viejo MA, Bru C, et al. Sonographic assessment of regional fat in HIV-1-infected people. Lancet 2000; 356(9239):1412–1413.
11. Tsiodras S, Mantzoras C, Hammer S, Samore M. Effects of protease inhibitors on hypergylcemia, hyperlipidemia, and lipodystrophy. Arch Intern Med 2000; 160(13):2050–2056.
12. Ridolfo AL, Gervasoni C, Bini T, Galli M. Body habitus alterations in HIV-infected women treated with combined antiretroviral therapy. AIDS Patient Care STDS 2000; 14(11):595–601.

13. Meyer S. Lipodystrophy In Patients With HIV. Dietitian's Edge 2001; 2(2):18–19.
14. Schwenk A, Breuer JP, Kremer G, Romer K, et al. Risk factors for the HIV-associated lipodystrophy syndrome in a cross-sectional single-centre study. Eur J Med Res 2000 Oct 30; 5(10):443–448.
15. Lo JC, Mulligan K, Tai VW, Algren H, Schambelan M. "Buffalo hump" in men with HIV-1 infection. Lancet 1998 Mar 21; 35(9106):867–870.
16. Thiebaut R, Daucourt V, Mercie P, Ekouevi DK, et al. Lipodystrophy, metabolic disorders, and human immunodeficiency virus infection: Aquitaine Cohort, France, 1999. Clin Infect Dis 2000 Dec; 31(6):1482–1487.
17. Schwenk A, Beisenherz A, Kremer G, Diehl V, et al. Bioelectrical impedance analysis in HIV-infected patients treated with triple antiretroivral treatment. Am J Clin Nutr 1999 Nov; 70(5):867–873.
18. Ledru E, Christeff N, Patey O, de Truchis P, et al. Alteration of tumor necrosis factor-alpha T-cell homeostasis following potent antiretroviral therapy: contribution to the development of human immunodeficiency virus-associated lipodystrophy syndrome. Blood 2000; 95(10):3191–3198.
19. Hardy H, Esch LD, Morse GD. Glucose disorders associated with HIV and its drug therapy. Ann Pharmacother 2001; 35(3):343–351.
20. Chang E, Tetreault D, Liu Y, Beall G. The effects of antiretroviral protease inhibitors on serum lipid levels in HIV-infected patients. J Am Diet Assoc 2001; 101(6):687–689.
21. Bonnet E, Ruidavets JB, Tuech J, FerriEres J, et al. Apoprotein C-III and E-containing lipoparticles are markedly increased in HIV-infected patients treated with protease inhibitors: association with the development of lipodystrophy. J Clin Endocrinol Metab 2001; 86(1):296–302.
22. Christeff N, Nunez EA, Gougeon ML. Changes in cortisol/DHEA ratio in HIV-infected men are related to immunological and metabolic perturbations leading to malnutrition and lipodystrophy. Ann N Y Acad Sci 2000; 917:962–970.
23. Heath KV, Hogg RS, Chan KJ, Harris M, et al. Lipodystrophy-associated morphological, cholesterol and triglyceride abnormalities in a population-based HIV/AIDS treatment database. AIDS 2001 Jan 26; 15(2):231–239.
24. Saint-Marc T, Partisani M, Poizot-Martin I, Bruno F, et al. A syndrome of peripheral fat wasting (lipodystrophy) in patients receiving long-term nucleo side analogue therapy. AIDS 1999; 13(13):1659–1667.
25. Hatano H, Miller KD, Yoder CP, Yanovski JA, et al. Metabolic and anthropometric consequences on interruption of highly active antiretroviral therapy. AIDS 2000; 14(13):1935–1942.
26. Reuters H. High-carbohydrate diet elevated triglyceride concentrations. Available at ipn. intelihealth.com. Accessed Jan 20, 2001.
27. Melroe NH, Kopaczewski J, Henry K, Heubsch J. Intervention for hyperlipidemia associated with protease inhibitors. J Assoc Nurses AIDS Care 1999; 10(5):109.
28. Lenhard JM, Croom DK, Weiel JE, Spaltenstein A, et al. Dietary fat alters HIV protease inhibitor-induced metabolic changes in mice. J Nutr 2000; 130(9):2361–2366.
29. Roubenoff R, Weiss L, McDermott A, Heflin T, et al. A pilot study of exercise training to reduce trunk fat in adults with HIV-associated fat redistribution. AIDS 1999; 13(11):1373–1375.

28

The Role of N-3 Fatty Acids in Preventing Coronary Artery Disease and Arrhythmias in AIDS Patients: A Hypothesis

Elizabeth H. Sheppard
Consultant, Tucson, Arizona, U.S.A.

INTRODUCTION

In recent years, there has been increasing incidence of coronary artery disease (CAD) within the AIDS patient population. As first noted in autopsies, the cardiac involvement in AIDS includes pericardial, myocardial, and endocardial abnormalities. Both bacterial and nonbacterial factors may be related to a variety of conditions including pericardial effusion, myocarditis, dilated cardiomyopathy, endocarditis, pulmonary hypertension, malignant neoplasm, and drug-related cardiotoxicity. Of particular interest and great concern are the cardiovascular toxic effects of the various antiretroviral medications that many HIV-infected patients regularly take. The role of antiretroviral therapy in the development of atherosclerosis and arrhythmias in these patients is unclear. However, as survival continues to improve due to aggressive treatment, it becomes increasingly important to address the prevention of CAD, not only for the patient's quality of life but also to avoid placing an additional burden on an already fragile immune system.

Since the first study in 1976 by Bang et al., of the antiatherosclerotic effects of a diet high in n-3 fatty acids, such as that eaten by the Greenland Eskimos, the role of n-3 fatty acids in preventing heart disease has been investigated (1). What role could n-3 fatty acids play in the prevention of CAD and arrhythmias in HIV-infected patients? That topic is the focus of this chapter.

INCIDENCE OF CORONARY ARTERY DISEASE AND HEART ARRHYTHMIAS IN AIDS PATIENTS

As antiretrovirus therapy in managing HIV infection becomes more complex, so do the long-term side effects of this therapy. Increasingly, autopsies of patients infected with HIV have revealed CAD—a condition in which the heart receives inadequate oxygen and becomes ischemic. This is typically induced by one of three mechanisms: the formation of atherosclerosis plaque, vascular spasm of the coronary arteries, or thromboembolism (2). Evidence of CAD in HIV-infected patients includes eccentric atherosclerosis, fibrosis of the tunica media of the coronary artery, and lesions typical of myocardial interstitial fibrosis (3).

Although the pathology of CAD in HIV patients is not known, several possible explanations have been suggested. Atherosclerosis seen in HIV-infected patients may be due to altered adhesion properties of the virus-infected monocytes and macrophages (3). Another explanation, suggested by Mattila et al., is that increased fibrinogen concentration, which has been proposed as a link between the inflammatory states of infection and increased risk for CAD, may cause a condition of hypercoagulability. This may, in turn, play a role in the pathogenesis of CAD (4). It has also been suggested that aggressive antiretroviral therapy, especially with protease inhibitors, may cause dyslipoproteinemia, which promotes atherosclerosis and atherothrombosis (5). Protease inhibitor therapy has been associated with increased cholesterol levels and triglycerides as risk factors for coronary artery disease (6). It is most likely that multiple factors facilitate the progression of CAD in HIV-infected patients.

In the largest study to date of myocardial infarctions associated with protease inhibitor therapy, Jutte et al., reporting from an HIV outpatient treatment facility, found five cases of myocardial infarctions within 6 months (4). All patients were on antiretroviral treatment and protease inhibitor therapy for a median of 10 months. When compared to a cohort of HIV patients receiving antiretroviral treatment but not protease inhibitors, the incidence of myocardial infarction was statistically significant by Fisher's exact test ($p = 0.025$). The patients on protease inhibitors showed rapid progression of atherosclerosis and hypertriglyceridemia. Hypertriglyceridemia is a common finding in AIDS and is independent of the wasting syndrome associated with AIDS (7). Jutte et al. suggest that protease inhibitors increase the HIV patient's risk for CAD and that there is a synergistic effect between altered lipid metabolism, hypercoagulability, and other precursors.

Table 1 Some Medications Used in HIV Patients That Cause Abnormal Electrocardiogram Waves

Medications	Treatment	Cardiovascular adverse effects
Amphotericin	Antifungal	Dilated cardiomypathy, hypertension, and bradycardia
Ganciclovir	Cytomegalovirus	Ventricular tachycardia
Interferon alpha	Antineoplastic, antiviral, and immunomodulator	Arrhythmia, myocardial infarction or ischemia, cardiomyopathy, sudden death, atrioventricular block, and congestive heart failure
Pentamidine	*Pneumocystis carinii*	QT prolongation and torsades de pointes
Pyrimethamine	*Toxoplasmosis*	QT prolongation
Trimethoprim/ sulfamethoxazole	*Pneumocystis carinii*	QT prolongation and torsades de pointes

Source: Ref. 3.

In addition to HIV patients' increased susceptibility to CAD, an area of concern for this population is drug-induced cardiotoxicity. Cardiotoxicity due to HIV medications induces such adverse cardiovascular effects as arrhythmia, bradycardia, and QT prolongation (Table 1) (3). A review by Sonnenblick et al. in 1991 found 44 cases in which arrhythmia was the most common manifestation of cardiotoxicity among patients taking interferon medications (8). This was specific to interferon alpha, which acts as an antineoplastic, antiviral, and immunomoduling agent. Other cardiotoxicities resulting from interferon therapy included cardiomyopathy, myocardial infarction, sudden death, atrioventricular block, and congestive heart failure. This review did reveal that the adverse effect of interferon usage was not related to the dose or duration of therapy. When this therapy was withdrawn, the adverse cardiac effects were reversed (3).

N-3 FATTY ACID IN THE PREVENTION OF CORONARY ARTERY DISEASE AND ARRHYTHMIAS

Many clinical and epidemiological studies have focused on determining the preventive effects of n-3 fatty acids in the development of CAD. In fact, more is known about the role of n-3 fatty acids in the prevention of CAD than in that any other disease (9). The n-3 fatty acid family includes α-linolenic acid (ALA; 18:3n-3) and its corresponding polyunsaturated fatty acids (PUFAs) eicosapentaenoic acid (EPA; 20:5n-3) and docosahexaenoic acid (DHA; 22:6n-3). ALA is considered an essential fatty acid because it cannot be formed in the body and must be provided by the diet. ALA can be converted to EPA and DHA, but ALA is not equal to the n-3 PUFAs in its biological effects. Both EPA and DHA are more rapidly incorporated into the plasma and membrane lipids and thus more rapid-acting than ALA (10). Therefore the majority of research studied the effects of fish or fish oil supplements, which is high in EPA and DHA, on patients with CAD. Fewer studies have been conducted regarding the effects of ALA in normal patients and patients with myocardial infarctions.

A main component of CAD is atherosclerosis, a complex disease involving the arterial walls. Its pathogenesis begins with a nonspecific injury to the artery endothelium. Monocytes, macrophages, platelets, and foam cells aggregate at the site of injury. The platelets release growth factor, which in turn causes smooth muscle migration and proliferation. Consequently, monocytes and macrophages are deposited in the vessel wall and cholesterol is deposited in the smooth muscle wall. These events lead to ground formation, ultimately causing the formation of plaque (9). As seen in Table 2, many of the factors relating to the development of arterial plaque can be reduced by n-3 fatty acids' interference with the atherogenic process (9). Some of the beneficial effects of n-3 fatty acids include reduced platelet aggregation, production of platelet-derived growth factor–like protein (PDGF), and platelet activating factor, all of which appear to play a role in the CAD seen in HIV-infected patients.

A recent randomized double-blind placebo-controlled study by Von Schacky et al. investigated the effect of n-3 fatty acids in the diet on the course of coronary artery atherosclerosis in humans (11). Angiograms were taken at baseline and at 2 years in 80 recipients of placebo and 82 recipients of fish oil. All patients had been previously diagnosed with CAD. Results showed that patients with CAD who

Table 2   The Effects of N-3 Fatty Acids on
Factors Involved in the Development of
Inflammation, Atherosclerosis, and Immune
Disease

↓ *Reduce or inhibit risk and/or precipitating factors*
Arachidonic acid
Platelet aggregation
Thromboxane A_2 formation
Monocyte and macrophage function
Leukotriene function (LTB_4)
Formation of platelet activating factors (PAF)
Toxic oxygen metabolites
Interleukin-1 formation (IL-1)
Formation of tumor necrosis factor (TNF)
Platelet-derived growth factor–like protein (PDGF)
Fibrinogen
Blood viscosity
Blood pressure
VLDL, LDL
Triglycerides
Lipoprotein (a)
↑ *Increase beneficial and/or protective factors*
Prostacyclin formation (PGI_2 + PGI_3)
Leukotriene B_5 (LTB_5)
Interleukin-2 (IL-2)
Endothelial-derived relaxing factor (EDRF)
Fibrinolytic activity
Red cell deformability
High-density lipoprotein (HDL)

Source: Ref. 10.

ingested 1.5 g/day of n-3 fatty acids for 2 years had less progression and more regression of CAD than those on placebo. The recipients of fish oil had fewer cardiovascular events ($p = 0.10$) and their loss of luminal diameter was less than that in the placebo group. The study concluded that eating fish twice a week or using a daily fish oil supplement was a beneficial addition to other treatments for the secondary prevention of CAD (11). Although, the subjects in this study did not have HIV, this research suggests the possibility of using n-3 fatty acid supplementation to reduce CAD in AIDS patients as well. The preventive advantage of a diet rich in n-3 fatty acids can also be observed in Japanese and Eskimos, both of which groups have lower rates of cardiovascular disorders than American—12, 7, and 45%, respectively (9).

In addition to displaying antiatherosclerotic potential, n-3 fatty acid has been shown to be antiarrhythmic in animals and recently in humans. A study by McLennan et al. have demonstrated, in rats, that when irreversible ventricular arrhythmias were induced by ligation of the coronary artery, they were completely prevented in those animals fed fish oil. This was in stark contrast to rats fed either saturated or monounsaturated fat, which had a high incidence of irreversible ventricular fibrillation (12).

Leaf et al. used these observations to explore the mechanisms for the anti-arrhythmic effects of n-3 fatty acids (13). The research they conducted suggests that the antiarrhythmic effects of n-3 fatty acid influence the electrophysiology of cardiac myocytes. N-3 PUFAs stabilize the electrical activity of cardiac myocytes by altering sarcolemmal ion channels. In modifying the sarcolemmal ions, a stronger electrical stimulus is required to induce an action potential. In addition, the cardiac myocyte refractory period is prolonged threefold (13).

The effectiveness of n-3 fatty acids in preventing arrhythmia is still being investigated, but so far the evidence has been promising. Three secondary prevention trials have been conducted regarding n-3 fatty supplementation acid to reduce ischemia-induced cardiac death. All studies showed encouraging results, with an inverse relationship between fish or fish oil consumption and reduced incidence of sudden cardiac death (13). Future studies may determine whether n-3 fatty acid can be used safely in HIV patients to reduce the incidence of arrhythmias, the primary cardiotoxic effect of certain HIV medications.

CONSIDERATIONS REGARDING N-3 FATTY ACID SUPPLEMENTATION IN AIDS PATIENTS

To date no studies have looked at the role of n-3 fatty acids in preventing CAD or arrhythmias in AIDS patients. The use of n-3 fatty acid supplementation in AIDS patients has been investigated in regards to improving immune function and preventing cachexia (14–17). Pichard et al. studied HIV-infected patients given arginine and n-3 fatty acid supplementation for 6 months. These supplements did help the HIV patients to gain weight and reduce gastrointestinal and anorexia symptoms but did not improve immunological parameters such as CD4 and CD8 cell counts (17).

In considering the supplementation of n-3 fatty acids in AIDS patients to prevent CAD and arrhythmia, the nutritional status and utilization of n-3 fatty acids must be regarded. In the study of Begin et al., lipid levels in AIDS patients were measured, and lower levels of C20 and C22 essential fatty acids of the n-3 family were found (18). It is believed that the altered availability of long-chain polyunsaturated fatty acid metabolites (LCPUFA) maybe related to HIV pathophysiology. Furthermore, HIV infection has been related to altered availability of certain essential fatty acids in a recent study of HIV-seropositive children (14).

Essential fatty acid metabolism appears to be affected by HIV infection, but the exact mechanism of these changes remains to be determined. Further research could help determine whether supplementary n-3 fatty acid in HIV-infected patients is effectively utilized. Future studies could include the use of stable, isotope-labeled fatty acids to determine the mechanism of alteration of n-3 fatty acids and other essential fatty acids in HIV infection. This would help to determine the relevance of n-3 fatty acid supplementation to reduce CAD and arrhythmia resulting from cardiotoxicity in AIDS patients.

As yet there is little evidence of adverse effects from n-3 fatty acid supplementation on cholesterol, glucose metabolism, or hemostatic function (19). It has been hypothesized that very large intakes of n-3 fatty acids could incite infection due to a weakened defense system, although there are no clinical data on this speculation (19). Moderate n-3 PUFA supplementation of 2 to 5 g/day results in benefits such as increased vasodilation and an antiaggregatory hemostatic profile but not in the increased bleeding tendency seen in larger doses (19). A daily intake of PUFAs below >10% of total energy appears to be safe. Another factor to consider regarding n-3 fatty acid supplementation in AIDS patients is the ratio of dietary vitamin E and n-3 fatty acids. Additional vitamin E is required in diets with higher levels of PUFAs to help prevent the oxidation of tissue PUFAs, especially if consumed in the form of fish oil.

CONCLUSIONS

The n-3 family of essential fatty acids—which include α-linolenic acid, eicosapentaenoic acid, and docosahexaenoic acid—promote hypolipidemic, antithrombic, vasodilatory, and anti-inflammatory effects (10). The use of n-3 fatty acid supplementation appears to be a promising avenue of secondary treatment to the prevention of CAD and arrhythmias. The role n-3 fatty acid supplementation could play in reducing the rising incidence of CAD in AIDS patients remains to be seen. However, using n-3 fatty acid as an adjuvant treatment in AIDS patients may prevent the overproduction of proinflammatory substances to avert such CAD provoking conditions as hypercoagulability and atherosclerosis.

Moreover, the recently discovered antiarrhythmic properties of n-3 fatty acids may be effective in preventing arrhythmia associated with interferon-induced cardiotoxicity and other medications used by HIV patients. N-3 fatty acid supplementation when taken in a moderate dosage of 2 to 5 g/day appears to be safe and have no side effects (19). Future research should focus on how the body infected with HIV metabolizes and utilizes essential fatty acid in order to determine the application of n-3 fatty acid supplementation in HIV patients to prevent CAD and heart arrhythmias.

REFERENCES

1. Bang H, Dyerberg J, Stoffersen E, Moncada S, Vane J. Eicosapentaenoic acid in the prevention of thrombosis and athersclerosis. Lancet 1978; 2:117–119.
2. Sherwood L. Human Physiology from Cells to System. 3d ed. Bellmont, CA: Wadsworth, 1997:265–304.
3. Rerkpattanapipat P, Wongpratparrut N, Jacobs L, Kotler M. Cardiac manifestations of acquired immunodeficiency syndrome. Arch Intern Med 2000; 160:602–608.
4. Jutte A, Schwenk A, Franzen C, Romer K, Diet F, Diehl V, Fatkenheuer G, Salzberg B. Increasing morbidity from myocardial infarction during HIV protease inhibitor treatment? AIDS 1999; 13:1796–1797.
5. Melroe H, Huebsh J. Severe premature coronary artery disease with protease inhibitors. Lancet 1998; 351:1328.
6. Carr A, Samaras K, Burton S. A syndrome of peripheral lipodystrophy, hyperlipidemia and insulin resistance in patients receiving HIV protease inhibitors. AIDS 1998; 12:F51–F58.

7. Grunfeld C, Kotler D, Hamadeh R, Tierney A, Wang J, Pierson R. Hypertriglyceridemia in aquired immunodeficiency syndrome. Am J Med 1989; 86:27–31.

8. Sonnenblick M, Rosin A. Cardiotoxicity of interferon: a review of 44 cases. Chest 1991; 99:557–561.

9. Simopolous A. Omega-3 fatty acids in health and disease and in growth development. Am J Clin Nutr 1991; 54:438–463.

10. Simopolous A. Essential fatty acids in health and chronic disease. Am J Clin Nutr 1999; 70:560S–569S.

11. Von Schacky C, Angerer P, Kothny W, Theisen K, Mudra H. The effect of dietary ω-3 fatty acids on coronary atherosclerosis: a randomized, double-blind, placebo-controlled trial. Ann Intern Med 1999; 130:554–562.

12. McLennan PL. Relative effects of dietary saturated, monounsaturated and polyunsaturated fatty acids in cardiac arrythmias in rats. Am J Clin Nutr 1993; 57:207–212.

13. Leaf A, Kang J, Xiao Y, Billman G, Voskuyl R. The antiarrhythmic and anticonvulsant effects of dietary n-3 fatty acids. J Membr Biol 1999; 172:1–11.

14. Decsi T, Koletzko B. Effects of protein-energy malnutrition and human immunodeficiency virus-1 infection on essential fatty acid metabolism in children. Nutrition 2000; 16:447–453.

15. Grunfeld C, Feingold K. The role of the cytokines, interferon alpha and tumor necrosis factor in the hyperglyceridemia and wasting of AIDS. J Nutr 1992; 122:749–753.

16. Kinsella J, Lokesh B, Broughton S, Whelan J. Dietary polyunsaturated fatty acids and eicosanoids: potential effects on the modulation of inflammatory and immune cells: an overview. Nutrition 1990; 6:24–44.

17. Pichard C, Sudre P, Karegard V, Yerly S, Slosman D, Delley V, Perrin L, Hirschel B. Swiss HIV Cohort Study, A randomized double-blind controlled study of 6 months of oral nutrition supplementation with arginine and Ω-3 fatty acids in HIV-infected patients. AIDS 1998; 12:53–63.

18. Begin M, Manku M, Horrobin D. Plasma fatty acid levels in patients with acquired immune deficiency syndrome and in controls. Prostaglandins Leukot Essent Fatty Acids 1989; 37:135–137.

19. Eritsland I. Safety considerations of polyunsaturated fatty acids. American Journal of Clinical Nutrition 2000; 71:197S–201S.

29

Cardiovascular Involvement in Simian AIDS in Nonhuman Primates

George G. Sokos and **Richard P. Shannon**
Allegheny General Hospital, Pittsburgh, Pennsylvania, U.S.A.

Angela A. L. Carville
New England Primate Research Center,
Southborough, Massachusetts, U.S.A.

INTRODUCTION

Over the course of the last decade, considerable strides have been made in the treatment of human immunodeficiency virus (HIV) infection, with resultant reductions in mortality and morbidity (1). Similarly, the clinical manifestations of HIV infection have changed dramatically over this period. The presenting signs and symptoms of immunodeficiency and associated opportunistic infections have been largely replaced by organ-specific involvement, such as nephropathy. More recently, as viral loads have been reduced, these clinical manifestations have further evolved to include adverse effects associated with antiretroviral agents, and cardiomyopathy has become increasingly recognized as clinical sequela of chronic retroviral infection.

Early estimates suggested that as many as 6% of all HIV-infected patients would have cardiovascular involvement and as many as 10 to 18% of seropositive individuals would have clinical evidence of left ventricular dysfunction (2). The development of dilated cardiomyopathy occurs in a poorly defined number of patients with HIV infection. With the increasing recognition of cardiovascular syndromes in HIV infection, numerous questions have been raised about the pathogenesis of HIV cardiomyopathy. In particular, cardiac myocytes and vascular endothelium do not appear to express the obligatory CD4 receptors and other coreceptors critical for productive HIV infection (3). How the HIV virus makes its way into the heart and, furthermore, how it inflicts its injury remains poorly understood.

To date, the study of HIV cardiomyopathy has been largely restricted to cohort studies in humans (4). These studies are frequently confounded by comorbid conditions that may themselves contribute to cardiovascular morbidity. Experimental transgenic murine models in which viral genes are expressed through recombinant technologies manifest some clinical signs of cardiovascular sequelae (5). However, these models are not associated with productive infection and do not closely mirror the human condition. Thus appropriate experimental animal models that manifest signs and symptoms of human AIDS, including cardiovascular involvement, seem most appropriate for the study of basic mechanisms in the pathogenesis of AIDS-related cardiomyopathy.

This chapter explores the role of experimental infection with simian immunodeficiency virus (SIV) in nonhuman primates as a suitable large animal model of AIDS cardiomyopathy. Our laboratory has extensive experience in this area. The insights and pathogenic mechanisms we have discerned are important in understanding the evolution of this complication in humans.

SIMIAN AIDS

The simian immunodeficiency virus (HTLV-II) is one of a class of lentiviruses that has a natural reservoir in African macaques and is closely related to the human immunodeficiency virus (HTLV-I) (6). These viruses, isolated first from rhesus macaques, have also been isolated in African green monkeys and sooty mangabeys. The virus appears to exist in a nonpathogenic reservoir against which the animals mount a robust antibody response. However, when the virus is experimentally introduced into Asian macaques, an immunodeficiency syndrome develops.

The clinical syndrome of simian AIDS following experimental infection in Asian macaques occurs within 6 to 8 weeks and includes the development of an acute transient maculopapular rash as well as visceral and axillary adenopathy. Over the course of many years of investigation, appropriate doses of the virus have been determined to ensure that no excess mortality associated with acute viral infection occurs, yet as many as 20% of infected Asian macaques will succumb following acute infection. However, those that survive develop chronic manifestations of the disease closely paralleling those seen in humans. These manifestations include weight loss, skeletal muscle wasting, superinfection with opportunistic organisms, and eventually the involvement of end organs, including the lung, brain, kidneys, intestines, and abdominal lymph nodes. Previous studies by King et al. (7) and Letvin et al. (6) first reported histopathological evidence of cardiac involvement in these nonhuman primates. However, these findings were largely left unexplored until more recent interest in cardiovascular abnormalities emerged (8).

The SIV virus shares with its human retroviral counterpart a specific tropism for bone marrow–derived cells. There is considerable controversy with respect to whether SIV infects cells not bearing CD4 receptors. The specificity of the CD4 molecule and the coreceptors CCR 5 and CXCR4 is critical for productive infection (9). Once these bone marrow–derived cells are infected with SIV, the immunological manifestations are considerable. Rhesus macaques that succumb within the first 6 months following SIV infection have no significant titers of anti-SIV antibody and no detectable virus-specific T-cell effector functions. Additionally, there are nonspecific qualitative and quantitative T-cell abnormalities. In contrast, the natural history of animals chronically infected with SIV is death within 1 to 2 years, ultimately determined by the frequency of opportunistic infection. The spectrum of opportunistic infections found in these animals closely resembles that observed in humans (i.e., *Pneumocystis carinii*, *Mycobacterium*, cytomegalovirus). In animals with chronic SIV infection, there is a prolonged clinical latency not unlike that observed in HIV infection. Immunological characteristics of the chronically infected animals include high antibody titers in response to the specific SIV strain used as well as early detectable virus-specific T-cell effector responses. This is consistent with previous experimental evidence suggesting that the ability to generate cytotoxic T-cell responses is associated with lower viral loads and a chronic, more protracted course. However, animals chronically infected with SIV, as is the case in humans with chronic HIV infection, eventually develop acute reductions in their CD4 lymphocyte count, and this remains the most useful marker of disease progression. While multiple organ system involvement has been noted in simian AIDS, only recently has there been convincing evidence of extensive functional as well as pathological cardiac involvement in this model (7). Our laboratory has studied the nature and extent of cardiac involvement in simian AIDS in an attempt to determine the pathogenesis of the cardiac injury.

CARDIOVASCULAR CONSEQUENCES OF ACUTE SIV INFECTION

Using cloned pathogenic virus ($SIV_{mac}239$), we have studied prospectively the consequences of acute retroviral infection on cardiac function by performing serial echocardiographic measurements of systolic and diastolic function (8). These measurements were taken prior to infection and at 6 weeks in a cohort of naive juvenile macaques. A similar age and sex matched cohort infected with $SIV_{mac}239$ Δ*nef*, a cloned virus with a knockout of the regulatory *nef* gene, which does not alter infectivity but limits viral replication, was used as an appropriate control (10,11). Animals infected with SIV Δ*nef* do not develop simian AIDS. In these studies, we have noticed no difference in left ventricular (LV) systolic function [baseline LV ejection fraction (LVEF) 73%, 6-week EF 71%] or LV chamber enlargement in either cohort (8). However, there was a significant difference in measured viral loads and a decline in CD4 cell count in the group infected with pathogenic strains of SIV compared to those infected with the Δ*nef* virus. The systemic viremia, as measured by recovery of the p27 antigen in the plasma, spiked at 2 to 4 weeks (0.2 to 2.7 ng p27/mL). No such antigenemia was manifest in the rhesus infected with SIV Δ*nef* virus. The CD4 cell counts declined by 50% in the pathogenic virus infected group, while there was no significant decline in the group infected with SIV Δ*nef*. It should be noted that the CD8+ T-cell subsets did not decline with acute viral infection. Thus, acute viral infection with pathological strains of SIV is not associated with functional or structural cardiovascular abnormalities.

CARDIOVASCULAR CONSEQUENCES OF CHRONIC SIV INFECTION

Our laboratory initially reported myocardial and vascular involvement in nonhuman primates chronically infected with $SIV_{mac}251$ or the cloned pathogenic virus $SIV_{mac}239$, which carries 93% sequence homology with the naturally occurring retrovirus. Both of these strains are associated with functional and histopathological cardiac abnormalities in approximately two-thirds of infected animals. LVEF was depressed significantly in rhesus monkeys chronically infected with pathogenic strains of SIV compared to those infected with SIV Δ*nef*. This was associated with contractile dysfunction and ventricular dilatation, as evidenced by increases in LV end-systolic volume and LV end-diastolic volume, respectively (Fig. 1).

To examine the underlying histopathological basis for the decline in LV function observed following chronic SIV infection, we conducted a systematic review of all myocardial samples harvested from 45 rhesus macaques that had succumbed to chronic simian AIDS following infection with $SIV_{mac}251$ or $SIV_{mac}239$. Cardiac histopathological lesions were evident in two-thirds of tissues examined, Lymphocytic myocarditis, which was found in 60% of the samples, was the most commonly encountered active histopathological lesion. The lymphocytic infiltrates included CD8- and CD4-positive cells. In approximately one-third of the cases examined, multinucleated cells were seen and stained positive for CD68 marker, indicative of macrophages (Fig. 2). The development of multinucleated cells in lymphocytic infiltrates has been seen in association with viral strains that have a particular affinity for CXCR4 coreceptor (12). The emergence of syncytial-inducing (SI) strains of SIV is the result of frequent viral mutations, particularly the error-prone reverse transcriptase activity, and lack of proofreading mechanisms during reverse transcription of viral RNA (12). A second, commonly encountered pathological lesion included extensive acellular areas of myocardial replacement fibrosis (Fig. 3).

In an attempt to determine why certain animals chronically infected with pathological strains of SIV develop cardiac involvement, we examined several clinical parameters. There were no significant differences in age (5.9 years), duration of infection (22 months), or body weight (5.5 kg). Notably, animals with simian AIDS that demonstrated cardiac involvement had lower viral loads, higher CD4 cell counts (867/µL versus 27/µL), and fewer opportunistic infections (33 versus 78%), which is consistent with their increased longevity. The higher CD4 counts in rhesus macaques with cardiac involvement are consistent with the finding of CD4+ T lymphocytes in the observed inflammatory lesions. Taken together, these data suggest that the relative maintenance of immunological responses may be an

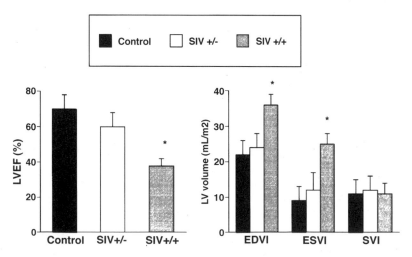

Figure 1 The effects of simian AIDS on LV structure and function. Compared to control, SIV-infected rhesus macaques had cardiac involvement, lower ejection fraction, and dilatated ventricles ($p < 0.5$).

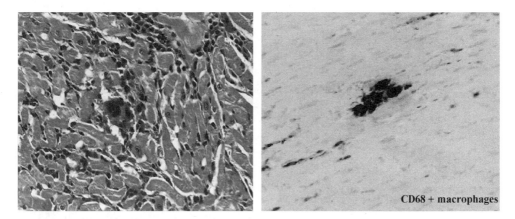

Figure 2 Lymphocytic myocarditis in a rhesus chronically infected with $SIV_{mac}251$ (left). The multinucleated synctial cell stains positive for the CD68 epitope, consistent with macrophage lineage.

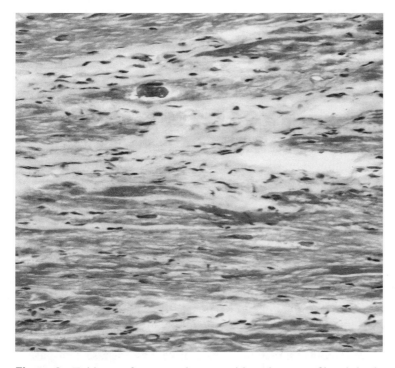

Figure 3 Evidence of myocyte dropout with replacement fibrosis in rhesus myocardium with chronic myocardial injury.

important feature in predisposing animals with simian AIDS to lymphocytic myocarditis and eventual replacement fibrosis.

ROLE OF RETROVIRAL INFECTION OF CARDIOMYOCYTES IN SIV CARDIOMYOPATHY

In order to better understand the pathogenesis of lymphocytic myocarditis, we examined myocardial samples harvested from these animals to determine the presence of retrovirus. A prerequisite for infection by HTLV-I or HTLV-II is the presence of CD4 receptor on target cells. Efficient infection also requires the presence of co-receptors, either CXCR4 or CCR5. In our population survey of SIV-infected animals, SIV viral remnants were found in the myocardium of approximately 45% of chronically infected animals. We employed a DNA riboprobe and subsequently a more sensitive RNA riboprobe. Colocalization techniques were used to identify the cellular constituents in which the virus resided. Using immunofluorescence probes, differential interference contrast, and confocal microscopy, we demonstrated that SIV always colocalized to CD4+ cells. In the presence of inflammatory infiltrates, the CD4+ cells bearing SIV were commonly macrophages, identified by the CD68+ epitope. In the absence of inflammation, SIV viral remnants colocalized to cardiac dendritic cells that also express the CD4 epitope. In no instance was the virus identified in cardiac myocytes. Taken together, these data suggest that SIV is frequently found in the myocardium of rhesus macaques chronically infected with SIV. When inflammatory infiltrates are observed, the virus localizes to tissue macrophages. When inflammation is absent, the virus localizes to cardiac dendritic cells. Thus, cardiac myocytes do not appear to be the primary target of SIV infection in the heart.

MECHANISM OF MYOCYTE CELL DEATH

In the presence of active inflammation in cardiac samples harvested from chronically infected animals with SIV, we next sought to identify the mechanisms of cellular injury. In the presence of active inflammation, we observed increased expression of Fas ligand on CD4+ T lymphocytes (Fig. 4). In addition, we found an upregulation of the Fas receptor on cardiac myocytes. This was associated with upregulation of active zymogens of caspases 2 and 3, indicative of the activation of Fas-FasL signaling in mediating cardiac myocyte apoptosis. Subsequent Tunel staining and DNA fragmentation studies prove that there was a marked increase in cellular apoptosis among myocyte and nonmyocyte populations within cardiac samples harvested from animals with chronic SIV infection. Taken together, these data indicate that active inflammation results in myocytic apoptosis mediated through the Fas-FasL pathway. We have subsequently shown that TNF-α and NOS2 are upregulated in the setting of chronic infection. Thus, active inflammation mediated as a consequence of SIV infection is associated with upregulation of cytokines, which increase the expression of Fas and FasL on appropriate cellular constituents. These, in turn, activate apoptotic cellular signaling cascades involving caspase 2/caspase 3, resulting in myocyte apoptosis.

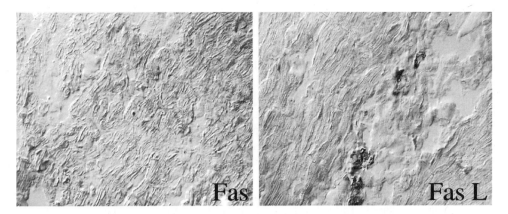

Figure 4 Immunohistochemical staining for Fas L on activated T cell and Fas receptor on cardiac myocytes in myocardium from a rhesus monkey with chronic SIV infection and lymphocytic myocarditis.

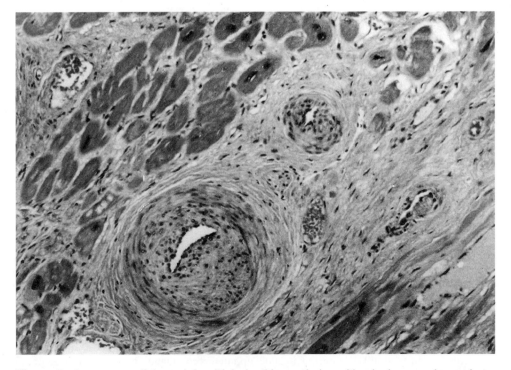

Figure 5 Intramyocardial arteriole with intimal hyperplasia and luminal encroachment in an area of chronic myocardial injury. These vascular lesions are characteristic of coronary arteriopathy observed with chronic SIV infection.

VASCULAR LESIONS IN SIV CARDIOMYOPATHY

Perhaps the most surprising observation made in these studies was the evidence of active vascular inflammation and vascular remodeling present in approximately one-third of animals with SIV-related cardiomyopathy (3). These vascular lesions take the form of cardiovascular infiltrates characterized by CD4 and CD8 + T cells. There were associated intimal and smooth hyperplastic responses culminating in the development of extensive intimal hyperplasia with luminal encroachment, which resulted in a reduction of luminal cross section. In acute inflammation, these vessels were sometimes seen obstructed with active thrombus (Fig. 5). Taken together, this histopathological substrate suggests that vascular inflammation and coronary arteritis may contribute substantially to myocyte cell death through an mechanism mediated by ischemia. Importantly, additional pathological surveys suggest that these vascular lesions are also present in pulmonary and renal arteries, suggesting a systemic vascular inflammation. The nature and extent of these cellular infiltrates in the process of vascular remodeling is currently the subject of ongoing investigation.

SUMMARY

SIV cardiomyopathy in nonhuman primates provides a unique and appropriate model of active retroviral infection associated with myocardial injury. Our findings indicate that cardiac involvement is commonly observed in chronically infected animals. Animals that appear to be predisposed include those with relative maintenance of immunological responsiveness, higher CD4 counts, and fewer opportunistic infections, which is consistent with the emergence of cardiomyopathy as a late manifestation of the syndrome. Our data suggest strongly that SIV does not infect cardiac myocytes but rather that cardiac myocytes are injured inadvertently by associated active inflammation, although the triggering events remain to be elucidated. Furthermore, myocardial injury appears to be mediated through a Fas-FasL (CD95/APO-1)–dependent pathway and associated cardiac myocyte apoptosis. Finally, we have verified a high incidence of coronary vascular involvement of SIV infection in nonhuman primates. This important observation may shed light on the predisposition of humans to vascular events that have recently been recognized with the widespread use of highly active antiretroviral agents. These observations underscore the importance of the nonhuman primate model that we have studied with SIV-related diseases.

REFERENCES

1. Yeni PG, Hammer SM, Carpenter CC, Cooper DA, Fischl MA, Gatell JM, Gazzard BG, Hirsch MS, Jacobsen DM, Katzenstein DA, Montaner JS, Richman DD, Saag MS, Schechter M, Schoole RT, Thompson MA, Vella S, Volberding PA. Antiretroviral treatment for adult HIV infection in 2002: updated recommendations of the International AIDS Society–USA Panel. JAMA 2002; 288(2):222–235.
2. Ferguson DW, Volpp BD. Cardiovascular complications of AIDS. Heart Dis Stroke 1994; 3:388–394.

3. Shannon RP. SIV cardiomyopathy in non-human primates. Trends Cardiovasc Med 2001; 11:242–246.
4. Roldan EO, Moskowitz L, Hensley GT. Pathology of the heart in acquired immunodeficiency syndrome. Arch Pathol Lab Med 1987; 111:943–946.
5. Hanna Z, Kay DG, Cool M, et al. Transgenic mice expressing human immunodeficiency virus type 1 in immune cells develop a severe AIDS-like disease. J Virol 1998; 72:121–132.
6. Letvin NL. Animal models for AIDS. Immunol Today 1990; 92:322–326.
7. Letvin NL, King NW. Immunologic and pathologic manifestations of the infection of rhesus monkeys with simian immunodeficiency virus of macaques. J AIDS 1990; 3:1023–1040.
8. Shannon RP, Simon MA, Geng JY, et al. Dilated cardiomyopathy associated with simian AIDS in non-human primates. Circulation 2000; 101:185–193.
9. Damas JK, Eiken HG, Oie E, et al. Myocardial expression of CC- and CXC-chemokines and their receptors in human end-stage heart failure. Cardiovasc Res 2000; 47:778–787.
10. Bourgault I, Chirat F, Tartar A, et al. Simian immunodefiency virus as a model for vaccination against HIV. Induction in rhesus macaques of GAG- or NEF- specific cytotoxic T lymphocytes by lipopeptides. J Immunol 1994; 152:2530–2537.
11. Reiger DA, Desrosiers RC. The complete nucleotide sequence of a pathogenic molecular clone of simian immunodefiency virus. AIDS Res Hum Retrovir 1990; 6:1221–1231.
12. Van Rij RP, Blaak H, Visser JA, et al. Differential co-receptor expression allows for independent evolution of non-syncytium-inducing and syncytium inducing HIV-1. J Clin Invest 2000; 106:1039–1052.

30

Cardiac Disease in HIV-1 Tg Animals

Paul Jolicoeur, Ping Yue, Zaher Hanna, Marie-Chantal Simard, and Denis G. Kay
Clinical Research Institute of Montreal, Montreal, Quebec, Canada

INTRODUCTION

The acquired immunodeficiency syndrome (AIDS) is induced by the human immu-nodeficiency virus (HIV-1) and represents a multiorgan disease (1–3). A major feature of the disease is the progressive loss of CD4 + T-cells with lymphadenopathy, thymic atrophy, and destruction of the architecture of lymphoid organs. Other significant AIDS-related phenotypes include lung disease (lymphocytic interstitial pneumonitis) (4,5), renal disease (interstitial nephritis, segmental glomerulosclerosis) (6–8), wasting (9,10), peripheral (11) and central (12–15) neurodegenerative diseases, hematological disorders (16), and cardiac disease. Such cardiac disease is now recognized as a relatively frequent complication of HIV-1 infection and is characterized by a pro-gressive dilated cardiomyopathy sometimes accompanied by compensatory cardiac hypertrophy and functional loss. A variety of histopathological lesions have been observed in hearts of HIV-1 infected individuals, the most common being cardio-myocyte necrosis, often with fibrosis. Mononuclear cell infiltration is often observed with these lesions but may be absent. Several reviews have appeared on the clinical and pathological aspects of the AIDS-associated cardiomyopathy (17–25).

The pathogenesis of AIDS-associated cardiac disease is not at all clear at the moment and animal models will undoubtedly improve our understanding of its cellular and molecular basis. Rhesus macaques infected with an HIV-1–related lentivirus, the simian immunodeficiency virus (SIV), have been among the most widely used animal models for HIV-1 infection and AIDS (26,27). Cardiac disease develops in SIV-1 infected macaques (28), and study of this simian model of cardiac disease is likely to shed light on its pathogenesis. Fortunately, cardiac disease has, in the last few years, been found to develop in transgenic (Tg) mice or rats expressing HIV-1 gene products. The present review focuses on these Tg animal models.

CARDIAC DISEASE IN HIV-1 Tg MICE OR RATS

Two models of HIV-1 Tg mice [Tg26 (29) and CD4C/HIV (30)], one model of SIV Tg mice (31) and one model of HIV-1 Tg rats (32) have been reported to develop cardiomyopathy.

Tg26 Mice

A review of the main characteristics of the cardiomyopathy developing in Tg26 mice has recently been published (33). These Tg mice harbor an HIV-1 genome (strain NL4-3) deleted of *gag* and *pol* sequences (34). Transgene viral RNA is expressed under the regulation of the HIV-1 long terminal repeat (LTR) promoter and is widespread. The highest expression was documented in skin, muscle, and tail but was also detectable in thymus, intestine, kidney, eye, brain, and spleen (34,35). However, heart, liver, pancreas, and lung did not express the transgene (36). Hemizygous Tg26 mice develop a severe renal disease, as well as skin and ocular diseases (34,37,38), but they do not show signs of CD4+ T-cell loss. Signs of renal disease (proteinuria) are seen early, by day 20 to 25 after birth (36,39).

Intriguingly, novel phenotypes [cachexia, growth retardation, lymphoproliferation with an increased number of splenic CD4+ and CD8+ T-cells, thymic atrophy, and early death (40)] were also observed in Tg26 mice homozygous for the transgene. Differences in transgene expression between homo- and heterozygote Tg26 mice were not found in kidney, spleen, and thymus but were mainly observed in lymph nodes, suggesting that some and perhaps all the novel phenotypes may not be related to transgene expression. The appearance of novel phenotypes in homozygote Tg-positive animals suggests the presence of a recessive host mutation induced by the chromosomal insertion of the transgene. This type of mutation is not rare during the construction of Tg mice (41–48).

It was recently reported that hemizygous Tg26 mice show cardiac dysfunction and reduced cardiac expression of sarcoplasmic calcium ATPase (SERCA2) but no histological heart lesions as compared to normal non-Tg mice (29,49). "Decreases in the first derivative of the maximal change in left ventricular (LV) systolic pressure with respect to time (+dP/dt)" and "an increased half-time of relaxation and ventricular relaxation ($-dP/dt$)" were reported in these Tg mice as compared to normal control mice (25,49).

CD4C/HIV Tg Mice

The CD4C/HIV Tg mice (50,51) express HIV-1 gene products under the regulation of the CD4C regulatory sequences from the human CD4 gene. Expression is targeted in CD4+ T cells (both immature $CD4^+CD8^+$ thymic T cells, and mature CD4+ T cells) and in cells of the myeloid lineage (macrophages, Kupffer cells, and dendritic cells). The CD4C/HIV Tg mice develop an AIDS-like disease very similar to human AIDS: weight loss/failure to thrive, wasting, early death, progressive and preferential loss of CD4+ T cells, thymic atrophy, lymphadenopathy, increased B-cell numbers, increased numbers of CD8+ T cells, inversion of the CD4/CD8 ratio, activation of T and B cells, production of autoantibodies, expansion of spleen marginal zone, impaired germinal center formation, lung disease (lymphocytic interstitial pneumonitis), kidney disease (interstitial nephritis, segmental glomerulosclerosis), and cardiac disease (30,50–52).

The cardiac disease of CD4C/HIV Tg mice consists of histopathological lesions and functional abnormalities (30). Heart enlargement was frequent in the early back crossing on the C3H background [from (C3H × C57BL/6)F2] but less so as inbreeding into the C3H background progressed. The lesions represent multifocal areas of myocytolysis (Fig. 1), sometimes associated with myocarditis. In the C3H background, calcifications also occur. In addition, both focal and diffuse interstitial fibrosis (detected by Sirius red staining) is observed in the heart of these Tg mice. CD4C/HIV Tg cardiomyocytes are decorated with endogenous immunoglobulin (Ig), which could represent antiheart autoantibodies. However, no disturbance of the dystrophin-associated glycoprotein (DAG) complex could be documented (Fig. 2).

Two functional abnormalities were detected in these Tg mice (30). The coronary vasculature of CD4C/HIV Tg mice showed signs of enhanced vasospasm under stress or hypoxia. This arteriospasm affected mainly the medium and small coronary vessels. Echocardiography also revealed functional defects: an increased systolic left ventricular internal dimension and a decrease of the fractional shortening, ejection fraction, stroke volume, and cardiac output, indicating compromised LV function.

Interestingly, the functional cardiac defects and the cardiac lesions may have a distinct pathogenesis, as both phenotypes tend to segregate independently during inbreeding on the C3H background. We noticed, indeed, that the penetrance of histopathological cardiac lesions in CD4C/HIV Tg mice decreased to ~20 to 25% after inbreeding (>10 generations), while the penetrance of the functional abnormalities detected by echocardiography was high (30).

CD4C/SHIV-nef^{SIV}

Tg mice expressing SIV nef under the CD4C regulatory sequences were also generated (31). These CD4C/SHIV-nef^{SIV} Tg mice develop an AIDS-like disease very similar to that of CD4C/HIV Tg mice except that the kidney and cardiac diseases were more severe and that a thymic developmental defect was observed. Heart enlargement was very severe in CD4C/SIV Tg mice during early breeding on the C3H background.

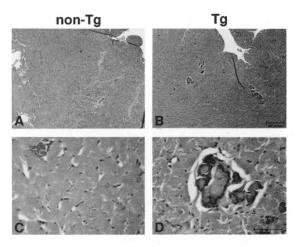

Figure 1 Cardiac pathology in CD4C/HIV^{MutB} Tg mice. Heart sections from non-Tg (A,C) and Tg (B,D) mice shown at low (A,B) and higher (C,D) power. Note the multifocal lesions in the left ventricular wall of Tg heart, consisting of myocytolysis with calcifications. Scale bar in B (for A,B) represents 250 μ*M* and in D (for C,D) represents 50 μ*M*. (Counterstain, hematoxylin and eosin.)

non-Tg   Tg   non-Tg   Tg

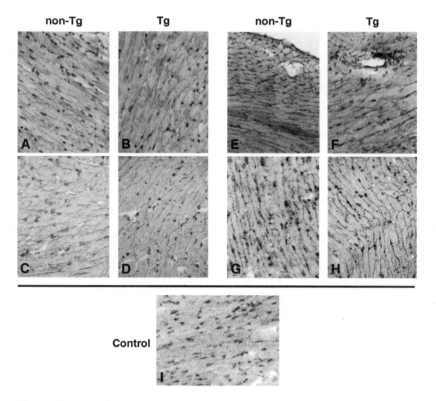

Control

Figure 2 The dystrophin-associated glycoprotein (DAG) complex is intact in the heart of CD4C/HIV Tg mice. To assess the integrity of the DAG complex, immunohistochemistry was performed with antibodies against some of its component proteins—namely dystrobrevin (A,B), γ (C,D), ε (E,F), and α-(G,H)-sarcoglycans—on heart sections from non-Tg (A,C,E,G) or Tg (B,D,F,H) hearts. No differences between the staining patterns for any of these proteins could be discerned between non-Tg and Tg animals. (I) Secondary antibody control (for α-sarcoglycan). No sarcolemmal immunoreactivity was detected with any of the secondary antibodies utilized. [Magnification (all panels): ×100. Counterstain: hematoxylin.]

Histopathological lesions in the hearts of these mice were also multifocal and were similar to those found in CD4C/HIV Tg mice. Data from echocardiography analysis are not yet available for these Tg mice.

HIV-1 Tg Rats

The HIV Tg rats harbor an HIV-1 genome (strain NL4-3) with a deletion of gag-pol sequences similar to that of Tg26 mice (32). Expression is controlled by the viral LTR and was documented in lymph nodes, thymus, liver, kidney, and spleen. Tg rats developed several AIDS-like phenotypes: weight loss, neurological abnormalities (gliosis, neuronal cell death, capillary changes), interstitial pneumonia, lymphade-nopathy, kidney disease (tubulointerstitial nephritis, glomerulolosclerosis), follicular hyperplasia of spleen and expansion of marginal zone, abnormal T-helper functions, and cardiac disease. The Tg rats also exhibit some phenotypes usually not encountered in HIV-1–infected individuals (cataracts, skin lesions). Unfortunately, the status of the CD4+ T-cell numbers was not reported.

The cardiac disease of Tg rats consisted of myocardial inflammation (necrosis, mononuclear cell infiltrate, and vascular abnormalities) and endocarditis. The penetrance of this phenotype was not specified.

PATHOGENESIS OF CARDIAC DISEASE IN HIV-1 Tg ANIMALS

One of the striking features of the cardiac disease developing in CD4C/HIV or CD4C/SHIV-nef[SIV] Tg mice, and possibly in HIV Tg rats, is the fact that it is induced distally by the expression of HIV-1 or SIV gene products in cells of the immune system, most likely by an indirect mechanism (30–32). This contrasts significantly with a number of other models of cardiomyopathy in mice (and in humans) in which disturbances (enhanced or decreased expression, mutation) of expression of structural proteins of cardiomyocytes themselves are primarily involved in development of cardiac diseases (53–61).

Two main populations of immune cells express the transgene in CD4C/HIV or CD4C/SHIV-nef[SIV] Tg mice through the CD4C promoter: CD4+ T cells (both immature CD4+CD8+ thymic T cells and mature CD4+ T cells) and cells of the myeloid lineage (macrophages, Kupffer cells, and dendritic cells) (50,51,62,63). In theory, reprogramming of any of these cell subpopulations by HIV-1 or SIV Nef could be responsible for initiating the cascade of events leading to the various cardiac lesions and cardiac dysfunctions observed. Experiments are in progress to determine the identity of the transgene-expressing cell population(s) responsible for eliciting these cardiac phenotypes.

The most obvious proximal cause of the cardiac disease in CD4C/HIV, CD4C/SHIV-nef[SIV], Tg26 Tg mice, and HIV Tg rats could be the kidney disease that develops in these strains and is associated with moderately elevated blood pressure (hypertension), as documented at least in the CD4C/HIV Tg mice (Paradis et al., in preparation). Hypertension could contribute to at least some of the functional cardiac defects observed in CD4C/HIV and Tg26 Tg mice. However, in CD4C/HIV Tg mice bred on the C3H background, we have noticed a segregation of the cardiac lesion phenotype and kidney disease (30), suggesting that kidney disease may not be responsible or may not be sufficient to induce the cardiac lesions. This notion is reinforced by the observation that in Tg 26 mice, severe kidney disease is not associated with cardiac lesions (29).

Another likely contributing factor to the cardiac disease of CD4C/HIV and CD4C/SHIV-nef[SIV] Tg mice is the presence of immunoglobulin (Ig) decorating the cardiomyocytes in these Tg mice (30,31). These may represent antiheart autoantibodies. Heart disease induced by antiheart antibodies has been described in humans (64) and in animal models (65). We have also reported that these CD4C/HIV and CD4C/SHIV-nef[SIV] Tg mice produce elevated anti-DNA antibodies (31,52).

Finally, a vascular problem may represent another proximal cause of the multifocal lesions observed in CD4C/HIV Tg mice. A vasospasm affecting mainly the medium and small cardiac vessels and enhanced under hypoxia and stress was documented in these Tg mice (30). This type of mechanism could explain the multifocal nature of the lesions.

WHAT HAVE WE LEARNED ABOUT HIV-1 CARDIOMYOPATHY FROM HIV-1 Tg ANIMALS?

From the few models of Tg animals available, already important knowledge about the HIV-1 associated cardiomyopathy has emerged.

First, this cardiomyopathy is likely to be caused by HIV-1 itself, directly or indirectly, and not by opportunistic infections. Indeed, Tg26 mice develop cardiac disease despite the fact that they do not show loss of CD4+ T-cells, while CD4C/HIV, CD4C/SHIV-nef[SIV] Tg mice and HIV Tg rats develop cardiac disease in SPF facilities in absence of obvious opportunistic infection.

Second, since Tg26 develop functional cardiac abnormalities in absence of loss of CD4+ T cells, it appears that T-cell impairment may not be required to elicit such dysfunctions. Rather, perturbation of cells of the myeloid lineage by HIV-1 gene products may affect the heart.

Third, cardiac disease develops in Tg26 mice (29) and HIV-1 Tg rats (32) that do not express HIV-1 Gag and Pol proteins and in CD4C/HIV[MutG] (30) and CD4C/SHIV-nef[SIV] (31) Tg mice expressing only Nef. Therefore, Gag and Pol proteins are not involved in the development of cardiac disease in these animals, and it appears that Nef harbors a major determinant of cardiac disease, at least in mice. In view of the fact that the several phenotypes of the AIDS-like disease of CD4C/HIV (51) closely mimic those in human AIDS, Nef is also likely to represent a major pathogenic factor for human hearts as well.

Fourth, in CD4C/HIV Tg mice, cardiac disease arises in the absence of detectable expression of HIV-1 in cardiomyocytes or coronary vasculature (30). Therefore expression of HIV-1 in cardiomyocytes or blood vessels may not be required either in humans for the development of an HIV-1–associated cardiomyopathy.

Fifth, in Tg26 mice, the presence of the HIV-1 transgene appears to synergize with antiretroviral therapy to induce cardiac dysfunction and cardiomyocyte damage (29,49), indicating that the apparent cardiac toxicity of drug therapy in individuals with AIDS may, at least in part, be influenced by the metabolic milieu generated by HIV-1 infection itself.

Sixth, in CD4C/HIV and CD4C/SHIV-nef[SIV] Tg mice, cardiomyopathy develops as a consequence of expression of Nef in cells of the immune system (CD4[+] T-cells or cells of the myeloid lineage) (30,31). This suggests that reprogramming of some immune cells by Nef induces an environment that predisposes to cardiac disease. It is conceivable that other cardiac diseases in individuals not infected by HIV-1 may also originate from specific disturbances of some of their immune CD4+ T cells or myeloid cell subpopulations. These immune alterations could represent specific mutations or infection by other microbes mimicking molecularly the action of Nef in these cells. This could be independent of bonafide cytotoxic T-cell (CTL) response or of antiheart autoantibodies generally thought to be responsible for cardiomyopathy after viral or bacterial infection.

CONCLUSION

Despite the fact that cardiac disease was recognized only recently as a consequence of HIV-1 expression in Tg animals, it is already apparent that these models mimic quite closely the human cardiac diseases arising in HIV-1 infected individuals with AIDS. It is expected that a study of these models will shed light on the pathogenesis of this human cardiomyopathy and hopefully will lead to a better therapy and ultimately to its prevention.

ACKNOWLEDGMENTS

Work in the authors' laboratory was supported by grants to Paul Jolicoeur from the Canadian Institute of Health Research and from the National Heart, Lung and Blood Institute, National Institutes of Health (HL-59846).

REFERENCES

1. Levy JA. Pathogenesis of human immunodeficiency virus infection. Microbiol Rev 1993; 57:183–289.
2. Pantaleo G, Graziosi C, Fauci AS. New concepts in the immunopathogenesis of human immunodeficiency virus infection. N Engl J Med 1993; 328:327–335.
3. Fauci AS, Pantaleo G, Stanley S, Weissman D. Immunopathogenic mechanisms of HIV infection. Ann Intern Med 1996; 124(7):654–663.
4. McSherry GD. Human immunodeficiency-virus-related pulmonary infections in children. Semin Respir Infect 1996; 11:173–183.
5. Clarke JR, Robinson DS, Coker RJ, Miller RF, Mitchell DM. Role of the human immunodeficiency virus within the lung. Thorax 1995; 50:567–576.
6. Rappaport J, Kopp JB, Klotman PE. Host virus interactions and the molecular regulation of HIV-1: role in the pathogenesis of HIV-associated nephropathy. Kidney Int 1994; 46:16–27.
7. Seney FD Jr, Burns DK, Silva FG. Acquired immunodeficiency syndrome and the kidney. Am J Kidney Dis 1990; 16(1):1–13.
8. Wenzel UO, Stahl RA. Chemokines, renal disease, and HIV infection. Nephron 1999; 81(1):5–16.
9. Grunfeld C. What causes wasting in AIDS? N Engl J Med 1995; 333:123–124.
10. Strawford A, Hellerstein M. The etiology of wasting in the human immunodeficiency virus and acquired immunodeficiency syndrome. Semin Oncol 1998; 25(2:suppl 6):76–81.
11. Simpson DM, Olney RK. Peripheral neuropathies associated with human immunodeficiency virus infection. Neurol Clin 1992; 10:685–711.
12. Price RW, Brew B, Sibtis J, Rosenblum M, Scheck AC, Cleary P. The brain in AIDS: central nervous system HIV infection and AIDS dementia complex. Science 1988; 239:586–592.
13. Gendelman HE, Persidsky Y, Ghorpade A, Limoges J, Stins M, Fiala M, Morrisett R. The neuropathogenesis of the AIDS dementia complex. Aids 1997; 11(suppl A):S35–S45.
14. Glass JD, Johnson RT. Human immunodeficiency virus and the brain. Annu Rev Neurosci 1996; 19:1–26.
15. Price RW. Neurological complications of HIV infection. Lancet 1996; 348(9025):445–452.
16. Moses A, Nelson J, Bagby GC Jr. The influence of human immunodeficiency virus-1 on hematopoiesis. Blood 1998; 91(5):1479–1495.
17. Acierno LJ. Cardiac complications in acquired immunodeficiency syndrome (AIDS): a review. J American Coll Cardiol 1989; 13(5):1144–1154.
18. Anderson DW, Virmani R. Emerging patterns of heart disease in human immunodeficiency virus infection. Hum Pathol 1990; 21(3):253–259.

19. Dacso CC. Pericarditis in AIDS. Cardiol Clin 1990; 8(4):697–699.

20. Ferguson DW, Volpp BD. Cardiovascular complications of AIDS. Heart Dis Stroke 1994; 3(6):388–394.

21. Herskowitz A. Cardiomyopathy and other symptomatic heart diseases associated with HIV infection. Curr Opin Cardiol 1996; 11:325–331.

22. Kaul S, Fishbein MC, Siegel RJ. Cardiac manifestations of acquired immune deficiency syndrome: a 1991 update. Am Heart J 1991; 122(2):535–544.

23. Michaels AD, Lederman RJ, MacGregor JS, Cheitlin MD. Cardiovascular involvement in AIDS. Curr Probl Cardiology 1997; 22(3):109–148.

24. Lipshultz SE. Cardiology in AIDS. New York: Chapman & Hall, 1998.

25. Lewis W. Cardiomyopathy in AIDS: a pathophysiological perspective. Progr Cardiovasc Dis 2000; 43(2):151–170.

26. Desrosiers RC, Letvin NL. Animal models for acquired immunodeficiency syndrome. Rev Infect Dis 1987; 9:438–446.

27. Desrosiers RC, Ringler DJ. Use of simian immunodeficiency viruses for AIDS research. Intervirology 1989; 30:301–312.

28. Shannon RP, Simon MA, Mathier MA, Geng YJ, Mankad S, Lackner AA. Dilated cardiomyopathy associated with simian AIDS in nonhuman primates. Circulation 2000; 101(2):185–193.

29. Lewis W, Haase CP, Raidel SM, Russ RB, Sutliff RL, Hoit BD, Samarel AM. Combined antiretroviral therapy causes cardiomyopathy and elevates plasma lactate in transgenic AIDS mice. Lab Invest 2001; 81:1527–1536.

30. Kay DG, Yue P, Hanna Z, Jothy S, Tremblay E, Jolicoeur P. Cardiac disease in transgenic mice expressing human immunodeficiency virus-1 nef in cells of the immune system. Am J Pathol 2002; 161:321–335.

31. Simard M-C, Chrobak P, Kay DG, Hanna Z, Jothy S, Jolicoeur P. Expression of simian immunodeficiency virus nef in immune cells of transgenic mice leads to a severe AIDS-like disease. J Virol 2002; 76:3981–3995.

32. Reid W, Sadowska M, Denaro F, Rao S, Foulke J Jr, Hayes N, Jones O, Doodnauth D, Davis H, Sill A, O'Driscoll P, Huso D, Fouts T, Lewis G, Hill M, Kamin-Lewis R, Wei C, Ray P, Gallo RC, Reitz M, Bryant J. An HIV-1 transgenic rat that develops HIV-related pathology and immunologic dysfunction. Proc Natl Acad Sci USA 2001; 98(16):9271–9276.

33. Lewis W. AIDS cardiomyopathy: physiological, molecular and biochemical studies in the transgenic mouse. Ann N Y Acad Sci 2002; 946:46–56.

34. Dickie P, Felser J, Eckhaus M, Bryant J, Silver J, Marinos N, Notkins AL. HIV-associated nephropathy in transgenic mice expressing HIV-1 genes. Virology 1991; 185:109–119.

35. Bruggeman LA, Thomson M, Nelson PJ, Kopp JB, Rappaport J, Klotman PE, Klotman ME. Patterns of HIV-1 mRNA expression in transgenic mice are tissue-dependent. Virology 1994; 202:940–948.

36. Dickie P. Nef modulation of HIV type 1 gene expression and cytopathicity in tissues of HIV transgenic mice. AIDS Res Hum Retrovir 2000; 16(8):777–790.

37. Dickie P. HIV type 1 nef perturbs eye lens development in transgenic mice. AIDS Res Hum Retrovir 1996; 12(3):177–189.

38. Kopp JB, Klotman ME, Adler SH, Bruggeman LA, Dickie P, Marinos NJ, Eckhaus M, Bryant JL, Notkins AL, Klotman PE. Progressive glomerulosclerosis and enhanced renal accumulation of basement membrane components in mice transgenic for human immunodeficiency virus type 1 genes. Proc Natl Acad Sci USA 1992; 89:1577–1581.

39. Kajiyama W, Kopp JB, Marinos NJ, Klotman PE, Dickie P. Glomerulosclerosis and viral gene expression in HIV-transgenic mice: role of nef. Kidney Int 2000; 58(3):1148–1159.

40. Santoro TJ, Bryant JL, Pellicoro J, Klotman ME, Kopp JB, Bruggeman LA, Franks RR,

Notkins AL, Klotman PE. Growth failure and AIDS-like cachexia syndrome in HIV-1 transgenic mice. Virology 1994; 201:147–151.

41. Covarrubias L, Nishida Y, Mintz B. Early postimplantation embryo lethality due to DNA rearrangements in a transgenic mouse strain. Proc Natl Acad Sci USA 1986; 83:6020–6024.

42. Covarrubias L, Nishida Y, Terao M, D'Eustachio P, Mintz B. Cellular DNA rearrangements and early developmental arrest caused by DNA insertion in transgenic mouse embryos. Mol Cell Biol 1987; 7:2243–2247.

43. Keller SA, Liptay S, Hajra A, Meisler MH. Transgene-induced mutation of the murine steel locus. Proc Natl Acad Sci USA 1990; 87:10019–10022.

44. McNeish JD, Scott WJ Jr, Potter SS. Legless, a novel mutation found in PHT1-1 transgenic mice. Science 1988; 241:837–839.

45. Wagner EF, Covarrubias L, Stewart TA, Mintz B. Prenatal lethalities in mice homozygous for human growth hormone gene sequences integrated in the germ line. Cell 1983; 35:647–655.

46. Weiher H, Noda T, Gray DA, Sharpe AH, Jaenisch R. Transgenic mouse model of kidney disease: insertional inactivation of ubiquitously expressed gene leads to nephrotic syndrome. Cell 1990; 62:425–434.

47. Woychik RP, Stewart TA, Davis LG, D'Eustachio P, Leder P. An inherited limb deformity created by insertional mutagenesis in a transgenic mouse. Nature 1985; 318:36–40.

48. Xiang X, Benson KF, Chada K. Mini-mouse: disruption of the pygmy locus in a transgenic insertional mutant. Science 1990; 247:967–969.

49. Lewis W, Grupp IL, Grupp G, Hoit B, Morris R, Samarel AM, Bruggeman L, Klotman PE. Cardiac dysfunction occurs in the HIV-1 transgenic mouse treated with zidovudine. Lab Invest 2000; 80(2):187–197.

50. Hanna Z, Kay DG, Cool M, Jothy S, Rebai N, Jolicoeur P. Transgenic mice expressing human immunodeficiency virus type 1 in immune cells develop a severe AIDS-like disease. J Virol 1998; 72:121–132.

51. Hanna Z, Kay DG, Rebai N, Guimond A, Jothy S, Jolicoeur P. Nef harbors a major determinant of pathogenicity for an AIDS-like disease induced by HIV-1 in transgenic mice. Cell 1998; 95:163–175.

52. Poudrier J, Weng X, Kay DG, Paré G, Calvo EL, Hanna Z, Kosko-Vilbois MH, Jolicoeur P. The AIDS disease of CD4C/HIV transgenic mice shows impaired germinal centers and autoantibodies and develops in the absence of IFN-γ and IL-6. Immunity 2001; 15:173–185.

53. Kushwaha SS, Fallon JT, Fuster V. Restrictive cardiomyopathy. N Engl J Med 1997; 336(4):267–276.

54. Marban E. Cardiac channelopathies. Nature 2002; 415(6868):213–218.

55. Seidman JG, Seidman C. The genetic basis for cardiomyopathy: from mutation identification to mechanistic paradigms. Cell 2001; 104(4):557–567.

56. Towbin JA, Bowles KR, Bowles NE. Etiologies of cardiomyopathy and heart failure. Nat Med 1999; 5(3):266–267.

57. Curran ME. Molecular basis of inherited cardiac arrhythmias. In: Chien K, ed. Molecular Basis of Cardiovascular Disease. Philadelphia: Saunders, 1999:302–311.

58. Keating MT, Sanguinetti MC. Molecular and cellular mechanisms of cardiac arrhythmias. Cell 2001; 104(4):569–580.

59. Hemler ME. Dystroglycan versatility. Cell 1999; 97(5):543–546.

60. Straub V, Campbell KP. Muscular dystrophies and the dystrophin-glycoprotein complex. Curr Opin Neurol 1997; 10(2):168–175.

61. Towbin JA. The role of cytoskeletal proteins in cardiomyopathies. Curr Opin Cell Biol 1998; 10(1):131–139.

62. Hanna Z, Simard C, Jolicoeur P. Specific expression of the human CD4 gene in mature

CD4+ CD8− and immature CD4+ CD8+ T cells, and in macrophages of transgenic mice. Mol Cell Biol 1994; 14:1084–1094.

63. Hanna Z, Rebai N, Poudrier J, Jolicoeur P. Distinct regulatory elements are required for faithful expression of human CD4 in T-cells, macrophages and dendritic cells of transgenic mice. Blood 2001; 98:2275–2278.

64. Cetta F, Michels VV. The autoimmune basis of dilated cardiomyopathy. Ann Med 1995; 27(2):169–173.

65. Huber SA. Autoimmunity in myocarditis: relevance of animal models. Clin Immunol Immunopathol 1997; 83(2):93–102.

31

Murine AIDS and HIV-1 Dementia

Mohsen Araghi-Niknam
University of Minnesota, Minneapolis, Minnesota, U.S.A.

HIV-1–associated dementia (HAD) involves nearly 15 to 20% of patients infected with AIDS (1). It is known as a metabolic encephalopathy induced by viral infection of brain mononuclear phagocytes (MPs) (perivascular and parenchymal brain macrophages/microglia) and continues through paracrine-amplified, inflammatory, and neurotoxic reactions. HAD has been defined clinically by the impediment of concentration, distorted cognition, slowness of movement, and behavioral changes (2). In the central nervous system, macrophages and resident microglia constitute a cellular reservoir of HIV-1, presenting a safe haven for virus, so that we will likely observe virus and host-coded producing neurotoxins in HAD (3). The neurotoxic activity has been characterized in many experiments via N-methyl aspartate (NMDA) receptors (4,5). Many researchers have reported that the probable causes are as follows: the virion protein toxin candidates NTox (6), platelet activating factor (7), tumor necrosis factor alpha (TNF-α) (8), quinolinate (9), Tat (10), gp120 (11), and gp41 (12). Furthermore, the strength of these toxins is in HIV-infected macrophage secretions, cerebrospinal fluid, or most likely within the brain tissues of subjects infected with HIV-1.

GABAERGIC NEURONS IN MURINE AIDS

Many of the retrolentiviruses—including HIV-1, LPBM-5 (murine AIDS), simian immunodeficiency virus, and caprine arthritis encephalitis virus, feline immunodeficiency virus (FIV) are characterized by neurological and neuropathological changes in the brain, and to varying degrees the biochemical basis for these diseases have been proposed as causes of murine dementia (13–17). Investigators have reported that neuropathological and metabolic consequences of FIV infection induced neuronal loss and glial activation. They have suggested that changes occurred after about 13 months postinfection and frontal brain tissue glutamate levels were significantly elevated, whereas neuronal glutamic acid decarboxylase (GAD) expression was significantly reduced and glial fibrillary acidic protein (GFAP) levels markedly increased in infected animals as compared with controls (18). Therefore, the retroviral infection would lead to unique morphological alterations in the brain, where there would be increased glutamatergic activity, possibly due to reduced GAD levels in GABAergic neurons. Haemophilus influenzae–infected Balb-C mice showed a significant increase in GFAP, as brain tissue GAD level declined significantly as age increased (19).

MACROPHAGES AND ASTROCYTES IN NEUROLOGICAL DISEASES

Researchers have suggested that macrophages/microglia, which constitute some 12% of cells in the central nervous system (CNS) (20), are the main immune effector cells and basic contributors to antigen presentation, phagocytosis, and secretion of cytokines, complement components, and especially the excitatory amino acids, including glutamate, nitric oxide, and oxidative radicals (21–23).

Macrophages and microglia have long been known to be involved in both developmental and pathophysiological changes—for instance, the dormant microglia as well as macrophages within normal mature CNS, whereas activated nonphagocytic cells play a significant role in CNS inflammation and the reactive phagocytic microglia in both infection and trauma. Macrophages as well as microglia have been suggested to secrete class I and II major histocompatibility complex (MHC) antigens, Fc receptors (I to III), complement receptors (CR1, CR2, and CR4), α_2 integrins, intercellular adhesion molecule 1 (ICAM-1), and costimulatory molecules B7-1 and B7-2 (24–31).

However, within the CNS, astrocytes contribute significantly to autoimmune diseases of the CNS and are a part of the blood-brain barrier (BBB), situated closely to endothelial cells and producing cytokines, which also introduce antigens to T cells (32). Cultured astrocytes are suggested to release following molecules with neurotrophic properties; ciliary neurotrophic factor (CNTF); glial-derived growth factor (GDGF); and nerve growth factor (NGF), including both class I and class II MHC antigens in reply to activation by interferons (33,34). Therefore both astrocytes and macrophages have both destructive and protective roles in the neuropathogenesis of HAD.

MICROGLIA AND ASTROCYTES IN HIV-1–ASSOCIATED DEMENTIA

HIV-1–associated dementia (HAD) has been suggested as a main basis of dementia in HIV-1–infected patients 20 to 59 years old, whereas symptomatic HIV-1 infected patients' brains may also present associated dementia (35). As a subcortical dementia, HAD is described by behavioral disorders (mania at the outset, apathy, and emotional liability); progressive motor abnormalities (tremor, gait ataxia, and a deficit in fine motor movements); cognitive impairments such as mental slowing, forgetfulness, and poor concentration (36–39); and neuronal loss, dendritic injury, and vacuolization (40).

A multicenter AIDS Cohort Study reported that 7% of HIV-infected patients acquired HAD within 12 months of the diagnosis of AIDS while 14% did within 2 years of AIDS onset (41). Since HIV-1 infection of the brain occurs in the very early phases of HIV-1 infection and contributes to invasion of the CNS via viremia, the initial genetic products of such infection would be seen in the cerebrospinal fluid (42–44).

Neuropathological features of the HIV-1–infected brain in infected adult individuals include multinucleated giant cells resulting from the combination of infected as well as uninfected cells (45) and scattered white matter pallor along fibers and microglial cells (36,37).

Since the macrophages provide viral reservoir in HAD (31), they contribute significantly to the neuroinvasiveness and penetration HIV-1 into the CNS (32). Although the virus seems to initiate the disease, there is no correlation between the infiltration of microphages/microglia and viral load in the blood. It has therefore been difficult to show the involvement of HIV-1 in the progression of HAD. As a result, other mechanisms secondary to virus infection—such as passage of monocytes and lymphocytes into the brain, activation of astrocytes, and production and release of inflammatory cytokines—need further attention. Animal models such as murine AIDS provide ample opportunities and serve as a good way of initiating experiments to enhance our understanding of the suggested mechanisms. In such animal models, tissues from spleen as well as brain can supplement each other in defining the viral infection through mitogenesis of both type 1 and 2 T-helper cells (Th1-and Th-2) and subsequent cytokine release (13,46), whereas the brain tissue samples in later murine AIDS would provide ample evidence to support the changes in neurotransmitter synthesis and synthesis of neurotoxin as a result of assault brought upon by retroviral infection.

HIV-1 encephalitis is associated with the immune activation of glial cells and contributes to changed secretory functions (47–51). Therefore, the immune system products ultimately bring the BBB barrier permeability and secretions of adhesion molecules on microglials and endothelial cells. Then adhesion molecules facilitate transendothelial migration of microglials (52).

The microglia and astrocytes in brain tissues of HIV-1–infected individuals release cytokines (specifically IL-1, IL-6, TNF, IFNs), reactive oxygen species (ROS), and neurotoxins, bringing about significant harmful effects on neurotransmitter actions as well as neuronal loss and leukoencephalopathy (53–55). These neurotoxins include nitric oxide (NO), and quinolinic acid (QUIN), tumor necrosis factor (TNF), arachidonic acid, and platelet activating factors (PAF), (56–64). All neurons, macrophages, and endothelial cells will synthesize NO, and this is reported to be associated with NMDA-type glutamate-initiated neurotoxicity (65).

Wesselingh et al. have reported very high levels TNF mRNA secretion by microglia as well as oligodendrocytes within the CNS subcortical regions of those HAD individuals infected with HIV-1 virus (66). QUIN is known as an extremely excitotoxic molecular marker of HIV neurological disease and a chief contributor to the pathogenesis of neuronal injury in both blood and brain associated with systemic and neurological disorder (59,60,67). In HAD, increased levels of gamma interferon (INF-α) lead to induction of indoleamine 2,3-dioxygenase and consequently increased QUIN synthesis (68).

The microglia/macrophages, as chief CNS cells, can produce HIV-1 and recognize early viral life-cycle markers in astrocytes. HIV-1–infected astrocytes are imperfect and would not induce considerable HIV protein synthesis (50,69–74).

The HIV-1–infected astrocytes mainly generate regulatory HIV-1 proteins, including Rev, Nef, and Tat (50,69–74). Studies have indicated that Rev, Nef, and Tat, along with other HIV-1 proteins like gp120, and gp41, are neurotoxic (62). Moreover, Tat protein could possibly affect some other cellular mechanisms. Tat triggers the nuclear factor-κB (NF-κB), protein kinase C, and cAMP-dependent protein kinase pathways (75,76). In turn, the astrocytes can generate MCP-1 through NF-κB d in (77) and cytokine secretions via endothelial cells under PKC pathway influence (78). Also, gp120 precisely influences not only neurons but also glia by attaching to the CD4/CCR5 receptor complex, activating PKC pathway, extracellular-regulated kinase (ERK), and eventually c-Jun N-terminal kinase (JNK) (79,80). Thus, HIV-1 proteins are involved in the activation and modification of several signaling pathways.

Macrophages and microglia interacting with astrocytes play an important role in HAD pathogenesis. Researchers have reported that, through these interactions, neurotoxic activities are affected and the secretion of viral proteins as well as production of cytokines such as IL-1, TNF, and arachidonic acid and its metabolites all are increased (63,81,82). It is suggested that the effects of cytokine secretion within the brain result from in situ production and communication within the brain (61).

Since the BBB may become harmed through TNF secretion in the brain, it can then allow HIV proteins and other cytokines to enter from the periphery (83). Therefore the direct mechanism of neurotoxicity is the upregulation of these viral neurotoxins, which can prevent the uptake of excitatory amino acids (e.g., glutamate) and other neuronal support functions by astrocytes (84,85). Increased glutamate, a sign of degenerative neuronal changes as well as neuronal loss in HAD, has been shown to induce a significant reduction of GAD expression in neurons of infected animals compared to controls (86,87).

ROLE OF GAD IN AIDS

Major absence in the GAD synthetic ability has been shown to contribute to the absence in GABA availability, which is the main inhibitory neurotransmitter in the mammalian CNS. GAD is responsible for the conversion of glutamate to GABA and is a marker for GABAergic neurons (88). A key shortage in GABA could affect vital biological functions such as locomotion, learning, reproduction, and circadian rhythms (88). GAD is a chief rate-limiting enzyme that modulates GABA synthesis from a pool of L-glutamate. In the mature brain, GAD is present in two major isoforms—GAD65 and GAD67—the products of two independently regulated genes located on chromosomes 2 and 10, respectively (89). GAD65 is a predominant GABA synthetic enzyme in rat and mouse brains (90,91), whereas GAD67 is the main form in the human brain (92).

GAD65 enzymatic activity is spread to axon terminals and is membrane-bound, while it contributes to vesicular synthesis of GABA (93). GABA vesicular synthesis is synchronized by firing neurons requiring synaptic input (94,95). On the contrary, GAD67 appears to be more determined in interneurons and neurons that fire tonically (96), is cytoplasmic, and is involved in nonvesicular GABA release (97).

Therefore, GAD67 is involved in the synthesis of GABA for general metabolic activity, while GAD65 is involved in synaptic transmission (98). Levels of GAD expression can be modulated posttranscriptionally by GABA itself. Moreover, glutamate can stimulate carrier-mediated nonvesicular GABA release via upregulation of GAD67 (88). Thus, glutamate agonists and antagonists can regulate GABA release by respectively increasing or decreasing GAD67 expression (88). For example, electrolytic lesions of glutamate afferents from the parafasicular nucleus of thalamus to the striatum (99) and chronic blockade of striatal NMDA receptors by dizocilpine (100) cause reductions in GAD67 mRNA levels in the respective target tissues.

The macrophages as well as microglia are both neurotoxic to astrocytes as neuroprotective in the neuropathogenesis of HAD (101). Since the astrocytes generate neurotrophic factors such as bFGF and NGF (102–104), they have a significant role in neuroregeneration within the CNS. Astrocytes could be considered neuroprotective by activating neurotoxic mechanisms (105,106). The regulatory task of astrocytes in HIV-1 encephalitis is to intensify the overexpression of eicosanoids, platelet activating factor, and TNF through activated HIV-1–infected monocytes. Therefore, astrocytes and macrophages present toxic as well as defensive properties in HIV-1–associated CNS disorders.

MICROGLIA/MACROPHAGES BALANCE WITH ASTROCYTES AND EFFECTS ON TH1/TH2

Th1 and Th2 are considered well-established signs of immune responses, as reported in studies of murine AIDS (13,46). The machinery that controls the balance of Th1 and Th2 cells consists in cytokine regulation (13,46). For instance, IL-12, produced by both microglia and macrophages, is vital to the growth of the immune response, mainly in the differentiation of Th precursor cells into the Th1 phenotype (107), while IL-4–endorsing Th2 cells increase. In HAD, a probable balance among macrophages and microglia on the one hand, with astrocytes on the other hand, provide an immune response, as well as Th1/Th2 secretions (108).

Stimulation of Th1 and Th2 by macrophages, microglia, and astrocytes relies on the MHC class II and CD40 molecules presence on their surface, as seen in murine AIDS spleen tissues (13,46). The macrophages as well as the microglia expressing MHC class II encourage myelin basic protein–reactive CD4+ T cells to produce IFN-α and TNF-α (109). After exposure to IFN-α and/or LPS, T cells express CD40 and activate Th1 responses. Resting human microglia/macrophages constitutively express proteins such as B 7-2, which may downregulate Th1 secretion. Th1 cells provoke prostaglandin release via the macrophages and microglia by a negative feedback mechanism, in turn preventing activities of Th1 cell responses. Activated macrophages, microglia, and Th1 cells, upon antigen presentation in the CNS, release IFN-α, which causes the astrocytes to generate PGE_2 and thus contributes to the control of all these cells activities (macrophages, microglia, and Th1 cells) (110). Moreover, autoreactive T cells play a key role in the pathogenesis of experimental encephalopathy, an animal model of HAD.

ROLE OF ASTROCYTES, MACROPHAGES/MICROGLIA ON CNS

Activation of microglia and macrophages in the inflammatory process of HAD may contributes directly to myelin damage via cytokine production, metalloproteinases, free-radical generation, and phagocytosis. Reactive astrocytes provide for axonal regrowth through release of both cytokines and neurotrophic factors (110). Astrocytes produce nerve growth factor (NGF), possibly avoiding the development of encephalopathy by expressing functional IL-4 receptors and secreting NGF upon exposure to IL-4 (111).

Astrocytes seem to provide ample protection in neurons by releasing glutamate and contributing to remyelination by secreting trophic factors such as glial cell line–derived neurotrophic factor (GDNF) and basic fibroblast growth factor (bFGF) (110). Astrocytes induce apoptosis of infiltrating inflammatory cells such as CNS-activated T cells (112). Immunohistochemical studies in HIV-1–infected postmortem brain tissues suggest infection of macrophages and microglia to be related to the apoptosis in neurons and macrophages/microglia (113–115).

APOPTOSIS IN HAD

Neurodegeneration, a typical mark of AIDS dementia, is usually linked via neuronal apoptosis in the brains of the pediatric as well as mature HIV-1 infected subjects. Studies have shown neuronal loss to be a chronic, progressive process that produces symptoms only years after seroconversion (113,116,117). Researchers have provided evidence of excessive glutamate, HIV-1 envelope glycoprotein, Tat, Vpr, cytokines (IL-1, TNF, IFN), NO, and other cellular factors released by HIV-1–infected macrophages (HIV/macrophage-induced neurotoxicity) (81,63,82).

The experimental evidence proposes that the above factors may contribute to toxicity through direct or indirect N-methyl-D-aspartate (NMDA)-type glutamate receptors (4,118,119). The effects of apoptotic HIV proteins are suggested to occur in chemokine receptors (49,77,120) through the following pathways in initiating apoptosis: death receptor–mediated (TNF-α and Fas) so-called extrinsic pathway, and mitochondrial-mediated intrinsic pathway (121–123), both of which eventually join through activating downstream effector caspases. Usually the intrinsic pathway is stopped through the Bcl-2 family of proteins (Bcl-2 and Bcl-xL) (123).

Bcl-2 proteins contribute to modulation of the neuronal apoptosis via brain injuries (124–126). However, their role in HIV-1-induced neuronal apoptosis needs to be studied further. Bcl-2 protein family members comprise the proapoptosis proteins—namely, Bax and the antiapoptosis proteins Bcl-2 and Bcl-xL (127,128). While induction of Bax-expression in neurons is linked to apoptosis (124,125,127,129–132) the induction of Bcl-2 or Bcl-xL expression may inhibit neuronal apoptosis caused via a different intrinsic pathway, namely mitochondrial-mediated injuries, including NMDA receptor overactivation (133–136). In some other cell types, induction of mitochondrial damage by activating the extrinsic pathway seems to happen by cleavage of another proapoptotic Bcl-2 family member called Bid (137,138).

Macrophages/microglia react to brain injuries by releasing LFA-1, ICAM-1, MHC class II molecules, phagocytosis, and cytotoxicity, which are downregulated through astrocytic factors that deactivate antigen-presenting cells within the CNS (139). IFN-/LPS-stimulated macrophages and microglia release IL-12, p75, and p40 are said to be significantly declined in coculture with astrocytes, demonstrating the regulatory role of astrocytes in the secretion of IL-12 via microglia (140). It is also suggested that astrocyte stimulation through LPS generates IL-10, which, in turn, acts as an anti-inflammatory cytokine (140). IL-10 prevents microglia and macrophage antigen-presenting activities, T-cell proliferation, and cytokine synthesis by Th1 cells.

The astrocytes in the pathogenesis of HAD can also inhibit endotoxin-induced NO production by microglia/macrophages and secretion of TGF-1, which facilitate microglia and macrophage apoptosis. These findings suggest that, in vivo, astrocytes could suppress microglia and macrophages and restrict the dissemination of the inflammatory reaction within brain parenchyma. Therefore neurologists may want to challenge this inconsistency so as to identify those cellular, biochemical, and phenomenological factors that may be beneficial in treatment of HAD patients.

ROLE OF REELIN IN BRAIN

Neural crest–derived cells will differentiate into numerous derivatives, including neurons, melanocytes (pigment cells of the skin and iris), and peripheral nerve glia, called satellite cells and Schwann cells (141). The fate of neural crest cells, as with other embryonic cell types, becomes progressively restricted as development proceeds. Neural crest cells that form the dorsal root ganglia (DRG) normally develop into sensory neurons, satellite cells, and Schwann cells.

The mammalian neocortex consists of six different layers, each of which would belong to morphologically different neuronal categories. In 1999, Takahashi and coworkers, through 5-bromodeoxyuridine (BrdU) studies (142), exposed the laminar destiny of cortical neurons born at different stages of embryonic development. Cortical neurons grow and differentiate in the ventricular zone (VZ) lining the lateral ventricle, then move toward the marginal zone (MZ) on the surface of the developing cortex, and finally initiate maturation. Because the later cohorts always pass the previously created cells next to the MZ, the early nerve cells eventually will be positioned in the deep layers, and the later ones in the superficial layers.

It has been suggested that this embryonic developmental progression will be arranged by the reelin signaling pathway. Reelin is a large extracellular matrix protein that is released by Cajal-Retzius neurons in the MZ (143). The reelin gene–deficient mouse, reeler, establishes an acute irregularity of neuronal positioning in the CNS (144). Further studies involving labeling experiments with [³H] thymidine have indicated general inversion of the birth-date gradient within the cortical plate (145). Other mutant mice, called yotari (146), and scrambler (147), are reported to have the same phenotype as reeler. The gene accountable for yotari as well as scrambler is shown to be Dab-1, encoding an intracellular phosphoprotein including the phosphotyrosine-binding (PTB) domain (148,149).

Other researchers have reported that reelin forms a homomeric complex (150) by functioning through a phosphorylation of specific tyrosines on Dab1 (149,151). Very low density lipoprotein receptor (VLDLR) and apolipoprotein receptor 2 (ApoER2), have also been recognized as the reelin receptors. As the extracellular domains bind to reelin protein directly (152,153) and their intracellular domains bind to Dab1 (154). Cadherin-related neuronal receptors (CNRs) (155) and alpha3-beta1 integrin (156) have been suggested to bind reelin. The normal cortical development begins with a neuroepithelium. This lasts until about E11 in the mouse, followed by a transient stage called preplate. When the first postmitotic neurons migrate to the periphery of the telencephalon they form a loose, horizontal network. The appearance of the cortical plate is the next stage. It occurs in mice at E13-E14 while in humans it appears at the 7th or 8th gestational week. In normal mice and all mammals, as far as we know, neurons are generated close to the ventricle. Most glutamatergic cells migrate radially from the ventricular zone, along radial cells, whereas most GABAergic neurons are generated in the ganglionic eminences, the primordium of the striatum, and gain access to the cortex by tangential migration. At the end of migration, cortical neurons form a dense, radially organized structure called the cortical plate. The cortical plate is very dense in normal animals and this compact cell layer splits the preplate into two components. Some preplate derivatives settle externally in the marginal zone, whereas others settle below the cortical plate and form the subcortical plate. In reeler mice and mice homozygous for mutations in members of the reelin pathway, neurons are generated at the normal time, at the normal place, and in normal numbers. They first migrate normally, but something goes wrong at the end of migration. The neurons of the reeler mouse cortical plate differentiate normally. They even connect normally. However, instead of assuming a radial architectonic organization, they develop an abnormal, distorted orientation.

The role of reelin in HAD and animal models such as murine AIDS has not been studied. The retroviruses LPB-M5 have been a leading model to study HIV-1 and HAD where it can be used in studying possible treatments of HAD disorders in humans. Murine AIDS caused by LPB-M5 retroviral infection has been studied as HAD animal models where significant immune dysregulation correlated with similarities reported in HIV associated dementia (157). Neurological disorders in HAD are characterized clinically with difficulty by concentration, slowness of movement, altered cognition, and behavioral changes (158).

Although the reelin molecular pathway signaling has been introduced, further studies on the reelin biological function, its mechanisms and causes of the abnormal cortical development are desired. This review found no evidence that reelin played any role in the progression of HAD and AIDS. Therefore, further studies in animal models resembling immunoreactivity in HIV-1 such as murine AIDS, may provide more knowledge in brain development changes that occur in HIV-infected newborns. This will furthermore enhance our skills in proposing mechanisms through reelin pathways and possible treatment(s) that would benefit neonatal infected patients as well as older HAD-infected individuals.

CYTOKINES IN BRAIN

Interleukin-1 (IL-1) and tumor necrosis factor (TNF) are important proinflammatory cytokines that are rapidly released in response to most viral infections. IL-1 and TNF encourage cytokine flow by provoking synthesis of themselves, other cytokines, and some disseminating second messengers in both autocrine as well as paracrine as in systemic tissue (159). Exogenous IL-1 has been reported to provoke self-secretion within cultured human microglia and astrocytes (157). It stimulates TNF, IL-6, GM-CSF, and TGF-1 release (160–161) in vitro by glia. They have suggested that IL-1 microinfusion into the cerebral ventricle did significantly increase mRNA levels for the whole IL-1 cytokine family, including TNF and TGF-1 (162), where they will induce astrocytosis (163).

In animal experiments, the endogenous IL-1 provokes release of IL-6 (164) inducing fever, a major indication of immune response to infection in rodent brain (165). IL-1 and TNF were also reported to cause COX2 and iNOS release, where inhibition of these enzymes changed more physiological actions of exogenous IL-1 and TNF, such as those seen in sleep and body temperature. Microinfusion of IL-1Ra, prostaglandin, or NO synthesis inhibitors into the attenuated IL-1 induced fever

(166). These data suggest that the prostaglandins and NO produced would eventually spread cytokine signals within brain parenchyma, inducing fever and consequently neuroendocrine activation. Cytokine signals would then spread throughout the brain via molecular flow that develops circulating IL-1α in the brain. IL-1α and TNF propagate the cytokine signal through the brain astrocytosis. The seizure propagation creates a well-defined spatio-temporal pattern that can be discerned by cerebral blood flow or glucose metabolism. Ipsilateral contralateral hippocampus-amygdala, the rest of the limbic system striatum sensory motor cortex lower brain centers thalamus septum parietal cortex (167).

The cytokine release signals are similar to those in epileptogenic seizure activity, depending on where in the brain they are initiated. IL-1 and TNF are generated via neurons where the immune reactivity is perceived (168). This implies that the cytokines continue to stay cell-bound and will not spread to trigger other cells. Spatial patterns of brain injury and seizure induce c-Fos expression. Then c-Fos binds c-Jun to form activation factor-1 (AP-1), a transcription factor, inducing upregulation of expression of IL-1, TNF, as well as some other genes (168,169). This suggests that AP-1 could initiate cytokine signals in neurons.

ASTROCYTES, GFAP, AND CYTOKINES

Following brain injuries through neurodegeneration, astrocytic proliferation takes place where there is an increase in cytokine release along with growth factors and glial fibrillary acidic protein (GFAP). GFAP, a cell-specific marker for reactive astrocytes is an intermediate filament protein whose expression in the CNS is restricted to astrocytes and related cells and glutamate transporters specific to astrocytes. Astrocytes preserve normal brain physiology by regulating both sodium and potassium ion homeostasis around neurons through neutralizing or removing excess chemicals from the extracellular space, particularly glutamate, which increases in HAD. A disturbance in astrocytic function can therefore have a significant effect in certain disorders of the CNS.

The astrocytes may dynamically regulate leukocyte entry into normal or injured CNS parenchyma as well as secrete both pro- and anti-inflammatory cytokines (170,171) and proteins that will extracellularly affect different cell types and nerve fiber migration (172–174). Therefore, it is been concluded that astrocytosis disrupts leukocyte trafficking within the CNS parenchyma, which signifies a possible pathogenic mechanism for CNS inflammatory responses. It has been reported that within CNS, the neural myelination was disrupted in mutant mice where astrocytic functions had been disturbed by ablation of the GFAP gene (175). Thus, the astrocytes have a key role in maintenance as well as development within CNS myelination. Even though astrocytes maintain neurite development and perhaps are vital in some nerve fibers growing in adults (176), researchers have concluded that following CNS injury the reactive astrocytes are a main barrier to the renewal of damaged axons.

As a result of CNS insults, cellular injury is brought on by numbers of endogenous chemicals, which can result in neurotoxic damage. The molecules comprise glutamate, dopamine, NO, and other transmitter candidates usually seen within intercellular communication. These include reactive oxygen species produced as byproducts of metabolism or part of the inflammatory response and cytokines.

Astrocytes are supposed to present endogenous mechanisms of neuroprotection as they encounter such molecules, however, they can also lead to formation of other toxicants. The astrocytes have the following activities: generating glutamate transporters vital in glutamate removal from extracellular space of the CNS (177), releasing enzymes significant in the defense against oxidants, and ROS exclusion (178).

On the contrary, astrocytes also release NO synthase and can produce potentially neurotoxic levels of NO, and have the capacity to produce numerous pro- and anti-inflammatory cytokines (105,170,171), the effects of which can be mixed on neuronal function. CNS injury causes increased levels of extracellular glutamate (179), and the ablation of astrocytes adjacent to brain injury in transgenic mice is associated with pronounced neuronal cell death, which can be prevented by glutamate-receptor antagonists, indicating that glutamate excitotoxicity contributed to the neuronal death. Thus, astrocyte loss or dysfunction represents a potentially significant cause of neuronal degeneration. Astrocyte dysfunction may, in addition to influencing neuronal survival or degeneration after CNS insults, have more subtle effects on neuronal function that could lead to neuronal dysfunction at the cellular, systems, and ultimately behavioral levels by influencing extracellular levels of glutamate or potassium, or through altered production of cytokines (180).

The AIDS-dementia complex represents a potential human correlate of astrocytic dysfunction and failure. Astrocyte infection with human immunodeficiency virus (HIV) (181) may lead to the production of neurotoxic molecules (182). Also, astrocyte failure could account for at least some of the neuropathological changes and disturbances in neurological function associated with HIV infection of the brain (183–185), as predicted on the basis of the cellular and molecular ablation studies in experimental animals summarized here.

CONCLUSION

The parameters controlling and regulating HIV-1 dementia include continuous recruitment of T cells from the periphery to the CNS, elevated TNF-α messenger RNA in microglia and astrocyte secretion—along with exogenous IL-1, TNF-α, and TGF-1–decreased synaptic and dendritic density along with reduced glutamate decarboxylase levels in GABAergic neurons. These findings now suggest that inflammatory cytokines such as TNF-α and IL-1, by activating caspases with neurons via TNF-α receptor-1 (TNFR1), in turn can trigger caspase-8 activation in neuronal apoptosis. Furthermore, this process may induce important synergistic roles in HIV-1 dementia neuropathology.

REFERENCES

1. van de Bovenkamp M, Nottet H, Pereira CF. Interactions of human immunodeficiency virus-1 proteins with neurons: possible role in the development of human immunodeficiency virus-1-associated dementia. Eur J Clin Invest 2000; 32(8):619.
2. Anderson E, Zink W, Xiong H, Gendelman HE. HIV-1-associated dementia: a metabolic encephalopathy perpetrated by virus-infected and immune-competent mononuclear phagocytes. J AIDS 2002; 31(suppl 2):S43–S54.

3. Gendelman HE, Persidsky Y, Ghorpade A, Limoges J, Stins M, Fiala M, Morrisett R. The neuropathogenesis of the AIDS dementia complex. AIDS 1997; 11(suppl A):S35–S45.

4. Giulian D, et al. Study of receptor-mediated neurotoxins released by HIV-1-infected mononuclear phagocytes found in human brain. J Neurosci 1996; 16:3139–3153.

5. Ushijima H, Perovic S, Leuck J, Rytik PG, Muller WE, Schroder HC. Suppression of PrP (Sc)- and HIV-1 gp120 induced neuronal cell death by sulfated colominic acid. J Neurovirol 1999; 5(3):289–299.

6. Giulian D, Yu J, Li X, Tom D, Li J, Wendt E, Lin SN, Schwarcz R, Noonan C. Study of receptor-mediated neurotoxins released by HIV-1-infected mononuclear phagocytes found in human brain. J Neurosci 1996; 16(10):3139–3153.

7. Gelbard HA, Nottet HS, Swindells S, Jett M, Dzenko KA, Genis P, White R, Wang L, Choi YB, Zhang D. Platelet-activating factor: a candidate human immunodeficiency virus type 1-induced neurotoxin. J Virol 1994; 68(7):4628–4635.

8. Achim CL, Heyes MP, Wiley CA. Quantitation of human immunodeficiency virus, immune activation factors, and quinolinic acid in AIDS brains. J Clin Invest 1993; 91(6):2769–2775.

9. Chao CC, Hu S, Gekker G, Lokensgard JR, Heyes MP, Peterson PK. U50,488 protection against HIV-1-related neurotoxicity: involvement of quinolinic acid suppression. Neuropharmacology 2000; 39(1):150–160.

10. Magnuson DS, Knudsen BE, Geiger JD, Brownstone RM, Nath A. Human immunodeficiency virus type 1 tat activates non-N-methyl-D-aspartate excitatory amino acid receptors and causes neurotoxicity. Ann Neurol 1995; 37(3):373–380.

11. Kaul M, Garden GA, Lipton SA. Pathways to neuronal injury and apoptosis in HIV-associated dementia. Nature 2001; 410:988–994.

12. Adamson DC, McArthur JC, Dawson TM, Dawson VL. Rate and severity of HIV-associated dementia (HAD): correlations with Gp41 and iNOS. Mol Med 1999; 5(2):98–109.

13. Araghi-Niknam M, Liang B, Zhang Z, Ardestani SK, Watson RR. Modulation of immune dysfunction during murine leukaemia retrovirus infection of old mice by dehydroepiandrosterone sulphate (DHEAS). Immunology 1997; 90(3):344–349.

14. Epstein LG, Gendelman HE. Human immunodeficiency virus type 1 infection of the nervous system: pathogenetic mechanisms. Ann Neurol 1993; 33:429–436.

15. Gray F, Lescs MC, Keohane C, Paraire F, Marc B, M. Early brain changes in HIV infection: neuropathological study of 11 HIV seropositive, non-AIDS cases. J Neuropathol Exp Neurol 1992; 51:3–11.

16. Lipton SA, Gendelman HE. Dementia associated with the acquired immunodeficiency syndrome. N Engl J Med 1995; 332:934–940.

17. Dandekar S, Gardner MB. Neurobiology of simian and feline immunodeficiency virus infections. Brain Pathol 1991; 1:201–212.

18. Power C, Moench T, Peeling J, Kong P, Langelier T. Feline immunodeficiency virus causes increased glutamate levels and neuronal loss in brain. Neuroscience 1997; 77(4):1175–1185.

19. Fatemi SH, Laurence J, Araghi-Niknam M, Sidwell RW. Prenatal viral infection increases GFAP in brains of Balb-C neonatal mice. Proc Am Coll Neuropsychopharmacol. In press.

20. Benveniste EN. Role of macrophage/microglia in multiple sclerosis and experimental allergic encephalomyelitis. J Mol Med 1997; 75:165–173.

21. Banati RB, Gehrmann J, Schubert P, Kreutzberg GW. Cytotoxicity of microglia. Glia 1993; 7:111–118.

22. Gordon S. The macrophage. Bioessays 1995; 17:977–986.

23. Gehrmann J, Matsumoto Y, Kreutzenberg GW. Microglia: intrinsic immunoeffector cell of the brain. Brain Res Rev 1995; 20:269–287.

24. Walker DG, Kim SU, McGeer PL. Complement and cytokine gene expression in cultured microglia derived from postmortem human brains. J Neurosci Res 1995; 40:478–493.

25. Shrikant P, Weber E, Jilling T, Benveniste EN. ICAM-1 gene expression by glial cells: differential mechanisms of inhibition by interleukin-10 and interleukin-6. J Immunol 1995; 155:1489–1501.

26. Panek RB, Benveniste EN. Class II MHC gene expression in microglia: regulation by the cytokines IFN-α TNF-α and TGF-β. J Immunol 1995; 154:2846–2854.

27. Frei K, Siepl C, Groscurth P, Bodmer S, Schwerdel C, Fontana A. Antigen presentation and tumor cytotoxicity by interferon-treated microglial cells. Eur J Immunol 1987; 17:1271–1278.

28. Suzumura A, Mezitis SGE, Gonatas NK, Silberberg DH. MHC antigen expression on bulk isolated macrophage-microglia from newborn mouse brain: induction of Ia antigen expression by α-interferon. J Neuroimmunol 1987; 15:263–278.

29. Williams K, Ulvestad E, Antel JP. B7/BB-1 antigen expression on adult human microglia studied in vitro and in situ. Eur J Immunol 1994; 24:3031–3037.

30. De Simone R, Giampaolo A, Giometto B, Gallo P, Levi G, Peschle C. The costimulatory molecule B7 is expressed on human microglia in culture and in multiple sclerosis acute lesions. J Neuropathol Exp Neurol 1995; 187:175–187.

31. Williams K, Bar-Or A, Ulvestad E, Olivier A, Antel JP, Yong VW. Biology of adult human microglia in culture: comparisons with peripheral blood monocytes and astrocytes. J Neuropathol Exp Neurol 1992; 51:538–549.

32. Fontana A, Fierz W, Wekerle H. Astrocytes present myelin basic protein to encephalitogenic T-cell lines. Nature 1984; 307:273–276.

33. Merrill JE, Jonakait GM. Interactions of the nervous and immune systems in development, normal brain homeostasis, and disease. FASEB J 1995; 9:611–618.

34. Kraus E, Schneider-Schaulis S, Miyasaka M, Tamatani T, Sedgwick J. Augmentation of major histocompatibility complex class I and ICAM-I expression on glial cells following measles virus infection: evidence for the role of type-1 interferon. Eur J Biochem 1992; 22:175–182.

35. Janssen RS, Nwanyanwu OC, Selik RM, Stehr-Green JK. Epidemiology of human immunodeficiency virus encephalopathy in the United States. Neurology 1992; 42:1472–1476.

36. Ragin AB, Storey P, Cohen BA, Epstein LG, Edelman RR. Whole brain diffusion tensor imaging in HIV-associated cognitive impairment. AJNR Am J Neuroradiol 2004; 25(2):195–200.

37. Maher JS, Choudhri O, Halliday W, Power C, Nath A. AIDS dementia complex with generalized myoclonus. Mov Disord 1997; 12:593–597.

38. Major EO, Rausch D, Marra C, Clifford D. HIV-associated dementia. Science 2000; 288:440–442.

39. Mirsattari SM, Berry ME, Holden JK, Ni W, Nath A, Power C. Paroxysmal dyskinesias in patients with HIV infection. Neurology 1999; 52:109–114.

40. McGeer EG, McGeer PL. The role of the immune system in neurodegenerative disorders. Mov Disord 1997; 12:855–858.

41. McArthur JC, Hoover DR, Bacellar H. Dementia in AIDS patients: incidence and risk factors. Neurology 1993; 43:2245–2252.

42. Resnick L, Berger JR, Shapshak P, Tourtellotte WW. Early penetration of the blood-brain-barrier by HIV. Neurology 1988; 38:9–14.

43. Achim C, Masliah E, Heyes MP, Sarnacki PG. Macrophage activation factors in the brains of AIDS patients. J Neurol AIDS 1996; 1:1–16.

44. Michaels J, Sharer LR, Epstein LG. Human immunodeficiency virus type 1 (HIV-1) infection of the nervous system: a review. Immunodefic Rev 1988; 1:71–104.
45. Masliah E, Nianfeng G, Achim CL, DeTeresa R, Wiley CA. Patterns of neuro-degeneration in HIV encephalitis. J Neuro-AIDS 1996; 1:161–173.
46. Araghi-Niknam M, Zhang Z, Jiang S, Call O, Eskelson CD, Watson RR. Cytokine dysregulation and increased oxidation is prevented by dehydroepiandrosterone in mice infected with murine leukemia retrovirus. Proc Soc Exp Biol Med 1997; 216(3):386–391.
47. Wesselingh SL, Power C, Glass JD, Tyor WR, McArthur JC, Farber JM, et al. Intracerebral cytokine messenger RNA expression in acquired immunodeficiency syndrome dementia. Ann Neurol 1993; 33:576–582.
48. Tyor WR, Glass JD, Griffin JW, Becker PS, McArthur JC, Bezman L, et al. Cytokine expression in the brain during the acquired immunodeficiency syndrome. Ann Neurol 1992; 31:349–360.
49. Conant K, et al. Induction of monocyte chemoattractant protein-1 in HIV-1 Tat-stimulated astrocytes and elevation in AIDS dementia. Proc Natl Acad Sci USA 1998; 95:3117–3121.
50. Nuovo GJ, Alfieri ML. AIDS dementia is associated with massive, activated HIV-1 infection and concomitant expression of several cytokines. Mol Med 1996; 2:358–366.
51. Vitkovic L, da Cunha A, Tyor WR. Cytokine expression and pathogenesis in AIDS brain. In: Price RW, Perry SW, eds. HIV, AIDS and the Brain. New York: Raven Press, 1994:203–222.
52. Nottet HS, Bar DR, van Hassel H, Verhoef J, Boven LA. Cellular aspects of HIV-1 infection of macrophages leading to neuronal dysfunction in vitro models for HIV-1 encephalitis. J Leuk Biol 1997; 62:107–116.
53. Navia BA, Jordan BD, Price RW. The AIDS dementia complex: I Clinical features. Ann Neurol 1986; 19:517–524.
54. Johnson RT, McArthur JC, Narayan O. The neurobiology of human immunodeficiency virus infections. FASEB J 1988; 2:2970–2981.
55. Boven LA, Gomes L, Hery C, Gary F, Verhoef J, Portegies P. Increased peroxynitrite activity in AIDS dementia complex: implications for the neuropathogenesis of HIV-1 infection. J Immunol 1999; 162:4319–4327.
56. Snyder S. Nitric oxide: first in a new class of neurotransmitters? Science 1992; 257:494–496.
57. Barbaro G, Di Lorenzo G, Soldini M, Giancaspro G, Grisorio B, Pellicelli AM, D'Amati G, Barbarini G. Clinical course of cardiomyopathy in HIV-infected patients with or without encephalopathy related to the myocardial expression of tumor necrosis factor-alpha and nitric oxide synthase. AIDS 2000; 5, 14(7):827–838.
58. Heyes MP, Brew BJ, Martin A, Price RW, Salazar AM, Sidtis JJ, Yergey JA, Mouradian MM, Sadler AE, Keilp. Quinolinic acid in cerebrospinal fluid and serum in HIV-1 infection: relationship to clinical and neurological status. Ann Neurol 1991; 29(2):202–209.
59. Heyes MO, Brew BJ, Satio K. Inter-relationships between quinolinic acid, neuroactive kynurenis, neopterin and 2-microglobulin in cerebrospinal fluid and serum of HIV-1 infected patients. J Neuroimmunol 1992; 40:71–80.
60. Heyes MP, Mefford IN, Quearry BJ, Dedhia M, Lackner A. Increased ratio of quinolinic acid to kynurenic acid in cerebrospinal fluid of D retrovirus-infected rhesus macaques: relationship to clinical and viral status. Ann Neurol 1990; 27:666–675.
61. Heyes MP, Rubinow D, Lane C, Markey SP. Cerebrospinal fluid quinolinic acid concentrations are increased in acquired immune deficiency syndrome. Ann Neurol 1989; 26:275–277.
62. Nath A, Geiger J. Neurobiological aspects of human immunodeficiency virus infection: neurotoxic mechanisms. Prog Neurobiol 1998; 54:19–33.

63. Genis PM, Jett EW, Bernton T, Boyle HA, Gelbard K, Dzenko. Cytokines and arachidonic metabolites produced during human immunodeficiency virus (HIV)-infected macrophage-astroglia interactions: implications for the neuropathogenesis of HIV disease. J Exp Med 1992; 176:1703–1718.

64. Dawson VL, Dawson TM, London ED, Bredt DS, Snyder SH. Nitric oxide mediates glutamate neurotoxicity in primary cortical structures. Proc Natl Acad Sci USA 1991; 88:368–371.

65. Wilt SG, Milward E, Zhou JM, Nagasato K, Patton H. In vitro evidence for a dual role of tumor necrosis factor-alpha in human immunodeficiency virus type 1 encephalopathy. Ann Neurol 1995; 38:483–486.

66. Wesselingh SL, Takahashi K, Glass JD, McArthur JC, Griffin JW, Griffin DE. Cellular localization of tumor necrosis factor mRNA in neurological tissue from HIV-infected patients by combined reverse transcriptase/polymerase chain reaction in situ hybridization and immunohistochemistry. J Neuroimmunol 1997; 74:1–8.

67. Heyes MP, Saito K, Crowley S. Quinolinic acid and kynurenine pathway metabolism in inflammatory and non-inflammatory neurological disease. Ann Neurol 1992; 115:1249–1273.

68. Byrne GI, Lehman LK, Kirschbaum JG, Borden EC. Induction of tryptophan degradation in vitro and in vivo: a gamma-interferon-stimulated activity. J Interferon Res 1986; 6:389–396.

69. Nuovo GJ, Gallery F, MacConnell P, Braun A. In situ detection of polymerase chain reaction-amplified HIV-1 nucleic acids and tumor necrosis factor-alpha RNA in the central nervous system. Am J Pathol 1994; 144:659–666.

70. Saito Y, Sharer LR, Epstein LG. Overexpression of Nef as a marker for restricted HIV-1 infection of astrocytes in postmortem pediatric central nervous tissues. Neurology 1994; 44:474–487.

71. Tornatore C, Chandra R, Berger JR, Major EO. HIV-1 infection of subcortical astrocytes in the pediatric central nervous system. Neurology 1994; 44:481–487.

72. Takashashi K, Wesselingh SL, Griffin DE, McArthur JC. Localization of HIV-1 in human brain using polymerase chain reaction/in situ hybridization and immunocytochemistry. Ann Neurol 1996; 39:511–705.

73. Bagasra O, Lavi E, Bobroski L. Cellular reservoirs of HIV-1 infection in the central nervous system of infected individuals: identification by the combination of in situ polymerase chain reaction and immunohistochemistry. AIDS 1996; 10:573–585.

74. Ranki A, Nyberg M, Ovod V. Abundant expression of HIV Nef and Rev proteins in brain astrocytes in vivo is associated with dementia. AIDS 1995; 9:1001–1008.

75. Conant K, Ma M, Nath A, Major EO. Extracellular human immunodeficiency virus type 1 Tat protein is associated with an increase in both NF-kappa B binding and protein kinase C activity in primary human astrocytes. J Virol 1996; 70:1384–1389.

76. Zidovetzki R, Wang JL, Chen P, Jeyaseelan R, Hofman F. Human immunodeficiency virus Tat protein induces interleukin 6 mRNA expression in human brain endothelial cells via protein kinase. AIDS Res Hum Retrovir 1998; 14:825–833.

77. Conant K, Garzino Demo A, Nath A, McArthur JC, Halliday W, Power C. Induction of monocytes chemoattractant protein-1 in HIV-1 Tat-stimulated astrocytes and elevation in AIDS dementia. Proc Natl Acad Sci USA 1998; 95:3117–3121.

78. Chen P, Mayne M, Power C, Nath A. The Tat protein of HIV-1 induces tumor necrosis factor-alpha production. Implications for HIV-1-associated neurological diseases. J Biol Chem 1997; 272:22385–22388.

79. Wyss-Coray T, Masliah E, Toggas SM, Rockenstein EM, Brooker MJ, Lee HS. Dysregulation of signal transduction pathways as a potential mechanism of nervous system alterations in HIV-1 gp 120 transgenic mice and humans with HIV-1 encephalitis. J Clin Invest 1996; 97:789–798.

80. Lannuzel A, Barnier JV, Hery C, Huynh VT, Guibert B, Gary F. Human immuno-deficiency virus type 1 and its coat protein gp 120 induce apoptosis and activate JNK and ERK mitogen-activated protein kinases in human neurons. Ann Neurol 1997; 42:847–856.

81. Fiala M, Rhodes RH, Shapsak P, Nagano I, Martinez-Maza O, Diagne A. Regulation of HIV-1 infection in astrocytes: expression of Nef, TNF- and IL-6 is enhanced in coculture of astrocytes and macrophages. J Neurovirol 1996; 2:158–166.

82. Hopkins SJ, Rothwell NJ. Cytokines and the nervous system: I Expression and recognition. Trends Neurosci 1995; 18:83–88.

83. Fiala M, Looney DJ, Stins M. TNF- opens a paracellular route for HIV-1 invasion across the blood brain barrier. Mol Med 1997; 3:553–564.

84. Dreyer EB, Lipton SA. The coat protein gp 120 of HIV-1 inhibits astrocyte uptake of excitatory amino acids via macrophage arachidonic acid. Eur J Neurosci 1995; 7:2502–2507.

85. Fine SM, Angel RA, Perry SW. Tumor necrosis factor alpha-inhibits glutamate uptake by primary human astrocytes—implications for pathogenesis of HIV-1 dementia. J Biol Chem 1996; 271:15303–15306.

86. Koirala TR, Nakagaki K, Ishida T, Nonaka S, Morikawa S, Tabira T. Decreased expression of MAP-2 and GAD in the brain of cats infected with feline immunodeficiency virus. Tohoku J Exp Med 2001; 195(3):141–151.

87. Fatemi SH, Laurence J, Araghi-Niknam M, Sidwell RW. GFAP and GAD 65 & 67 kDa proteins are increased brains of neonatal BALB-C mice following viral infection in utero. Schizophrenia Research. In press.

88. Soghomonian JJ, Martin DL. Two isoforms of glutamate decarboxylase. Trends Pharmacol Sci 1998; 19(12):500–505.

89. Erlander MG, Tilakaratne NJ, Feldblum S, Patel N, Tobin AJ. Two genes encode distinct glutamate decarboxylases. Neuron 1991; 7(1):91–100.

90. Izzo E, Auta J, Impagnatiello F, Pesold C, Guidotti A, Costa E. Glutamic acid decarboxylase and glutamate receptor changes during tolerance and dependence to benzodiazepines. Proc Natl Acad Sci USA 2001; 98(6):3483–3488.

91. Liu CP, Jiang K, Wu CH, Lee WH, Lin WJ. Detection of glutamic acid decarboxylase-activated T cells with I-Ag7 tetramers. Proc Natl Acad Sci USA 2000, (26):14596–14601.

92. Guidotti A, Auta J, Daavis JM, Di-Giorgi-Gerevini V, Dived Y, Grayson DR, Impagnatiello F, Pandey G, Pesold C, Sharma R, Uzunov D, Costa E, DiGiorgi Gerevini V. Decrease in reelin and glutamic acid decarboxylase67 (GAD67) expression in schizophrenia and bipolar disorder: a postmortem brain study. Arch Gen Psychiatry 2000; 57(11):1061–1069.

93. Soghomonian JJ, Laprade N. Glutamate decarboxylase (GAD67 and GAD65) gene expression is increased in a subpopulation of neurons in the putamen of Parkinsonian monkeys. Synapse 1997; 27(2):122–132.

94. Esclapez M, Tillakaratne NJ, Kaufman DL, Tobin AJ, Houser CR. Comparative localization of two forms of glutamic acid decarboxylase and their mRNAs in rat brain supports the concept of functional differences between the forms. J Neurosci 1994; 14(3 Pt 2):1834–1855.

95. Feldblum S, Erlander MG, Tobin AJ. Different distributions of GAD65 and GAD67 mRNAs suggest that the two glutamate decarboxylases play distinctive functional roles. J Neurosci Res 1993; 34(6):689–706.

96. Esclapez M, Tillakaratne NJ, Kaufman DL, Tobin AJ, Houser CR. Comparative localization of two forms of glutamic acid decarboxylase and their mRNAs in rat brain supports the concept of functional differences between the forms. J Neurosci 1994; 14(3 Pt 2):1834–1855.

97. Reetz A, Solimena M, Matteoli M, Folli F, Takei K, De Camilli P. GABA and pancreatic

beta-cells: colocalization of glutamic acid decarboxylase (GAD) and GABA with synaptic-like microvesicles suggests their role in GABA storage and secretion. EMBO J 1991; 10(5):1275–1284.

98. Martin DL, Rimvall K. Regulation of gamma-aminobutyric acid synthesis in the brain [review]. J Neurochem 1993; 60(2):395–407.

99. Corda MG, Lecca D, Piras G, Di Chiara G, Giorgi O. Biochemical parameters of dopaminergic and GABAergic neurotransmission in the CNS of Roman high-avoidance and Roman low-avoidance rats. Behav Genet 1997; 27(6):527–536.

100. Qin ZH, Zhang SP, Weiss B. Dopaminergic and glutamatergic blocking drugs differentially regulate glutamic acid decarboxylase mRNA in mouse brain. Brain Res Mol Brain Res 1994; 21(3-4):293–302.

101. Mallat M, Chamak B. Brain macrophages: neurotoxic or neurotrophic effector cells? Leuk Biol 1994; 56:416–422.

102. Boven LA, Middel J, Portegies P, Verhoef J, Jansen GH, Nottet HS. Overexpression of nerve growth factor and basic fibroblast factor in AIDS dementia complex. J Neuroimmunol 1999; 3690:154–162.

103. Pechan PA, Chowdhury K, Siefert W. Free radicals induce gene expression of NGF and bFGF in rat astrocyte culture. Neuroreport 1992; 3:469–472.

104. Ballabriga J, Pozas E, Planas AM, Ferrer I. BFGF and FGFR-3 in reactive astrocytes, and FGFR-3 in reactive microglia. Brain Res 1997; 752:315–318.

105. Mucke L, Eddleston M. Astrocytes in infectious and immune-mediated diseases of the central nervous system. FASEB J 1993; 7:1226–1232.

106. Rosenberg PA. Accumulation of extracellular glutamate and neuronal death in astrocyte-poor cortical cultures exposed to glutamine. Glia 1991; 4:91–100.

107. Scott P. IL-12: initiation cytokine for cell-mediated immunity. Science 1993; 23:547-549.

108. Xiao B-G, Link H. Is there a balance between microglia and astrocytes in regulating Th1/Th2-cell responses and neuropathologies? Trends Immunol Today 1999; 20:477–479.

109. Ford AL, Foulcher E, Lemckert FA, Sedgwick JD. Microglia induces CD4 T lymphocyte final effector function and death. Exp Med 1996; 184:1737–1745.

110. Oh LY, Yong VW. Astrocytes promote process outgrowth by adult human oligodendrocytes in vitro through interaction between bFGF and astrocyte extracellular matrix. Glia 1996; 17:237–253.

111. Awatsuji H, Furukawa Y, Hirota M, Murakami Y, Nii S, Furukawa S. Interleukin-4 and -5 as modulators of nerve growth factor synthesis/secretion in astrocytes. J Neurosci Res 1993; 34(5):539–545.

112. Pender MP, Rist MJ. Apoptosis of inflammatory cells in immune control of the nervous system: role of glia. Glia 2001; 36:137–144.

113. Dore GJ, et al. Trends in incidence of AIDS illnesses in Australia from 1983 to 1994: the Australian AIDS cohort. J AIDS Hum Retrovir 1997; 16:39–43.

114. Glass JD, Fedor H, Wesselingh SL, McArthur JC. Immunocytochemical quantitation of human immunodeficiency virus in the brain: correlations with dementia Ann. Neurol 1995; 38:755–762.

115. Combadiere C, et al. Identification of CX3CR1. A chemotactic receptor for the human CX3C chemokine fractalkine and a fusion coreceptor for HIV-1. J Biol Chem 1998; 273:23799–23804.

116. Lazarini F, et al. Differential signaling of the chemokine receptor CXCR4 by stromal cell-derived factor 1 and the HIV glycoprotein in rat neurons and astrocytes. Eur J Neurosci 2000; 12:117–125.

117. Liu Y, et al. Uptake of HIV-1 Tat protein mediated by low-density lipoprotein receptor-related protein disrupts the neuronal metabolic balance of the receptor ligands. Nat Med 2000; 6:1380–1387.

118. Everall IP, et al. Cortical synaptic density is reduced in mild to moderate human immunodeficiency virus neurocognitive disorder. HNRC Group, HIV Neurobehavioral Research Center. Brain Pathol 1999; 9:209–217.

119. Adle-Biassette H, et al. Neuronal apoptosis does not correlate with dementia in HIV infection but is related to microglial activation and axonal damage. Neuropathol Appl Neurobiol 1999; 25:123–133.

120. Ellis RJ, et al. Cerebrospinal fluid human immunodeficiency virus type-1 RNA levels are elevated in neurocognitively impaired individuals with acquired immunodeficiency syndrome. HIV Neurobehavioral Research Center Group. Ann Neurol 1997; 42:679–688.

121. Asensio VC, Campbell IL. Chemokines in the CNS: plurifunctional mediators in diverse states. Trends Neurosci 1999; 22:504–512.

122. Cinque P, et al. Elevated cerebrospinal fluid levels of monocyte chemotactic protein-1 correlate with HIV-1 encephalitis and local viral replication. AIDS 1998; 12:1327–1332.

123. Meucci O, Fatatis A, Simen AA, Miller RJ. Expression of CX3CR1 chemokine receptors on neurons and their role in neuronal survival. Proc Natl Acad Sci USA 2000; 97:8075–8080.

124. Gartner S. HIV infection and dementia. Science 2000; 287:602–604.

125. Adle-Biassette H, et al. Neuronal apoptosis in HIV infection in adults. Neuropathol Appl Neurobiol 1995; 21:218–227.

126. Hesselgesser J, et al. Neuronal apoptosis induced by HIV-1 gp120 and the chemokine SDF-1 is mediated by the chemokine receptor CXCR4. Curr Biol 1998; 8:595–598.

127. Bonfoco E, Krainc D, Ankarcrona M, Nicotera P, Lipton SA. Apoptosis and necrosis: two distinct events induced, respectively, by mild and intense insults with N-methyl-D-aspartate or nitric oxide/superoxide in cortical cell cultures. Proc Natl Acad Sci USA 1995; 92:7162–7166.

128. Lipton SA. Treating AIDS dementia. Science 1997; 276:1629–1630.

129. Ellis RJ, et al. Neurocognitive impairment is an independent risk factor for death in HIV infection. San Diego HIV Neurobehavioral Research Center Group. Arch Neurol 1997; 54:416–424.

130. Masliah G, Ge N, Achim CL, Hansen LA, Wiley CA. Selective neuronal vulnerability in HIV encephalitis. J Neuropathol Exp Neurol 1992; 51:585–593.

131. Chapman GA, et al. Fractalkine cleavage from neuronal membranes represents an acute event in the inflammatory response to excitotoxic brain damage. J Neurosci 2000; 20:RC87.

132. Toggas SM, Masliah E, Rockenstein EM, Rall GF, Abraham CR, Mucke L. Central nervous system damage produced by expression of the HIV-1 coat protein gp120 in transgenic mice. Nature 1994; 367:188–193.

133. Ferrando S, et al. Highly active antiretroviral treatment in HIV infection: benefits for neuropsychological function. AIDS 1998; 12:F65–F70.

134. Lipton A, Gendelman HE. Dementia associated with the acquired immunodeficiency syndrome. N Engl J Med 1995; 332:934–940.

135. Tong N, et al. Neuronal fractalkine expression in HIV-1 encephalitis: roles for macrophage recruitment and neuroprotection in the central nervous system. J Immunol 2000; 164:1333–1339.

136. Wyss-Coray T, et al. Dysregulation of signal transduction pathways as a potential mechanism of nervous system alterations in HIV-1 gp120 transgenic mice and humans with HIV-1 encephalitis. J Clin Invest 1996; 97:789–798.

137. Petito CK, Roberts B. Evidence of apoptotic cell death in HIV encephalitis. Am J Pathol 1995; 146:1121–1130.

138. Brew BJ, et al. Quinolinic acid production is related to macrophage tropic isolates of HIV-1. J Neurovirol 1995; 1:369–374.

139. von Zahn J, Moller T, Kettenmann H, Nolte C. Microglial phagocytosis is modulated by pro- and anti-inflammatory cytokines. Neuroreport 1997; 8:3851–3856.

140. Aloisi F, Penna G, Cerase J, Menendez I, Adorini L. IL-12 production by central nervous system microglia is inhibited by astrocytes. Immunology 1997; 159:1604–1612.

141. Le Douarin NM, Kalcheim C. The Neural Crest. 2d ed. New York: Cambridge University Press, 1999.

142. Moriki T, Takahashi T, Hiroi M, Yamane T, Hara H. Histological grade in invasive ductal carcinoma of breast correlates with the proliferative activity evaluated by BrdU: an immunohistochemical study including correlations with p53, c-erbB-2 and estrogen receptor status. Pathol Int 1996; 46(6):417–425.

143. D'Arcangelo G, Miao GG, Chen SC, Soares HD, Morgan JI, Curran T. A protein related to extracellular matrix proteins deleted in the mouse mutant reeler. Nature 1995; 374(6524):719–723.

144. Alter M, Liebo J, Desnick SO, Strommer B. The behavior of the reeler neurological mutant mouse. Neurology 1968; 18(3):289.

145. Caviness VS Jr. Neocortical histogenesis in normal and reeler mice: a developmental study based upon [3H] thymidine autoradiography. Brain Res 1982; 256(3):293–302.

146. Yoneshima H, Nagata E, Matsumoto M, Yamada M, Nakajima K, Miyata T, Ogawa M, Mikoshiba K. A novel neurological mutant mouse, yotari, which exhibits reeler-like phenotype but express CR-50 antigen/reelin. Neurosci Res 1997; 29(3):217–223.

147. Sweet HO, Bronson RT, Johnson KR, Cook SA, Davisson MT. Scrambler, a new neurological mutation of the mouse with abnormalities of neuronal migration. Mamm Genome 1996; 7(11):798–802.

148. Sheldon M, Rice DS, D'Arcangelo G, Yoneshima H, Nakajima K, Mikoshiba K, Howell BW, Cooper JA, Goldowitz D, Curran T. Scrambler and yotari disrupt the disabled gene and produce a reeler-like phenotype in mice. Nature 1997; 16, (389 (6652):730–733.

149. Howell BW, Hawkes R, Soriano P, Cooper JA. Neuronal position in the developing brain is regulated by mouse disabled-1. Nature 1997; 16, 389(6652):733–737.

150. Utsunomiya-Tate N, Kubo K, Tate S, Kainosho M, Katayama E, Nakajima K, Mikoshiba K. Reelin molecules assemble together to form a large protein complex, which is inhibited by the function-blocking CR-50 antibody. Proc Natl Acad Sci USA 2000; 15, 97(17):9729–9734.

151. Keshvara L, Benhayon D, Magdaleno S, Curran T. Identification of reelin-induced sites of tyrosyl phosphorylation on disabled. J Biol Chem 2001; 276(19):16008–16014.

152. Hiesberger T, Trommsdorff M, Howell BW, Goffinet A, Mumby MC, Cooper JA, Herz J. Direct binding of Reelin to VLDL receptor and ApoE receptor 2 induces tyrosine phosphorylation of disabled-1 and modulates tau phosphorylation. Neuron 1999; 24(2):481–489.

153. D'Arcangelo G, Homayouni R, Keshvara L, Rice DS, Sheldon M, Curran T. Reelin is a ligand for lipoprotein receptors. Neuron 1999; 24(2):471–479.

154. Trommsdorff M, Borg JP, Margolis B, Herz J. Interaction of cytosolic adaptor proteins with neuronal apolipoprotein E receptors and the amyloid precursor protein. J Biol Chem 1998; 273(50):33556–33560.

155. Senzaki K, Ogawa M, Yagi T. Proteins of the CNR family are multiple receptors for Reelin. Cell 1999; 99(6):635–647.

156. Dulabon L, Olson EC, Taglienti MG, Eisenhuth S, McGrath B, Walsh CA, Kreidberg JA, Anton ES. Reelin binds alpha3beta integrin and inhibits neuronal migration. Neuron 2000; 1:33–44.

157. Lee SC, Liu W, Dickson DW, Brosnan CF, Berman JW. Cytokine production by human fetal microglia and astrocytes. Differential induction by lipopolysaccharide and IL-1 beta. J Immunol 1993; 150:2659–2667.

158. Baumann H, Gauldie J. The acute phase response. Immunol Today 1994; 15:74–80.

159. Arzt E, Stalla GK. Cytokines: autocrine and paracrine roles in the anterior pituitary. Neuroimmunomodulation 1996; 3:28–34.

160. Vitkovic L, Chatham JJ, da Cunha A. Distinct expressions of three cytokines by IL-1-stimulated astrocytes in vitro and in AIDS brain. Brain Behav Immun 1995; 9:378–388.

161. Da Cunha A, Jefferson JA, Jackson RW, Vitkovic L. Glial cell-specific mechanisms of TGF-beta 1 induction by IL-1 in cerebral cortex. J Neuroimmunol 1993; 42:71–85.

162. Plata-Salaman CR, Ilyin SE. Interleukin-1beta (IL-1beta)-induced modulation of the hypothalamic IL-1beta system, tumor necrosis factor-alpha, and transforming growth factor-beta1 mRNA in obese (fafa) and lean (FaFa) Zucker rats: implications to IL-1beta feedback systems and cytokine-cytokine interactions. J Neurosci Res 1997; 49:541–550.

163. Da Cunha A, Jefferson JJ, Tyor WR, Glass JD, Jannotta FS, Vitkovic L. Control of astrocytosis by interleukin-1 and transforming growth factor-beta 1 in human brain. Brain Res 1993; 631:39–45.

164. Chai Z, Gatti S, Toniatti C, Poli V, Bartfai T. Interleukin (IL)-6 gene expression in the central nervous system is necessary for fever response to lipopolysaccharide or IL-1 beta: a study on IL-6-deficient mice. J Exp Med 1996; 183:311–316.

165. Gourine AV, Rudolph K, Leon LR, Kluger MJ. Effect of interleukin-11 on body temperature in afebrile and febrile rats. Neuroimmunomodulation 2000; 1:8–12.

166. Lin JH, Lin MT. Inhibition of nitric oxide synthase or cyclo-oxygenase pathways in organum vasculosum laminae terminalis attenuates interleukin-1 beta fever in rabbits. Neurosci Lett 1996; 208:155–158.

167. Goto Y, Araki T, Kato M, Fukui M. Propagation of hippocampal seizure activity arising from the hippocampus: a local cerebral blood flow study. Brain Res 1994; 634: 203–213.

168. Tchélingérian J, Le Saux F, Pouzet B, Jacque C. Widespread neuronal expression of c-Fos throughout the brain and local expression in glia following a hippocampal injury. Neurosci Lett 1997; 226:175–178.

169. Tchélingérian J, Quinonero J, Booss J, Jacque C. Localization of TNF alpha and IL-1 alpha immunoreactivities in striatal neurons after surgical injury to the hippocampus. Neuron 1993; 10:213–224.

170. Mucke ML. Molecular profile of reactive astrocytes implications for their role in neurological disease. Neuroscience 1993; 54:15–36.

171. Ransohoff RM, Tani M. Do chemokines mediate leukocyte recruitment in post-traumatic CNS inflammation? Trends Neurosci 1998; 21:154–159.

172. Blakemore WF, Crang AJ. The relationship between type-1 astrocytes, Schwann cells and oligodendrocytes following transplantation of glial cell cultures into demyelinating lesions in the adult rat spinal cord. J Neurocytol 1989; 18:519–528.

173. Grumet M, Flaccus A, Margolis RU. Functional characterization of chondroitin sulfate proteoglycans of brain: interactions with neurons and neural cell adhesion molecules. J Cell Biol 1993; 120:815–824.

174. Davies SJA, Fitch MT, Memberg SP, Hall AK, Raisman G, Silver J. Regeneration of adult axons in white matter tracts of the central nervous system. Nature 1997; 390:680–683.

175. Liedtke W, Edelmann W, Bieri PL, Chiu F, Cowan NJ, Kucherlapati R. GFAP is necessary for the integrity of CNS white matter architecture and long-term maintenance of myelination. Neuron 1996; 17:607–615.

176. Gage FH, Olejniczak P, Armstrong DM. Astrocytes are important for sprouting in the septohippocampal circuit. Exp Neurol 1988; 102:2–13.

177. Rothstein JD, Martin L, Levey AI, Dykes-Hoberg M, Jin L, Wu D. Localization of neuronal and glial glutamate transporters. Neuron 1994; 13:713–725.

178. Wilson JX. Antioxidant defense of the brain: a role for astrocytes. Can J Physiol Pharmacol 1997; 75:1149–1163.

179. Faden AI, Demediuk P, Panter SS, Vink R. The role of excitatory amino acids and NMDA receptors in traumatic brain injury. Science 1989; 244:798–800.

180. Licinio J, Wong ML. The role of inflammatory mediators in the biology of major depression: central nervous system cytokines modulate the biological substrate of depressive symptoms, regulate stress-responsive systems, and contribute to neurotoxicity and neuroprotection. Mol Psychiatry 1999; 4:317–327.

181. Fiala M, Rhodes RH, Shapshak P. Regulation of HIV-1 infection in astrocytes: expression of Nef, TNF-alpha and IL-6 is enhanced in coculture of astrocytes with macrophages. J Neurovirol 1996; 2:158–166.

182. Toggas SM, et al. Central nervous system damage produced by expression of the HIV-1 coat protein gp120 in transgenic mice. Nature 1994; 367:188–193.

183. Glass JD, Johnson RT. Human immunodeficiency virus and the brain. Annu Rev Neurosci 1966; 19:126.

184. Glass JD, Fedor H, Wesselingh SL, McArthur JC. Immunocytochemical quantitation of human immunodeficiency virus in the brain: correlations with dementia. Ann Neurol 1995; 38:755–762.

185. Combs CK, Johnson DE, Cannady SB, Lehman TM, Landreth GE. Identification of microglial signal transduction pathways mediating a neurotoxic response to amyloidogenic fragments of beta-amyloid and prion proteins. J Neurosci 1999; 19:928–939.

Index